Queueing Theory

Second Edition

Lester Lipsky

Queueing Theory

A Linear Algebraic Approach

Second Edition

Springer

Lester Lipsky
Professor Emeritus
Department of Computer Science
and Engineering
University of Connecticut
Storrs, CT 06268-2155
lester.lipsky@uconn.edu

First South Asian Edition 2019

ISBN: 978-1-4939-9116-7

ISBN: 978-1-4419-2386-8 e-ISBN: 978-0-387-49706-8
DOI 10.1007/978-0-387-49706-8

Mathematics Subject Classification (2000): 60XX, 68XX, 90XX, 60K25, 60J27, 90B22, 60K05

The first edition of this book was first published by: Macmillan (now Pearson Publications, Inc.)

springer.com

Printed in India by Replika Press Pvt. Ltd.

Dedication

To my wife, Sue, with whom each day is
fresh and new, a truly Markovian relationship.

A Path to Discovery

Theories of the known which are described by different ideas, may be equivalent in all their predictions and are hence scientifically indistinguishable. However, they are not psychologically identical when trying to move from that base into the unknown. For different views suggest different kinds of modifications which might be made. Therefore, a good scientist today might find it useful to have a wide range of viewpoints and mathematical expressions of the same theory available to him. This may be asking too much of one person. The new students should as a class have this. If every individual student follows the same current fashion in expressing and thinking about the generally understood areas, then the variety of hypotheses being generated to understand the still open problems is limited. Perhaps rightly so, ... BUT if the truth is in another direction, who will find it?

Richard P. Feynman

So spoke an honest man, the outstanding intuitionist of our age and a prime example of what may lie in store for anyone who dares to follow the beat of a different drum.

Julian Schwinger

From a special issue on Richard Feynman (who died on 15 February 1988) in Physics Today, February 1989. Feynman's quote (slightly paraphrased here) was taken from his Nobel lecture in June 1965.

[Note: Feynman and Schwinger shared the Nobel prize with S. Tomonaga in 1965 for their work on quantum electrodynamics in the late forties. Working independently, and using radically different methods, they ended up with mathematically equivalent theories. Schwinger and Tomonaga were the "mainstreamers," but everyone calculates using Feynman's method to this day.]

Contents

Preface to Second Edition

We have a habit in writing articles published in scientific journals to make the work as finished as possible, to cover up all the tracks, to not worry about the blind alleys or describe how we had the wrong idea first, and so on. So there isn't any place to publish, in a dignified manner, what we actually did in order to get to do the work.
Richard P. Feymann, Nobel Lecture, 1965.

When the first edition of this book first appeared, there were few books that covered Linear Algebraic Queueing Theory (LAQT), all at a higher level. At that time I made the claim that this would become the approach of choice. Now, some 15 years later, the claim has largely been realized, particularly in problems concerning semi-Markov processes and system reliability. The prediction that because transient phenomena could now be expressed in a computationally manageable form, this subject would also become more important, seems to be slowly coming true as well. Many research papers have been published, resulting in several books containing collections of these papers, mostly on computational methods, as in for instance, [STEWART95], [CHAK-ALFA97]i, and [LATOUCHETAYLOR00]. The monograph by Latouche and Ramaswami (leaders in the field) [LATOUCHE-RAM99] covers the subject well, but at a higher level. (Their title, *Introduction to Matrix Analytic Methods ...* could be modified to *Introduction to Advanced Matrix Analytic Methods ...*[†].) Yet no new book at the intermediate level has emerged that takes a linear algebraic approach. That is, when possible, theorems are proven by matrix algebraic manipulation, rather than using explicit properties of matrices or probabilistic arguments. Therefore, an updated version of the original is needed.

This second edition, in addition to making many corrections and improvements, is larger by a third than the first edition. The increase in size reflects the growing recognition of the importance of processes that generate unboundedly large variances or long-range autocorrelation, as seen in CPU times, file sizes, telecommunications traffic, finance, and insurance claims. Thus an extensive amount of material has been added to Chapter 3 describing a broad set of ME functions. In particular there is an entire section on power-tail (PT), or Pareto distributions (they form a proper subset of the heavy-tailed distributions), including a section showing how they can be represented by ME distributions within the Markovian structure, even though they have infinite moments. They are then used in Chapters 4 and 5 to study queues with

[†]A definition of *elementary,* or *introductory* is: "that which the author understands." *Advanced* means: "that which the author is not sure about," whereas *intermediate* is: "that which the author figured out while writing the book."

PT service times, and to see how PT renewal processes affect system times.

A new Chapter 8 has been added that covers Semi-Markov processes (SMP), an important topic that is used extensively in queueing models of performance from system reliability to telecommunications systems to performance of computer clusters to inventory problems in operations research. We first give a formal mathematical description of the properties of SMPs and the related Markov Renewal Processes (MRP). Several detailed examples are then presented, each with a different state-space construction. We then look at some *ON-OFF* models used in modeling telecommunications traffic.

The old Chapter 8 is now Chapter 9, and includes a new section on how to deal with networks of nonexponential servers.

Acknowledgments

When I decided to write a second edition in 2000 I realized that the original text, written in DITROFF, would have to be translated to LaTeX. Lucky for me that my friend, Dr. Michael Greiner, willingly took on the task of writing the translator and overseeing its execution by Michael Schneider. Without their efforts I might still be doing the translation by hand. I must thank my friends at Technical University of Munich, Prof. Eike Jessen and Dr. Manfred Jobmann, for their longtime support and encouragement from the time I spent my sabbatical year at TUM in 1994. Manfred has carefully read the original and now the final version and has found more errata than I can afford to pay at $1 per error. Don Costello invited me to give a series of lectures and then encouraged me to write the second edition with expanded coverage of heavy-tailed distributions. Thanks to former Dean Amir Fagri and the School of Engineering at UCONN, and my department chair, Reda Ammar, for providing funding and a sabbatical so I could work on the book and hire Justin Besiglio and Robert Sheahan to produce many of the figures herein. In the last two years, Robert and Feng Zhang have generated the rest of the graphs and helped with the formatting of the book. I don't know how I can show proper appreciation of their extraordinary efforts. Thanks to my former students, Jisung Woo, Steve Thompson, Marwan Sleiman, Sarah Tasneem, Cindy Siriwong, Gehan Verasinghe and the many students who have taken my LAQT course but whose names have slipped from my grasp, for sharing in the proofreading. Special thanks to my former students and present collaborators, Hans-Peter Schwefel, Pierre Fiorini, Ahmed Mohamed, and Imad Antonios for their invaluable input. Prof. Søren Asmussen provided valuable suggestions on making tighter definitions, in particular on defining *heavy-tailed* distributions and their subsets. I also want to thank Peter Kühl for spending so much time editing the entire book, as well as other suggestions for improving the text. Any errors that remain are mine alone. My thanks to Springer-Verlag for their offer to publish the book, and thanks most of all to my wife, Sue, for persevering through it all.

Storrs, CT, April 2008 Lester Lipsky

Preface to First Edition

"Necessity is the mother of invention" is a misleading proverb. "Necessity is the mother of temporary fixups" is much nearer to the truth. The basis of the growth of modern invention is science, and science is largely the outgrowth of intellectual curiosity.
Alfred North Whitehead

At least 50 worthwhile books on queueing theory have been written in the last 35 years. Two or three times as many books have been published in which queueing theory and Markov chains play an important part. Most of these books, even the older ones, are still useful for understanding at least some part of the subject. Why, then, should yet another book be published? The answer, simply, is that there is no book (or even collection of papers) that covers intermediate queueing theory using what I call "Linear Algebraic Queueing Theory" (LAQT). There are in fact only two books which use a linear algebraic approach, both by Marcel Neuts [NEUTS81] and [NEUTS89], and both of them are written for experts in the field. I waited five years for someone to write a book that could be used for a first or second course in the subject (never do anything if someone else is going to do it), but to no avail. So in 1988 I started to write it myself.

The reason that LAQT should become familiar to novices as well as to those who are already knowledgeable in intermediate and advanced queueing theory is that any problems that can be cast into a matrix-vector format can easily be adapted to make use of the high-speed parallel and vector processors available today. Also, many problems in queueing theory that traditionally are solved by unrelated mathematical techniques can now be solved in a consistent integrated fashion. This allows for better physical insight. But, most important, many system performance measures that are normally ignored because of their computational and formulational difficulties can be dealt with easily in LAQT. Some examples are: properties of the busy period, departure processes, first-passage times, residual times, distinctions between what an observer sees and what a customer sees, and compound processes in general. Each of these topics is treated here without requiring prior knowledge of the reader. This book makes the following claim. "Any problem that can be solved for exponential servers can somehow be extended to treat nonexponential servers." Of course, it remains to be seen whether the future will vindicate this optimism.

Many decisions had to be made before this book could be written. First, who is the intended audience? There are a half a dozen disciplines that claim queueing theory as one of their "bread-and-butter" techniques. Applied probability, computer science, electrical engineering, management science, operations research, systems engineering, and even physics lay claim to various parts of this subject as their own, each with its own terminology. Because I dabble in all these fields, I decided to try to write a generic book that could be understood by all. The terms used are defined in relation to customers arriving at, being served by, and departing from subsystems, from the different viewpoints of the customer and of an outside (sometimes random) observer. The mental image one gets is of humans being served by mechanical objects, while being observed by other human beings.

Another decision to be made was the level at which to present the material, namely, as a first or second course in queueing theory, as a reference book for practitioners, or as a monograph for would-be researchers in the field. Once again, I decided to try to aim for all. There is no reason why this material cannot be taught to mathematically mature college seniors or new graduate students who have already had courses in linear algebra and probability theory, but have not necessarily had any queueing theory. Unfortunately this would have required that the first two chapters be expanded to more than twice their present size without ever mentioning LAQT. There are already many books available that give an excellent introduction to queueing theory. Therefore I opted for either a first course, where the student already has had some background in Markov processes and elementary queueing theory, or a second course. For instance, many students in computer science and electrical engineering take a course in applied probability covering material such as that in Chapters 7 and 8 of Trivedi's book [TRIVEDI82]. Alternately, many courses in performance modeling (e.g., courses using [MOLLOY89] or [LAZOWSKAETAL84]) are adequate to serve as an introduction to this book.

We assume that the reader is already familiar with matrix theory. However, except for such elementary formulas as that defining matrix multiplication, we do not expect the student to have any particular theorem at his or her fingertips. Therefore background information is introduced as needed. There is no special section put aside for reviewing linear algebra. We assume the same about the reader's knowledge of integral and differential calculus (in particular, Taylor's series and l'Hospital's rule) and elementary probability theory. For those whose mathematics is a bit rusty, we recommend that an elementary text in each of these areas be kept handy. But worry not; for all the mathematical content, this is not a rigorous text. It is a "why and how to" book. Whenever we would like a matrix to have a particular property, we assume it is so, whether or not we can prove it.

The material is rather densely packed, so several readings and rereadings may be necessary for the less experienced queueing theorist, particularly because there are numerous definitions in the text, and definitions do not usually stick in one's mind without some effort. This problem is reduced somewhat by the book's layout. We are inclined to introduce an idea in one chapter, and then use it again in a subsequent section, but in a more intricate way. We have done our best to give explicit reference to material previously discussed.

For Instructors and Practitioners

One might say that the "father" of LAQT is Victor Wallace, who in the 1960s introduced the concept of Quasi Birth-Death (QBD) processes and proved that there exists a matrix geometric solution for a large class of such systems, including the open G/G/C queue [WALLACE69]. His presentation, although motivated by queueing theory [WALLACE72], was couched in terms of abstract Markov chains, and so was acknowledged, but was not picked up as a practical way of dealing mathematically, conceptually, or computationally with specific problems in elementary or intermediate queueing theory.

The first researcher actually to take this viewpoint in solving problems specific to queueing theory was Marcel Neuts, who in the mid-1970s introduced *PHase* distributions [NEUTS75] and showed that they had matrix representations which could be manipulated algebraically, while operating on state vectors corresponding to the queue length probabilities (one vector for each value of n, the queue length). He strongly argued that a matrix formulation could more easily be handled by computers than could integration or differentiation [NEUTS81]. Also, since so many problems seemed to have a recursive solution, algorithms for their numerical evaluation became straightforward. However, he and his students concentrated most of their efforts attacking hitherto unsolved problems, and thus remained too abstract to be appreciated by the practical users (as I was then) of queueing theory. It seemed as though this was just another one of the many techniques one might use to solve a small set of problems.

This researcher became interested in the subject in the late 1970s in studying the problem of what happens to a subnetwork of exponential servers when the number of customers who can be active simultaneously is restricted. My students and I soon realized that if the subsystem was restricted to one active customer, then that subsystem was equivalent to a single server with a nonexponential (Coxian, or Kendall [KENDALL64], or RLT, or matrix exponential) distribution. Then, after John Carroll reduced the balance equations from second-order to first-order difference equations [CARROLL79], we independently, and virtually simultaneously with Neuts, found the explicit matrix geometric solution to M/G/1 and G/M/C queues. The two papers appeared back-to-back in the May-June 1982 issue of *Operations Research* [CARROLLLIPVDL82], [NEUTS82]. I consider this to be the true beginning of LAQT, for then it became clear that many seemingly diverse problems could be solved using one technique and one viewpoint.

It is interesting to realize that the basis for LAQT was established by Erlang himself [ERLANG17] when he represented a single server by a series of exponential stages, but linear algebra was not in vogue at the turn of this century, so queueing theory had to be developed entirely within the framework of what is called "modern analysis." The "method of stages" is really a part of LAQT, distorted so it could fit into the classical view, whereas D. R. Cox's work in the 1950s [COX55], showing iin effect that "every pdf can be approximated arbitrarily closely by a function whose Laplace transform can be written as the ratio of two polynomials (RLT functions)" is really the basis for claiming that there exists a linear algebraic formulation of every problem which can be formulated otherwise.

You might question whether LAQT really is a peer to the standard variety of queueing theory. Well, for decades now, it has been standard technique in various areas of applied mathematics to replace differential operators on a solution function by an equivalent linear operator on a vector in Hilbert space. In fact, the pair of representations of quantum theory, Werner Heisenberg's *matrix mechanics* and Erwin Schrödinger's *wave mechanics*, is the prime example of this duality. The proof by John von Neumann that they are mathematically equivalent is closely related to Cox's completeness statement in extending A. K. Erlang's method of stages to include all functions with rational Laplace transforms [Cox55]. Fortunately for physics, linear algebra was a known quantity by the 1920s, so the two viewpoints grew together and have become so intertwined that the typical quantum practitioner switches from one to the other and back again with little difficulty. A similar statement can be made about *linear control theory*. Both of those disciplines deal with functions of complex variables, even though what is actually observed must be real. If physicists can talk about the *charm* of *quarks*, which can never be seen outside their nuclear home, and electrical engineers can have imaginary currents, surely our customers should be allowed to travel with negative probabilities and complex service times from one phase to another, as long as they remain inside one subsystem or another, and as long as all observable entities are real.

The reader should avoid mapping this material onto already familiar techniques, at least until Chapter 4 has been covered. By then you will see the power and elegance of this methodology, as well as its usefulness, and be able to "switch back and forth without difficulty." Furthermore, because most solutions are in terms of matrix operations rather than integrals, or roots of equations, highly efficient algorithms for both single and parallel computer systems can easily be written. There are several mathematical tool kits readily available (e.g., MATLAB, Mathematica, Maple) that execute matrix equations directly.

Organization

The book is laid out by chapter in order of increasing complexity of structure. There is more than enough material for a two-semester course, but a one-semester first course or a one-semester second course can easily be fashioned.

In Chapter 1 we make a quick survey of those topics normally connected to Markov chains. Chapter 2 starts out as a continuation of Chapter 1 by using the Chapman-Kolmogorov equations to set up the M/M/1 queue. But we soon switch to the simpler and intuitively more satisfying view associated with steady-state transition diagrams. Every queueing system is made up of two subsystems, each of which contains one exponential server. In Chapter 3 we show that by adding structure to a subsystem we give it a nonexponential (called *Matrix Exponential*, ME) service time distribution. In Chapter 4 we combine the ideas of the two previous chapters to study the M/G/1 queue (i.e., one nonexponential and one exponential subsystem). As long as our system is closed (finite population of customers), there is no difference between an M/G/1//N loop and a G/M/1//N loop. But if the population is increased unboundedly, one or the other server will saturate. So, if the nonexponential server is the faster one, we have the open M/G/1 queue as given in Chapter 4. However, in Chapter 5 we assume that the exponential server is faster, and derive the properties of an open G/M/1 queue.

In Chapter 6 two or more customers can independently be active at once in one subsystem, the M/G/C system. This increases the complexity of the mathematics required, as well as the computational complexity and sizes of matrices. But it also enormously increases the range of problems that can be solved, the so-called "generalized M/G/C systems." In Chapter 7 we revert to one active customer per subsystem, but now both subsystems have structure, and we are dealing with a G/G/1//N loop. This leads to a different increase in complexity, requiring a *direct product* of vector spaces, which we must first discuss before actually finding the steady-state solution.

Finally, in Chapter 8 we try to give a linear algebraic formulation that does not depend upon a physical interpretation of individual states. As such, it acts as a review of the book.

The chapters are all structured in more or less the same way, with obvious deviations because of the material. First we find the closed steady-state solution. Then we "open" the loop by increasing the customer population unboundedly. Then we look at certain specialized topics (e.g., load-dependent servers, renewal theory, comparison with other methods). Finally we explore the transient behavior of the appropriate queue.

A one-semester first course would cover Chapter 1 and the steady-state parts of Chapters 2, 3, 4, and 5. Depending on the background of the students, the instructor might add some descriptive material to Chapters 1 and 2.

Assuming that students have already had a course in queueing theory, but not one that covered LAQT, a one-semester second course would skim through Chapter 1 and the first part of Chapter 2. But then Section 2.3 must be covered in earnest, as must the first part of Chapter 3. Except for the material on residual times, which must be covered, Section 3.5 can be omitted. Most of Chapters 4 and 5 should be covered, but the instructor can skip Chapter 6 if desired and go directly to Chapter 7. However, Chapter 6 is potentially of great practical importance, therefore the instructor may prefer to skip Chapter 7 instead. Chapter 9 can be put in or left out, as per taste.

A two-semester course can be given that combines the two one-semester courses in the order just described, or one can go sequentially from beginning to end, skipping those topics which seem inappropriate. However, one cannot study Section 6.5, for example, without first covering the related material in Chapters 2, 4, and 5.

Acknowledgments

I would like to thank Professor Howard Sholl and BECAT of the University of Connecticut for continued support in the technical creation of this book. In particular, Anthony Guzzi has rewritten DITROFF[†] so it actually does what it is supposed to do (at least on my workstation). His devotion to my needs has been beyond the call. Also, I thank John Marshall and Sue Zajac[*] for keeping the system up (most of the time) and the secretaries (Jean, Sue, Ruth, Sandi, and Sherry) for keeping me up (most of the time). To my former students, now collaborators, Appie van de Liefvoort (University of Missouri-KC), Aby Tehranipour (Eastern Michigan University), and Yiping Ding (now at BGS Systems, Inc.), I give thanks for technical advice in the various chapters where they are experts. Thanks to Seva nanda Adari, Jinzhu (Jim) Chen, and Houzhong Yan for reading the first draft and pointing out how ideas could be made clearer. I thank the students who were in my class in the fall of 1990 (Somnath Deb, Sharad Garg, Rudi Hackenberg, Chengdong Lu, Jim Moriarty, Carolyn Pe, and Cien Xu), who used the second version of this book and searched for errors of content. Siddhartha Roy and Dilip Tagare meticulously went through the final draft, searching for errors of all kinds (and they found many). Dilip and Ed Bigos were also responsible for generating most of the graphs. To Professors Joseph Macek (University of Tennessee); George Nagy (Rensselaer Polytechnic Institute); Don Costello and Sharad Seth (University of Nebraska); Don Towsley (University of Massachusetts); Victor Wallace (University of Kansas); and Arnie Russek (my thesis advisor), Jim Galligan, and Krishna Pattipati (all of the University of Connecticut), thanks for useful critical comments. I must also thank Macmillan Publishing Company's Ed Maura for taking the initiative in inviting me to do the book, John Griffin who oversaw the project from cover to cover, the unknown proofreader who went through the text with the devotion of a mother combing her daughter's hair, and especially Leo Malek who was determined that this would be a good-looking book. Thanks to Erikson/Dillon Art services for creating such fine figures and page layout, and finally, Janet Pecorelli and the American Mathematical Society's printing service in Providence, RI, for producing such high-quality galley proofs at short notice.

Storrs, CT, November 1991 Lester Lipsky

[†]DITROFF is a registered trademark of AT&T.

[*]As of May 4, 1996, now known as Sue Marie Lipsky.

Chapter 1

INTRODUCTION

The ultimate Markov observation:
"Today is the first day of the rest of your life."

This author is often asked what queueing theory is. First we state that *queueing* is the only word in the English language with five successive vowels (there is an alternative spelling that deletes the second *e*, but it is obviously inferior) and that a queue is a line of customers waiting to be served, such as one sees in banks, supermarkets, and fast-food outlets. More often than not, the questioner will interrupt to say, "You've been doing a bad job, and common sense would tell us how to do things better." Of course we have not even begun to explain where the theory comes in ("So, you're in queueing?"). The goal of a mathematical modeler (the class of researchers to which queueing theorists belong) is to describe and understand what is really going on, for only then can someone (not necessarily the modeler) make an informed decision on what should be done to improve things. You, the reader, presumably already know what a queue is and will have the patience to learn some of the theory, particularly that related to our Linear Algebraic Approach to Queueing Theory (LAQT), which doesn't show up until Chapter 3.

1.1 Background

Any system in which the available resources are not sufficient to satisfy the demands placed upon them at all times is a candidate for queueing analysis. This is quite a general statement, but in this treatise we have tried to keep our picture as simple and as explicit as possible. We deal with ***subsystems*** (or ***service centers***), denoted by S_1, S_2, …, S_m. Customers then wander from one subsystem to another, perhaps forever. We are not so ambitious as to consider in detail more than two subsystems at a time, but we do allow each subsystem to have one or more servers in it, where each server is itself made up of one or more stages, or phases. But we are getting ahead of ourselves with such detail.

1.1.1 Basic Formulas

What can we say about such systems? What do we know? Well, the single most important rule is ***Little's formula*** (1.1.2) [LITTLE61], which we now describe. Consider an arbitrary subsystem, as shown in Figure 1.1.1. Customers

L. Lipsky, *Queueing Theory*, DOI 10.1007/978-0-387-49706-8_1,

come and go and wander from one service center to another. An outside observer can count the number of customers who enter that subsystem over a period of time t, symbolizing that count by $N(t)$. The same customers may

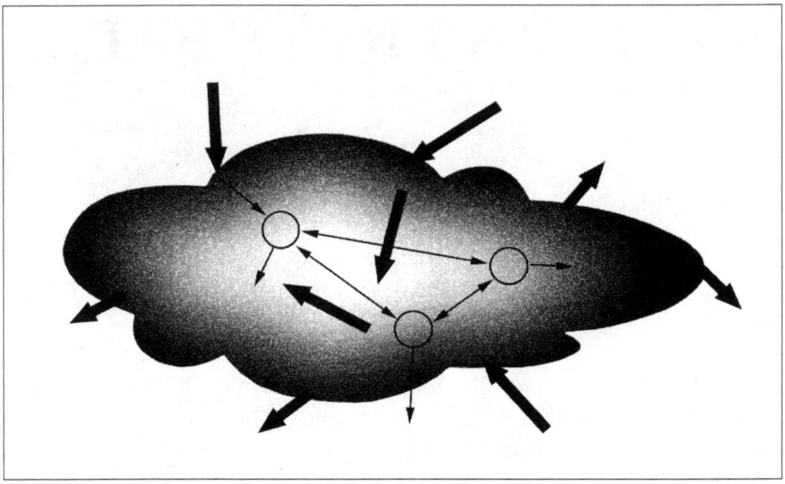

Figure 1.1.1: Arbitrary subsystem of servers. Any number of customers may enter the subsystem (therefore, it is *open*) and travel from one server to another repeatedly before leaving. Customers are not marked, therefore if one leaves and reenters, he is counted twice.

have come and gone more than once, but they are counted each time. After a very long period of time, we would suppose that the difference between the number who have arrived and the number who have left is negligible compared to either (no one stays forever). Then the observer might find that the measured ***arrival rate***, $N(t)/t$, approaches a constant,

$$\Lambda := \frac{N(t)}{t}$$

after a very long time t. †

"How long is *very long*?" is an important question, so it pays to pause for a moment to discuss it. Mathematicians and statisticians have a procedure for dealing with this; they say, "In the limit as t goes to infinity," or

$$\Lambda = \lim_{t\to\infty} \frac{N(t)}{t} . \tag{1.1.1a}$$

Because it actually *is* important, we discuss seriously what is really meant by this limit. A mathematician would assume that $N(t)$ is a monotonic, non-

†The symbol ":=", as used in expressions of the form

$$A \;:=\; B,$$

means "symbol A is defined by expression B." In such cases, A is (almost surely) appearing for the first time.

decreasing function of t that is the same from day to day. His definition of (1.1.1a), as you may recall, is the following.

Definition 1.1.1

If for all $\varepsilon > 0$, there exists a t_o such that for all $t > t_o$, the following is true

$$\left| \frac{N(t)}{t} - \Lambda \right| < \varepsilon ,$$

then (1.1.1a) is true in the mathematical sense. (We use $|X|$ to denote absolute value of X.) □[†]

On the other hand, the outside observer, as she counts the arriving customers, would note that $N(T)$ is a stochastic function (also monotonic nondecreasing) that varies from day to day. Her definition of (1.1.1a) is the following:

Definition 1.1.2

If for all δ and $\varepsilon > 0$, there exists a t_o such that for all $t > t_o$, the following is true,

$$\mathbf{Pr}\left(\left| \frac{N(t)}{t} - \Lambda \right| > \varepsilon \right) < \delta,$$

then (1.1.1a) is true in the probabilistic sense. (The symbol $\mathbf{Pr}(X)$ stands for the phrase "the probability that the expression represented by X is true.") □

The additional assumption (in both cases) is that the underlying conditions do not change from day-to-day, even though, for the observer, the count will be different each day. Depending on the context, we mean one or the other definition when we write something like (1.1.1a). The reader should spend a few moments reviewing these two ideas.

We now return to our discussion of ***Little's formula***. As a second measurement, our observer could keep track of how long each customer spends in the subsystem, for each visit, calling it x_i for the i-th visitor. Then the average time spent in the subsystem by a typical customer is given by

$$\bar{T} = \frac{1}{N(t)} \sum_{i=1}^{N(t)} x_i \qquad (1.1.1b)$$

for very large t (as $t \to \infty$).

As a third measurement, or set of measurements, our observer might at random times count how many customers are in the subsystem, and call it n_i. (We were rather flippant in the use of ***random times***. By that we mean the random observer takes measurements at times that are separated by intervals that are independent and taken from the same exponential distribution, the definition of a Poisson process.) If she does this often enough, say, m times, she

[†]Symbol □ designates end of definition.

can claim that the average number of customers in S (or the ***queue length*** at S) up to any time is given by

$$\bar{q} = \frac{1}{m}\sum_{i=1}^{m} n_i \,. \tag{1.1.1c}$$

If m and t are large enough Little's formula relates these three measurements by the simple formula

$$\bar{q} = \Lambda\bar{T}. \tag{1.1.2}$$

Little published his proof in 1961 [LITTLE61], but it was not satisfactory, and several papers were published subsequently, including S. Stidham's "Last Word" in 1974 [STIDHAM74]. But even that was unsatisfactory to F. J. Beutler who "Revisited" it in 1980 [BEUTLER83]. Since then, rigorous proofs have been published for specific systems (see e.g. [GLYNN-WHITT93] and [ASMUSSEN03]). To this day it is more likely to be called Little's formula instead of Little's theorem or Little's law. Even so, it is used broadly and widely, and no counterexamples of consequence have surfaced. See [KLEINROCK75] or [MOLLOY89] for a constructive (and instructive) proof .

Little's formula tells us that given any two of the performance parameters, the third parameter is uniquely determined by (1.1.2). In other words, the three measurements, in principle, are not independent of each other. In fact, Little's formula is true even if $\bar{T}$, $\bar{q}$, and Λ do not approach a limit, just as long as $n_i/N(t) << 1$. In studying real-world systems, cautious experimenters will usually measure all three parameters and then use Little's formula to check for self-consistency and/or reliability of data. In mathematical modeling the limit as t goes to infinity can be taken correctly, therefore (1.1.2) holds exactly (except for some pathological systems that we ignore here).

The second most important formula, and the first one always derived in any discussion of queueing systems, is the steady-state solution of the open M/M/1 queue. We derive and discuss this in Chapter 2, but for now we merely look at the result. Suppose that customers arrive randomly and independently of each other to a lone server and that the average rate at which they arrive is given by the parameter λ. Suppose further that the time between arrivals is a random number taken from the exponential distribution, with mean $\bar{x}_2 = 1/\lambda$ and that the arrivals are independent of each other. This is known as a *Poisson arrival process*, which we run across again and again throughout the book. Let X be the random variable (r.v.) denoting the time needed by a customer once he gets to be served. The actual time he needs is also taken from an exponential distribution, but with mean $\bar{x}_1$. We have thus described the M/M/1 queue. The M stands for "Memoryless", or "Markovian" (nobody seems to know which†), and means for us that the process being represented by M comes

†However, according to Peter Kühl (University of Basel, Switzerland), D. G. Kendall first introduced the symbols, M, D, and G in order to indicate various distributions of the generation time of bacteria [KENDALL52]. The following year Kendall applied this notation, supplemented with GI, for characterizing queueing systems [KENDALL53]. He used M for *Markovian*, D for *Deterministic*, G for *G*eneral, and GI for *General Independent*. Kendall never used the term, memoryless. In fact, Kühl points out that using M for *M*emoryless is a misnomer. Instead, if used at all, ML should be used for *MemoryLess*.

from an exponential distribution. The first symbol, [A], in ***Kendall notation*** [KENDALL53]

$$\mathrm{A/B/}C$$

describes the arrival process, the second symbol, [B], describes the service distribution, and the third symbol, [C], tells us how many servers there are in the subsystem. Thus we have a Poisson arrival process [A = M] to a single [$C = 1$] exponential server [B = M].

We next define the ***utilization factor*** (or ***utilization parameter***) to be

$$\rho := \lambda \bar{x}_1 = \frac{\bar{x}_1}{\bar{x}_2}\,. \tag{1.1.3}$$

Suppose, for instance, that customers need 9 minutes of service, on average, and that they are arriving at the rate of 6 per hour (or 10 minutes between arrivals, on average); then $\rho = 0.9$, and we would expect our server to be busy 90% of the time. Therefore, it will be idle $1 - \rho = 0.1$, or 10% of the time. In Chapter 2, Equation (2.1.6b), we show that

$$\bar{q} = \frac{\rho}{1-\rho}\,, \tag{1.1.4a}$$

and from Little's formula

$$\mathbb{E}[T] = \frac{\bar{q}}{\lambda} = \frac{\bar{x}_1}{1-\rho}\,. \tag{1.1.4b}$$

According to these formulas, the average customer (remember, a very large number of customers has gone through) will arrive at a queue that already has nine other customers in it (including the one in service) and will have to wait 90 minutes (on average) from the time he arrives at the subsystem to the time he leaves. This behavior is represented in Figure 1.1.2 by the curve labeled M/M/1.

Before going on, we must clarify what is meant by "will see, on average," because in this case an arriving customer will see more than nine customers in the queue one-third of the time, and one-third of the time he will see three or fewer. In fact, he will see exactly nine customers less than 4% of the time. Actually we are still being loose with our words. What we really mean is that "a customer will find nine customers in the queue with a probability less than 0.04." More rigorously, we write the following:

$$\mathbb{P}\mathbf{r}(N = 9) < 0.04.$$

For averages, we use the following definition.

Definition 1.1.3

Let N be a random variable denoting the number of customers an arriving customer finds in the queue. Then the ***mean number of customers*** is given by

$$\mathbb{E}[N] := \sum_{n=0}^{\infty} n\,\mathbb{P}\mathbf{r}(N = n), \tag{1.1.5a}$$

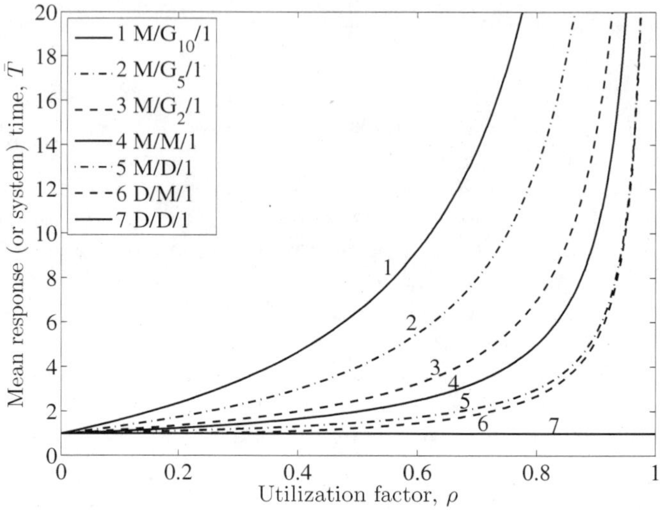

Figure 1.1.2: Steady-state mean response times for various single-server queues. The horizontal axis is the utilization factor ρ from (1.1.3). The average arrival rate must be smaller than the service rate ($\rho < 1$), otherwise the queue will back up indefinitely. All but two of the curves represent queues with Poisson arrivals, for which (1.1.6) is applicable. The squared coefficients of variation for the various service time distributions are $C_v^2 = 0$ (M/D/1), $C_v^2 = 1$ (M/M/1), and $C_v^2 = 2, 5, 10$ (worse than exponential, G_2, G_5, G_{10}). The other two curves have *deterministic* arrivals (the time between successive arrivals is constant) corresponding to the D/M/1 and D/D/1 queues, respectively. It is clear that all the curves blow up at $\rho = 1$.

where for any function of N we say that

$$\mathbf{E}[f(N)] := \sum_{n=0}^{\infty} f(n)\mathbf{Pr}(N = n), \tag{1.1.5b}$$

is the ***expected value*** (or ***expectation value***) of $f(n)$. We also use "***average value***" although it has a broader meaning in everyday usage. It is common notation in queueing theory books to use $\bar{q}$ for $\mathbf{E}[N]$. We do so here. □

Because the precise terminology is so bulky, we tend to use the vague expressions that we hope we have clarified in this section. The reader should always be prepared to insert the precise wording when necessary.

Returning to the M/M/1 queue, we see an apparent contradiction. From an outside observer's (e.g., manager's) viewpoint, the server is idle (dawdling) 10% of the time, whereas from a customer's point of view, the queue is (almost) always very long. The explanation has to do with the unpredictability of arrivals and time for service, for sometimes customers will seem to come in bunches, and sometimes one customer will require far more than the average service time. For instance, the probability that 2 or more customers will arrive

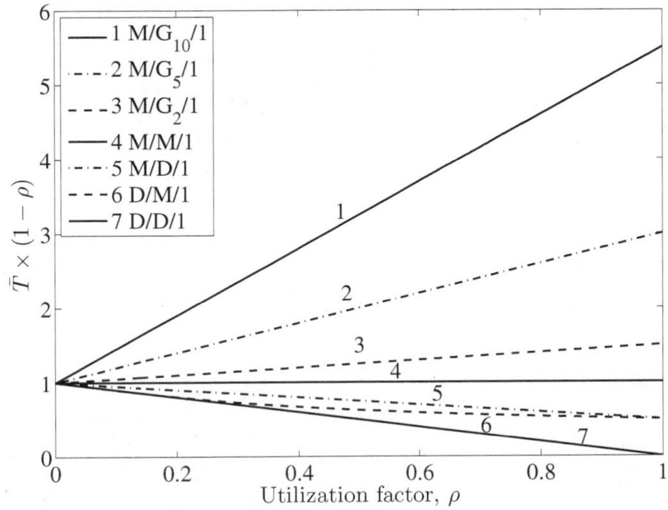

Figure 1.1.3: $T \times (1 - \rho)$ versus ρ for the same service distributions as in Fig 1.1.2. All but the D/M/1 queue (6) are straight lines, and all are finite at $\rho = 1$.

in one mean interarrival time, is greater than 26% $\mathbf{Pr}(n \geq 2) = 2/e]$, and 13% $(1/e^2)$ of the customers will need more than twice the mean service time. These large fluctuations will cause the queue to back up at times. Once the queue backs up, it will be difficult for it to drain quickly. As an example, suppose that at some time there are 10 customers at S. Then it will take about 90 minutes (on average) to service them. But in that time, approximately 9 new customers will arrive, and it will take another 81 minutes to satisfy them. So on and on it goes. The inverse question, "How long will it take to get 10 customers in the queue in the first place?" is also important. After all, some systems may not exist long enough to reach their steady state. In this case, (2.3.3b) tells us that we can expect over 13 hours to elapse before an observer will find 10 customers in the queue, and over 80 customers will have come and gone by then. We look at this transient behavior very closely throughout the book.

This very simplest of systems tells us that if you try to keep your server busy most of the time, you will have to pay for it in vastly degraded service to your customers. This has nothing to do with overworking your servers and thereby making them less efficient or tired or lazy. Nor is it due to the arrival of an unexpectedly large group of customers all at once. It is due entirely to the irregularity and unpredictability of arrivals and service demands. More complicated or more sophisticated or more realistic systems share this behavior; that is, they all depend on the term $1/(1-\rho)$. Unfortunately, these explanations are not intuitively satisfying to the typical observer, despite their validity. Somehow, people always say, "If I were in charge, I would do things better." Even people who are in charge say it, but they say, "If I *really* were in charge ...." This only points out all the more strongly that we, the human species, have extremely poor intuition concerning statistically fluctuating phenomena. This is all the more reason to have mathematical models to protect us from our faulty feelings. That is why the M/M/1 queue is so important even though it oversimplifies almost all real systems. However inaccurate it is, it is far more reliable than our intuition, because it contains that ubiquitous denominator, $1-\rho$.

What, then, can be done to improve service? Obviously, more servers can be added (i.e., go to an M/M/C queue in Section 2.1.5, where C is the number of customers who can be served simultaneously), if more money is available. Alternatively, the behavior of the customers can be controlled for example, by not permitting them to demand much more service time than the average customer gets. ("Sorry, your time is up".)† In the early 1930s, F. Pollaczek [POLLACZEK30] and A. Y. Khinchine [KHINCHINE32] separately studied the steady-state M/G/1 queue (the G means that the service distribution is *General*; i.e., it can be almost anything) and derived what has come to be known as the P-K formula, which we discuss in detail in Chapter 4. That formula [Equations (4.2.6)] shows that the mean number of customers waiting for service (including the one being served) depends only on their arrival rate λ, and the mean ($\bar{x} = \mathbf{E}[X]$) and *variance* ([$\sigma^2 := \mathbf{E}[X^2] - \bar{x}^2$) of the service time distribution. It is usually expressed in terms of the *squared coefficient of variation*, $C_v^2 := \sigma^2/\bar{x}^2$, as given here.

$$\bar{q} := \mathbf{E}[N] = \rho + \frac{\lambda^2}{1-\rho} \cdot \frac{\mathbf{E}[X^2]}{2} = \frac{\rho}{1-\rho} + \frac{\rho^2}{1-\rho} \cdot \frac{C_v^2 - 1}{2}, \tag{1.1.6a}$$

The mean system time comes from Little's formula (1.1.2), using $\rho = \lambda\bar{x}$ and $\Lambda = \lambda$:

$$\mathbf{E}[T] = \frac{\bar{q}}{\lambda} = \bar{x} + \frac{\lambda}{1-\rho} \cdot \frac{\mathbf{E}[X^2]}{2} = \frac{\bar{x}}{1-\rho} + \frac{\rho\bar{x}}{1-\rho} \cdot \frac{C_v^2 - 1}{2}. \tag{1.1.6b}$$

These reduce to Equations (1.1.4) when $C_v^2 = 1$. Equation (1.1.6a) shows that even if every customer were given exactly the same amount of service time (i.e., $C_v^2 = 0$), the mean queue length would only be reduced to half, and $1-\rho$ is still in its denominator. Furthermore, if no constraint were placed on the customers with the greatest demands, the mean queue length (and mean waiting time) could become arbitrarily large (i.e., when $C_v^2 \gg 1$). That is, there is no upper bound on how bad it could get. The mean system time from Equation (1.1.6b) for $C_v^2 = 0$ is plotted in Figure 1.1.2 with the label *best of Poisson arrivals* (M/D/1). The *worse cases* are for various values of C_v^2 greater than 1. There is no *worst* case, because we can always find a service distribution with a larger C_v^2.

A more convenient way to compare system times is to look at $g(\rho) := (1-\rho)\mathbf{E}[T]$, for this function does not blow up as ρ approaches 1. In fact, for

†Note, however, that if this is done, not only will the fluctuations be reduced, but the mean service time will be reduced as well. Customers will not necessarily get what they came for.

M/G/1 queues, from (1.1.6b)

$$g(\rho) = \bar{x} + \rho\bar{x} \cdot \frac{C_v^2 - 1}{2}.$$

That is, $g(\rho)$ is a straight line with $g(0) = \bar{x}$ for all service time distributions, and $g(1) = \bar{x}(C_v^2 + 1)/2$. This is seen in Figure 1.1.3. For G/M/1, and other queues, $g(\rho)$ is not a straight line, but for well-behaved systems $g(1)$ is still finite, as seen by the D/M/1 queue, labelled 6.

One way to modify the performance of a single steady-state queue is to control the arrival pattern of customers by, for instance, scheduling them to come at 10-minute intervals, as doctors and dentists do. In Chapter 5 we look at the G/M/1 queue and see that even if customers come exactly at their appointed times, the waiting time, [from Equation (5.1.7c)], will again only be cut approximately in half (again with a variant of $1 - \rho$ in its denominator), because of the uncertainty of how long service will take. This is shown in Figures 1.1.2 and 1.1.3 with the curve labeled *best of exponential servers* (D/M/1) [COHEN82].

Only complete control of both arrivals and service times will yield the desired efficiency of no waiting. This is shown in Figure 1.1.2 by the horizontal line labeled *ideal* (D/D/1). But in that case, will the customers get anything near what they came for? The job of queueing theorists is to analyze systems with given, or possible, performance characteristics as described by their arrival and service distributions. Optimally, we would prefer to leave the arrival and service demands (needs) alone and change the inanimate system characteristics. We leave it to the CEOs, politicians, management consultants, and other (so-called) efficiency experts to modify or control customer and server behavior to suit their goals.

Since the early 1970s, networks of queues have been studied and applied to numerous areas in computer science and engineering with a high degree of success. The basis for this success was due to Jackson [JACKSON63] and Gordon and Newell [GORDON-NEWELL67], who showed that certain classes of steady-state queueing networks with any number of service centers could be solved using a ***product-form solution***. Subsequently, Buzen [BUZEN73] showed that the ominous-looking formulas the previous researchers had derived were actually computationally manageable, and thereafter the performance analysis of queueing networks began to blossom into a research field of its own. The theory has ultimately been extended to include, for instance, multiple classes, other service time distributions if the queueing discipline is not first-come, first-served (FCFS), and state-dependent routing [BASKETETAL75]. ***Jackson networks***, as they are now called, have been so successful in so many areas that it is hard to see where they do not apply. Their success lies in their ability to fit the measurements of any given queueing network. The reason is that the product-form solution has enough free parameters in it to fit anything (see Section 4.4.4). They also contain, hidden within them, the all-important denominator $1 - \rho$. The fact that it is hidden within the complex formalism can be valuable, because questioners are then unlikely to say "I can do better." One is far less likely to argue with the output of a sophisticated computer program that requires an enormous amount of data input than with an algebraic formula or the verbal arguments of an "expert."

But the ability of Jackson networks to predict is an open question. It is important to emphasize that *they do not apply to systems where there are population size constraints*, or to *non-steady-state systems*, or *nonexponential servers with FCFS queueing discipline.* This book therefore goes in a direction orthogonal to that covered by Jackson networks. Only in Chapters 4 and 6 do we discuss the connection. We show in Section 4.4.4 in what sense they are not valid for FCFS M/G/1 queues. In Section 6.2.4 we introduce *generalized* M/G/C//N networks and show that they reduce to (single-class) Jackson networks only when $N \leq C$. The meaning of all this becomes clear as the reader goes through the book. At the moment it is only important for those already familiar with Jackson networks to realize that there is much in queueing theory that is not covered by Jackson networks.

As you might surmise from this discussion, just about everything that has been done in queueing theory has assumed the steady state. Very little is known about transient behavior, for one of two reasons. We do not know which of these two statements is valid:

1. Transient behavior is unimportant; therefore, it is not studied.

2. Transient behavior is too difficult to measure and analyze; therefore, it is declared to be unimportant.

A growing number of researchers (including this author) have "declared" that transient behavior should be considered important (see, e.g., [NEUTS77]); therefore, we devote a considerable amount of space and effort in each chapter to its analysis. If it should no longer prove too difficult to study, perhaps more researchers will agree that it is important.

1.1.2 Markov Property

The reader is not expected to know anything special about Markov chains, the property that Markov introduced and built on in 1907 [MARKOV07]. It is, however, an important underpinning of the approach expounded here. There are many books that cover this in detail at multiple levels, from basic (e.g., [GROSS-HARRIS98], [TRIVEDI02], and [KLEINROCK75], and many more) to advanced (e.g., [HEYMAN-SOBEL82], [FELLER71], and [ASMUSSEN03]). We assume that the reader already has some passing knowledge of the subject, but we introduce concepts as needed.

We first describe what we mean by a *state*. A complete specification of a system or subsystem is collectively called a state. No two states can have the same complete specification; therefore, they must differ in at least one aspect. For example, for the purposes of coin-flipping, a coin can be in only one of two states, heads or tails. Two coins, collectively, can be in one of three states, HH, HT, or TT. So after the flips we could say (assuming it is true) that "the system is in state HT." We also use the word to describe the probability that the flips will result in one state or another. That is, we could say before the flips (or without having seen the results) that "the system is in state $\mathbf{p}$," where

$$\mathbf{p} = [\,0.25\,,\ 0.50\,,\ 0.25\,],$$

corresponding to the probability for each of the three states to occur. If we must make a distinction, we will call the former a ***pure state***, and the latter a ***composite state***. We will also refer to the triplet of values, $\mathbf{p}$, as a ***state vector***. Now you might ask if HT is completely specified, because it could have been ht or th. From the coin flipping game point of view, or if we cannot tell which coin is which, there is only the one ***external state***, HT, but it has two ***internal states***. The other two external states, HH and TT, have only one internal state each. The set of internal states corresponding to an external state is referred to as its *state space*. Thus we say that

$$\Xi_{HT} \;:=\; \{\,ht\,,\,th\,\}$$

or that "ht is an element of Ξ_{HT}," written

$$ht\ \in \Xi_{HT}\,.$$

If this seems confusing, it should become clearer over time, because we use these terms regularly. For instance, suppose that we are studying a subsystem, represented by the symbol S. If we could look inside we would see, say, three exponential servers (which we call *phases*). Next suppose that only one customer can be inside the subsystem at a time, and there are five customers there altogether (one inside and four outside). Then we say that the subsystem is in external state [5] and that the system has three internal states. We might write $\Xi_5 = \{1, 2, 3\}$.

In general, the sum of probabilities of being in a set of internal states with the same external state will be the probability of being observed in that external state. This is quite analogous to the terms "sample" and "event" used in many probability texts, where an event is a set of samples, and the probability of an event is the sum (or integral) of probabilities over the sample points [TRIVEDI02]. In our case, the external states are mutually exclusive, and the internal states (sample points) may not be individually measurable or even physically meaningful (we may not always be allowed to look inside S). Even so, we use the rather picturesque description of customers meandering, sometimes with negative probabilities, through networks of exponential servers (phases), whose service times may be complex numbers. Even if this annoys the realist within each of us, it helps us to picture and remember the process being discussed and to distinguish it from similar processes that might also be of interest. But in the end, the mathematical conclusions must be correct if the theory is to be meaningful.

Suppose that a system can be completely described as being in one of a countable (either finite or infinite) number of states. The set of states is discrete, thus the system cannot gradually go from one state to another. Therefore at a later time it will hop to another of those states. In time, then, the history of the system can be described by a sequence of states. Such a sequence is called a ***chain***. The Markov property states that the probability that the system will be in a particular state at the next moment of time (i.e., after the next hop) depends only on the state it is in now, not where it was previously. A ***Markov chain*** is a sequence of states generated by a process that satisfies the Markov property. This abstract idea becomes meaningful once we look at some simple systems. For now we give the formal definition of a discrete Markov chain.

Definition 1.1.4

Let Ξ be a countable set of states. Furthermore, let $\mathcal{S} = \{I_o, I_1, I_2, \ldots, I_n, \ldots\}$ be a discrete sequence of random variables, each of which takes its values from Ξ. In general we might expect that the value I_n takes on would depend on the values taken by I_o through I_{n-1}. But if

$$\mathbb{P}\mathbf{r}(I_n = \ell_n \mid I_o = \ell_o, I_1 = \ell_1, \cdots, I_{n-1} = \ell_{n-1})$$

$$= \mathbb{P}\mathbf{r}(I_n = \ell_n \mid I_{n-1} = \ell_{n-1}),$$

where $\ell_k \in \Xi$, then $\mathcal{S}$ is a ***discrete Markov chain***. □

Although not all aspects of queueing theory are described by Markov processes, there are few known analytical techniques that go beyond the Markov property. Thus we should say a few words about the so-called *memoryless* property. Only a system with one state is truly memoryless. (See Section 1.2.1). A system can be extended to include pseudostates that serve the purpose of "remembering" some of the past. It is not uncommon to construct such states even though they are not observable, as long as the formalism is maintained.

The question then is: "what is a non-Markovian system?" This can be answered in the following way. In general, a system's future behavior depends on its entire past history and thus it must "remember" everything. A Markovian system, on the other hand, can remember only a part of its history and thus must discard old information as new events occur. Two points follow directly from this idea. First, for short amounts of time (depending on the size of the state space), a Markovian model would be an excellent representation of a non-Markovian system.

Over long periods of time, however, a Markovian system will forget its initial state and thus would be a poor approximation for those systems that do depend on their initial state.

1.1.3 Notation, Pronouns, Examples

The following notational standards are adhered to as closely as possible. All matrices (two-subscripted arrays) are represented by boldface capital letters (e.g., $\mathbf{M}$), while their components are noted in either of two ways, M_{ij} or $(\mathbf{M})_{ij}$, depending on the context. Similarly, all vectors (single-subscripted arrays) are represented by boldface lowercase letters [e.g., $\mathbf{v}$ has components v_i or $(\mathbf{v})_i$]. Row vectors and column vectors play distinctly different roles in the formalism presented here. As in many books on matrix theory, the symbol "$'$", means ***transpose***, but we are always interested in an object or its transpose, never both, so $\mathbf{v}'$ always denotes a column vector. Sometimes we discuss a set of vectors or matrices, such as $\{\mathbf{v_1}, \mathbf{v_2}, \mathbf{v_3}\}$. In this case, the subscripts are also set in boldface type. So the j-th component of the i-th vector is $(\mathbf{v_i})_j$.

We also strictly adhere to the following convention on the use of pronouns. We are always talking about "customers", the "author", ***random observer*** (or ***outside observer***), "servers" (or "service centers" or "subsystems"), and the "reader". To minimize the ambiguity, we always refer to the reader as "you"; a customer is "he"; an observer (random or outside) is "she;" and a "server" (service center, or subsystem), is "it." Thus the following statement has an unambiguous meaning: "***We*** point out to ***you*** that ***she*** sees ***him*** enter ***it***." Translation: "The reader should note that the observer sees the customer enter the subsystem." However she may not be able to see what he does after he enters (although she might figure out what he is *probably doing*).

All equations, definitions, figures, examples, and exercises are numbered in sequence by chapter and section (but not subsection). Thus "Figure 2.3.4" is the fourth figure in Section 2.3. Also, "(4.1.13d)" is the fourth [d] equation in the thirteenth set of equations in Section 4.1, whereas "Equations (4.1.13)" refers to all four of (4.1.13a), (4.1.13b), (4.1.13c), and (4.1.13d). Note that an object such as "(4.1.13)" without a qualifier always refers to an equation. Otherwise we say "Definition 4.5.7," and so on. Since lemmas are really theorems, and both can have corollaries, we have chosen to number them together in a single sequence. Thus we have Lemma 4.2.1, Theorem 4.2.2, and Corollary 4.2.2, but no Theorem 4.2.1. Clearly, Corollary 4.2.2 is a corollary to Theorem 4.2.2.

To help the reader quickly locate a word or phrase from the index, such objects usually appear on the page referenced in ***bold-faced, italic font***. This is particularly true if the term is defined or extensively discussed there.

We have given many examples throughout the book, most of them involving numerical computation, invariably summarized by a family of curves in a graph. Most of the exercises we have asked the student to perform are proofs or other mathematical manipulations. The examples can easily be made into exercises by having the student redo the example using a different distribution function. In a class environment, each student can be assigned a different function. Then a comparison study can be made by the class as a whole to see how the different functions affect the particular phenomenon being studied.

1.2 Distribution Functions Over Time

We use the word ***system*** in referring to a closed entity, one in which customers neither enter nor leave. Yet we often use ***closed system*** to retain clarity. On the other hand, a ***subsystem*** is one to which customers come and go. The simplest of all subsystems has only one state, with at most one customer. Then that state is either occupied or unoccupied. In the next two sections we show how such a simple system evolves in time, where we assume that events could occur at any time (continuous) or at equally spaced moments (discrete).

1.2.1 Exponential Distribution (Continuous Time, t)

We start with a single customer and a single subsystem S. Let $R(t)$ be the probability that the customer is in the subsystem at time t, where t is a continuous parameter. Assume that at $t = 0$ he definitely was there [$R(0) = 1$]. We can also think of $R(t)$ as the probability that he left after t. That is

$$R(t) = \mathbb{P}\mathbf{r}(T > t),$$

where T is the random variable denoting the time he leaves S. The probability that he will still be in S at a time $t + \delta$ is equal to the probability that he was there at time t, [$R(t)$], times the probability that he is still there a time δ later, [$R(\delta|t)$], that is, $R(t + \delta) = R(t) \times R(\delta|t)$. Now, whatever else $R(\delta|t)$ is, it must have $R(0|t) = 1$, and if we assume that it is a smooth function, it is expandable in a Maclaurin series, $R(\delta, t) = 1 - \mu(t)\delta + O(\delta^2)$, where μ may depend on t (but not on δ). At this point we make the memoryless assumption that $R(x|t)$ does not depend on its second argument [i.e., $R(x|t_1) = R(x|t_2)$], thus making μ a constant. Then

$$R(t + \delta) = R(t)[1 - \mu\delta + O(\delta^2)].$$

Subtracting $R(t)$ from both sides of this equation and dividing by δ, we get

$$\frac{R(t + \delta) - R(t)}{\delta} = -\mu R(t) + O(\delta).$$

Next let δ go to 0 and get

$$\frac{dR(t)}{dt} = -\mu R(t). \tag{1.2.1a}$$

It is well known, and can be proven by direct substitution, that the solution of (1.2.1a) is

$$R(t) = e^{-\mu t}, \tag{1.2.1b}$$

an exponential function.

Let us pause here to discuss some notational difficulties and conventions. First we enumerate some well-known terms from probability theory. As already mentioned, $R(t)$ is the probability that the event being awaited has not yet occurred by time t (or equivalently, will occur after time t), and is often called the ***reliability function*** for the subsystem. The probability that it will have occurred by t is

$$F(t) := \mathbb{P}\mathbf{r}(T \le t) = 1 - R(t) \tag{1.2.2a}$$

and is called the ***Probability Distribution Function*** (**PDF**), (or simply ***distribution function***) with derivative

$$f(t) := \frac{dF(t)}{dt} \tag{1.2.2b}$$

called the ***probability density function*** (**pdf**) (or simply ***density function***). Because $R(t) = 1 - F(t)$, $R(t)$ is also known as the ***complementary distribution function*** and is often denoted as $\bar{F}(t)$.

A slight terminology problem shows up when we deal with functions. For instance, is $f(x)$ different from $f(t)$? If one is thinking of the function as a whole (i.e., the entire set of points $\{(x, f(x))|0 \le x < \infty\}$, or equivalently $\{t, f(t) \mid 0 \le t < \infty\}$, they are the same set. In other words, the graphs of the two expressions are the same curve. Therefore, the notation $f(\cdot)$ is often used to mean that any symbol could go inside the parentheses. Extending the confusion, we often write

$$\bar{t} := \int_0^\infty t\, f(t)\, dt,$$

but t is a dummy variable, so this integral is the same as

$$\int_0^\infty x\, f(x)\, dx$$

(or any other symbol), which we would be inclined to represent by $\bar{x}$. We see then, that the important information is the f, not the variable symbol. Also, the bar notation can be ambiguous. The situation gets even more complicated when we are dealing with several functions at the same time. To get around this (and for other reasons), random variables are used to denote possible values of a given function. One now says rthe following.

Definition 1.2.1

Let T be a ***random variable***, distributed according to $f(t)$ [or $f(x)$, or even $f_T(x)$]. Then we can write

$$\mathbb{E}[T] \;:=\; \int_0^\infty tf(t)\, dt \;=\; \int_0^\infty xf(x)\, dx. \tag{1.2.3a}$$

(Random variables are always capital letters.) In words, we read this as: "The ***expected value*** (or ***expectation value***) of T is equal to $\cdots$." When we are dealing with time variables, the expected value is often referred to as the ***mean lifetime***, or ***mean service time***, or simply, ***lifetime***. In general, we can write

$$\mathbb{E}[T^n] := \int_0^\infty t^n f(t)\, dt. \tag{1.2.3b}$$

We read this as: "The expected value of T^n" or "the n-th moment of $f(t)$." This notation extends to any function as

$$\mathbb{E}[h(T)] := \int_0^\infty h(t)\, f_T(t)\, dt, \tag{1.2.3c}$$

The symbol $\mathbb{E}[X]$ is a different object, because X must be a random variable distributed according to a different function, perhaps $g(x)$ or $f_X(x)$, or even $f_X(t)$. □

It is common practice to use $\bar{t}$ for $\mathbf{E}[T]$. We often do that here, but will generally avoid expressions such as $\bar{t^2}$. Also, both letters, x and t, will be used as the time variable. We try our best not to use $\bar{x}$ and $\bar{t}$ in the same context.

Another much used function is the ***variance***, symbolized by σ^2 and defined by

$$\sigma^2 := \mathbf{E}\left[(T - \mathbf{E}[T])^2\right] = \int_0^\infty (t - \bar{t})^2 f(t)\, dt \tag{1.2.4a}$$

which can be shown to be equal to

$$\sigma^2 = \mathbf{E}[T^2] - \mathbf{E}[T]^2 = \mathbf{E}[T^2] - \bar{t}^2. \tag{1.2.4b}$$

The ***standard deviation*** of $f(t)$ is symbolized by σ, which satisfies the obvious, $\sigma := \sqrt{\sigma^2}$. In words, σ is a measure of the *spread* about the mean; the smaller σ is, the narrower the distribution. We usually deal with functions that are defined only for positive t, therefore a relative width is often useful. Hence we have the ***coefficient of variation***, whose square is defined by

$$C_v^2 = \frac{\sigma^2}{(\mathbf{E}[T])^2}. \tag{1.2.4c}$$

We hope this discussion has not brought on more confusion than it has allayed. We have found that trivial notational problems such as these often prevent understanding of expressions with which the reader would otherwise have no trouble.

Let us return to where we were before the pause. Continuing from (1.2.1b) and (1.2.2a), the pdf for the exponential distribution is

$$f(t) = -\frac{dR(t)}{dt} = \mu\, e^{-\mu t}. \tag{1.2.5a}$$

The mean lifetime for the process is

$$\mathbf{E}[T] := \int_0^\infty t\, f(t)\, dt = \int_0^\infty t\, \mu\, e^{-\mu t}\, dt = \frac{1}{\mu}. \tag{1.2.5b}$$

The reciprocal of the mean lifetime, in this case μ, is interpretable as the ***service rate***, or the rate of leaving. The n-th moment for the exponential distribution is

$$\mathbf{E}[T^n] = \frac{n!}{\mu^n}. \tag{1.2.5c}$$

The variance is $\sigma^2 = 1/\mu^2$ and the squared coefficient of variation $C_v^2 = 1$.

Finally, we show that exponential distributions have the memoryless property [the reverse of what we did to get (1.2.1)]. Let T be the random variable denoting the time that the subsystem stops being active. Suppose that the subsystem has been actively servicing the customer for some time, t. What is the probability that it will continue to be active more than a further time x? By definition

$$R(t + x) = \mathbf{Pr}(T > t + x).$$

That is, $R(x+t)$ is the probability that activity will last longer than $t+x$, and $R(t)$ is the probability that it will last longer than t. From the rule of conditional probabilities for any two events A and B we have

$$\mathbb{Pr}(A \mid B) = \frac{\mathbb{Pr}(A \cap B)}{\mathbb{Pr}(B)}.$$

(Read: "probability that A occurs, given that B occurs.") Let A be the event that the process finished after time $t+x$ ($T > x+t$), and let B be the event that the process ended after time t ($T > t$). Clearly, $A \cap B = A$, $\mathbb{Pr}(A) = R(t+x)$ and $\mathbb{Pr}(B) = R(t)$, so

$$\mathbb{Pr}(T > t+x \mid T > t) = \frac{R(t+x)}{R(t)}. \tag{1.2.6a}$$

If $R(t) = e^{-\mu t}$, as given by (1.2.1b), then

$$\mathbb{Pr}(T > t+x \mid T > t) = \frac{e^{-\mu(t+x)}}{e^{-\mu t}} = e^{-\mu x}. \tag{1.2.6b}$$

This tells us that the time remaining does not depend on how long the process has already been active. The exponential distribution is the only distribution with this property. Clearly it is ***memoryless***.

The assumption at the beginning of this section that $R(x \mid t)$ is independent of t (we assume that μ is independent of t) is also known as memoryless. Each implies the other. We use this idea to get another expression of memoryless. Independence of the past tells us that $\mathbb{Pr}(T > t+x \mid T > t) = \mathbb{Pr}(T > x) = R(x)$. Thus (1.2.6a) becomes $R(x) = R(t+x)/R(t)$, or

$$R(t+x) = R(t)\, R(x). \tag{1.2.6c}$$

This is known as the ***semigroup property***† (see, for instance, [FELLER71]). The exponential function (with any value for μ) is the only scalar function of a single continuous variable that satisfies (1.2.6c).

Exercise 1.2.1: Prove that $e^{-\mu t}$ for any μ is the unique solution to (1.2.6c) in the following way. Subtract $R(x)$ from both sides of the equation, divide by x, take the limit as $x \to 0$, and let $R'(0) = -\mu$, thereby yielding (1.2.1a).

1.2.2 Geometric Distribution (Discrete Time, *n*)

Suppose that events can occur only at discrete moments of time, such as at the tick of a clock, and suppose that the subsystem stays busy at each tick

† A semigroup is a set $\boldsymbol{S}$ whose elements satisfy the following. Let $A, B, C \in \boldsymbol{S}$. Then $AB \in \boldsymbol{S}$ (closure) and $(AB)C = A(BC)$ (associative law).

with probability p. If $R_o = 1$, then $R_1 = p$ and $R_2 = pR_1 = p_2$. In general, the probability R_n that it will still be busy by the n-th step is equal to $p \cdot R_{n-1}$, from which it follows that

$$R_n = p^n. \tag{1.2.7a}$$

R_n is the discrete analogue of $R(t)$, so we could call it the ***discrete reliability function***. The analogue to $f(t)$ (sometimes called the ***probability mass function*** or *discrete density function*), symbolized by f_n, is the probability that the server will finish in exactly n steps. It is known that b_n is the ***geometric distribution***, or the negative binomial distribution of order 1, but we calculate it here by doing the analogue of differentiation:

$$f_n = R_{n-1} - R_n = (1-p)p^{n-1}. \tag{1.2.7b}$$

Let N be the random variable denoting the number of steps taken before completion. Then

$$\mathbb{E}[N] = \sum_{n=1}^{\infty} n\, f_n = (1-p) \sum_{n=1}^{\infty} n\, p^{n-1} = \frac{1}{1-p}. \tag{1.2.7c}$$

Equation (1.2.1b) and Equations (1.2.5) are much closer to Equations (1.2.7) than it would seem by superficial examination. Suppose that although time is a continuous parameter, the system of Section 1.2.1 is examined only at regular intervals, as with the cinema or video. Let δ be the time between snapshots. Then $t = n\delta$. Using this in (1.2.1b), we get

$$R(t) = e^{-\mu n \delta} = \left(e^{-\mu\delta}\right)^n. \tag{1.2.8a}$$

Let $p = e^{-\mu\delta}$; then $R(t) = R_n$. At least as far as the reliability function is concerned, a discrete time system is indistinguishable from a continuous-time system in which observations are made at regular intervals. Equations (1.2.5b) and (1.2.7c) do not yield identical values, but the following inequality is satisfied.

$$\delta\,(\mathbb{E}[N] - 1) < \mathbb{E}[T] < \delta\,\mathbb{E}[N]. \tag{1.2.8b}$$

The proof follows directly by substituting for p and letting $u = \mu\delta$. Then (1.2.8b) converts [after multiplying all terms by $(e^{u-1})/\delta$] to the inequality

$$1 < \frac{e^u - 1}{u} < e^u, \qquad \text{for } u > 0.$$

Equation (1.2.8b) says that the uncertainty in $\mathbb{E}[T]$, when measured to the nearest (rounded up) multiple of δ, is less than one time unit, which is as close as a discrete and continuous system can come to each other. This is true even for more general systems, where the strict inequality may be replaced by $\leq$.

1.3 Chapman-Kolmogorov Equations

We now consider a system that has many states of possible existence. In Chapter 2, when we deal with queues the states are explicitly described. For now it is sufficient to consider a state to be one possible complete specification of the system's condition. The system can be in one and only one state at a time, and in the course of time it will change from one state to another. The set of all possible states is called the *state space.* Probability books often identify these with *samples* in a *sample space.* If the space is finite, or at most countably infinite, we have a *discrete state space.* We are interested exclusively in systems with discrete state spaces. As our system evolves in time, it must "jump" from one state to the next, because there is no continuum of states in a discrete space to match the continuous time parameter. A sequence of such states is called a *chain*, and if the Markov property holds, we have a *Markov chain.* Of course, time can be continuous or discrete, giving a ***continuous Markov chain*** or ***discrete Markov chain.*** If the state space is uncountable, change ***chain*** to ***process.***

1.3.1 Continuous Time

As with most expositions purporting to start from scratch, the first few sections are overladen with definitions. Let i and j take on positive integer values, corresponding to the possible states of the system. Then

Definition 1.3.1

$\Xi \ := \{i \mid i \textit{ is a state of the system}\}$. We read this as: "$\Xi$ is the set of all i, such that i is a state of the system." We also call i a ***pure state*** of the system. If Ξ is a finite set of states with, say, m members (i.e., $m = |\Xi|$), we can write $1 \leq i \leq m$, or $i \in \Xi$ (i is an element of Ξ). □

Next, define the following.

Definition 1.3.2

$\pi_i(t)$:= *probability that the system will be in state* $i \in \Xi$ *at time* t. $\boldsymbol{\pi}(t)$ is an m-dimensional row vector whose i-th component is $\pi_i(t)$, and is called the ***state probability vector*** or just the ***probability vector.*** $\boldsymbol{\pi}(0)$ is referred to as the ***initial state of the system.*** □

We often say that "the system is in state $\boldsymbol{\pi}$" when we mean that "the system is in state $i \in \Xi$ with probability π_i." If a distinction between the two ideas is necessary, we say that the system is in ***composite state*** $\boldsymbol{\pi}$, as opposed to *pure state* i. In this case, $\pi_j = \delta_{ij}$, where δ is defined as follows.

Definition 1.3.3

The ***Kronecker delta*** has the values

$$\delta_{ij} = \begin{cases} 0 & \text{for} \quad i \neq j \\ 1 & \text{for} \quad i = j \end{cases} .$$

It can be thought of as the ij-th component of the identity matrix. □

The movement of the system from state to state is governed by the following.

Definition 1.3.4

P_{ij} := probability that the system will jump to $j \in \Xi$ upon leaving state $i \in \Xi$. The matrix $\boldsymbol{P}$, defined by $(\boldsymbol{P})_{ij} = P_{ij}$, is called a ***transition matrix*** *if $P_{ij} \geq O$ and $\sum_{j=1}^{m} P_{ij} \leq 1$ for all i and j.* It is also referred to as a ***Markov matrix*** or a ***stochastic matrix*** if $\sum_{j=1}^{m} P_{ij} = 1$. If $\sum_{j=1}^{m} P_{ij} < 1$ for some i, then $\boldsymbol{P}$ is called a ***substochastic matrix***. Formally we follow Definition 1.1.4 and write

$$P_{ij} = \mathbb{P}\mathbf{r}(I_n = j \mid I_{n-1} = i).$$

We assume that transition probabilities are independent of how long the process was running. That is, $\boldsymbol{P}$ is independent of n, (i.e., the number of steps that have already been made). This is known as a ***stationary process*** [FELLER71]. □

Because a system, by definition, is closed, the sum of probabilities of all possible jumps must be 1. That is,

$$\sum_{j=1}^{m} P_{ij} = 1. \tag{1.3.1a}$$

By introducing the special row vector,

$$\boldsymbol{\epsilon} := [\ 1,\ 1,\ 1,\ \cdots\ ,\ 1\ ],$$

with $\boldsymbol{\epsilon}'$ being the ***transpose*** (i.e., column vector) of $\boldsymbol{\epsilon}$, (1.3.1a) can be rewritten in matrix form as

$$\boldsymbol{P}\boldsymbol{\epsilon}' = \boldsymbol{\epsilon}'. \tag{1.3.1b}$$

Many matrices in this book have this property so we give it a special name.

Definition 1.3.5

Any matrix that satisfies (1.3.1b) is called an ***isometric matrix***. Thus $\boldsymbol{P}$ is *isometric*. Using an extended view of the definition, we can say that $\boldsymbol{\epsilon}'$ itself is isometric, because its row sum (only one term) is 1. In Section 3.4.2 we give an extended rationale for this nomenclature when we show that many formulas are invariant to isometric transformations.
□

Note that (1.3.1b) is a matrix equation, whereas (1.3.1a) looks explicitly at the components. The reader need not be concerned at the moment with the subtle distinction we are trying to makei here. However, as the book evolves, we will tend to ignore the properties of the individual matrix elements. It is the matrix as a whole that operates on the system's present state vector and changes it to the future state vector. Therefore, we almost never make use of the property $P_{ij} > 0$. However, we are always concerned to see if a matrix is isometric, for this is an algebraic property of the matrix. When we prove that a square matrix is isometric, the reader is welcome to think of it as being a stochastic matrix, but we seldom prove it.

We next derive the generalization of (1.2.1a), keeping in mind that the system can go to any state, including the one it is in presently, or one it previously visited. However, not only is there more than one server, but there are two time parameters. t is the time from when the process began being observed, and x is the time since the last event occurred. Without the memoryless assumption, it would be almost impossible to find a solvable analytic formulation. Therefore, $R_i(\delta|t, x)$ (the probability that the system will be in state i at time $t + \delta$, given that it was in state i at time t and has been there continuously for a time interval x) reduces to $R_i(\delta)$. With this understood, we have

$$\pi_i(t + \delta) = \pi_i(t)R_i(\delta) + \sum_j \pi_j(t)[1 - R_j(\delta)]P_{ji} + O(\delta^2).$$

In words, the probability that the system will be in state i at time $t + \delta$, $[\pi_i(t+\delta)]$, is equal to the probability that it was in state i at time t $[\pi_i(t)]$, and has remained there for time δ $[R_i(\delta)]$, plus the sum of probabilities that it was in some other state, j (including i), at time t $[\pi_j(t)]$, left that state within the interval δ, $[1 - R_j(\delta)]$, and went to i $[P_{ji}]$, plus multiple transitions $[O(\delta^2)]$. As with the derivation of (1.2.1a), replace R_i with its Taylor expansion, subtract $\pi_i(t)$ from both sides of the equation, divide by δ and take the limit for δ goes to 0, and get

$$\frac{d\pi_i(t)}{dt} = \sum_j \pi_j(t)\mu_j P_{ji} - \pi_i(t)\mu_i. \tag{1.3.2a}$$

This is one form of the ***Chapman-Kolmogorov (C-K) equation***. It can be expressed more elegantly as a matrix equation in the following way. We have already defined the row vector:

$$\boldsymbol{\pi}(t) := [\pi_1(t), \pi_2(t), \cdots],$$

and now introduce a diagonal matrix.

Definition 1.3.6

$(\boldsymbol{M})_{ij} = \mu_i\delta_{ij}$, *where* δ_{ij}, *is the Kronecker delta* defined above. In other words, $\boldsymbol{M}$ is a diagonal matrix, with diagonal elements $M_{ii} = \mu_i$, where μ_i is the rate of leaving state i. $\boldsymbol{M}$ is called the ***completion rate matrix***. It is also referred to as the ***holding rate matrix***, but that term is not used here. □

We now can rewrite (1.3.2a) as

$$\frac{d\boldsymbol{\pi}(t)}{dt} = \boldsymbol{\pi}(t)\boldsymbol{M}\boldsymbol{P} - \boldsymbol{\pi}(t)\boldsymbol{M} = -\boldsymbol{\pi}(t)\boldsymbol{Q}, \tag{1.3.2b}$$

where the ***transition rate matrix*** (also called the ***infinitesimal rate matrix***, or simply ***rate matrix***) $\boldsymbol{Q}$, is defined by

$$\boldsymbol{Q} := \boldsymbol{M}(\boldsymbol{I} - \boldsymbol{P}). \tag{1.3.2c}$$

Although equivalent to the usual definition (most researchers define $-\boldsymbol{Q}$ as the transition rate matrix), $\boldsymbol{Q}$ is given in a somewhat different form because we have separated the process of leaving a state [$\boldsymbol{M}$] from that of deciding which state to go to next [$\boldsymbol{P}$]. This is most useful to us in succeeding chapters. $\boldsymbol{M}$ governs the time between events and $\boldsymbol{P}$ controls what happens when an event occurs. Thus we can look at the behavior of systems conditioned by the occurrence of specific events. For instance, in Chapter 4 we not only study the steady-state probabilities of finding an M/G/1 queue in a given state, but also analyze the probabilities of being in a given state after a departure or after an arrival.

Let us define $\mathbf{o}$ to be the row vector of all 0s. It is clear from (1.3.1b) and (1.3.2c) that $\boldsymbol{Q}\,\boldsymbol{\epsilon}' = \mathbf{o}'$, so upon multiplying (1.3.2b) from the right with $\boldsymbol{\epsilon}'$, it follows that

$$\frac{d}{dt}[\boldsymbol{\pi}(t)\,\boldsymbol{\epsilon}'] = 0. \qquad (1.3.2d)$$

In other words, $\boldsymbol{\pi}(t)\,\boldsymbol{\epsilon}'$ is a constant that we may presume to be 1 for all t, because

$$\left[\boldsymbol{\pi}(t)\boldsymbol{\epsilon}'\right]_{t=o} = \sum_i \pi_i(0) = 1$$

This is no more than would be expected in a closed system.

The solution to (1.3.2b), another form of the C-K equation, is the matrix equivalent of (1.2.1b), namely

$$\boldsymbol{\pi}(t) = \boldsymbol{\pi}(0)\boldsymbol{G}(t), \qquad (1.3.2e)$$

where

$$\boldsymbol{G}(t) = \exp(-t\,\boldsymbol{Q}). \qquad (1.3.3a)$$

Some explanation is required, however. Only multiplication, addition and subtraction of matrices are defined. Division is replaced by taking the inverse, if it exists. Therefore, a function of a matrix must be defined in terms of these primitives. So, in general, any function of a matrix is formally defined by a Maclaurin series expansion, satisfying:

Theorem 1.3.1: Let $f(t)$ be any function of t whose Maclaurin series converges for all $|\,t\,| < r$ (its radius of convergence), and let ξ be the spectral radius of any square matrix, $\mathbf{X}$. If $\mathbf{X}$ is of finite dimension, then

$$\xi := \max_i |\,\lambda_i\,|,$$

where the λs are the eigenvalues of $\mathbf{X}$. The matrix function $f(t\mathbf{X})$ is well defined by the Maclaurin expansion of $f(\cdot)$, for all $t < r < \xi$. Note that $f(\cdot)$ takes on the algebraic structure of its argument. If its argument is a scalar [t] then $f(t)$ is a scalar. If its argument is a square matrix [$\mathbf{X}$] then $f(\mathbf{X})$ is a square matrix, with the same dimension.■†

†The symbol ■ designates the end of a theorem, lemma, or corollary.

For example,

$$\exp(-t\mathbf{X}) := \mathbf{I} - t\mathbf{X} + \frac{t^2}{2!}\mathbf{X}^2 - \frac{t^3}{3!}\mathbf{X}^3 + \cdots . \qquad (1.3.3b)$$

The radius of convergence for the exponential function is infinite, so (1.3.3b) is valid for all t.

Corollary 1.3.1: Let $f(t)$ be any function of t whose Maclaurin series converges for all $| t |< r$. Then $f(t\mathbf{X})$ commutes with $\mathbf{X}$ whenever $f(t\mathbf{X})$ is defined. That is,

$$f(t\mathbf{X})\mathbf{X} = \mathbf{X}f(t\mathbf{X})$$

for all $| t |< r/\xi$, as defined in Theorem 1.3.1. ■

> **Exercise 1.3.1:** Use (1.3.3b) to show that (1.3.2e) satisfies (1.3.2b).

Because $\boldsymbol{Q}\boldsymbol{\epsilon}' = \mathbf{o}'$, it is a straightforward step using (1.3.3b), to show that

$$\boldsymbol{G}(t)\boldsymbol{\epsilon}' = \boldsymbol{\epsilon}' \quad \text{for all } t, \qquad (1.3.4a)$$

so $\boldsymbol{G}(t)$ is an isometric matrix. It can also be shown that if $\boldsymbol{P}$ is a stochastic matrix, then $\boldsymbol{G}(t)$ is also, but only for $t \geq 0$. That is, $[\boldsymbol{G}(t)]_{ij} \geq 0$ if $t \geq 0$. (It is dangerous to try to go backward in time.)

One cannot take it for granted that all relations in elementary algebra follow through for matrix algebra. For instance,

Theorem 1.3.2: Let $\mathbf{A}$ and $\mathbf{B}$ and be two square matrices of the same dimension, then

$$\exp[t(\mathbf{A}+\mathbf{B})] = \exp(t\mathbf{A})\exp(t\mathbf{B}) \quad \text{for all } t, \text{ iff } \mathbf{A}\,\mathbf{B} = \mathbf{B}\,\mathbf{A}.$$

(iff stands for *if and only if*). We restate for emphasis: if $\mathbf{A}$ and $\mathbf{B}$ do not commute, the equation is not valid. ■

> **Exercise 1.3.2:** Prove Theorem 1.3.2 by direct substitution of the appropriate Taylor expansions.

It is clear from (1.3.3a) that $\mathbf{G}(t)$ is the operator that translates a system directly from time 0 to time t. Theorem 1.3.2 allows the most familiar form of the C-K equation to be written:

$$\boldsymbol{G}(s+t) = \boldsymbol{G}(s)\boldsymbol{G}(t). \qquad (1.3.4b)$$

Remember that $\boldsymbol{G}(t)$ is an isometric matrix (think "transition matrix") whose elements change with t. Comparing with (1.2.6c), we see that $\boldsymbol{G}(t)$ also satisfies the ***semigroup*** property, but here, $\boldsymbol{G}$ is a matrix function of t.

Exercise 1.3.3: Let

$$\boldsymbol{M} = \begin{bmatrix} 1 & 0 \\ 0 & 2 \end{bmatrix} \quad \text{and} \quad \boldsymbol{P} = \begin{bmatrix} 0 & 1 \\ 1 & 0 \end{bmatrix}.$$

Find $\boldsymbol{G}(t)$. Show that it is a transition matrix. What is $\boldsymbol{G}(t)$ in the limit as t goes to infinity?

1.3.2 Discrete Time

The discrete-time analogue of (1.3.2b) is self-evident from the definition of the transition matrix $\boldsymbol{P}$. Let $\pi_{\mathbf{d}}(n)$ be the vector whose i-th component is the probability that the system will be in state i at step n. Then

$$\boldsymbol{\pi_d}(n) = \boldsymbol{\pi_d}(n-1)\boldsymbol{P} = \boldsymbol{\pi_d}(0)\boldsymbol{P}^n. \tag{1.3.5a}$$

The discrete analogue to $\boldsymbol{G}(t)$ is $\boldsymbol{G_d}(n) = \boldsymbol{P}^n$. The obvious analogue to (1.3.4b) is

$$\boldsymbol{G_d}(n+m) = \boldsymbol{G_d}(n)\boldsymbol{G_d}(m). \tag{1.3.5b}$$

As in Section 1.2, if a continuous-time system is observed only at integral multiples of some time interval δ, that system is indistinguishable from a discrete-time system with transition matrix

$$\boldsymbol{P_d} = \boldsymbol{G_d}(1) = \boldsymbol{G}(\delta) = \exp(-\delta\boldsymbol{Q}).$$

Although every $\boldsymbol{Q}$ maps onto some $\boldsymbol{P_d}$, not every transition matrix can be expressed in this way. In general, all elements of $\boldsymbol{P_d}$ will be greater than 0, unless:

1. The graph associated with $\boldsymbol{Q}$ is made up of two or more disjoint subgraphs (this would be the case iff 1 is a multiple eigenvalue of $\boldsymbol{Q}$). We would then say that $\boldsymbol{Q}$ is ***reducible***.
2. There exists a state, or set of states, that are ***transient***, (i.e., states that cannot be reached from, but can reach, the rest of the network).

If it is possible to get from state i to state j at all, then $(\boldsymbol{P_d})_{ij} > 0$ and in fact, is of order δ^n, where n is the number of steps it takes to get there. One might say that for every $\boldsymbol{Q}$, the matrix $\boldsymbol{P_d} = \exp(-\delta\boldsymbol{Q})$ exists, but we cannot say the inverse for every $\boldsymbol{P}$. ["log $(\boldsymbol{P})$" (whatever that is) does not necessarily exist for a given $\boldsymbol{P}$, because $\log(x)$ does not have a Maclaurin expansion, although $\log(1+x)$ does.]

Exercise 1.3.4: A simple example of both (1) and (2) is given by

$$\boldsymbol{P} = \begin{bmatrix} 0 & 1 & 0 & 0 \\ 0 & 1 & 0 & 0 \\ 0 & 0 & 0 & 1 \\ 0 & 0 & 1 & 0 \end{bmatrix}.$$

Find the eigenvalues and eigenvectors of $\boldsymbol{P}$. Clearly, states 1 and 2 are disjoint from 3 and 4, and state 1 is transient.

1.3.3 Time-Dependent and Steady-State Solutions

As you may have seen from Exercise 1.3.3, (1.3.2e) is not as explicitly useful as it seems. More useful solutions of this are covered in depth in the literature. We discuss it slightly here, enough to see how $\boldsymbol{\pi}(t)$ varies with time, and do some examples in detail in Chapter 2. First we review a little matrix theory.

1.3.3.1 Some Properties of Matrices

The ***eigenvalues*** of a matrix (also called ***proper values***, or ***characteristic values***) $\mathbf{X}$ are the roots of its ***characteristic equation***,

$$\phi(\lambda) \ :=\mid \lambda\mathbf{I} - \mathbf{X} \mid = 0, \tag{1.3.6}$$

where $| \cdot |$ denotes the *determinant* of any square matrix. In other words, λ_i is an eigenvalue of $\mathbf{X}$ if and only if it is a root of $\phi(\lambda)$ [i.e., $\phi(\lambda_i) = 0$]. If $\mathbf{X}$ is of finite dimension, say m, then $\phi(\lambda)$ is a polynomial of degree m, with m roots. If a particular root appears more than once, it is a ***multiple root***, and we say there is a ***degeneracy*** in that eigenvalue. Otherwise, it is a ***simple root***.

Corresponding to each λ_i is at least one ***left eigenvector*** and one ***right eigenvector*** (also called ***proper vector***), satisfying the following.

$$\mathbf{u_i X} = \lambda_i \mathbf{u_i} \quad \text{and} \quad \mathbf{X\,v_i'} = \lambda_i \mathbf{v_i'}. \tag{1.3.7a}$$

For any square matrix the number of right eigenvectors belonging to each eigenvalue is greater than or equal to one, and less than or equal to the degree of multiplicity of that root. If the number of eigenvectors belonging to a given eigenvalue is strictly less than the degree of multiplicity of that root, then the matrix is said to be a ***defective matrix***. There are as many left as there are right eigenvectors, and they satisfy the following ***orthogonality condition***:

$$\mathbf{u_i v_j'} = 0 \quad \text{for} \quad \lambda_i \neq \lambda_j. \tag{1.3.7b}$$

This condition guarantees that eigenvectors belonging to different eigenvalues are automatically linearly independent. The general case can be treated with some difficulty, but for now assume that the λ_i's are distinct. Then the set of left (or right) eigenvectors forms a complete set. That is, every m-dimensional row (column) vector can be written as a linear combination of left (right) eigenvectors. Then we say that each eigenvector is a ***basis vector***, and the set of left (right) eigenvectors is a ***basis set*** for all row (column) vectors.

It can also be assumed that

$$\mathbf{u_i v_i'} = 1. \tag{1.3.7c}$$

Note that each $\mathbf{u_i}$ is a row vector with m components $[(\mathbf{u_i})_k, 1 \le k \le m]$ and that each $\mathbf{v_i'}$ is a column vector, also with m components. Consider the $m \times m$ matrices

$$(\mathbf{U})_{ik} := (\mathbf{u}_i)_k$$

and

$$(\mathbf{V})_{ki} := (\mathbf{v_i'})_k.$$

Equations (1.3.7) imply that $\mathbf{U}$ and $\mathbf{V}$ are inverses of each other, (i.e., $\mathbf{U\,V} = \mathbf{V\,U} = \mathbf{I}$).

If all the eigenvalues of $\mathbf{X}$ are distinct, the ***spectral decomposition theorem*** states that (where m is the dimension of $\mathbf{X}$)

$$\mathbf{X} = \sum_{i=1}^{m} \lambda_i \mathbf{v_i'}\,\mathbf{u_i} \quad \text{and} \quad \mathbf{I} = \sum_{i=1}^{m} \mathbf{v_i'}\,\mathbf{u_i}. \tag{1.3.8a}$$

Note that whereas

$$\mathbf{u_i}\,\mathbf{v_j'} = \sum_{k=1}^{m} (\mathbf{u_i})_k\,(\mathbf{v_j'})_k$$

(***inner, dot*** or ***scalar product***) is a scalar, the object $\mathbf{v_j'}\,\mathbf{u_i}$ (***outer product***) is an m-dimensional matrix of rank 1, where all rows are proportional to each other and to $\mathbf{u_i}$. That is, $(\mathbf{v_j'}\,\mathbf{u_i})_{kl} = (\mathbf{v_j'})_k\,(\mathbf{u_i})_l$. It follows from the orthogonality conditions above that

$$\mathbf{X}^k = \sum_{i=1}^{m} \lambda_i^k \mathbf{v_i'}\,\mathbf{u_i} \tag{1.3.8b}$$

and more generally,

$$f(t\mathbf{X}) = \sum_{i=1}^{m} f(t\lambda_i)\mathbf{v_i'}\,\mathbf{u_i}, \tag{1.3.8c}$$

where $f(x)$ is any function expressible in a Maclaurin series. Theorem 1.3.1 follows directly from this.

We make a final comment in this section that will be useful in Chapter 3. Each of the eigenvectors, $\mathbf{u_i}$ and $\mathbf{v_i'}$ of (1.3.7a) is determined by a homogeneous equation. Thus if $\mathbf{u_i}$ satisfies (1.3.7a) so does $c\mathbf{u_i}$, where $c \ne 0$. Similarly with $c'\mathbf{v_i'}$. The product of the constants can be determined by (1.3.7c). That is, let $\bar{\mathbf{u}}_\mathbf{i}$ and $\bar{\mathbf{v}}_\mathbf{i}'$ be the computed solutions to (1.3.7a) for eigenvalue λ_i, but

$\bar{\mathbf{u}}_\mathbf{i}\,\bar{\mathbf{v}}'_\mathbf{i} = d \neq 1$. In order to satisfy (1.3.7a), we must multiply each of them by a constant, and fix those constants by satisfying

$$c\bar{\mathbf{u}}_\mathbf{i}\, c'\bar{\mathbf{v}}'_\mathbf{i} = c\,c'\,d = 1.$$

This only determines the product of the two constants. Usually one fixes c or c' in some arbitrary manner and then determines the other. In Chapter 3 we have reason to use the following normalization formula. Determine c by satisfying, if possible, $c\bar{\mathbf{u}}_\mathbf{i}\,\boldsymbol{\epsilon}' = 1$, and then let $c' = 1/c\,d$. By doing this, the matrix $\mathbf{U}$, defined above as the matrix whose rows are the $(\mathbf{u}_\mathbf{i})$s, is isometric, and thus so is $\mathbf{V}$. There can be a problem here, because sometimes $\bar{\mathbf{u}}_\mathbf{i}\,\boldsymbol{\epsilon}' = 0$, so one cannot solve for c in this way. In the application we have in mind this will not be a burden, but rather will allow us to reduce the dimension of $\mathbf{X}$.

1.3.3.2 How a System Approaches Its Steady State

Recall that for the transition rate matrix $\boldsymbol{Q}\,\boldsymbol{\epsilon}' = \mathbf{o}' = 0\,\boldsymbol{\epsilon}'$, so $\boldsymbol{\epsilon}'$ is a right eigenvector of $\boldsymbol{Q}$ with eigenvalue 0. Every eigenvalue must have a left eigenvector as well. We have assumed that all eigenvalues are distinct, therefore a unique $\boldsymbol{\pi}$ satisfying

$$\boldsymbol{\pi}\,\boldsymbol{Q} = \mathbf{o} \quad \text{and} \quad \boldsymbol{\pi}\,\boldsymbol{\epsilon}' = 1 \tag{1.3.9a}$$

exists and is known as the ***steady-state*** ($s.s$) ***vector*** or ***equilibrium vector***. Because the order in which eigenvalues and eigenvectors are labeled is arbitrary, let $\lambda_1 = 0$, $\mathbf{u}_\mathbf{1} = \boldsymbol{\pi}$, and $\mathbf{v}'_\mathbf{1} = \boldsymbol{\epsilon}'$. Then (1.3.3a) and (1.3.2e) become

$$\boldsymbol{G}(t) = \boldsymbol{\epsilon}'\,\boldsymbol{\pi} + \sum_{i=2}^{m} e^{-t\lambda_i}\mathbf{v}'_\mathbf{i}\,\mathbf{u}_\mathbf{i}, \tag{1.3.9b}$$

and [where $\alpha_i := \boldsymbol{\pi}(0)\mathbf{v}'_\mathbf{i}$]

$$\boldsymbol{\pi}(t) = \boldsymbol{\pi} + \sum_{i=2}^{m} \alpha_i\, e^{-t\lambda_i}\,\mathbf{u}_\mathbf{i}. \tag{1.3.9c}$$

Recall from the theory of complex variables that if z is a complex number, then $z = x + iy$, where x and y are real numbers. $x := \Re(z)$ is the *real part* of z, $y := \Im(z)$ is the *imaginary part*, $(\pm i)^2 = -1$, and $\mid z^2 \mid := (x+iy)(x-iy) = x^2 + y^2$. Therefore,

$$\mid e^{-z} \mid = \mid e^{-x} e^{-iy} \mid = \mid e^{-x} \mid\mid e^{-iy} \mid = e^{-x},$$

because $e^{\pm iy} = \cos y \pm i \sin y$, and $\mid e^{\pm iy} \mid = \sqrt{\cos^2 y + \sin^2 y} = 1$. It follows that if $\Re(\lambda_j) > 0$ for all $j > 1$ (which is the case for transition rate matrices as defined so far),

$$\lim_{t\to\infty} \mathbf{G}(t) = \boldsymbol{\epsilon}'\,\boldsymbol{\pi} \tag{1.3.10a}$$

and

$$\lim_{t\to\infty} \boldsymbol{\pi}(t) = \boldsymbol{\pi}. \tag{1.3.10b}$$

Clearly, the asymptotic behavior of $\boldsymbol{\pi}(t)$ is independent of its initial state, $\boldsymbol{\pi}(0)$. We summarize all this in a theorem.

Theorem 1.3.3: Let a system S have m states. The time spent in state i is exponentially distributed with parameter μ_i. Let $\boldsymbol{\pi}(t)$, $\boldsymbol{P}$ and $\boldsymbol{M}$ be as described in Definitions 1.3.2, 1.3.4, and 1.3.6, respectively. Define $\boldsymbol{Q}$ as in (1.3.2c). Then $\boldsymbol{\pi}(t)$ evolves in time according to (1.3.9c). It approaches its limit $\boldsymbol{\pi}$ as t approaches ∞. $\boldsymbol{\pi}$ satisfies (1.3.9a), which can be rewritten in the following way.

$$\boldsymbol{\pi M} = \boldsymbol{\pi M\, P}.$$

This is called the (vector) ***steady-state balance equation*** (or just ***vector balance equation***, and $\boldsymbol{\pi}$ is the ***steady-state vector***. This equation has the following physical interpretation. $\pi_i \mu_i$ (the i-th component of vector $\boldsymbol{\pi M}$) is the *probability rate* of leaving state i. $\sum_{j=1}^{m} \pi_j\, \mu_j\, P_{ji}$ (the i-th component of the vector $\boldsymbol{\pi M\, P}$) is the probability rate of entering state i from all other states. The equality of the two flows, together with $\boldsymbol{\pi \epsilon'} = 1$, uniquely determines $\boldsymbol{\pi}$. ■

Before going on, we note that if the set of states can be partitioned into two subsets, such that there is no way to get from one subset to the other, then $\lim_{t\to\infty} \boldsymbol{\pi}(t)$ depends on the probability that the system began in one subset or the other. But this also implies that the eigenvalue 0 is degenerate, and there are at least two left eigenvectors with eigenvalue 0, call them $\boldsymbol{\pi_1}$ and $\boldsymbol{\pi_2}$. In other words, $\lim_{t\to\infty} \boldsymbol{\pi}(t) = a\boldsymbol{\pi_1} + (1-a)\boldsymbol{\pi_2}$. It is not hard to see that if such a partition exists, we can treat both subsets independently and solve them separately. Therefore, we can assume that our system is connected (i.e., ***irreducible***), so the 0 eigenvector $\boldsymbol{\pi}$ is unique.

The question, "How long will it take to get to the asymptotic region?" is not easy to answer, but one rule of thumb involves the ***relaxation time*** (*RT*) [Morse58], (also called the settling time) defined by

$$\frac{1}{RT} := \min_{i=2}^{m} [\Re(\lambda_i)]. \tag{1.3.11}$$

In words, list the real parts of all the eigenvalues of $\boldsymbol{Q}$. (They all must be positive, or else we are in trouble.) Pick the smallest one. Then the reciprocal of that number is RT. If t is much greater than RT, we can expect that $\boldsymbol{\pi}(t)$ will be close to $\boldsymbol{\pi}$. For t small enough, the system is said to be in a ***transient region*** and displays transient behavior. But as t gets larger, the difference between $\boldsymbol{\pi}(t)$ and $\boldsymbol{\pi}$ eventually becomes small. Look at the following string of inequalities for the k-th component of their difference.

$$|[\boldsymbol{\pi}(t) - \boldsymbol{\pi}]_k| = \left| \sum_{i=2}^{m} \alpha_i e^{-t\lambda_i} (\mathbf{u_i})_k \right| \leq \sum_{i=2}^{m} |\alpha_i|\, |(\mathbf{u_i})_k|\, \exp[-t\,\Re(\lambda_i)]$$

$$\leq e^{-t/RT} \sum_{i=2}^{m} |\alpha_i|\, |(\mathbf{u}_i)_k| = Ce^{-t/RT}.$$

We see that the upper bound of the difference drops at least by a factor of e for each time unit RT, but C could be enormous, so it could take a long time before the actual difference $|\boldsymbol{\pi}(t) - \boldsymbol{\pi}|$ shows this behavior.

Equations (1.3.10) can be interpreted in the following way. Set the system of interest going and wait some time longer than RT before determining the state of the system. The probability that it is in state k is close to π_k. But one observation is meaningless, so more data must be taken. After the measurement, the system continues to evolve as though it just started in the measured state. Thus one must wait another long time before measuring it again.

This is not a particularly efficient way to validate (1.3.10b). Consider, instead, the conceptual experiment of setting up a large number of identical systems (sometimes called an ***ensemble***), let them all run simultaneously, and observe the state each is in after a time t. The fraction of them that are in state k should be close to $[\boldsymbol{\pi}(t)]_k$. The different systems are perpetually changing state, but after a long period of time, the fraction of systems that leave a state in some small time interval is the same as the fraction that enter that state in the same time interval. Therefore, the fraction of systems that are in state k no longer changes, i.e. the ensemble is in its steady state.

A more practical viewpoint is available. Suppose that one wishes to know the fraction of time a system spends in each state over a long period of time T. This would correspond to the time average of $\boldsymbol{\pi}(t)$,

$$\bar{\boldsymbol{\pi}}(T) := \frac{1}{T}\int_0^T \boldsymbol{\pi}(t)dt = \boldsymbol{\pi}(0)\bar{\boldsymbol{G}}(T), \tag{1.3.12a}$$

where

$$\bar{\boldsymbol{G}}(T) := \frac{1}{T}\int_0^T \exp(-t\boldsymbol{Q})dt = \frac{1}{T}\int_0^T \left[\boldsymbol{\epsilon}'\boldsymbol{\pi} + \sum_{i=2}^{m} e^{-t\lambda_i}\mathbf{v}_i'\mathbf{u}_i\right] dt$$

$$= \boldsymbol{\epsilon}'\boldsymbol{\pi} + \sum_{i=2}^{m} \mathbf{v}_i'\mathbf{u}_i \left[\frac{1-e^{-T\lambda_i}}{T\lambda_i}\right]. \tag{1.3.12b}$$

Again, as long as $\Re(\lambda_i) > 0$,

$$\lim_{T\to\infty} \bar{\boldsymbol{G}}(T) = \boldsymbol{\epsilon}'\boldsymbol{\pi} \tag{1.3.13a}$$

and

$$\lim_{T\to\infty} \bar{\boldsymbol{\pi}}(T) = \boldsymbol{\pi}, \tag{1.3.13b}$$

the same as their unbarred counterparts in (1.3.10).

> **Exercise 1.3.5:** Prove that $(\boldsymbol{\epsilon}'\boldsymbol{\pi})^2 = \boldsymbol{\epsilon}'\boldsymbol{\pi}$. More generally, show that for any two vectors satisfying $\mathbf{u}\mathbf{v}' = 1$ it follows that $(\mathbf{v}'\mathbf{u})^2 = \mathbf{v}'\mathbf{u}$. Matrices that have this property are said to be ***idempotent***.

Note that whereas $\boldsymbol{G}(t)$ and $\boldsymbol{\pi}(t)$ converge exponentially to their asymptotic limits according to Equations (1.3.9) (which may be a very long time if

RT is very large), $\bar{\boldsymbol{G}}(T)$ and $\bar{\boldsymbol{\pi}}(T)$ approach their limits much more slowly, as $1/T$ and Equations (1.3.12). That is, although the initial state has little influence on the long-term behavior of a system, its effect on the time average of system behavior lingers on.

As an aside, it is interesting to note that researchers in discrete simulation methods usually throw away the first 100 or more data points if they want their results to converge more rapidly to the steady state. Accumulated simulation statistics are equivalent to $\bar{\boldsymbol{\pi}}(T)$. One is led to question the significance of the steady-state $\boldsymbol{\pi}$, for those systems that run only for a time T comparable to, or less than, RT. In the succeeding chapters we discuss other parameters that describe relatively short-term behavior of queueing systems.

Discrete systems behave in a manner similar to continuous systems with one exception, namely those that are ***periodic***. Intuitively, these are systems that have at least one state to which the system returns in exactly n, $n > 1$ steps. These correspond to transition matrices that have at least one eigenvalue with modulus 1, other than 1 itself.

We now turn our attention to Equations (1.3.5), and as in the continuous case, let λ_i be the set of eigenvalues of $\boldsymbol{P}$, while $\mathbf{u_i}$ and $\mathbf{v}'_\mathbf{i}$ are its left and right eigenvectors, respectively. Note that except for $\mathbf{v}'_\mathbf{1} = \boldsymbol{\epsilon}'$, these objects are different from those for $\boldsymbol{Q}$ in the continuous case. Also, $\lambda_1 = 1$, and $\boldsymbol{\pi_d} = \mathbf{u_1}$ satisfies

$$\boldsymbol{\pi_d}\boldsymbol{P} = \boldsymbol{\pi_d} \quad \text{and} \quad \boldsymbol{\pi_d}\,\boldsymbol{\epsilon}' = 1 \tag{1.3.14a}$$

and is not the same $\boldsymbol{\pi}$ as that defined in (1.3.9a), although they are closely related.

Exercise 1.3.6: Prove that the $\boldsymbol{\pi}$ in (1.3.9a), when right-multiplied by $\boldsymbol{M}$, is a constant times the $\boldsymbol{\pi_d}$ in (1.3.14a). That is, $\boldsymbol{\pi}\mathbf{M} = c\pi_\mathbf{d}$.

The limit of (1.3.5a) as n goes to infinity can be evaluated with the aid of the spectral decomposition theorem. Inserting (1.3.8a) (with $\boldsymbol{P}$ replacing $\boldsymbol{Q}$) into (1.3.5a) leads to

$$\lim_{n\to\infty} \boldsymbol{\pi_d}(n) = \lim_{n\to\infty} \boldsymbol{\pi_d}(0)\boldsymbol{P}^n = \boldsymbol{\pi_d}(0) \lim_{n\to\infty} \left[\boldsymbol{\epsilon}'\,\boldsymbol{\pi_d} + \sum_{i=2}^{m} \lambda_i^n \mathbf{v}'_\mathbf{i}\mathbf{u_i}\right]$$

$$= \boldsymbol{\pi_d} + \sum_{i=2}^{m} [\boldsymbol{\pi_d}(0)\mathbf{v}'_\mathbf{i}] \left[\lim_{n\to\infty} \lambda_i^n\right] \mathbf{u_i}. \tag{1.3.14b}$$

Clearly, if $|\, \lambda_i \,| < 1$ for $i > 1$, then $\lim_{n\to\infty} \lambda_i^n = 0$ and

$$\lim_{n\to\infty} \boldsymbol{\pi_d}(n) = \boldsymbol{\pi_d}. \tag{1.3.14c}$$

Similarly, again with $|\, \lambda_i \,| < 1$,

$$\lim_{n\to\infty} \boldsymbol{P}^n = \boldsymbol{\epsilon}'\boldsymbol{\pi_d}. \tag{1.3.14d}$$

As already mentioned, although all irreducible chains have only one eigenvalue equal to 1, they can have other eigenvalues whose modulus is 1. For example, the $\boldsymbol{P}$ in Exercise 1.3.3 has eigenvalues +1 and -1. When this is the case, the limit as n goes to infinity of λ_i^n does not exist for some i, so $\boldsymbol{\pi_d}(n)$ has no limit [unless $\boldsymbol{\pi_d}(0)\mathbf{v}_i' = 0$]. In other words, there may be no steady state.

What, then, does $\boldsymbol{\pi_d}$ mean? The answer comes from the discrete-time average equivalent to Equations (1.3.12). Define

$$\bar{\boldsymbol{G}}_{\boldsymbol{d}}(N) := \frac{1}{N}\left(\boldsymbol{I} + \boldsymbol{P} + \cdots + \boldsymbol{P}^{N-1}\right) = \boldsymbol{\epsilon}'\boldsymbol{\pi_d} + \frac{1}{N}\sum_{k=0}^{N-1}\left(\sum_{i=2}^{m}\lambda_i^k \mathbf{v}_i'\mathbf{u}_i\right)$$

$$= \boldsymbol{\epsilon}'\boldsymbol{\pi_d} + \frac{1}{N}\sum_{i=2}^{m}\mathbf{v}_i'\mathbf{u}_i\left(\sum_{k=0}^{N-1}\lambda_i^k\right)$$

or

$$\bar{\boldsymbol{G}}_{\boldsymbol{d}}(N) = \boldsymbol{\epsilon}'\boldsymbol{\pi_d} + \frac{1}{N}\sum_{i=2}^{m}\mathbf{v}_i'\mathbf{u}_i\left(\frac{1-\lambda_i^N}{1-\lambda_i}\right). \tag{1.3.15a}$$

Clearly, as long as $|\lambda_i| \leq 1$ (the term corresponding to $\lambda_i = 1$ has already been excluded), we can write

$$\lim_{n\to\infty}\frac{1-\lambda_i^n}{n(1-\lambda_i)} = 0,$$

so

$$\lim_{n\to\infty}\bar{\boldsymbol{G}}_{\boldsymbol{d}}(n) = \boldsymbol{\epsilon}'\boldsymbol{\pi_d} \tag{1.3.15b}$$

even for cyclic chains. We see, then, that the "average" interpretation for $\boldsymbol{\pi_d}$ still holds, even though there may be no steady state. Is it disturbing that discrete chains have at least one property that continuous chains do not have? This dilemma can be resolved by the following argument. Discrete chains assume that exactly n transitions have occurred by time n, whereas for continuous t, even after a relatively short time, one cannot be sure exactly how many steps have occurred. So even if the system is cyclic in the physical sense, one cannot be sure how many cycles have occurred. This carries over to the discrete chain if one loses track of the exact number of steps. For instance, suppose that a system has been running for 10,000 units of time, take or leave a few. Then the average of $\boldsymbol{\pi_d}(n)$ over those few would be $\boldsymbol{\pi_d}$. Mathematically, suppose that our system has a cycle of length $k > 1$, so that

$$\lim_{n\to\infty}\left[\boldsymbol{\pi_d}(n+j) - \boldsymbol{\pi_d}(n)\right] = 0$$

only if j is a multiple of k. Then

$$\boldsymbol{\pi_d} = \lim_{n\to\infty}\frac{1}{k}\sum_{j=1}^{k}\boldsymbol{\pi_d}(n+j).$$

Exercise 1.3.7: Let (where $0 < a < 1$)

$$\boldsymbol{P} = \begin{bmatrix} 0 & a & 1-a \\ 1 & 0 & 0 \\ 1 & 0 & 0 \end{bmatrix}.$$

Find all the eigenvalues and eigenvectors of $\boldsymbol{P}$, solve for $\boldsymbol{\pi_d}(n)$, and show that for large n, $\frac{1}{2}[\boldsymbol{\pi_d}(n) + \boldsymbol{\pi_d}(n+1)]$ approaches $\boldsymbol{\pi_d}$.

Despite the fact that there was much matrix theory in this chapter, we have not yet touched upon what is meant by LAQT. That must wait until Chapter 3. From now on we consider only continuous-time systems. It should not be inferred from this that discrete-time systems are less utilitarian. There is some belief, in fact, that they could be more useful. Some day we may try to treat the queueing world as a movie in discrete time.

Chapter 2

M/M/1 QUEUE

I'm sure that I've never been in a queue as slow as this.
Any Customer, Anywhere, Anytime

Nobody goes there anymore. It's too crowded.
Yogi Berra

The M/M/1 queue, the simplest and most elementary of all queues, is covered it here in some detail. But what we discuss differs from that covered in the usual first course in queueing theory, and we use different techniques to accomplish our goals. Our purpose is threefold. First, we want to connect Chapter 1 with queueing theory and familiarize the reader with our terminology. Second, we want to set up points of view and techniques that are used in later chapters when LAQT is finally introduced. Third, we want to reinforce the view that the behavior of a queueing system in the transient or small time region may be important more often than we have thought heretofore, and that it is possible to study that region realistically and perform calculations relatively easily, in fact, in some cases with the same ease (or difficulty) as with the steady state.

All systems treated in this book are ***closed***. That is, there is always a fixed number of customers in the system. Each system is made up of two subsystems that interact with each other exclusively by exchanging customers. If N, the fixed number of customers, is large enough, we show that one of the subsystems must become saturated ($\mathbb{P}\mathbf{r}$(subsystem is idle) $\rightarrow 0$). It then becomes a steady source of customers to the other subsystem. ***Open systems***, then, are those where N is so large that one of the subsystems is continuously fed by the other which is at full capacity (almost) all the time. We make this clear in what follows.

2.1 Steady-State M/M/1-Type Loops

Consider the system shown in Figure 2.1.1. It is made of two subsystems, called S_1 and S_2. At any time, S_1 has n customers, S_2 has k customers, and the system as a whole has $N = n + k$ customers. In this chapter both S_1 and S_2 are memoryless and thus have exponential service time pdfs of the form $\mu \exp(-\mu x)$ and $\lambda \exp(-\lambda x)$, respectively (which from a formal point of view

L. Lipsky, *Queueing Theory*, DOI 10.1007/978-0-387-49706-8_2,

means that each external state has only one internal state, but more of that in Chapter 3). The system is completely specified at any time if n and k are known. Since N is fixed, k is known if n is known, so the states of the system can be labeled by $n = 0, 1, 2, \ldots N$ (i.e., there are $N + 1$ states).

The notation $M_2/M_1/1//N$ corresponds to Figure 2.1.1 in the following way. First assume that S_1 has a shorter mean service time than S_2. The first symbol $[M_2]$ indicates that S_2 is memoryless or Markovian or exponential, or equivalently, has only one internal state. M_1 says the same thing about S_1. The third position, containing the number "1", means that S_1 can serve only one customer at a time. The space between the third and fourth slashes tells us that there is no limit as to how many customers can be in the queue at S_1. If there had been a number there, S_1 would have had a ***finite waiting room*** or ***finite buffer***. We look at this *slot* when discussing the *customer loss* problem. The last symbol N indicates that there are a total of N customers in the system. Some books assume that S_2 has N identical servers, so all customers at S_2 can be served simultaneously, as in the ***machine minding model*** (also known as ***machine repairman model***) or in a ***time-sharing system***. This is discussed in detail in Section 2.1.4, and again in Section 6.3.5.

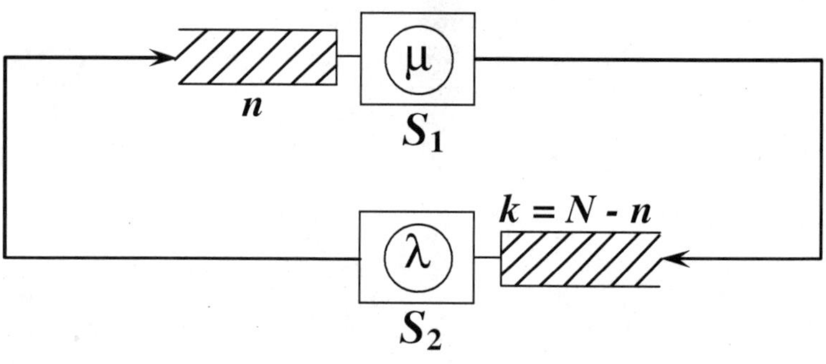

Figure 2.1.1: Closed loop made up of two subsystems, S_1 and S_2. The number of customers at S_1 (including the one in service) is n, and k is the number at S_2. Their sum $N = k + n$ is fixed, thus the system is closed.

Recall from Equations (1.3.2) that the completion rate matrix, $\boldsymbol{M}$, is diagonal, where M_{ii} is the rate at which the system leaves state i given that it is in state i. Here i stands for the integer pair $(n, N - n)$, so, for instance, for $n = 0$, all customers are at S_2, and because only one can be served at a time, $M_{00} = \lambda$. Similarly, when all the customers are at S_1 $(n = N)$, no customers can be served at S_2, so $M_{NN} = \mu$. However, for n in between, both subsystems are servicing customers, so the total departure rate is the sum of two service rates, namely, $M_{ii} = \mu + \lambda$. We prove this by deriving the density function for the first subsystem to complete service. First let $R_1(x) = \exp(-\mu x)$ be the probability that S_1 will still be unchanged at time x. Similarly, let $R_2(x) = \exp(-\lambda x)$. Then $R_1(x)R_2(x) = \exp[-(\mu + \lambda)x]$ is the probability that both S_1 and S_2 are unchanged at time x. Next define

$$B_<(x) := 1 - R_1(x)R_2(x)$$

as the probability that at least one of the subsystems has done something by time x. Then

$$b_<(x) := \frac{d}{dx}B_<(x) = (\mu + \lambda)e^{-(\mu+\lambda)x}$$

is the desired pdf. Therefore the process in which one of two things can happen is exponentially distributed, with service (departure in this case) rate $(\mu + \lambda)$.

In summary, the completion rate matrix looks like

$$\boldsymbol{M} = \begin{bmatrix} \lambda & 0 & 0 & \cdots & 0 \\ 0 & \mu+\lambda & 0 & \cdots & 0 \\ 0 & 0 & \mu+\lambda & \cdots & 0 \\ \vdots & \vdots & \vdots & \cdots & \vdots \\ 0 & 0 & 0 & \cdots & \mu \end{bmatrix}. \tag{2.1.1a}$$

The transition matrix $\boldsymbol{P}$ from Equations (1.3.1) has the following values. For $n = 0$, the only thing that can happen is for a customer to leave S_2 and go to S_1, so $P_{01} = 1$. Similarly, $P_{N,N-1} = 1$. For all other n, one of two things could happen. Either a customer could leave S_2 and go to S_1, or the reverse. In the first case the system would go from state n to $n + 1$, and in the other case the system would go from n to $n - 1$. The probability that one would happen over the other is proportional to the separate subsystems' (servers') service rates, μ and λ. In other words, $P_{n,n+1} = \lambda/(\mu + \lambda)$. We show this by evaluating the probability that S_2 will finish before S_1. This will occur if S_2 finishes around time t $[b_2(t)dt]$ while S_1 is still running $[R_1(t)]$ for any $t > 0$ (integrate over t). This gives us

$$\mathbf{Pr}(S_2\text{will finish before } S_1) = \int_0^\infty b_2(t)R_1(t)dt$$

$$= \int_0^\infty \lambda e^{-\lambda t}e^{-\mu t}dt = \lambda \int_0^\infty e^{-(\mu+\lambda)t}dt = \frac{\lambda}{\mu + \lambda}. \tag{2.1.1b}$$

What we have just shown is important enough to be summarized in a theorem.

> **Theorem 2.1.1:** Let X_1 and X_2 be independent random variables having exponential distribution functions with rates μ and λ, respectively. Then the PDF for the first one to finish, given that both have already started, but have not finished, by time $x = 0$, is also exponentially distributed, with parameter $\mu + \lambda$. That is, let
>
> $$X = \min[X_1, X_2].$$
>
> Then
>
> $$\Pr(X < x) := B_<(x) = 1 - e^{-(\lambda+\mu)x},$$

and

$$b_<(x) = (\mu + \lambda)e^{-(\lambda+\mu)x}.$$

Furthermore, $\Pr(X_2 < X_1)$ is given by (2.1.1b). Because both X_1 and X_2 are exponentially distributed, these results do not depend upon which server started first. ■

The entire $\boldsymbol{P}$ matrix is the following.

$$\boldsymbol{P} = \begin{bmatrix} 0 & 1 & 0 & 0 & \cdots & 0 & 0 & 0 \\ \frac{\mu}{\mu+\lambda} & 0 & \frac{\lambda}{\mu+\lambda} & 0 & \cdots & 0 & 0 & 0 \\ 0 & \frac{\mu}{\mu+\lambda} & 0 & \frac{\lambda}{\mu+\lambda} & \cdots & 0 & 0 & 0 \\ \vdots & \vdots & \vdots & \vdots & \cdots & \vdots & \vdots & \vdots \\ 0 & 0 & 0 & 0 & \cdots & 0 & \frac{\lambda}{\mu+\lambda} & 0 \\ 0 & 0 & 0 & 0 & \cdots & \frac{\mu}{\mu+\lambda} & 0 & \frac{\lambda}{\mu+\lambda} \\ 0 & 0 & 0 & 0 & \cdots & 0 & 1 & 0 \end{bmatrix}. \tag{2.1.1c}$$

Finally, $\boldsymbol{Q} = \boldsymbol{M}(\boldsymbol{I} - \boldsymbol{P})$ can easily be calculated to give us

$$\boldsymbol{Q} = \begin{bmatrix} \lambda & -\lambda & 0 & 0 & \cdots & 0 & 0 & 0 \\ -\mu & \mu+\lambda & -\lambda & 0 & \cdots & 0 & 0 & 0 \\ 0 & -\mu & \mu+\lambda & -\lambda & \cdots & 0 & 0 & 0 \\ \vdots & \vdots & \vdots & \vdots & \ddots & \vdots & \vdots & \vdots \\ 0 & 0 & 0 & 0 & \cdots & \mu+\lambda & -\lambda & 0 \\ 0 & 0 & 0 & 0 & \cdots & -\mu & \mu+\lambda & -\lambda \\ 0 & 0 & 0 & 0 & \cdots & 0 & -\mu & \mu \end{bmatrix}. \tag{2.1.1d}$$

This procedure of calculating $\boldsymbol{Q}$ in two steps rather than directly, as is usually done, seems cumbersome, but its utility becomes clear in later chapters.

$\boldsymbol{Q}$ matrices of the form in (2.1.1d) (i.e., those that are tridiagonal) generate what are known as ***birth-death processes***. In general, if the states can be linearly ordered, and transitions only occur between neighboring states (i.e., given that the system is in state n, it can only go to $n-1$, n, or $n+1$), then we have a birth-death process. This can be generalized in the following way. Suppose that the states of the system can be partitioned into subsets that are linearly ordered as $\{\Xi_o, \Xi_1, \Xi_2, \ldots, \Xi_{n-1}, \Xi_n, \Xi_{n+1}, \ldots\}$. If transitions can only occur between adjacent sets, we have a ***Quasi Birth-Death* (QBD) *process*** [WALLACE69]. The $\boldsymbol{Q}$ matrix for a QBD process looks like (2.1.1d), except that each of the elements is itself a matrix. All the processes discussed in this book are QBD. This means leaving out such topics as bulk arrival processes, a typical topic in other queueing theory books.

2.1.1 Time-Dependent Solution for $N = 2$

The time-dependent solution for $N = 1$ was actually done in Exercise 1.3.3. The next simplest nontrivial case is $N = 2$. Here

$$\boldsymbol{Q} = \begin{bmatrix} \lambda & -\lambda & 0 \\ -\mu & \mu+\lambda & -\lambda \\ 0 & -\mu & \mu \end{bmatrix}. \tag{2.1.2}$$

Obviously, $\boldsymbol{\epsilon}'$ ($\boldsymbol{\epsilon} = [1, 1, 1]$) is a right eigenvector of $\boldsymbol{Q}$ with eigenvalue 0, and it is not hard to find its companion, the left eigenvector with eigenvalue 0 [i.e., $\boldsymbol{\pi}(2)\boldsymbol{Q} = \mathbf{o}$]. One proves by direct substitution that

$$\boldsymbol{\pi}(2) = \frac{1}{1+\rho+\rho^2}[1,\ \rho,\ \rho^2],$$

where $\rho = \lambda/\mu$ and $\boldsymbol{\pi}\boldsymbol{\epsilon}' = 1$. The components of the total probability vector $[\boldsymbol{\pi}(2)]_j$ are the steady-state probabilities of finding $(j-1)$ customers at S_1. Put colloquially, after a long time, a random observer who may come along will find $j-1$ customers at S_1 with probability $[\boldsymbol{\pi}(2)]_j$. The eigenvalues of $\boldsymbol{Q}$ satisfy the polynomial equation coming from Equations (1.3.6),

$$\phi(\beta) = \beta^3 - 2(\mu+\lambda)\beta^2 + (\mu^2 + \mu\lambda + \lambda^2)\beta = 0. \tag{2.1.3a}$$

The roots of this equation are (for convenience we let the indices take on values 0 to $N = 2$ rather than the convention used in Chapter 1)

$$\begin{aligned} \beta_o &= 0 \\ \beta_1 &= \mu(1+\rho+\sqrt{\rho}) \\ \beta_2 &= \mu(1+\rho-\sqrt{\rho}). \end{aligned} \tag{2.1.3b}$$

β_o is the root corresponding to the steady-state solution, whereas $\beta_1$and β_2 moderate the transient behavior. Now $\beta_2 < \beta_1$, so the relaxation time from Equations (1.3.11) is $1/\beta_2$. Because the time units are arbitrary, we must establish some comparison to learn something from the formula. One convenient time unit to use in this case is the mean time for a single customer to go around the loop once, unimpeded. A simple way to do this is to let $1/\mu + 1/\lambda = 1$; then, from Equations (1.3.11),

$$RT(\rho) = \frac{\rho}{(1+\rho)(1+\rho-\sqrt{\rho})}.$$

In this case it should be easy to see that RT is maximal when $\rho = 1$ and that $RT(\rho) = RT(1/\rho)$. We examine the general case in Section 2.2, but we note that these results are typical.

Exercise 2.1.1: For a cycle time of 1 ($1/\mu + 1/\lambda = 1$) show that the formula above is true, and draw a graph of RT versus ρ. When is RT a maximum? Prove that $RT(\rho) = RT(1/\rho)$.

Exercise 2.1.2: Find all the left and right eigenvectors of $\boldsymbol{Q}$ and verify that Equations (1.3.8a) are satisfied. Construct $\boldsymbol{G}(t)$ from (1.3.9a), and then $\boldsymbol{\pi}(t; 2)$, where $\boldsymbol{\pi}(0; 2)$ is one of [1 0 0], or [0 1 0], or [0 0 1].

2.1.2 Steady-State Solution for Any N

The steady-state solution for the M/M/1//N queue is, of course, well known and is shown in every book that discusses queueing theory to any extent. We discuss it briefly here to show how one goes from closed to open systems. Our assumption in this section is that S_2 is load independent. That is, the service rate of S_2 is the same irrespective of how many customers are in its queue.

From (1.3.9) and (1.3.10), the steady-state solution of our loop satisfies $\pi \boldsymbol{Q} = \mathbf{o}$, which from (1.3.2c) is the same as $\boldsymbol{\pi} \boldsymbol{M} = \boldsymbol{\pi} \boldsymbol{M} \boldsymbol{P}$. (See Theorem 1.3.3 for a summary.) These equations are referred to as the steady-state ***balance equations***. In the notation of Chapter 1, the left-hand side $(\pi_i\, \mu_i)$ is interpreted as the probability rate of leaving state i, and the right-hand side is the probability rate of entering state i. And, of course, they are equal when a system reaches its steady state.

At this point it is advantageous for us to change our notation, to be consistent with succeeding chapters, where $\boldsymbol{\pi}$ takes on a different meaning. The abstract state i stands for there being $n = i - 1$ customers at S_1, we therefore define the following.

Definition 2.1.1

$r(n; N)$:= *steady-state probability that there are n customers at* S_1, *where N is the (fixed) number of customers in the system overall.* Then $r(n; N)$ replaces $[\boldsymbol{\pi}(N)]_i \quad (n = i - 1)$ everywhere. □

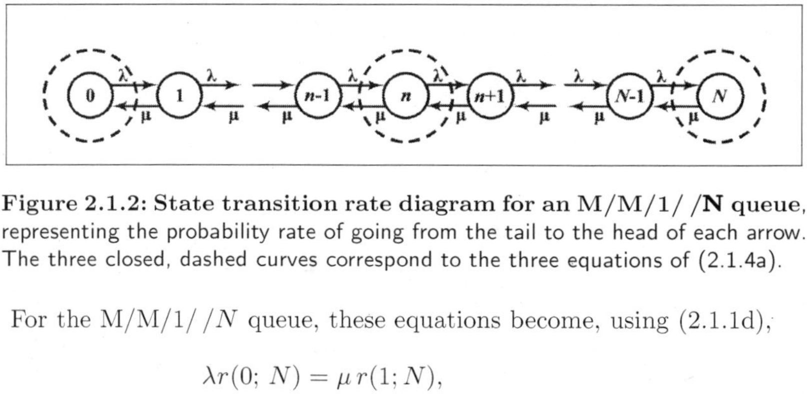

Figure 2.1.2: State transition rate diagram for an M/M/1/ /N queue, representing the probability rate of going from the tail to the head of each arrow. The three closed, dashed curves correspond to the three equations of (2.1.4a).

For the M/M/1//N queue, these equations become, using (2.1.1d),

$$\begin{aligned} \lambda r(0;\, N) &= \mu\, r(1; N), \\ (\mu + \lambda) r(n;\, N) &= \lambda r(n-1;\, N) + \mu\, r(n+1;\, N), \\ \mu\, r(N;\, N) &= \lambda\, r(N-1;\, N), \end{aligned} \tag{2.1.4a}$$

where $0 < n < N$. It is common to represent these equations graphically by what are called ***state transition rate diagrams*** (or simply ***transition diagrams***), as shown in Figure 2.1.2. Each arrow corresponds to going from the state represented by the circle at the tail to the state represented by the circle at the head, with probability rate equal to the probability of being at the tail times the rate corresponding to the arrow. Every closed curve encompassing part of the graph represents a valid balance equation, where the sum of the rates represented by the arrows going into the loop equals the sum of the rates leaving the loop. In particular, each closed loop enclosing only one state (circle) yields one of the equations in (2.1.4a).

In any case, the solution to (2.1.4a) is well known to be

$$r(n;N) = \frac{\rho^n}{K(N)}, \qquad 0 \leq n \leq N, \tag{2.1.4b}$$

where

$$K(N) := \sum_{n=0}^{N} \rho^n = \frac{1-\rho^{N+1}}{1-\rho} \qquad (\rho \neq 1). \tag{2.1.4c}$$

The proof follows by substituting (2.1.4b) into (2.1.4a). Equation (2.1.4c) follows from the requirement that $\sum_{n=0}^{N} r(n;N) = 1$. For future reference, observe that $K(N)$ satisfies the recurrence relation

$$K(N) = 1 + \rho K(N-1). \tag{2.1.4d}$$

When $\rho = 1$, $r(n;N) = 1/(N+1)$ for all n. That is, the steady-state probability for all queue lengths is the same. Yet if the system initially had all its customers at S_1, it would be a long time indeed before a majority of them would be found at S_2. Of course, for very large N, and after a long period of time, we are unlikely to find the system in any particular state. Thus the steady-state solution, if anything, is warning our random observer to be wary of any conclusions concerning the behavior of a system that are based on short-term observations. We look at this again in Section 2.3.

Example 2.1.1: In Figure 2.1.3 we have plotted the steady-state queue length probabilities for the M/M/1//20 queue for various values of ρ. Notice that when $\rho < 1$, $r(n;20)$ is a monotonically decreasing function of n, and when $\rho > 1$, it is a monotonically decreasing function of $N - n$. As you might expect, the curves labeled $\rho = 0.5$ and $\rho = 2$ are mirror images of each other. The most significant feature of these curves is that they are so broad, particularly when ρ is near 1. It is best to think of $r(n;N)$ as being the fraction of time that n customers will be at S_1 over a very very long period of time. ▲[†]

What is often of interest in closed systems is the activity of each of the servers. The probability that a server is busy is equivalent to the fraction of time it is busy over a long period of time. This, in turn, determines the amount of "work" done per unit time by that server. Now suppose that customers somehow enter our closed loop, travel around until they have received a total of T_i units of service from S_i ($i = 1, 2$), and then leave, being replaced instantly by a statistical clone. By definition, $T_1/T_2 = \rho$. Next define the steady-state probabilities.

Definition 2.1.2

$P_i(N)$:= *steady-state probability that* S_i, $i = 1, 2$, *is busy, given that*

[†]Symbol ▲ designates the end of the example

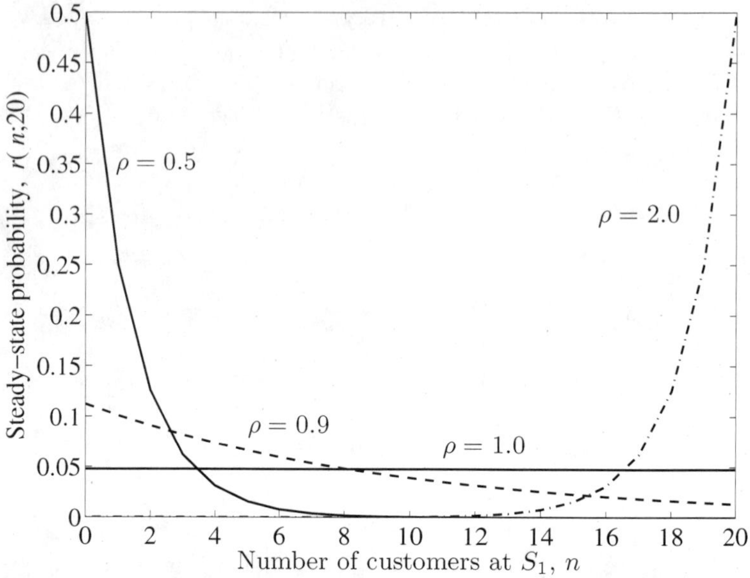

Figure 2.1.3: Steady-state probabilities $r(n;20)$ that there will be n customers at or in S_1, for $\rho = 0.5, 0.9, 1,$ and 2. The curves for $\rho = 0.5$ and 2 are mirror images of each other. Also, the curve for $\rho = 1$ is a constant; that is, all queue lengths are equally likely. These observations are not necessarily true for more general queues. Equations (2.1.4b) and (2.1.4c or d) are used to compute the values plotted.

there are N customers in the loop. Then

$$\Lambda(N) := \frac{P_i(N)}{T_i} \tag{2.1.5a}$$

is the rate at which customers enter and leave the loop, and is independent of i. $\Lambda(N)$ can be referred to as the ***system throughput***. In fact, this formula is valid for networks of any number of servers, as long as customers do not have the option of using a different server if the one they want is busy, and if the servers are not load dependent. □

$P_1(N)$ is 1 minus the probability that S_1 is idle, so from (2.1.4b) with $n = 0$, and (2.1.4d),

$$P_1(N) = 1 - r(0;N) = 1 - \frac{1}{K(N)} = \frac{K(N)-1}{K(N)} = \rho\frac{K(N-1)}{K(N)}. \tag{2.1.5b}$$

Similarly, from (2.1.4c),

$$P_2(N) = 1 - r(N;N) = \frac{K(N)-\rho^N}{K(N)} = \frac{K(N-1)}{K(N)}. \tag{2.1.5c}$$

Then, because $\rho = T_1/T_2$, we show that the throughput as seen at S_1 is the same as that seen at S_2:

$$\Lambda(N) = \frac{P_1(N)}{T_1} = \frac{1}{T_2}\frac{K(N-1)}{K(N)} = \frac{P_2(N)}{T_2}. \tag{2.1.5d}$$

Example 2.1.2: We can understand the throughput behavior by looking at Figure 2.1.4, which shows $\Lambda(N)$ as a function of N for several values of ρ. Note that $\Lambda(N;\rho) = \Lambda(N;1/\rho)$. In all cases, $\Lambda(N)$ saturates as N becomes increasingly large, and we see behavior typical of even more complicated queueing systems. That is, $\Lambda(N+1) > \Lambda(N)$ for all N, but

$$[\Lambda(N+2) - \Lambda(N+1)] < [\Lambda(N+1) - \Lambda(N)].$$

This is the law of diminishing returns. "Adding yet one more customer to the system will increase throughput, but the increase will not be as much as it was in adding the previous customer." Finally,

$$\lim_{N\to\infty} [P_1(N) + P_2(N)] = 1 + \rho, \qquad \text{for } \rho \leq 1.$$

That is, in general, only one server will saturate, and the other will be busy only a fraction of the time. Only when $\rho = 1$ will both servers approach full capacity with ever-increasing N. ▲

Exercise 2.1.3: Prove that the limit given in the preceding equation is indeed true. What is the limit when ρ is greater than 1? Also prove that $\Lambda(N;\rho) = \Lambda(N;1/\rho)$ when $T_1 + T_2 = 1$.

2.1.3 Open M/M/1 Queue ($N \to \infty$)

We can find the open system solution by doing the following. When $\rho < 1$, Equations (2.1.4) retain their meaning for large N. In this case,

$$\lim_{N\to\infty} K(N) = \frac{1}{1-\rho},$$

so

$$r(n) := \lim_{N\to\infty} r(n;N) = (1-\rho)\rho^n \tag{2.1.6a}$$

and

$$\lim_{n\to\infty} r(n) = 0.$$

That is, when N is very large, the probability that S_2 will be idle is negligible, so it is continually serving customers whose interdeparture times are exponentially distributed. Each new customer starts up in the same way the previous one did, so S_2 becomes a steady Poisson process of arrivals to S_1.

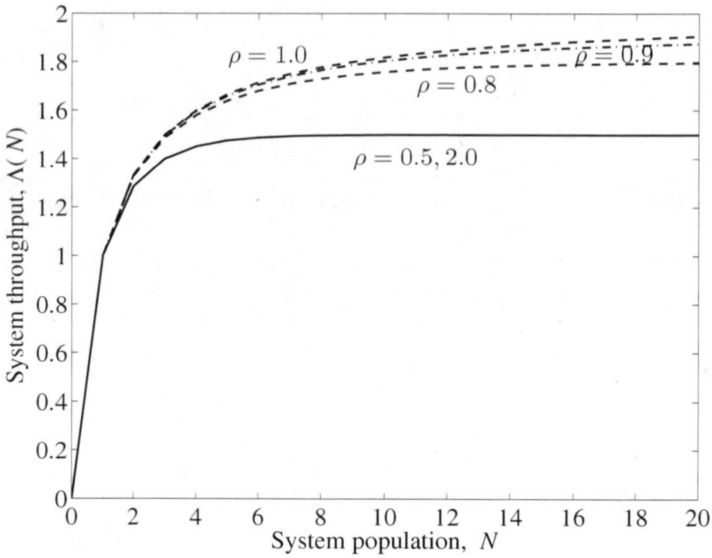

Figure 2.1.4: Throughput for steady-state M/M/1//N queues, where the total resource time needed for a customer to go around once is $T_1 + T_2 = 1$. The curves for $\rho = 0.5$ and $\rho = 2$ are identical because ρ and $1/\rho$ yield the same system with S_1 and S_2 interchanged. All the curves will saturate (become horizontal) if N is made large enough. Use Equations (2.1.5c), (2.1.5d), and (2.1.4d).

Thus we have the equivalent of an open M/M/1 queue, with a mean queue length of

$$\bar{q}_s := \sum_{n=1}^{\infty} n\, r(n) = (1-\rho) \sum_{n=1}^{\infty} n\, \rho^n = \frac{\rho}{1-\rho}. \tag{2.1.6b}$$

When $\rho > 1$ it follows from (2.1.4c) that $1/K(N)$ becomes vanishingly small for very large N, and thus for small n, $r(n; N)$ is essentially zero. Now S_1 is never idle and becomes a Poisson source for S_2. One would expect a certain duality between S_1 and S_2, which indeed is the case. Simply interchange 1 and 2, and thus replace ρ by $1/\rho$.

It is also interesting to evaluate the asymptotic throughput of our loop. We are thus interested in [from (2.1.5d)]

$$\lim_{N\to\infty} \Lambda(N) = \frac{1}{T_2} \frac{K(N-1)}{K(N)}.$$

We have already noted that when $\rho < 1$, $K(N)$ approaches $(1-\rho)^{-1}$, but from (2.1.4c), $K(N)$ grows as ρ^N when ρ is greater than 1. This leads easily to the following limiting values.

$$\lim_{N\to\infty} \Lambda(N) = \frac{1}{T_2} \quad \text{for } \rho \le 1$$

and

$$\lim_{N\to\infty} \Lambda(N) = \frac{1}{T_2}\frac{1}{\rho} = \frac{1}{T_1} \quad \text{for } \rho \geq 1.$$

In other words, we have proven what should be obvious. The throughput of the system is bounded by the maximal throughput of the slower server, the ***bottleneck***. The two equations can be summarized by

$$\lim_{N\to\infty} \Lambda(N) = \min\left(\frac{1}{T_1}, \frac{1}{T_2}\right). \tag{2.1.6c}$$

A perhaps more interesting question to answer is: how long will a customer be at S_1, both waiting for and being served? This turns out to be easy to answer once the mean queue length is known. The relevant expression, ***Little's formula***, which we introduced in (1.1.2), existed for many years before being proven under certain conditions by J. D. C. Little in 1961 [LITTLE61]. Recall that it is valid for any subsystem that has been in operation long enough so that the number of customers who have come and gone is far greater than the number presently there or who were there originally. Restated simply,

$$\bar{q}_s = \Lambda \bar{T}_s, \tag{2.1.7a}$$

where Λ is the mean arrival rate to (and departure rate from) the subsystem and $\bar{T}_s$ is the mean time spent there by each customer. In our case, $\Lambda = \lambda$ and $\rho = \lambda/\mu$, so from (2.1.6b), we have proven (1.1.4b)

$$\bar{T}_s = \frac{\bar{q}_s}{\lambda} = \frac{\bar{x}}{1-\rho}, \tag{2.1.7b}$$

where $\bar{x} = 1/\mu$ is the mean service time of S_1. Note that if $\rho = 0$ (no customers waiting at all), the mean time a customer remains in the system is the expected $\bar{x}$, and as with the mean queue length, the time a customer must wait grows unboundedly as ρ approaches 1.

It is useful to tighten up our terminology somewhat. Often, one wishes to make a distinction between the time spent waiting for service and the time in service. We use the term ***system time*** or ***total time*** spent in, say, S_1 as the time spent by a customer from the moment he enters S_1's queue until he leaves that subsystem. In a closed loop, this also corresponds to the time interval from the moment the customer leaves S_2 until he returns. For that reason, this time interval is also called the ***response time*** for S_1. We use the three terms interchangeably, tending to prefer the first two when discussing open systems, whereas the latter tends to be used more in dealing with time-sharing systems.

In many applications, the time spent being served is considered useful, and only the time spent waiting in the queue is wasted. This time is called both ***queueing time*** and ***waiting time***. We try to use the latter term, for there is some ambiguity here when load-dependent servers are considered (see the following section and Section 5.4), or when we consider "generalized M/G/C systems" in Chapter 6, for then it is not always clear when waiting ends and service begins. We often talk about ***queue length***, or the *number of customers* *in the queue*, and when we do, we invariably mean "the number of customers at, or in, S_i," that is, including those being served.

If only one customer can be served at a time, and the performance of S_1 is the same no matter how many customers are in its queue, the steady-state mean system time $\bar{T}_s$ and mean waiting time $\bar{T}_w$ are related by the simple relation

$$\bar{T}_s = \bar{T}_w + \bar{x}_1. \tag{2.1.7c}$$

From Little's formula, the number in the queue and the number in S_1 are related by the slightly strange formula

$$\bar{q}_s = \bar{q}_w + \rho. \tag{2.1.7d}$$

The reason ρ appears instead of 1 is that sometimes there is no one waiting when someone is being served. It is pleasant to realize that (2.1.7c) and (2.1.7d) are true for any distribution, but the reader should be careful to observe the restrictions as stated in the beginning of this paragraph.

2.1.4 Buffer Overflow and Cell Loss for M/M/1/N Queues

An important problem in designing systems with queues involves deciding how much space should be provided to accommodate waiting customers. We look at this issue in two ways. First consider that a ***waiting room*** is made up of a ***primary buffer*** that can accommodate, say N_1 customers, and a secondary buffer, or ***backup buffer***, that can hold as many as needed. An example of this might be a cache interfacing a bulk storage device with a communications channel. Then the question is the following.

(1) What is the probability that an arriving customer will not be able to fit into the primary buffer, or in other words, will the ***buffer overflow***?

One could instead assume that there is only a primary buffer, with no backup. Then an arriving customer, seeing a full buffer, would give up and disappear, or what is mathematically equivalent, return to the queue at S_2. The question then is the following.

(2) What is the probability that an arriving customer will be rejected from the queue at S_1?

The first case corresponds to an M/M/1 queue, and the second corresponds to an M/M/1/N_1/N queue. The latter expression requires some interpretation. If $N_1 < N$ and we are to assume that customers arriving at a full queue would have to instantly return to the end of the queue at S_2, then S_2 is always busy, so N might just as well be ∞. For this reason, the M/M/1/N queue is considered to be open even though the population at S_1 is always less than or equal to N_1.

If, on the other hand, $N_1 \geq N$ the buffer can never be full to an arriving customer. Therefore,

$$\mathrm{M/M/1}/N_1/N \equiv \begin{cases} \mathrm{M/M/1}/N_1 & \text{for} \quad N_1 < N \\ \mathrm{M/M/1}//N & \text{for} \quad N_1 \geq N \end{cases}$$

In general, the solutions for M/G/1//N loops are very similar to those for M/G/1/N queues. The difference becomes significant in Section 5.3 when we compare the G/M/1//N and G/M/1/N queues, but we give a short explanation here. When a customer arrives at an M/M/1/N queue that already has N customers, the arriving customer is turned away. Each subsequent arrival will be turned away until S_1 has a completion. Given that the arrival process is a Poisson process, the time for the next arrival is exponentially distributed, but now starting at the time of the departure, having no memory of the previous arrival. The M/M/1//N loop behaves in the following way. If all N customers are at S_1, there can be no further arrivals until S_1 has a completion. After such a completion, S_2 can service its new arrival, thereby preparing a new arrival for S_1. We see that shutting off the arrival process has the same effect as turning away arrivals, but only if the arrival process is memoryless, that is, Poisson.

Cases (1) and (2) both talk about an ***arriving customer***, whereas we have given solutions for a random observer $[r(n)]$. Therefore we must introduce some new variables.

Definition 2.1.3

$a(n;\, N)$:= *probability that a customer arriving at S_1 in an M/M/1//N loop will see n customers already in the queue, including the one in service.* By this definition, it must be that

$$a(N;\, N) = 0.$$

After all, the arriving customer is one of the N customers in the system, so he can see at most $N - 1$ customers before him at S_1. □

We give similar definitions for the M/M/1/N queue, using ***f*** (for ***finite buffer***) as the distinguishing marker.

Definition 2.1.4

$r_f(n;\, N)$:= *probability that a random observer will see n customers at or in S_1 for an M/M/1/N queue.*

$a_f(n;\, N)$:= *probability that a customer arriving at an M/M/1/N queue will see n customers already in the queue, including the one in service.* By this definition, $a_f(N;\, N)$ is the probability that an arriving customer will be turned away (i.e., the ***customer loss*** probability). If we were dealing with the tranmission of packets or cells in telecommunications we would call this ***packet loss probability*** or ***cell loss probability***. □

In Chapters 4 and 5 we give a more rigorous argument for the following equations, but for the systems of interest here the following arguments are sufficient. Because we are looking at Poisson arrivals, each arriving customer has no knowledge of when the previous customer arrived, therefore he will see the same thing that a random observer does, except that he cannot see N customers already in thc queue. Therefore,

$$a(n;\, N) = \begin{cases} c(N)\, r(n;\, N) & \text{for } 0 \le n < N \\ 0 & \text{for } n = N \end{cases}.$$

The sum of the $a(n;\, N)$'s must be 1, therefore it follows that $c(N) = (1 - \rho^{N+1})/(1-\rho^N)$. We can now summarize the steady-state properties of the M/M/1//N queue in the following theorem.

Theorem 2.1.2: The steady-state probabilities of finding n customers in an M/M/1//N loop are given by Equations (2.1.4), namely,

$$r(n; N) = \frac{\rho^n}{K(N)}, \qquad 0 \le n \le N,$$

where $K(N) = N + 1$ for $\rho = 1$, and for $\rho \neq 1$

$$K(N) := \sum_{n=0}^{N} \rho^n = \frac{1-\rho^{N+1}}{1-\rho} = 1 + \rho K(N-1).$$

The probability that a customer arriving at S_1 will find n customers already there is given by

$$a(n;\, N) = \frac{1-\rho}{1-\rho^N}\rho^n \quad \text{for } 0 \le n < N, \tag{2.1.8a}$$

and $a(N;\, N) = 0$. For $\rho = 1$, $a(n;\, N) = 1/N$. In other words, $a(n;\, N) = r(n;\, N-1)$ for $n < N$.

The probability that an arriving customer will see $N_1 \le n < N$ or more customers already in the queue (***overflow probability***) is given by:

$$P_o(N_1;\, N) := \sum_{n=N_1}^{N-1} a(n;\, N) = \frac{\rho^{N_1} - \rho^N}{1-\rho^N}. \tag{2.1.8b}$$

For $\rho < 1$ the open M/M/1 queue steady-state probabilities, from (2.1.6a) and (2.1.8a), are

$$a(n) = r(n) = \lim_{N\to\infty} r(n;\, N) = (1-\rho)\rho^n. \tag{2.1.8c}$$

Here, the arriving customer and the random observer see the same queue lengths.

The mean queue length, from (2.1.6b) is

$$\bar{q}_s = \frac{\rho}{1-\rho}$$

and the mean system time, from (2.1.7b), is

$$\bar{T}_s = \frac{\bar{x}}{1-\rho},$$

where $\rho = \lambda/\mu$ and $\bar{x} = 1/\mu$. Also,

$$P_o(N_1) := \lim_{N\to\infty} P_o(N_1;\, N) = \rho^{N_1}. \tag{2.1.8d}$$

We have used the subscript ***o*** to denote primary buffer ***o***verflow. ■

The steady-state solutions for the $M/M/1/N_1$ queue are easy to write down, because an arriving customer in a Poisson arrival process sees the same thing as the random observer, even if the finite buffer is full. Therefore, we have the following.

Theorem 2.1.3: Systems with finite buffers have the following probabilities.

$$a_f(n;\, N_1) = r_f(n;\, N_1) = r(n;\, N_1) = \frac{1-\rho}{1-\rho^{N_1+1}}\rho^n. \qquad (2.1.9a)$$

These equations are valid for all ρ. The probability that an arriving customer will find the buffer full, and be turned away is given by:

$$P_f(N_1) = a_f(N_1;\, N_1) = \frac{1-\rho}{1-\rho^{N_1+1}}\rho^{N_1}. \qquad (2.1.9b)$$

In telecommunications systems, this is known as the ***cell loss probability*** or ***packet loss probability***.

The mean queue length, $\bar{q}_f(N_1)$, is

$$\bar{q}_f(N_1) := \sum_{n=1}^{N_1} n\, r_f(n;\, N_1)$$

$$= \frac{\rho}{1-\rho}\left[\frac{1 + N_1\rho^{N_1+1} - (N_1+1)\rho^{N_1}}{1-\rho^{N_1+1}}\right]. \qquad (2.1.9c)$$

Note that $\bar{q}_f(N_1)$ does not blow up at $\rho = 1$. In fact $\bar{q}_f(N_1|\rho = 1) = N_1/2$, and $P_f(N_1|\rho = 1) = 1/(N_1+1)$. In other words, a relatively small loss of cells can yield a manageable size queue. (Recall that the mean queue length for a queue with an infinite buffer, where no losses are allowed, is infinite when $\rho = 1$).

Let $T_f(N)$ be the random variable denoting the system time for a customer that is not rejected. Then

$$\mathbb{E}[T_f(N_1)] = \frac{1/\mu}{1-\rho}\left[\frac{1 + N_1\rho^{N_1+1} - (N_1+1)\rho^{N_1}}{1-\rho^{N_1}}\right]. \qquad (2.1.9d)$$

This last equation requires some explanation which we give in the following proof. ■

Proof: In order to get (2.1.9d) from (2.1.9c) using Little's formula, one must use the *effective* arrival rate to the queue. That is, one must include only those customers that are not turned away. That is,

$$\lambda_f(N_1) := \frac{\lambda}{1 - Pff(N_1)} = \frac{1-\rho^{N_1}}{1-\rho^{N_1+1}}\lambda.$$

Then (2.1.9d) follows from

$$\mathbb{E}[T_f(N_1)] = \frac{\bar{q}_f(N_1)}{\lambda_f(N_1)}.$$

An alternate proof is given as an exercise.

Note that the effective arrival process is no longer a Poisson process. In fact, it's no longer a renewal process. Observe that the customers are not thrown away randomly. If one is thrown away, then the next one is also likely to be lost. **QED**†

Exercise 2.1.4: Using (2.1.9b) and given a fixed value for the probability p_ℓ of customer loss, show that ρ must always be less than $1/(1-p_\ell)$ in order that $P_f(N) \leq p_\ell$, no matter how large N is. [See Equations (2.1.10) for a general proof.]

Exercise 2.1.5: One can derive (2.1.9d) directly from the definition of $a_f(n;\, N_1)$. The service distribution is exponential here, therefore the mean time remaining for the customer in service at the moment a new customer arrives is $1/\mu$, the same as from the beginning of service. If a customer arrives with $n < N$ already in the queue, then he must expect to wait $[(n+1)/\mu]$ units of time until all those in front and he himself are served. The probability that he will find n in the queue, given that he will be accepted, is given by $a_f(n;\, N_1 \,|\, \text{accepted}) := a_f(n;\, N_1)/[1 - P_f(N_1)]$ Then

$$\bar{T}_f(N_1) = \sum_{n=o}^{N_1-1} \left[\frac{n+1}{\mu}\right] a_f(n;\, N_1 \,|\, \text{accepted}).$$

Use this expression to derive (2.1.9d)

Before closing this section we compare $P_o(N_1)$ and $P_f(N_1)$ and discuss their uses and significance. First note that $P_f(N_1) < P_o(N_1)$ for every ρ, remembering that $P_o(N_1)$ is not defined for $\rho \geq 1$. The reason should be clear, because the finite buffer system throws away customers, and thus processes fewer of them than the overflow system for any given arrival rate. In exchange for this, the mean queue length and the mean waiting time for the customers is considerably reduced. For instance, let $\rho = 1$ and $N_1 = 10$. Then the mean queue length in the back-up buffer of the M/M/1 queue is infinite, but $\bar{q}_f(10) = 5$. This can be evaluated from (2.1.9c) by using L'Hospital's rule, or by recognizing that $a_f(n;\, N_1;\, \rho = 1) = 1/(N_1+1)\ \forall\, n$. We see, then, by throwing away one customer in 11, one allows the others to get decent service; that is, $\bar{T}_f(10;\, \rho = 1) = 5.5/\mu$.

† These letters stand for the time-honored Latin phrase *Quod Erat Demonstrandum*, whose translation is "which was to be demonstrated." **QEDdesignates the end of a proof.**

Maximum Cell Loss

Finite buffers can be a useful solution for systems where not all customers must be served. For instance, one may throw away 10% of the packets carrying telephone messages or video data over telecommunications networks, and still be able to recognize the audio or video signal. But as ρ approaches 2, half the customers have to be rejected, a circumstance that is not acceptable even for these examples. In any case, as ρ becomes larger, $\bar{q}_f(N_1)$ approaches N_1.

Suppose that a system can tolerate a maximum fractional loss of p_ℓ. Then there exists a maximum ρ_m above which even an infinite buffer will be inadequate. Consider a very large interval of time Δ. During that period, a total of $N_a(\Delta)$ customers will have arrived at the server, while $N_s(\Delta)$ customers will have been served. Their difference $N(\Delta)$ is the number waiting, or thrown away. In the limit as Δ becomes unboundedly large, all three must become unboundedly large. Because we are assuming a finite buffer, if the arrival rate is greater than the service rate, $N(\Delta)/\Delta$ must be the rate at which customers are lost. Therefore, $N(\Delta)/N_a(\Delta)$ must be the fraction that are lost. But

$$\lambda := \lim_{\Delta\to\infty} \frac{N_a(\Delta)}{\Delta} \quad \text{and} \quad \mu := \lim_{\Delta\to\infty} \frac{N_s(\Delta)}{\Delta}.$$

Therefore,

$$p_\ell > \lim_{\Delta\to\infty} \frac{N(\Delta)}{N_a(\Delta)} = \lim_{\Delta\to\infty} \frac{N_a(\Delta) - N_s(\Delta)}{N_a(\Delta)} = 1 - \frac{\mu}{\lambda} = 1 - \frac{1}{\rho}, \tag{2.1.10a}$$

and solving for ρ,

$$\rho < \rho_m = \frac{1}{1 - p_\ell}. \tag{2.1.10b}$$

Note that $\rho_m > 1$. Thus, as ρ approaches ρ_m, the buffer size needed to keep losses below p_ℓ goes to infinity, and excessive losses cannot be prevented. This is true for all load-independent single-server queues. For load-dependent, or multiple-server queues the concept of utilization must be generalized, but then an appropriate bound can be derived.

In many applications, no amount of loss is acceptable, as in the transmission of data or text over a communications channel. The formulas for $P_o(N_1)$ and $P_f(N_1)$ show that both are proportional to ρ^{N_1}, so to reduce the loss or overflow, one can either increase the buffer size, or decrease ρ by replacing the server with a faster one. If delay is not the critical factor, then increasing the buffer's capacity may be the cheaper solution. For instance, by doubling N_1, one gets $P(2\,N_1) \approx P(N_1)^2$. If $P(N_1)$ is already small, say 0.01, then $P(2\,N_1) \approx .0001$, very small indeed. Thus one often solves such problems by throwing buffer space at it. In Chapter 4 we show that for certain kinds of service time distributions, this solution will not work.

Exercise 2.1.6: Draw curves of $\bar{q}_f(N_1)$ as a function of $\rho = 0 \to 2$ for $N_1 = 10$, 20, and 40. Include $\bar{q}_s$ for $\rho = 0 \to 1$ for comparison.

Exercise 2.1.7: Suppose that a router has enough space to hold 20 packets, and that $\rho = 0.9$. What percentage of packets will be lost if there is no backup buffer? By how much must the service rate [μ] be increased to reduce losses by a factor of 10? How much buffer space must be added for the same reduction? Redo the problem for overflow to a backup buffer.

2.1.5 Load-Dependent Servers

The solutions for the M/M/1 queue can be extended without much difficulty to the M/M/C/ /N, and even somewhat more general, queues. Suppose that there are C identical exponential servers in S_1, each with service rate μ, feeding off a single queue. That is, as long as there are $n \geq C$ customers at S_1, all of the servers will be active, and as long as $n \leq C$, none of the customers will be waiting to be served. As we already know, if several exponential servers are busy, the probability rate for something to happen is the sum of their service rates. Therefore, we can define a service rate for S_1 that depends on the number of customers there. That is, let $\mu(n)$ be the service rate of S_1 when there are n customers there; then

$$\mu(n) = \begin{cases} n\,\mu & \text{for } n \leq C \\ C\,\mu & \text{for } n \geq C. \end{cases} \tag{2.1.11a}$$

We think of S_1 as a load-dependent server. Actually, the formulas we derive in this section do not depend on the explicit form we have just given the μ's; thus we can immediately generalize, and let $\mu(1)$, $\mu(2)$, and so on, be any positive numbers. The reader may think of S_i as a ***multiple server*** subsystem, or as a single server whose service rate changes (not necessarily by integral units) with change of queue length. See the end of this section for further notational discussion.

Another formulation, which we adopt here, is to introduce the ***load-dependence factor*** $\alpha_1(n)$, which is the ratio of service rates $\mu(n)$ and $\mu(1)$. By definition, $\mu(1) := \mu$, $\alpha_1(1)$ always equals 1, and $\alpha_1(n) = \mu(n)/\mu$, which for a subsystem with C identical servers gives the following.

$$\alpha_1(n) = \begin{cases} n & \text{for } n \leq C \\ C & \text{for } n \geq C. \end{cases} \tag{2.1.11b}$$

Clearly, $\mu(n) = \alpha_1(n)\mu$. Similarly, we can view S_2 as a load-dependent server, with load-dependence factor $\alpha_2(n)$. Then $\lambda(n) = \alpha_2(n)\lambda$. Next look at Figure 2.1.2. The arrow going from n to $n-1$ corresponds to the probability rate of going from n to $n-1$, which can happen only if there is a completion at S_1. The rate for this to happen is $\mu(n)$. Similarly, the arrow going from n to $n+1$

corresponds to an arrival from S_2, whose rate must be $\lambda(N-n)$. Then all the arrows pointing to the left should be labeled (reading from right to left)

$$\mu(N),\ \mu(N-1),\ \ldots,\ \mu(n+1),\ \mu(n),\ \mu(n-1),\ \ldots,\ \mu(1),$$

and those pointing to the right are labeled (reading, this time, from left to right)

$$\lambda(N),\ \lambda(N-1),\ \ldots,\ \lambda(N-n+1),\ \lambda(N-n), \lambda(N-n-1),\ \ldots,\ \lambda(1).$$

Before solving for the M/M/C//N loop, let us review the meaning of a *state transition-rate diagram*. If, as in Figure 2.1.2, a single node is encircled, the sum of the probability rates entering the circle minus the sum of those leaving must be zero in the steady state. Suppose, instead, that two adjacent nodes are enclosed together. Then the arrows connecting them would not be included in the balance equations. But this would yield the same as one would get by adding the single equations together. After all, each of the two arrows appears in each equation, once as leaving one node, and once as entering the other, canceling out when the two equations are added. In general, then, we can say that for *any* closed curve, what goes in must equal what goes out for the steady state to occur. Now consider the closed curve that encompasses all nodes from 0 to n. Only one arrow goes in, and one arrow goes out, so we have the simple set of first-order difference equations:

$$\lambda(N-n)r(n;N) = \mu(n+1)r(n+1;N) \quad \text{for } 0 \le n < N. \tag{2.1.12a}$$

In particular,

$$r(1;N) = \frac{\lambda(N)}{\mu(1)} r(0;N) \tag{2.1.12b}$$

and

$$r(2;N) = \frac{\lambda(N-1)}{\mu(2)} r(1;N) = \frac{\lambda(N)\,\lambda(N-1)}{\mu(1)\,\mu(2)} r(0;N). \tag{2.1.12c}$$

Next, following the notation of [GORDON-NEWELL67], let $\rho = \lambda/\mu$, $\beta_i(0) := 1$, and for $n > 0$,

$$\beta_i(n) := \alpha_i(n)\beta_i(n-1) = \alpha_i(1)\alpha_i(2)\cdots\alpha_i(n). \tag{2.1.13a}$$

For a subsystem with C identical servers, we have

$$\beta_i(n) := \begin{cases} n! & \text{for } n \le C \\ C!\,C^{n-c} & \text{for } n \ge C. \end{cases} \tag{2.1.13b}$$

Then with only a little trickery, the general solution becomes

$$r(n;\,N) = \frac{1}{K(N)} \frac{\rho^n}{\beta_1(n)\,\beta_2(N-n)}, \tag{2.1.14a}$$

where, owing to the fact that the sum of probabilities must be 1,

$$K(N) := \sum_{n=0}^{N} \frac{\rho^n}{\beta_1(n)\beta_2(N-n)}. \tag{2.1.14b}$$

The reader may recognize this as a discrete convolution of the reciprocals of the μ's and λ's.

Next consider a generalization of the throughput as defined in (2.1.5a). The probability that S_1 is busy no longer can yield the throughput, because its service rate depends on n. Therefore, it is somewhat more difficult to express for a load-dependent server, but turns out to be just as simple to compute. The rate at which S_1 serves customers depends on the distribution of the number in the queue. Then $\Lambda(N)$ is a weighted average of the $\mu(n)$'s:

$$\Lambda(N) = \sum_{n=1}^{N} \mu(n) r(n;N) = \sum_{n=1}^{N} \mu\, \alpha_1(n) r(n;N) = \frac{\mu}{K(N)} \sum_{n=1}^{N} \frac{\alpha_1(n)\rho^n}{\beta_1(n)\beta_2(N-n)}.$$

But $\alpha_1(n)/\beta_1(n) = 1/\beta_1(n-1)$ and $\mu\,\rho = \lambda$, so (change the summation variable from n to $n-1$)

$$\Lambda(N) = \frac{\lambda}{K(N)} \sum_{n=1}^{N} \frac{\rho^{n-1}}{\beta_1(n-1)\beta_2(N-n)} = \frac{\lambda K(N-1)}{K(N)}. \tag{2.1.15a}$$

This is identical to the throughput for the load-independent system described in (2.1.5d) with $\lambda = 1/T_2$, except that now $K(N)$ does not satisfy (2.1.4d). There is no simple recursive relationship among the $K(N)$s for arbitrary β's.

There are three different ways to "open up" our load-dependent system, two of which yield equivalent results. For the first way, merely let $\beta_2(n) = 1$ for all n. Then, if $\lambda/\mu(N)$ is less than 1 for large N, S_2 is a Poisson source to S_1 and we have the standard M/M/C queue when $\beta_1(n)$ satisfies (2.1.13b). That is, from Equations (2.1.14),

$$K := \lim_{N\to\infty} K(N) = \sum_{n=0}^{\infty} \frac{\rho^n}{\beta_1(n)} \tag{2.1.15b}$$

and

$$r(n) := \lim_{N\to\infty} r(n;N) = \frac{1}{K}\frac{\rho^n}{\beta_1(n)}. \tag{2.1.15c}$$

Actually, one can make a somewhat more general statement. If

$$\lambda_\infty := \lim_{N\to\infty} \lambda(N)$$

exists and $\lambda_\infty/\mu(N)$ is less than 1 for large N, everything still holds except that now $\rho = \lambda_\infty/\mu$.

A second approach is to argue that $\lambda(n)$ is really a function of N and n by way of their difference, $N-n$. That is, let

$$\bar{\lambda}(n) := \lim_{N\to\infty} \lambda(N-n)$$

and

$$K = \sum_{n=0}^{\infty} \frac{\rho^n}{\beta_1(n)\bar{\beta}_2(n)},$$

where $\bar{\alpha}_2(n) := \bar{\lambda}(n)/\bar{\lambda}(1)$, $\bar{\beta}_2(0) := 1$, and

$$\bar{\beta}_2(n) := \bar{\alpha}_2(n)\,\bar{\beta}_2(n-1).$$

The $\bar{\alpha}_2$s can be interpreted as a slowdown of the arrival process because of the increasing queue length, so this is referred to as an M/M/C queue with ***discouraged arrivals***. This may be a misnomer in some countries where consumer goods are scarce. In those places, we are told, arrival rates to queues actually increase with queue length. Mathematically, because K in this case is not a convolution, β_1 and $\bar{\beta}_2$ can be combined into a single load-dependent factor. However, for more general queues (e.g., M/G/C and G/M/C) the two must still be kept separate. The third view, which ends up being the same as the first, considers all customers, while they are at S_2, to act independently. That is, each customer spends a random amount of time at S_2, with mean Z, and then, independently of the other customers, goes to S_1. The completion rate is exactly $(N-n)/Z$. Z is called the ***think time***, or ***delay time***, and S_2 is called a ***think stage*** or ***time-sharing stage*** or ***delay stage***, as well as some other names. Clearly, as N goes to infinity, the arrival rate grows unboundedly, thereby swamping S_1. In reality, there never are an infinite number of potential customers, but there may be so many and they may stay at S_2 so long that n (the number at S_1) is always small compared to N, so the departure rate from S_2 is more or less constant. In mathematical terms, let Z grow unboundedly with N, and let

$$\lambda_\infty = \lim_{N\to\infty} \frac{N}{Z}.$$

This yields the same solution as case 1.

In all these cases we can make a statement that generalizes (2.1.6c). Let μ_∞ be the limiting value of $\mu(N)$; then

$$\lim_{N\to\infty} \Lambda(N) = \min(\mu_\infty, \lambda_\infty)\,. \tag{2.1.16}$$

Once again, the throughput of the system is bounded by the maximal capacity of its slowest server.

Example 2.1.3: The simplest example of a load-dependent queue is the M/M/2 queue. In this case, $\beta_1(n) = 2^{n-1}$, $\bar{\beta}_2(n) = 1$,

$$r(0) = \frac{2-\rho}{2+\rho},$$

and

$$r(n) = \frac{2}{K}\left(\frac{\rho}{2}\right)^n \quad \text{for } n > 0,$$

where

$$K = 2\,\frac{2+\rho}{2-\rho}.$$

We leave it for the reader in Exercise 2.1.8 below to show that

$$\bar{q}_s = \frac{4\rho}{4-\rho^2}, \quad \text{and} \quad \bar{T}_s = \frac{4\bar{x}}{4-\rho^2}.$$

Note that the queue doesn't blow up until ρ approaches 2. ▲

Finally, let us consider our open M/M/C queue, and let C go to infinity. Then S_1 is a place where customers arrive randomly, "hang around" for a while, $[1/\mu]$, and then leave. The number present at any time is distributed according to the Poisson distribution. Because $\beta_1(n) = n!$,

$$K = \sum_{n=0}^{\infty} \frac{\rho^n}{n!} = e^{\rho},$$

leading to

$$r(n) = \frac{\rho^n}{n!} e^{-\rho}. \tag{2.1.17}$$

This is just one of the many derivations of the Poisson distribution that start from different assumptions.

Observe that all the formulas are valid whether or not $\alpha(n)$ and $\mu(n)$ satisfy Equations (2.1.11). If they do, we retain the notation "M/M/C//N loop," including the system with a time-sharing subsystem, for which we use the notation "M/M/∞//N" or "M/M/C//C." If we wish to look at systems in which the α's are not necessarily integers but instead satisfy a weakened version of Equations (2.1.11), namely, for $n \leq C$, $\alpha_1(n) =$ anything > 0, but

$$\alpha_1(n) = \alpha_1(C) \quad \text{for } n \geq C,$$

then we would refer to it as a ***generalized M/M/C//N loop***. If the α's can be anything whatsoever, we use the notation, "M/M/X/ /N *loop*." To maintain a connection with the outside literature, we refer to all of these generically as "M/M/C*-type systems*," or, *systems with load-dependent servers*." We also adhere to this notation in dealing with more general distributions in Sections 4.4.4 and 5.4, and Chapter 6 (e.g., G/M/X and M/G/C queues). In Chapter 6, we also introduce the generalized M/G/C system.

Exercise 2.1.8: Consider systems (A) through (D) as described below. What are the formulas for their respective system times? Call them T_A, T_B, T_C, and T_D, respectively. Assume that the service rate for the base server is $\mu = 1$. Plot the four system times on the same graph as a function of $\lambda = \rho$, for $0 \leq \lambda < 2$. Of course, T_A blows up at $\lambda = 1$, but the other three have the same maximal capacity, and blow up at $\lambda = 2$.

Even the simple M/M/1 queue can have realistic practical applications. We present one in the following exercises. In most facilities it is generally true that the demand for a critical resource will always increase in time. This can be viewed in our simple world as an arrival rate λ that increases monotonically with time. Inevitably then, the system time, as given by (2.1.7b) will become intolerably long. Call this *System* (A). This leads to two questions: How can the service be improved? And for what value of λ should the improvement be implemented? We consider two possible changes for improvement: either add a second server, or replace the existing one by another that is faster. For simple analysis we assume that the new server is twice as fast. In the latter case, this is still an M/M/1 queue where $\mu \Rightarrow 2\mu$. Call this *System* (D). In the former case consider two possible implementations. Arriving customers come to a dispatching point, and are then randomly assigned (with equal probability) to either of the two servers, where they then queue for service. It can be shown that this is equivalent to having each server see a Poisson arrival stream, but with arrival rate $\lambda/2$. This yields two M/M/1 queues. Call this *System* (B). Finally, for *System* (C), customers queue up at the dispatching point, and are assigned to a processor as soon as it becomes idle. This is the M/M/2 described in this section. In Chapter 5 we present another dispatching option.

Exercise 2.1.9: Using the results of the previous exercise, show that $T_A > T_B > T_C > T_D$ for all $0 < \lambda < 2$. In fact, show that:

$$T_B = 2\,T_D \quad \text{and} \quad T_C = T_D + \frac{1}{2+\lambda}.$$

We seem to have shown that "twice as fast is always better than twice as much," but remember, we have only shown this for Poisson arrivals to exponential servers. In Chapter 6 we show that if the squared coefficient of variation, C_v^2 is large, this is not necessarily the case.

We have seen *how* a system might be improved, and now we look at the question as to *when* it would be cost effective to do so.

Exercise 2.1.10: Suppose that one single-speed server costs C dollars per hour to rent, and that each customer is paid S dollars per hour. Assume that when a customer is waiting for, or receiving service, his time is being wasted. Then at all times, on average, there are $\bar{q}_s$ customers wasting their time. The total cost then can be given as

$$\$_A = C + S\,\bar{q}_A(\lambda) \quad \text{and} \quad \$_I = 2C + S\,\bar{q}_I(\lambda),$$

where $I \in \{B, C, D\}$. We are assuming that the double-fast server costs as much as two single servers. Clearly, for λ very small, $\$_A$ is smaller than the other three, and it doesn't pay to upgrade. But $\$_A$ blows up at $\lambda = 1$ whereas the others don't blow up until $\lambda = 2$. Therefore, the curves must cross somewhere for $0 < \lambda < 1$. This must be true for any values of C and S. In fact, the crossing point depends only on their ratio, $r = S/C$. Make a graph of the four $\$_I$s for $0 \le \lambda < 1$ for $r = 0.1,\ 1.0,\ 10.0$, showing the crossings in each case. What are the values of λ_I at those points? Now draw three curves on the same graph of λ_I versus r.

2.1.6 Departure Process

Let us now consider one last steady-state process before moving on to the transient behavior of the M/M/1 queue. Suppose that an observer is sitting just downstream from S_1, measuring the time between departures, without knowing the state of the system. What would she expect to see? In other words, given that a customer has just left, what is the time until the next one leaves S_1? We are asking for the distribution of *interdeparture times*. First we give some appropriate definitions.

Definition 2.1.5

$X_d(N)$:=*r.v. denoting the time between departures for a steady-state M/M/1//N queue* (***interdeparture times***).

$$X_d := \lim_{N\to\infty} X_d(N)$$

$b_d(t;\,N) := b_{X_d(N)}(t) =$ density function for the process. □

This question was originally considered by P. J. Burke [BURKE56] and is easy enough to find out once we accept a theorem about M/M/1 queues that is be proven in Section 4.1.3, Theorem 4.1.4. This theorem states that for both open and closed M/M/1 queues, and more generally, M/G/1 (but *not* G/M/1) queues, the steady-state probability that a departing customer will leave n fellow customers behind at S_1 is the same as the steady-state probability of finding n there, except that he will never leave N customers behind, because he, at least, must be at S_2. Let $d(n;\,N)$ be this probability; then from (2.1.4b) we can write

$$d(n;N) = \frac{\rho^n}{c(N)}, \tag{2.1.18}$$

where $c(N)$ is found by summing over n, from 0 to $N-1$. Thus $c(N) = K(N-1)$ from (2.1.4c).

Now, as long as S_1 is busy, the density function for the departure of the next customer is simply the same as the pdf of S_1 (i.e., $\mu e^{-\mu t}$). But if S_1 is idle, our downstream observer must wait first for a customer to finish being served at S_2 and then be processed by S_1. This is the ***convolution*** of the two pdfs:

$$[b_1 \times b_2](t) := \int_0^t b_1(s) b_2(t-s) ds = \int_0^t b_1(t-s) b_2(s) ds,$$

which for two exponential distributions yields

$$\begin{aligned}[b_1 \times b_2](t) :&= \int_0^t \mu e^{-\mu s} \lambda e^{-\lambda(t-s)} ds = \mu\lambda e^{-\lambda t} \int_0^t e^{-(\mu-\lambda)s} ds \\ &= \frac{\mu\lambda}{\mu-\lambda}\left(e^{-\lambda t} - e^{-\mu t}\right).\end{aligned}$$

The overall distribution is the weighted average of the two possibilities. Recall that $\rho = \lambda/\mu$; then

$$\begin{aligned}b_d(t;N) &= d(0:N)[b_1 \times b_2](t) + [1 - d(0;N)]\mu e^{-\mu t} \\ &= \frac{1-\rho}{1-\rho^N}\frac{\lambda}{1-\rho}\left(e^{-\lambda t} - e^{-\mu t}\right) + \left(1 - \frac{1-\rho}{1-\rho^N}\right)\mu e^{-\mu t}.\end{aligned}$$

We can regroup the terms to get the following simple form.

$$b_d(t:N) = \frac{1}{1-\rho^N}\lambda e^{-\lambda t} - \frac{\rho^N}{1-\rho^N}\mu e^{-\mu t}. \tag{2.1.19a}$$

For the closed loop, the departure process is *not* a Poisson process, because the interdeparture times are not exponentially distributed. For the open queue, where $\rho < 1$ and $N \to \infty$, $b_d(t)$ *is* exponential. The mean time between departures is easy enough to get:

$$\mathbf{E}[X_d(N)] = \int_0^\infty t\, b_d(t:N)\, dt = \frac{1-\rho^{N+1}}{1-\rho^N}\frac{1}{\lambda}. \tag{2.1.19b}$$

We leave it to the following exercise to show that $\mathbf{E}[X_d(N)]$ is the reciprocal of the mean throughput given by (2.1.5d).

Exercise 2.1.11: Verify that (2.1.19b) is true, and show that $\mathbf{E}[X_d(N)] = 1/\Lambda(N)$.

Either from (2.1.19b) or from (2.1.6c), we have

$$\lim_{N\to\infty} \mathbf{E}[X_d(N)] = \max\left(\frac{1}{\lambda}, \frac{1}{\mu}\right). \tag{2.1.20a}$$

For the open queue, if ρ is less than 1, ($\lambda < \mu$), the mean departure rate from S_1 is the same as the mean arrival rate. But if ρ is greater than 1, the mean departure rate is governed by the service rate of S_1. We can now prove the well-known result, first given by P. J. Burke in 1956, that the departures from an open M/M/1 queue are exponentially distributed. Simply let N go to infinity on (2.1.19a),

$$\begin{aligned} b_d(t) := \lim_{N\to\infty} b_d(t;\, N) &= \lambda\, e^{-\lambda t} \quad \text{for } \rho < 1 \\ &= \mu\, e^{-\mu x} \quad \text{for } \rho > 1. \end{aligned} \tag{2.1.20b}$$

As long as ρ is less than 1, it is as though S_1 did not exist (exponential in $\to$ exponential out). We also see once again that S_2, with its unbounded number of customers, is a Poisson source for S_1. But if ρ is greater than 1, S_1 releases customers at its service rate and becomes a Poisson source for S_2. The symmetry of our loop would require this, anyway.

We must emphasize that this result (exponential in $\to$ exponential out, for an open, unsaturated M/M/1 queue) is indeed extraordinary. It is also valid for load-dependent (i.e., M/M/C) queues. Note however that it is not true for first-come first-served M/G/1 queues or even G/M/1 queues. It is not even true for closed M/M/1//N loops. We must be careful not to generalize too quickly from what we learn about the M/M/1 queue.

2.2 Relaxation Time for M/M/1//N Loops

For the rest of this chapter we examine systems for which not enough time has elapsed to declare that a system is in its steady state. We call this time range the ***transient region***. In principle we would like to solve the Chapman-Kolmogorov equations (1.3.2b), but in practice, if N is large, this is not an easy task. Aside from the M/M/1 queue, there are very few known analytic solutions to this equation. A rather ingenious solution for the open M/M/1 queue, where N is infinite, is given in [TAKACS62]. That may well be the only explicit solution for an infinite state-space, transient queueing system in existence. But even the existence of that solution does not help much, because it is so difficult to evaluate or interpret.* Therefore we must find some simpler ways of parameterizing transient behavior. For our initial view, we remind the reader of the discussion about relaxation times in Section 1.3.3 and (1.3.11).

*Takacs actually supplies two different forms for the solution, neither of which is easy to evaluate. Most texts list the second form, which involves an infinite sum of Bessel functions, but the first form turns out to be more useful (particularly in the region where the time parameter is neither very small nor very large) if one is comfortable with numerical integration.

In general, finding the eigenvalues of a matrix is not a trivial task, particularly if one wants to express them in terms of unspecified parameters rather than numerically. If the dimension of the matrix is small enough, as with (2.1.2) and (2.1.3), the eigenvalues can be found by straightforward, if tedious, methods. In the case of our $\boldsymbol{Q}$, one of the eigenvalues is zero, thus the characteristic equation can be written as degree N rather than $N+1$, the size of $\boldsymbol{Q}$. It is well known that no general formula (such as the quadratic equation) exists for the roots of polynomials of degree greater than four, nor can one ever be found. (If you have ever used the cubic or quartic formulas to get analytic expressions, you might be inclined to say that even four is too big.) Therefore, unless one is "lucky" (as with the zero eigenvalue), the task is hopeless for $N > 4$.

By a fortuitous stroke of good fortune, because the $\boldsymbol{Q}$ of (2.1.1c) is so repetitive, $\phi_N(\beta) = |\boldsymbol{Q} - \beta \boldsymbol{I}|$ satisfies a recurrence relation in N which turns out to be similar to that satisfied by Chebyshev polynomials of the second kind, from which all the eigenvalues can be obtained. The details can be found in [MORSE58]. As always, $\beta_o = 0$, and

$$\beta_k = \mu + \lambda + 2\sqrt{\mu\,\lambda}\,\cos\frac{k\pi}{N+1} \qquad \text{for } k = 1, 2, 3, \ldots, N. \tag{2.2.1a}$$

The smallest β is β_N, which therefore must be $1/RT$. As in Exercise 2.1.1, it is convenient to express the relaxation time in units of the time it takes a lone customer to make one cycle $(1/\mu + 1/\lambda)$. Then, recalling that $\rho = \lambda/\mu$, and $\cos[\pi N/(N+1)] = -\cos[\pi/(N+1)]$, we get the following expression for the ***normalized relaxation time***.

$$T(\rho,\, N) := \frac{\mu\lambda}{\mu + \lambda} RT = \frac{\rho}{(1+\rho)} \left(1 + \rho - 2\sqrt{\rho}\,\cos\frac{\pi}{N+1}\right)^{-1}. \tag{2.2.1b}$$

T is invariant to the replacement of ρ with $1/\rho$; that is, $T(\rho, N) = T(1/\rho, N)$.

Next, we look at $T(\rho, N)$ when N is very large. For $\rho \neq 1$, $T(\rho, N)$ has a finite limit as N goes to infinity. Thus the relaxation time for an open system (normalized so that $1/\mu + 1/\lambda = 1$) is

$$T(\rho) \;:=\; \lim_{N\to\infty} T(\rho, N) = \frac{\rho}{(1+\rho)(1-\sqrt{\rho})^2} = T(1/\rho). \tag{2.2.2a}$$

It is not hard to show that $T(\rho)$ approaches $0.5/(1-\rho)^2$ when ρ is close to 1 [FANGLIPSKY82]. As so often happens, $\rho = 1$ must be treated as a special case. We can either set $\rho = 1$, or let $N \to \infty$, but not both at the same time. $T(1, N)$ goes to infinity as $\mathrm{O}(N^2)$. We show this by setting ρ equal to 1 in (2.2.1b) to get

$$T(1, N) = \frac{1}{2}\left(2 - 2\cos\frac{\pi}{N+1}\right)^{-1} = \frac{1}{4}\left(1 - \cos\frac{\pi}{N+1}\right)^{-1},$$

and then use Maclaurin's expansion for $\cos x$ $[\cos x = 1 - x^2/2 + \mathrm{O}(x^4)]$:

$$T(1, N) = \frac{1}{4}\left[\frac{1}{2}\left(\frac{\pi}{N+1}\right)^2 + \mathrm{O}\left(\frac{1}{N^4}\right)\right]^{-1}$$

$$= \frac{1}{2}\left(\frac{N+1}{\pi}\right)^2 \left[1 + \mathrm{O}\left(\frac{1}{N^2}\right)\right]. \tag{2.2.2b}$$

Naturally, the relaxation time for an open system ($N = \infty$) is infinite when $\rho = 1$. That is, the system never reaches a steady state.

Example 2.2.1: Figure 2.2.1 summarizes what we have said about relax-

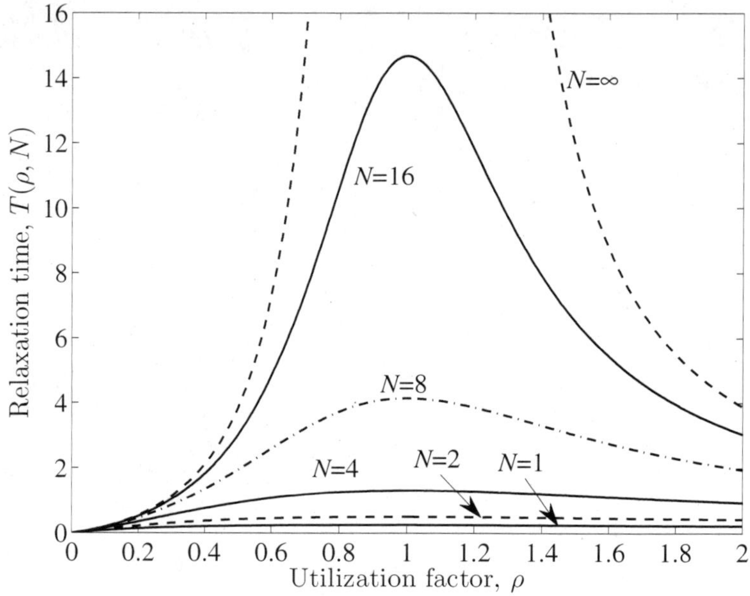

Figure 2.2.1: Relaxation time as a function of ρ for M/M/1//N queues, as given by (2.2.1b). $T(\rho, N)$ is in units of cycle time for one customer. All curves peak at $\rho = 1$, whereas at $\rho = 1$, $T(1, N)$ goes to infinity as N becomes increasingly large. For all values of ρ, the relaxation time increases with N.

ation times. What is most important is to observe that as systems get bigger (in this case, N larger) and more saturated (ρ close to 1), the time it takes to approach the steady-state solution grows as well. This puts into question the steady-state solution as a description of systems that are in existence for relatively short times. ▲

Example 2.2.2: Figure 2.2.2 presents the same information in a different way. Now N varies for fixed $\rho = 0.5, 0.9, 0.95$, and 1. As with the throughput curves, $T(\rho, N) = T(1/\rho, N)$, so $\rho = 2$ yields the same curve as $\rho = 1/2$. As $N \to \infty$, each curve approaches its limit as given by (2.2.2a), except, of course, for $\rho = 1$, which has no limit. ▲

Clearly, if ρ is close to 1, the relaxation time can be very large. However, if ρ is very small (or very large), $T(\rho, N)$ is small. This may be an underestimate of how long it takes a system to come close to its steady state. If all customers

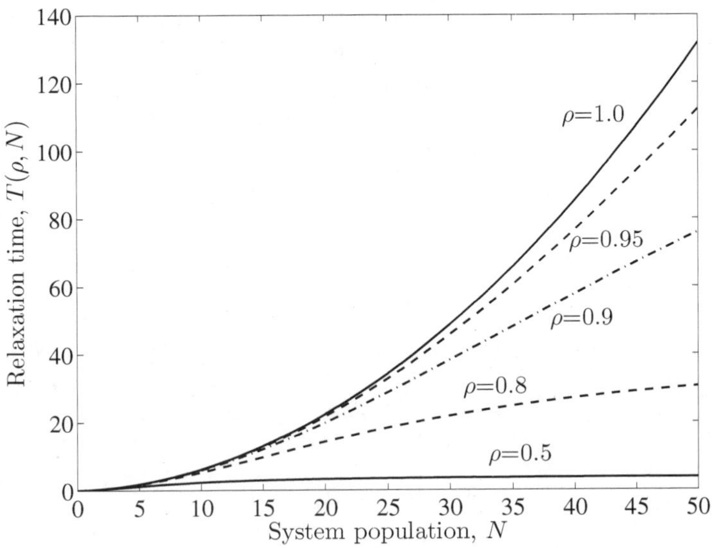

Figure 2.2.2: Relaxation times as a function of system population N for M/M/1/ /N loops. The RT's for ρ and $1/\rho$ are identical; therefore, we only show curves for $\rho \leq 1$. As $N \to \infty$, all curves except that for $\rho = 1$ will saturate.

are initially at the slower server, very few completions would have to occur to approach the steady state, because very few customers are ever likely to be at the faster server at any one time. Even so, the mean time for one slow server completion (in units of the cycle time) is $1/(1+\rho)$, which (for small ρ) is $1/\rho$ times larger than $T(\rho, N)$. On the other hand, if all the customers are initially at the faster server, the steady state cannot be approached until almost all of them have been served at least once. The mean time for this is of the order of $\rho N/(1+\rho)$. The two conditions together imply that

$$0 \leq RT \leq \frac{N}{\rho} T(\rho, N), \quad \text{for } \rho < 1. \tag{2.2.2c}$$

RT could be 0 if the system were initially in its steady state, which means that all queue lengths are possible from the beginning (i.e., we do not know anything).

2.3 Other Transient Parameters

In this section we introduce alternative ways (other than RT) of examining the transient region. We are pleased to find that some of the objects we needed for the steady-state solution are also used here. As with every Markov chain, only one thing at a time can happen in a queueing network; the evolution of the system in time is marked by a discrete sequence of events. We call the interval after one event up to and including the next event an ***epoch***.

This deviates from conventional use. Feller [FELLER71] prefers to use *epoch* to mean the time the event occured (not the interval). Sometimes, the time between events is called the ***sojourn time***.

Such sequences, or epochs, can be represented by *time-dependent state transition diagrams*. The technique described here is easily generalized to include nonexponential and even more general service centers, and that is done in succeeding chapters.

2.3.1 Mean First-Passage Times for Queue Growth

As a first application, we examine the time it takes for a queue to grow from 0 to some integer n. Such processes are referred to as *first passages*, and the average times for such events to take place are called ***mean first-passage times***, or simply ***first-passage times***. The points at which a Markov chain reaches each length for the first time are called ***ladder points***. All the things that happen from the time the queue reaches j to the time it reaches $j+1$ is said to have "occurred during the j-th epoch."

Looking at Figure 2.1.1, suppose that initially all the customers are at S_2; then in mean time $1/\lambda$ the first event occurs, corresponding to an arrival to S_1 (epoch 0 has ended). After that, one of two events can occur: either the customer at S_1 returns to S_2, or another customer from S_2 goes to S_1. The sequence of possible events grows factorially after that, and it becomes thoroughly impractical to enumerate all of them. However, if in any sequence the system returns to a state it was in previously, a recursive relation can be set up that may be solvable. This is known as a ***regenerative process*** [KINGMAN72]. We show how this works in this section and use it frequently in subsequent chapters. To apply this method, one must start with single jumps. So we define

Definition 2.3.1

$\tau_u(n) :=$ ***mean first-passage time*** *for the queue at* S_1 *to go from* n *to* $n+1$. The n-th epoch begins with n customers at S_1. Customers may leave and arrive in arbitrary order, but eventually there will be $n+1$ customers at S_1 for the first time (end of epoch n and beginning of epoch $(n+1)$. The mean time for this to happen is $\tau_u(n)$. The subscript ***u*** stands for ***u***p. (In subsequent sections we will have occasion to use ***d*** for ***d***own and ***m*** for ***m***ax.) □

Consider Figure 2.3.1. The circles on the lowest horizontal line correspond to the set of states the system can be in initially, which in the present case is labeled by the number of customers at S_1. The second horizontal line represents the state the system is in after one transition. The average time elapsed between the two lines depends on the initial state. Thus if the system started with all customers at S_2 [$n = 0$], the mean time for the first transition would be $1/\lambda$. Similarly, if all customers were initially at $S_1[n = N]$, the average time elapsed would be $1/\mu$. For all other initial states, the time would be $1/(\mu + \lambda)$. A straight arrow corresponds to a single direct transition, with the probability that it will occur written near it. For instance, the system can go

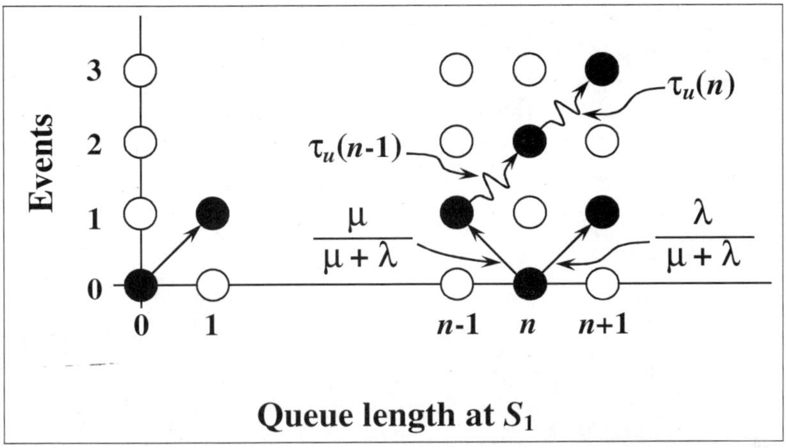

Figure 2.3.1: Time-dependent state transition diagram for a closed M/M/1/ /N loop, describing the mean time $[\tau_u(n)]$ for a queue to grow by one customer. See text for details.

from $n \to n+1$ in one step, with probability $\lambda/(\mu+\lambda)$, with a mean time delay of $1/(\mu+\lambda)$. A wavy arrow corresponds to the sum of all possible ways the system can get from the tail to the head for the first time, irrespective of the number of transitions taken. Thus the arrow labeled "$\tau_u(n)$" includes not only the direct transition $(n \to n+1)$, but also $(n \to n-1 \to n \to n+1)$, and $(n \to n-1 \to n-2 \to n-1 \to n \to n-1 \to n \to n+1)$ and the infinite number of other sequences that eventually lead to $n+1$.

Our ability to represent an infinite number of sequences by a single symbol is the key to setting up a soluble set of recursive relations. If the system starts with n at S_1, an event will occur in mean time $1/(\mu+\lambda)$. That event can be one of two things. Either the queue will go directly to $n+1$, or it will drop to $n-1$, in which case it will take time $\tau_u(n-1)$ to get back to n, and a further $\tau_u(n)$ to finally get to $n+1$. Mathematically we can write

$$\tau_u(n) = \frac{\lambda}{\mu+\lambda} \cdot \frac{1}{\mu+\lambda} + \frac{\mu}{\mu+\lambda}\left[\frac{1}{\mu+\lambda} + \tau_u(n-1) + \tau_u(n)\right],$$

where $\tau_u(0) = 1/\lambda$. For convenience, drop the subscript u when no confusion is likely to arise. The two terms without a τ in them combine to yield the following.

$$\tau(n) = \frac{1}{\mu+\lambda} + \frac{\mu}{\mu+\lambda}[\tau(n-1) + \tau(n)]. \tag{2.3.1a}$$

We interpret this as follows. It takes a mean time of $1/(\mu+\lambda)$ for something to happen. If the event was an arrival, we are done. The probability that it was not an arrival is $\mu/(\mu+\lambda)$, in which case the queue will have dropped back to $n-1$ and take a mean time of $[\tau(n-1)+\tau(n)]$ to first get back to n and then to $n+1$. Note that $\tau(n)$ appears on both sides of the equation, indicating that the system got back to where it started, and that is what we mean by a regenerative process. We derive equations for more complicated processes in just this way, so the reader should expect to return to this section for reference.

We next solve for $\tau(n)$ and get the following recursive equation.

$$\tau(n) = \frac{1}{\lambda}[1 + \mu\tau(n-1)], \quad \text{for } n > 0, \tag{2.3.1b}$$

and $\tau(0) = 1/\lambda$. By direct substitution into (2.3.1b) it follows that $\tau(1) = (1 + 1/\rho)/\lambda$ and $\tau(2) = (1 + 1/\rho + 1/\rho^2)/\lambda$. One can guess that the general expression for $\tau(n)$ is

$$\tau(n) = \frac{1}{\lambda}\sum_{j=o}^{n} \frac{1}{\rho^j}, \tag{2.3.2a}$$

which can be proven by induction to be the solution of (2.3.1b). †. Equation (2.3.2a) is the well-known (certainly by now) geometric series for which a closed-form expression exists.

$$\tau(n) = \frac{1}{\lambda}\sum_{j=0}^{n} \frac{1}{\rho^j} = \frac{1/\mu}{1-\rho}\left(\frac{1}{\rho^{n+1}} - 1\right) \quad \text{for } \rho \neq 1 \tag{2.3.2b}$$

and

$$\tau(n) = \frac{n+1}{\mu} \quad \text{for } \rho = 1. \tag{2.3.2c}$$

We are now ready to find the time it takes for a queue to grow to a given length.

Definition 2.3.2

$t_u(0 \to n)$:= *mean first-passage time for the queue at* S_1 *to grow from* 0 *to* n *customers.* The queue could drop to 0 many times before finally reaching the goal. □

This parameter satisfies the following.

$$t_u(0 \to n) = \sum_{j=0}^{n-1} \tau_u(j). \tag{2.3.3a}$$

After substituting Equations (2.3.2) into the above (and omitting the subscript u), the explicit expressions follow.

$$t(0 \to n) = \frac{1/\mu}{1-\rho}\left(\frac{1}{\rho^n}\frac{1-\rho^n}{1-\rho} - n\right) \quad \text{for } \rho \neq 1 \tag{2.3.3b}$$

† We interject a word or two about "guessing." If science were merely a sequence of deductions, we all would have already been replaced by computers. Research is a creative process. The imaginative scientist, mathematician, or engineer plays with the tools of the trade and regularly makes guesses at what is correct. (These guesses are often credited to intuition.) Most guesses that prove wrong never come to public light. You, the reader, only see the successes and thus may think that there is some secret process going on to which you will never be privy. Nonsense. The creative person who plays long enough with the relevant material will ultimately make many correct guesses. Remember, proof by induction does not require that we defend the source of the guess. It must only prove that the guess is correct (if it is).

and

$$t(0 \to n) = \frac{n(n+1)}{2\mu} \quad \text{for } \rho = 1. \tag{2.3.3c}$$

Equations (2.3.3) can be thought of as the mean rate at which a queue grows in time. For instance, we see from (2.3.3c) that for $\rho = 1$ and large n, $t(0 \to n)$ grows as n^2. We can get a different insight to this process by thinking of $t(0 \to n)$ as the independent variable. Then we see that n grows as the square root of t. This is quite similar to behavior of a ***random walk*** process, and is in fact a special type of random walk with a barrier. [FELLER71] considers such processes to be ***renewal processes***.

For $\rho < 1$, (2.3.3b) implies that $\mu t(0 \to n)$ approaches $(1/\rho)^n/(1-\rho)^2$ as n gets increasingly large. Considering n as the dependent variable, it follows that n grows as the $\log t$. This is indeed an extremely slow growth rate, for although all queue lengths are possible, when ρ is less than 1, long queue lengths take exponential time to be reached even once.

Finally, for $\rho > 1$, (2.3.3b) implies that $t(0 \to n)$ and n grow proportionally. This actually makes intuitive sense, whereas the two previous examples are a consequence of statistical fluctuations. Clearly, the arrival rate exceeds the service rate, so with every passing unit of time, customers who have yet to be served accumulate at S_1 in proportion to the difference between the arrival and service rates, namely $\mu(\rho - 1)$. Examples for all three cases are shown in Figure 2.3.2. Asymptotic behavior can be summarized by the following equations.

$$n(t) \to \frac{\log(\mu t)}{\log(1/\rho)} \quad \text{for } \rho < 1, \tag{2.3.4a}$$

$$n(t) \to \sqrt{2\mu t} \quad \text{for } \rho = 1, \tag{2.3.4b}$$

$$n(t) \to \mu t(\rho - 1) + \frac{1}{\rho - 1} \quad \text{for } \rho > 1. \tag{2.3.4c}$$

These three asymptotic forms are quite different, yet if ρ is close to 1, μt must be rather large before the three will look considerably different.

Example 2.3.1: It can be seen from Figure 2.3.2 that the closer ρ is to 1, the larger μt will be before (2.3.4a) or (2.3.4c) deviate from (2.3.4b). An interesting consequence of this is the following. In taking data of such a system (or an ensemble of such systems), an observer cannot measure very accurately what ρ is, without waiting an extremely long time. Also, note that even after 50 cycle times, the queue has not come anywhere near its steady-state mean queue length for $\rho > 0.9$. ▲

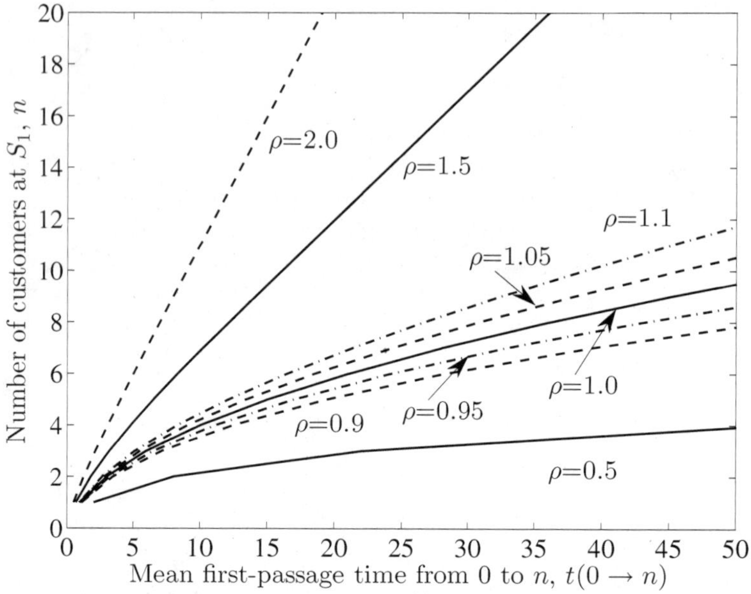

Figure 2.3.2: Number of customers versus mean first-passage time for the queue at S_1 to grow from 0 to n, $t(0 \to n)$, as given by Equations (2.3.3). Equations (2.3.4) show that when $\rho < 1$, n grows as $\log t$, but when $\rho > 1$, n grows linearly with t. Yet t must be very large for this behavior to become apparent if ρ is close to 1.

Exercise 2.3.1: An interesting variation of $t(0 \to n)$ is to find the mean number of arrivals before the queue reaches its steady-state mean queue length for the first time. Here ρ must be less than 1, and $\lambda t(0 \to n)$ is that quantity, for any n. Let n be $\bar{q}$ from (2.1.6b) and draw a curve of $\lambda t(0 \to \bar{q})$ versus ρ, for ρ between 0 and 1. How do these results compare with Figures 2.2.2 and 2.3.2?

2.3.2 *k*-Busy Period

A much-used view of queueing systems that does not require waiting for the steady-state is the ***busy period***. By definition, a busy period begins when a customer arrives at an empty subsystem and ends when a customer leaves behind an empty subsystem. Put differently, the busy period is the interval between idle periods. In general, one can imagine starting with k customers at S_1 and then have customers come and go until, eventually, the queue drains. This is known as the ***k-busy period***, with $k = 1$ being simply the busy period. A good insight into system behavior can often be gained by taking data over several busy periods, and comparing with analytical results. Unlike the steady state, each period has a well-defined beginning and end.

2.3.2.1 Mean Time of a Busy Period

The first parameter we consider is the mean time for the busy period. This can be calculated in a manner very similar to the preceding section. Whereas in that section we were interested in queue growth, here we are interested in queue-length reduction. We use the same symbols as before [τ and $t(0 \to n)$, etc.], and when a distinction between the two types is necessary, we use subscripts u for "up" and d for "down". Otherwise, the subscripts are omitted.

In analogy with Section 2.3.1, with the apparent added restriction that the queue never exceeds N, define the following.

Definition 2.3.3

$\tau_d(n; N)$:= ***mean first-passage time*** *for the queue at* S_1 *to* ***drop*** *from* n *to* $n-1$, *in an* M/M/1/ /N *loop*. Given that there are only N customers in the system, the queue can never exceed N. The process begins with n customers at S_1 and ends when the queue reaches $n-1$ for the first time and could have risen to N any number of times in that period of time. □

This actually is exactly analogous to Definition 2.3.1, because $\tau_u(n)$ includes the self-evident constraint that the queue can never drop below 0.

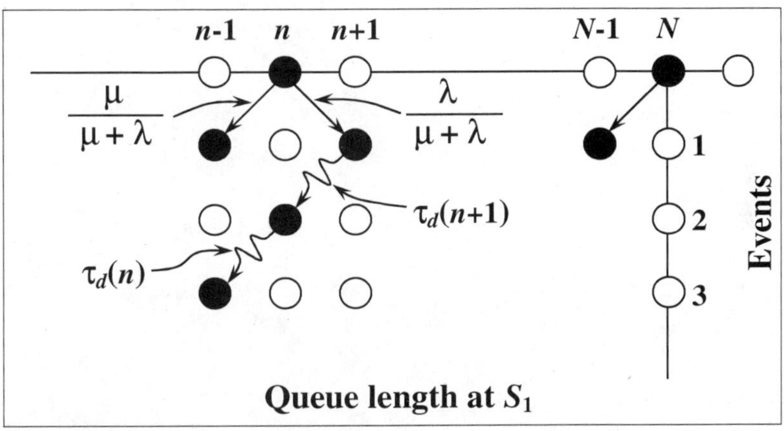

Figure 2.3.3: Time-dependent state transition diagram for a closed M/M/1/ /N loop describing the mean time [$\tau_d(n)$] for a queue to decrease by 1 customer. $\tau_d(1)$ is the mean busy period. See text for full details.

Figure 2.3.3 is similar to Figure 2.3.1, but now the τ_d-s are pointing toward lower lengths. As before, in mean time $1/(\mu+\lambda)$, something happens, and if that something is not a departure, then with probability $\lambda/(\mu+\lambda)$ it is an arrival that raises the queue length by 1, after which it will drift back down to n in time $\tau_d(n+1; N)$, and finally, to $n-1$ in further time, $\tau_d(n; N)$. This leads to (dropping the subscripts d)

$$\tau(n; N) = \frac{1}{\mu+\lambda} + \frac{\lambda}{\mu+\lambda}[\tau(n+1; N) + \tau(n; N)], \tag{2.3.5a}$$

where $\tau(N;N) = 1/\mu$. Making the substitution $\rho = \lambda/\mu$ and the usual rearrangements, we get

$$\mu\tau(n;N) = 1 + \rho\mu\tau(n+1;N). \tag{2.3.5b}$$

Directly substituting into (2.3.5b) for $n = N-1$ and $N-2$, it follows that $\mu\tau(N-1;N) = 1+\rho$, and $\mu\tau(N-2;N) = 1+\rho+\rho^2$. One can easily guess, and prove by induction, that

$$\tau(N-k;\,N) = \frac{1}{\mu}\sum_{i=0}^{k}\rho^i = \frac{1-\rho^{k+1}}{\mu(1-\rho)} \quad \text{for } \rho \neq 1 \tag{2.3.6a}$$

and

$$\tau(N-k;\,N) = \frac{k+1}{\mu} \quad \text{for } \rho = 1, \tag{2.3.6b}$$

where $k = N-n$. It is clear that when $\rho \geq 1$, τ_d grows unboundedly with N (and k), but when $\rho < 1$, then

$$\tau_d(n) := \lim_{N\to\infty} \tau_d(n;\,N) = \frac{1/\mu}{(1-\rho)}. \tag{2.3.6c}$$

We see then, that for an open system, the mean time for a queue to drop by 1 is the same for all n, a result that some might call obvious.

By definition, the mean time for a busy (1-busy) period is the same as the mean time to eventually go from $n=1$ to $n=0$. The *k-busy time* is defined as follows.

Definition 2.3.4

$t_d(k \to 0;\,N)$:= *the mean time for the* ***k-busy period*** *of an* M/M/1//*N loop*. The process begins with k customers at S_1, and ends when there are 0 customers there for the first time. □

First we have

$$t_d(1 \to 0;\,N) = \tau(1;\,N) = \frac{1-\rho^N}{\mu(1-\rho)} \quad \text{for } \rho \neq 1 \tag{2.3.7a}$$

and

$$t_d(1 \to 0;\,N) = \frac{N}{\mu} \quad \text{for } \rho = 1. \tag{2.3.7b}$$

As with the τ_ds, when $\rho \geq 1$, the mean extent of the busy period grows unboundedly with N, but when $\rho < 1$, the limit for $t_d(1 \to 0;\,N)$ exists and approaches [the same as (2.3.6c)]

$$t_d := t_d(1 \to 0) = t_d(1) = \frac{1/\mu}{(1-\rho)}. \tag{2.3.7c}$$

This expression looks familiar. It tells us that the mean busy period for an open M/M/1 queue is the same as its mean system time as given by (2.1.7b).

Actually, (2.3.7c) gives the mean time of a busy period for all open M/G/1 queues (but not G/M/1 queues), whereas the expression for the mean system time for M/G/1 queues [see (4.2.6e) and (4.2.6f)], is more complicated.

An expression for t_d can be derived in the following way. Any single server queue (open or closed) will alternate between busy and idle periods. Let T_i and X_i be the lengths of the i-th busy and idle periods, respectively. Then

$$R_b(m) := \frac{\sum_{i=1}^{m} T_i}{\sum_{i=1}^{m}(T_i + X_i)} \tag{2.3.7d}$$

is the fraction of time S_1 is busy during the first m cycles. As m gets very large, $(\sum T_i/m)$ approaches t_d, $(\sum X_i)/m$ approaches the mean idle time (call it t_I), and R_b approaches $1 - r(0,\, N) = \Pr(S_1 \text{ is busy})$. When we put this all together, we get

$$t_d = t_I \frac{1 - r(0,\, N)}{r(0,\, N)}. \tag{2.3.7e}$$

For every open single-server queue ($N \to \infty$), $r(0,\, N) \to 1-\rho$, and for Poisson arrivals, $t_I = 1/\lambda$. All this yields (2.3.7c).

In direct analogy with Equations (2.3.3) we see that the mean time for the k-busy period is

$$t_d(k \to 0; N) = \sum_{j=1}^{k} \tau_d(j; N) = \frac{1/\mu}{1-\rho} \sum_{j=1}^{k} (1 - \rho^{N-j+1}),$$

which after some straightforward manipulation yields

$$\mu\, t_d(k \to 0; N) = \frac{k}{1-\rho} - \frac{\rho^{N-k+1}}{(1-\rho)^2} + \frac{\rho^{N+1}}{(1-\rho)^2} \quad \text{for } \rho \neq 1 \tag{2.3.8a}$$

and

$$\mu\, t_d(k \to 0; N) = kN - \frac{k(k-1)}{2} \quad \text{for } \rho = 1. \tag{2.3.8b}$$

As with the τ_ds for open systems, the k-busy period is infinite when $\rho \geq 1$, but when $\rho < 1$,

$$\mu\, t_d(k \to 0) = \frac{k}{1-\rho}. \tag{2.3.8c}$$

This makes sense, because it takes a time $1/[\mu\,(1-\rho)]$ [or what is the same thing, $\rho/[\lambda(1-\rho)]$] for an open queue to drop by 1, so if there were k customers to start with, it should take k times $\lambda\rho/(1-\rho)$ to drop to 0.

2.3.2.2 Probability That Queue Will Reach Length k

Although the time for a busy period may be important, it is by no means the only parameter worth examining. From an experimental point of view, it is easy to measure, for instance, the number of busy periods in which a given queue length was reached or the maximum queue length reached. It is desirable, therefore, to be able to compute these quantities as well.

By now we should be getting pretty good at working with time-dependent state transition diagrams. Unfortunately we now have a new complication. All objects we looked at previously in this section were certain to happen. The busy period was certain to end (if $\rho \leq 1$), and all queue lengths will occur eventually. But now we have to worry whether a busy period will end before reaching a given queue length. Such processes are known as ***taboo processes*** (it is taboo - or tabu - to reach that given length) which we now define.

Definition 2.3.5

Let Ξ be the set of all possible states of a system. Let Ξ_1 and Ξ_2 be disjoint proper subsets of Ξ. That is, $\Xi_1 \cap \Xi_2 = \emptyset$ (empty). Also, let $\Xi_1 \cup \Xi_2 \subset \Xi$ (proper subset). That is, $\Xi_3 := \Xi - [\Xi_1 \cup \Xi_2] \neq \emptyset$ (not empty). In other words, Ξ_1, Ξ_2, and Ξ_3 form a ***partition*** of Ξ (every $s \in \Xi$ is in one, and only one of the Ξ_is). A ***taboo process*** is one that starts in some state $s_i \in \Xi_3$, and ends when the system finds itself in some state $s_f \in \Xi_1 \cup \Xi_2$. The process succeeded if $s_f \in \Xi_1$, and failed if $s_f \in \Xi_2$ (the taboo states). We are usually interested in $\mathbf{Pr}(s_f \in \Xi_1 \,|\, s_i \in \Xi_3)$ (i.e., the probability that the outcome was *good*). If Ξ_2 is empty then $\mathbf{Pr}(\cdot) = 1$, unless there is no way to get from s_i to Ξ_1, in which case $\mathbf{Pr}(\cdot) = \infty$, because by our definition, the process never ends. □

The next processes are examples of taboo processses.

The procedure for calculating probabilities for queue changes is similar to that for calculating the mean time for the change to occur. First we must calculate the probabilities for one step at a time, and then take the product of the probabilities (note that we take the sum of the step times) for the complete process. First define the following.

Definition 2.3.6

$W_u(n)$:= *probability that the queue at* S_1 *will go from* n *to* $n+1$ *during a busy period* (i.e., without going to 0). The process begins with n customers at S_1, and ends when the queue (including the active customer) either reaches $n+1$ or 0. The queue can fall and rise any number of times before the process ends.

This is a taboo process where $\Xi = \{s \,|\, 0 \leq s < \infty\}$, $\Xi_1 = \{s \,|\, s > n\}$, $\Xi_2 = \{0\}$ and $\Xi_3 = \{s \,|\, 0 < s \leq n\}$. The process starts with $s_i = n \in \Xi_3$, and ends when $s_f = n+1 \in \Xi_1$ (good) or when $s_f = 0 \in \Xi_2$ (bad). So $W_u(n) = \mathbf{Pr}(s_f \in \Xi_1 \,|\, s_i = n)$. The reader should decide if the taboo concept is helpful for understanding particular processes. □

The queue either goes up [with probability $\lambda/(\mu+\lambda)$], or goes down [$\mu/(\mu+\lambda)$], in which case it must eventually get back to n without first going to 0 [$W_u(n-1)$], and then get to $n+1$, [$W_u(n)$, another regenerative process]. The equation describing this is

$$W_u(n) = \frac{\lambda}{\mu+\lambda} + \frac{\mu}{\mu+\lambda}[W_u(n-1)W_u(n)]. \tag{2.3.9a}$$

This reorganizes to

$$W_u(n) = \rho[1 + \rho - W_u(n-1)]^{-1}, \tag{2.3.9b}$$

where $W_u(1) = \lambda/(\mu + \lambda) = \rho/(1+\rho)$. Our "great" experience with these things allows us to guess and prove by induction, with $K(0) = 1$, that

$$W_u(n) = \rho \frac{K(n-1)}{K(n)}, \tag{2.3.9c}$$

where $K(n)$ was defined in (2.1.4c) and satisfies the recursive and explicit formulas

$$K(n) = \sum_{j=0}^{n} \rho^j = 1 + \rho K(n-1) = \frac{1-\rho^{n+1}}{1-\rho} \quad \text{for } \rho \neq 1 \tag{2.3.10a}$$

and

$$K(n) = n + 1 \quad \text{for } \rho = 1. \tag{2.3.10b}$$

We will not always be so fortunate to find explicit expressions for more complicated queues.

As the final effort of this section, we calculate the probability that the queue will get at least to k during a busy period. This is the same as the following.

Definition 2.3.7

$W_u(1 \to k) :=$ *probability that the queue at* S_1 *will go from* 1 *to* k *before going to* 0. The process begins with one customer at S_1 and ends when the queue (including the active customer) reaches either k or 0. This is another taboo process. □

Then $W_u(1 \to 1) = 1$, and for $k > 1$,

$$W_u(1 \to k) = \prod_{n=1}^{k-1} W_u(n) := W_u(1)W_u(2)\cdots W_u(k-1), \tag{2.3.11a}$$

which due to (2.3.9c) gives us

$$W_u(1 \to k) = \frac{\rho}{K(1)} \rho \frac{K(1)}{K(2)} \rho \frac{K(2)}{K(3)} \cdots \rho \frac{K(k-2)}{K(k-1)}.$$

As long as ρ does not equal 1, this conveniently simplifies to

$$W_u(1 \to k) = \frac{\rho^{k-1}}{K(k-1)} = \frac{(1-\rho)\rho^{k-1}}{1-\rho^k}. \tag{2.3.11b}$$

For $\rho = 1$ we get the much simpler expression

$$W_u(1 \to k) = \frac{1}{k} \quad (\rho = 1). \tag{2.3.11c}$$

Note that (2.3.11a, b, and c) are valid for any customer population as long as $k \le N$. Thus they are valid for open systems as well. Observe that as might be expected if $\rho \le 1$, then $W_u(1 \to k)$ approaches 0 as k gets increasingly large. However, if $\rho > 1$, then

$$\lim_{k\to\infty} W_u(1 \to k) = \lim_{k\to\infty} \frac{(1-\rho)\rho^{k-1}}{1-\rho^k} = 1 - \frac{1}{\rho}. \tag{2.3.11d}$$

In other words, for an open system with $\rho > 1$, the probability that the queue will grow to infinity without the busy period ever ending is $1 - 1/\rho$. That is, the probability that a busy period will end is $1/\rho$. A process that is not guaranteed to end is sometimes referred to as having a ***defective probability distribution*** [FELLER71]. When $\rho = 1$, we have the interesting apparent contradiction that each busy period will surely end $[1 - W_u(1 \to \infty) = 1]$, but on average it will take an infinite amount of time to do so.

2.3.2.3 Maximum Queue Length During a Busy Period

The last property that we study in this chapter is the probability that S_1's maximum queue length in a busy period will be k. Call this $W_m(k; N)$, where N is the total number of customers in the system. To evaluate this, we not only use the W_u's of the preceding section, but we also evaluate the probabilities of coming down without ever exceeding $k < N$. So, define the following.

Definition 2.3.8

$W_d(n, k; N)$ = *probability that the queue at* S_1 *will go from* n *to* $n-1$ *without exceeding* k*, where* $N \ge k \ge n > 0$. The process begins with n customers at S_1 and ends when the queue either reaches $n-1$ or $k+1$. Put differently, $W_d(n, k; N)$ is also the probability that the queue will reach $n-1$ before going to $k+1$. For $k = N$, then, $W_d(n, N; N) = 1$, because it is certain that the queue will eventually drop by 1 from any n. This is yet another taboo process, where $\Xi_1 = \{j \mid j < n\}$, $\Xi_2 = \{j \mid k < j \le N\}$, and $\Xi_3 = \{j \mid n \le j \le k\}$. □

Next we recognize that for $k < N$,

$$W_d(k, k; N) = \frac{\mu}{\mu + \lambda} = \frac{1}{1+\rho}. \tag{2.3.12a}$$

For $n < k$, the recursive formulas are exactly analogous to (2.3.9), namely

$$W_d(n, k; N) = \frac{\mu}{\mu+\lambda} + \frac{\lambda}{\mu+\lambda}[W_d(n+1, k; N) W_d(n, k; N)],$$

which leads to

$$W_d(n, k; N) = [1 + \rho - \rho W_d(n+1, k; N)]^{-1}. \tag{2.3.12b}$$

The usual guess and proof by induction gives us an explicit expression for $W_d(n, k; N)$:

$$W_d(n, k; N) = \frac{K(k-n)}{K(k-n+1)} \quad \text{for } k < N. \tag{2.3.12c}$$

Notice that this expression is independent of N, as long as $k < N$. For $k = N$ it is clear that $W_d(N, N; N) = 1$, because the queue cannot grow beyond N. It follows from (2.3.12b) that if $W_d(n+1, N; N) = 1$, then $W_d(n, N; N)$ must also equal 1. Therefore,

$$W_d(n, N; N) = 1 \quad \text{for } 1 \leq n \leq N. \tag{2.3.12d}$$

This merely states the obvious, that a closed system will experience every queue length with certainty (not once, but over and over), and of course, irrespective of what ρ is. It is nice to know that our mathematics sometimes produces the expected. Remember, though, that (2.3.12d) is not necessarily true of open systems.

> **Exercise 2.3.2:** Given Equations (2.3.10) and (2.3.12a), prove by induction that (2.3.12c) is the unique solution of (2.3.12b).

Our next task is to calculate the object in the following definition.

Definition 2.3.9

$W_d(k \to 0; N) :=$ *probability that the queue at S_1 will drop from $k \to 0$ without ever exceeding k, in an* M/M/1//N *loop*. The process begins with k customers at S_1, and ends when it reaches either $k+1$ or 0. □

This must be the product of the probabilities of events cascading downward one stepat a time. Therefore, given that $K(0) = 1$, this is

$$W_d(k \to 0; N) = \prod_{n=1}^{k} W_d(n, k; N) = \frac{K(k-1)}{K(k)} \frac{K(k-2)}{K(k-1)} \cdots \frac{K(1)}{K(2)} \frac{K(0)}{K(1)}.$$

All but one of the terms cancel, leaving us with the simple formula

$$W_d(k \to 0; N) = \frac{1}{K(k)} = \frac{1-\rho}{1-\rho^{k+1}}, \tag{2.3.13a}$$

for $k = 1, 2, 3, \cdots, N-1$, with

$$W_d(N \to 0; N) = 1. \tag{2.3.13b}$$

This last equation must be true. Because it is impossible for the queue to exceed N, it must drain eventually.

Our final exercise is to calculate the probability described in this section's title. Clearly, this is equal to the probability that the queue at S_1 will reach k $[W_u(1 \to k)]$ and then drop to 0 without ever exceeding k $[W_d(k \to 0; N)]$. Therefore, we define for the M/M/1/ /N queue as follows.

Definition 2.3.10

$W_m(k; N) :=$ *probability that the queue at S_1 will reach a maximum of k during a busy period for an* M/M/1//N *queue*. The process begins with 1 customer at S_1, and ends when there are either $k+1$ or 0 customers there. The process is a success only if it ends with 0 customers, and the queue reaches k at least once during the interval. □

This turns out to be

$$W_m(k;N) = W_u(1 \to k)W_d(k \to 0;N)$$
$$= \frac{\rho^{k-1}}{K(k-1)}\frac{1}{K(k)} \quad \text{for } 1 \le k < N \tag{2.3.14a}$$

and

$$W_m(N;N) = W_u(1 \to N) = \frac{\rho^{N-1}}{K(N-1)}. \tag{2.3.14b}$$

Note that $W_m(k,N)$ does not depend on N as long as $k < N$; thus we can write that

$$W_m(k;N) = W_m(k;\infty) \quad \text{for } k < N.$$

The queue at S_1 must grow to some maximum length during a busy period, therefore it must follow that

$$\sum_{k=1}^{N} W_m(k;N) = 1. \tag{2.3.15}$$

This is shown to be true by recognizing that because $K(n) = 1 + \rho K(n-1)$,

$$W_m(k;N) = \frac{\rho^{k-1}}{K(k-1)K(k)} = \frac{\rho^{k-1}}{K(k-1)} - \frac{\rho^k}{K(k)}. \tag{2.3.16a}$$

Clearly, in validating that (2.3.16a) satisfies (2.3.15), the negative term of $W_m(k;N)$ exactly cancels the positive term of $W_m(k+1;N)$, and given that $W_m(N;N)$ has only a positive term, all terms cancel except the positive part of $W_m(1;N)$, which is $\rho^o/K(0) = 1$.

Equation (2.3.16a) tells us something else, which we should have suspected in the first place. Notice from (2.3.11b) that

$$W_m(k;N) = W_u(1 \to k) - W_u(1 \to k+1), \tag{2.3.16b}$$

but still, it is nice to know that we have derived it.

Example 2.3.2: As our truly final example for this chapter, we observe how $W_m(k;N)$ behaves when both k and N are very large. This is shown in Figure 2.3.4 for $N = 10$ and various values of ρ. Clearly, when $\rho < 1$, W_m goes to 0 as ρ^k. That is, the probability of reaching long queues becomes highly unlikely. Now, if $\rho = 1$, then $W_m(k;N) = 1/k(k+1)$ for $k < N$ and $W_m(N;N) = 1/N$. Thus very large queue lengths can be expected during a busy period, in fact, so large that it may take forever for some busy periods to end. ▲

Exercise 2.3.3: Evaluate $W_m(k;\infty)$ and $W_m(N;N)$ for all k for $N = 5$ and 20, and $\rho = 0.1$, 0.5, 0.9, 1, 1.1, and 2. Make sure that your numbers satisfy (2.3.15). How do your numbers compare with Figure 2.3.4?

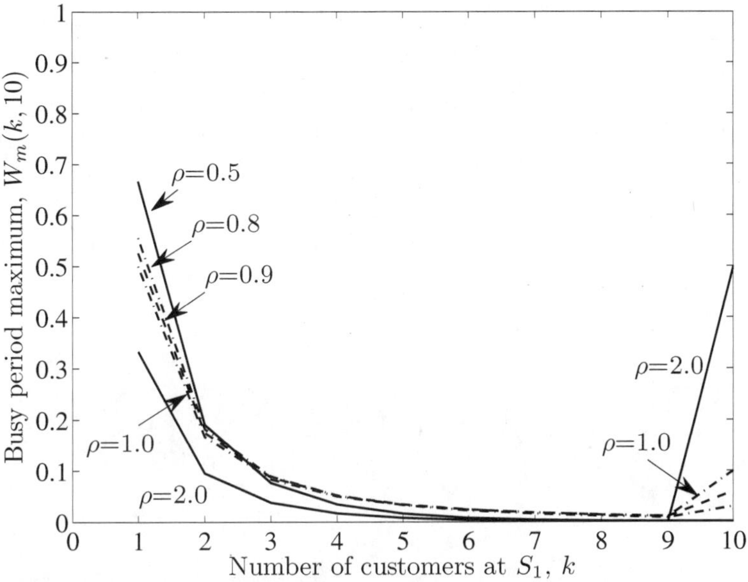

Figure 2.3.4: Probability $W_m(k; 10)$ that the queue at S_1 will reach a maximum of k during a busy period of an M/M/1//10 loop. Curves for $\rho = 0.5$, 0.8, 0.9, 1.0, and 2.0 are displayed. All the curves decrease for increasing k, except at $k = 10$. Given that $W_m(k; 10) = W_m(k; \infty)$ for all $k < 10$, $W_m(10; 10)$ corresponds to the probability that the open queue will exceed a length 9 during a busy period. At $k = 1, W_m(1; 10)$ decreases with ρ, but at $k = 10$, the reverse is true.

Perhaps the most interesting results for maximum queue length occur for $\rho > 1$. In this case $W_m(k; N)$ goes to 0 as $1/\rho^k$, just as it does for $\rho < 1$. But $W_m(N; N)$ approaches the finite limit, $1 - 1/\rho$. This, of course, is the probability that the busy period will never end in an open system. For those busy periods that do end (the probability of which is $1/\rho$), $W_m(k; \infty)$ is still the correct probability that k will be the maximum queue length.

Chapter 3

M. E. FUNCTIONS

I shall never believe that God plays dice with the universe
Albert Einstein

Einstein, stop telling God what to do.
Niels Bohr

God not only plays dice. He also sometimes throws the dice where they cannot be seen.
Stephen Hawking

We are now ready to give structure to the subsystems S_1 and S_2 . In Chapter 2 we assumed that each subsystem had only one internal state, which was equivalent to assuming that they were exponential servers. Now we assume that S_1 has m states, but defer consideration of S_2 until Chapter 4. Without loss of generality, a subsystem with m states can be viewed as a network of exponential ***phases***, or ***stages***, that can be accessed by only one customer at a time; the rest of the customers wait outside until the active one leaves. We show that such a subsystem is in turn equivalent to a single server whose pdf is certainly not exponential. In fact, every pdf that can be written as a finite sum of terms of the form $x^k \exp(-\mu x)$ (any number of terms with any nonnegative integer k, with any number of different μ's whose real part is positive) is equivalent to a subsystem of this form. We know that functions of this type can approximate every pdf arbitrarily closely in some sense. Therefore, we can say that the ***closure*** of this set (infinite sums) contains all (well, maybe almost all) pdfs. We also know that every one of these functions has a Laplace transform that can be written as a ratio of two polynomials. Such functions are said to have ***Rational Laplace Transforms*** (RLT).

3.1 Properties of a Subsystem, *S*

Once again, we must start with a series of definitions. Let our subsystem S be made up of a collection of phases as shown in Figure 3.1.1. The term *stage* is often used instead of *phase*, and if we are thinking of a subsystem made up of real components, each of these phases, or stages, would be an exponential server in its own right. The reader is welcome to think of them in this light, and indeed we talk of them as though they *are* real. However, in

L. Lipsky, *Queueing Theory*, DOI 10.1007/978-0-387-49706-8_3,

the long run they are merely meant to be mathematical building blocks for constructing the matrix operators we need for ***Linear Algebraic Queueing Theory*** (**LAQT**). Therefore, we (almost always) adhere to Neuts' convention and call them *phases* [NEUTS75], because that word is as far from the real thing as we can get.

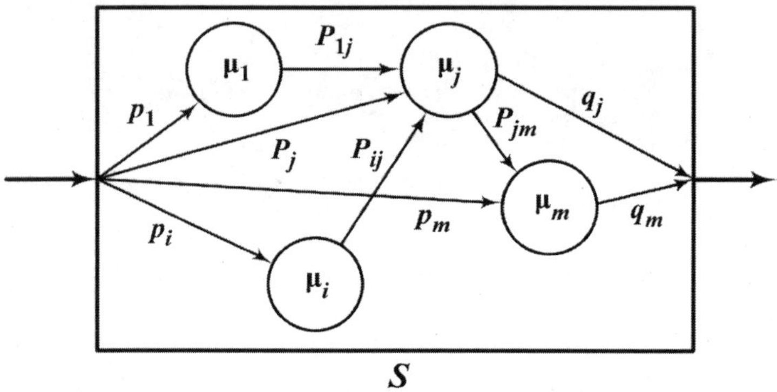

Figure 3.1.1: Typical subsystem S, with m phases, and where only one customer can be active at a time. $\mathbf{p}$ is the ***entrance vector***, whose i-th component is the probability that a customer, upon entering S, will go to phase i. $\mathbf{q}'$ is the ***exit vector***, whose i-th component is the probability that a customer, upon completing service at phase i, will leave S. $\mathbf{P}$ is the ***substochastic transition matrix***, whose ij-th component is the probability that a customer who has just finished service at i will go to j. Each phase has exponentially distributed completion time, with mean completion rate $\mu_i = (M)_{ii}$.

As in Section 1.3.1, $\mathbf{M}$ is the ***completion rate matrix*** whose diagonal elements are the completion rates of the individual phases in S. $\mathbf{P}$ is again the transition matrix where $[\mathbf{P}]_{ij} = P_{ij}$ is the probability that a customer will go from phase i to phase j when service is completed at i. However, now $\mathbf{P}$ is not isometric, because it does not satisfy (1.3.1b). Now it is possible for a customer to leave. We define an ***exit vector*** $\mathbf{q}'$, where $[\mathbf{q}']_i = q_i$, is the probability of leaving S when service is completed at i. It then follows that

$$\mathbf{P}\boldsymbol{\epsilon}' + \mathbf{q}' = \boldsymbol{\epsilon}'. \tag{3.1.1a}$$

If $\mathbf{q}' \neq \mathbf{o}'$ (with no negative components) and $P_{ij} \geq 0$, then $\mathbf{P}$ is said to be substochastic. Assume that for each i there exists a path to some j for which $q_j \neq 0$. This is equivalent to saying that no matter where a customer starts in S, he will eventually leave. It turns out to be equivalent to the statement that $(\mathbf{I} - \mathbf{P})$ has an inverse. We now show that if $(\mathbf{I} - \mathbf{P})$ has an inverse, the customer can always get out (eventually). Let x_i be the probability that a customer who started at phase i will eventually leave, and let $\mathbf{x}'$ be the column vector whose i-th component is x_i. Then we can say that the probability of leaving eventually is equal to the probability of leaving immediately $[q_i]$ plus the probability of going instead to some other phase j $[P_{ij}]$ and eventually leaving from there $[x_j]$. Mathematically, this is

$$x_i = q_i + \sum_{j=1}^{m} P_{ij} x_j,$$

or in matrix form (another regenerative process),

$$\mathbf{x}' = \mathbf{q}' + \mathbf{P}\mathbf{x}'.$$

This can be rewritten as $(\mathbf{I} - \mathbf{P})\mathbf{x}' = \mathbf{q}'$. If the inverse exists, there is only one solution to this equation. From (3.1.1a), we have

$$\mathbf{q}' = (\mathbf{I} - \mathbf{P})\boldsymbol{\epsilon}', \tag{3.1.1b}$$

so $\mathbf{x}' = \boldsymbol{\epsilon}'$. In other words, $x_i = 1$ for all i; that is, the customer can always get out. The converse is a little different. If the customer can always get out, we only need

$$\lim_{n \to \infty} \mathbf{P}^n \boldsymbol{\epsilon}' = \mathbf{o}',$$

which is a little weaker than requiring that $(\mathbf{I} - \mathbf{P})^{-1}$ exist. If $\mathbf{P}$ is substochastic, this must always be true. We avoid the rigorous mathematical issues underlying this by assuming that $(\mathbf{I} - \mathbf{P})$ has an inverse, and leave it at that. A necessary and sufficient condition for this to be true is for $\mathbf{P}$ to have no eigenvalue equal to 1, which physically implies that there are no closed loops and therefore no ***absorbing states*** (or ***sink states***) in S.

Finally we define the ***entrance vector*** $\mathbf{p}$ whose component p_i is the probability that upon entering S, a customer will go directly to phase i. Because the customer must go somewhere, $\sum_{i=1}^{m} p_i = 1$, or $\mathbf{p}\boldsymbol{\epsilon}' = 1$ ($\mathbf{p}$ is isometric, but $\mathbf{P}$ is not).

3.1.1 Mean Time to Leave S

We are now in a position to find the mean time it takes for a customer to meander through S and finally leave. Frequently, we extend this to subsystems where a direct physical picture is false, so we are really dealing with a mathematical analogy rather than a true physical situation. This is no different than talking about electrical currents of the form $\exp(i\,\omega\, t)$, rather than $\sin(\omega\, t)$.

Define $\boldsymbol{\tau}'$ to be that column vector whose component τ_i is the mean time it will take for a customer to leave S, given that he started at i. The path of the customer can be described by the following sequence. First the customer must be served by i, which on the average takes a time of $1/\mu_i = (\mathbf{M}^{-1}\boldsymbol{\epsilon}')_i$. Then either he leaves (with probability q_i, using no additional time) or he goes to phase j with probability P_{ij}. At this point it will take the customer a time τ_j to finally leave. Mathematically we have, in vector form,

$$\boldsymbol{\tau}' = \mathbf{M}^{-1}\boldsymbol{\epsilon}' + 0\mathbf{q}' + \mathbf{P}\boldsymbol{\tau}' = \mathbf{M}^{-1}\boldsymbol{\epsilon}' + \mathbf{P}\boldsymbol{\tau}'. \tag{3.1.2a}$$

Note both the similarities and differences between this equation and (2.3.1a) and (2.3.5a). In Chapter 2 the population of S could either increase or decrease, whereas here it can either decrease (the customer leaves) or stay the same. In all cases $\boldsymbol{\tau}'$ appears on both sides of the equation, but here $\boldsymbol{\tau}'$ is a column vector rather than a scalar, so (3.1.2a) stands for m equations involving the set of τ_is (i.e., the m components of $\boldsymbol{\tau}'$). As in Section 2.3.1, this is also a regenerative process, but with a difference. The subsystem need not return to the same state, but to any internal state while S is still active. All m unknowns can be found simultaneously by solving the matrix equation for $\boldsymbol{\tau}'$ [i.e., $\boldsymbol{\tau}' - \mathbf{P}\boldsymbol{\tau}' = (\mathbf{I} - \mathbf{P})\boldsymbol{\tau}' = \mathbf{M}^{-1}\boldsymbol{\epsilon}'$]. Given that $(\mathbf{I} - \mathbf{P})$ has an inverse,

$$\boldsymbol{\tau}' = (\mathbf{I} - \mathbf{P})^{-1}\mathbf{M}^{-1}\boldsymbol{\epsilon}' = [\mathbf{M}(\mathbf{I} - \mathbf{P})]^{-1}\boldsymbol{\epsilon}'.$$

We can now write in concise form,

$$\boldsymbol{\tau}' = \mathbf{V}\boldsymbol{\epsilon}', \tag{3.1.2b}$$

where, because they appear so often throughout this treatise, we define

$$\mathbf{B} := \mathbf{M}(\mathbf{I} - \mathbf{P}) \quad \text{and} \quad \mathbf{V} := \mathbf{B}^{-1}. \tag{3.1.3}$$

This important relation leads us to give $\mathbf{V}$ the name ***service time matrix***. Its individual components V_{ij} are interpretable as the mean time a customer spends at j (counting all visits to it) from the time he first visits i until he leaves S. $\mathbf{B}$, the inverse of $\mathbf{V}$ is of equal importance. $\mathbf{B}$ looks very similar to the transition rate matrix $\boldsymbol{Q}$, defined in Section 1.3.1, with the important major difference that $\boldsymbol{Q}$ describes an entire closed system, and $\boldsymbol{Q}\boldsymbol{\epsilon}' = \mathbf{o}'$, whereas $\mathbf{B}$ refers only to a subsystem, and $\mathbf{B}\boldsymbol{\epsilon}'$ definitely does not equal $\mathbf{o}'$. As shown below, $\mathbf{B}$ is the generator of the service time distribution, so we give it the name ***service rate matrix***. We also express the distributions of other processes in terms of matrices. Therefore, $\mathbf{B}$ is a ***process rate matrix***, and $\mathbf{V}$ is a ***process time matrix***.

As mentioned above, when a customer first enters S he goes to i with probability p_i, and then spends a total time τ_i in S before leaving. Let T be the random variable denoting the time a customer spends in S from the moment he enters to the moment he leaves. Then $\mathbb{E}[T]$ is the sum

$$\mathbb{E}[T] = \sum_{i=1}^{m} p_i\tau_i,$$

or in matrix form, using (3.1.2b), the mean service time of S is

$$\mathbb{E}[T] = \mathbf{p}\,\boldsymbol{\tau}' = \mathbf{p}\,\mathbf{V}\,\boldsymbol{\epsilon}'. \tag{3.1.4a}$$

Expressions where $\mathbf{p}$ appears on the left of a square matrix, followed by $\boldsymbol{\epsilon}'$ on the right, yielding a scalar value, are important and frequent enough to be given a special notation. Therefore, define

$$\Psi\,[\mathbf{X}] := \mathbf{p}\,\mathbf{X}\,\boldsymbol{\epsilon}', \tag{3.1.5}$$

where $\mathbf{X}$ is any square matrix. Then (3.1.4a) can be written as

$$\mathbb{E}[T] = \Psi[\mathbf{V}]. \tag{3.1.4b}$$

$\Psi[\cdot]$ is a ***linear operator***, in that it transforms square matrices into complex numbers (i.e., scalars) and has the following properties. Let α and β be any scalars, and let $\mathbf{X}$ and $\mathbf{Y}$ be any square matrices of the same size; then

$$\Psi[\alpha\mathbf{X} + \beta\mathbf{Y}] = \alpha\Psi[\mathbf{X}] + \beta\Psi[\mathbf{Y}].$$

It is also true that $\Psi[\cdot]$ commutes with integration; that is, for any matrix function of t,

$$\int \Psi[\mathbf{F}(t)]\, dt = \Psi\left[\int \mathbf{F}(t)\, dt\right].$$

Exercise 3.1.1: Consider S with two equal phases with completion rate μ. Assume that a customer always goes to phase 1 upon entering. After finishing at 1, he goes to 2, and after that, leaves. This produces what is called an ***Erlangian-2*** (E_2) ***distribution***. What are $\mathbf{p}$, $\mathbf{P}$, $\mathbf{q}'$, $\mathbf{M}$, $\mathbf{B}$, $\mathbf{V}$, $\boldsymbol{\tau}'$, and $\mathbb{E}[T]$?

Exercise 3.1.2: Again there are two phases in S, but with different completion rates, μ_1 and μ_2. Suppose that a customer, upon entering, goes to 1 with probability p_1, or to 2 (with probability $p_2 = 1 - p_1$), and then leaves when finished. This is known as a ***2-phase hyperexponential distribution***, with PDF $H_2(x)$ and pdf $h_2(x)$. In this case, what are: $\mathbf{p}$, $\mathbf{P}$, $\mathbf{q}'$, $\mathbf{M}$, $\mathbf{B}$, $\mathbf{V}$, $\boldsymbol{\tau}'$, and $\mathbb{E}[T]$?

The importance of $\mathbf{B}$ is displayed in the next sections.

3.1.2 Service Time Distribution of S

Once a customer enters a subsystem, his interaction with the outside world is suspended until he exits. An outside observer only sees a beginning and an end to service. One would expect that some density function exists that describes the time spent in S. This is in fact the case. First define the ***reliability matrix function***.

Definition 3.1.1

$[\mathbf{R}(t)]_{ij}$:= *probability that the customer is at phase j in S at time t, given that he was at phase i at time* 0. The associated vector function, $\mathbf{R}(t)\boldsymbol{\epsilon}'$, is a column vector whose i-th component is the probability that the customer will still be somewhere in S at time t, given that he started at phase i at time 0. □

The customer will be at phase j at time $t+\delta$ if:

1. He was there at time t $[R_{ij}(t)]$, and nothing happened in the interval δ $[1-\mu_j\delta]$; or
2. He was at another phase at time t, finished service $[M_{kk}\delta]$, and then went to j $[P_{kj}]$ in the interval δ; or
3. He made two or more transitions in the interval.

Mathematically, one can write

$$R_{ij}(t+\delta) = R_{ij}(t)(1-M_{jj}\delta) + \sum_{k=1}^{m} R_{ik}(t)M_{kk}P_{kj}\delta + \mathrm{O}\left(\delta^2\right),$$

or in matrix form (make sure you agree before going on),

$$\mathbf{R}(t+\delta) = \mathbf{R}(t)(\mathbf{I}-\mathbf{M}\delta) + \mathbf{R}(t)\mathbf{M}\mathbf{P}\delta + \mathrm{O}\left(\delta^2\right).$$

Next perform the usual procedure of subtracting $\mathbf{R}(t)$ from both sides, dividing both sides by δ, and then taking the limit as δ goes to zero. The expected result is

$$\frac{d\mathbf{R}(t)}{dt} = -\mathbf{R}(t)\mathbf{B}. \tag{3.1.6a}$$

The scalar equivalent of this differential equation has been seen before, in (1.2.1a). (See Section 1.3.1 for an analogous matrix equation). Its solution, remembering that $\mathbf{R}(0)=\mathbf{I}$, is

$$\mathbf{R}(t) = \exp(-t\mathbf{B}). \tag{3.1.6b}$$

This is the matrix equivalent of the reliability function defined in Section 1.2.1, thus we call it the ***reliability matrix function*** of S. Because of the form of this equation, we call a function that is generated by any finite $\mathbf{B}$, a ***matrix exponential* (ME) *function*** [LIEFVOORT87]. If it should have the properties of a probability distribution, it is called an ***ME distribution***. The definition is extended to include infinite matrices in Section 3.2.1. When we sum over all possible states (or phases) we get the vector $\exp(-t\mathbf{B})\boldsymbol{\epsilon}'$, whose i-th component is the probability that the customer is still in S at time t, given that he was at phase i at time 0. Now, if the customer first entered S at time 0, he would go to phase i with probability p_i. We can define a ***reliability vector function*** as follows.

Definition 3.1.2

$[\mathbf{r}(t)]_i := [\mathbf{pR}(t)]_i =$ *probability that a customer who entered S at time 0 will be at phase i at time t. The associated scalar probability that he will still be somewhere in S at time t is the sum over i.* That is, $R(t) := \mathbf{r}(t)\boldsymbol{\epsilon}' = \Psi[\mathbf{R}(t)]$. This is the ***reliability function*** for the r.v. T [see (3.1.7b) below]. □

$\mathbf{r}(t)$ is a row vector satisfying the following.

$$\mathbf{r}(t) := \mathbf{p}\mathbf{R}(t) = \mathbf{p}\exp(-t\mathbf{B}). \tag{3.1.7a}$$

The reliability function [the nonexponential generalization of (1.2.1b)] is the scalar function associated with $\mathbf{r}(t)$ and $\mathbf{R}(t)$, satisfying

$$R(t) = \mathbb{P}\mathbf{r}(T > t) = \mathbf{r}(t)\boldsymbol{\epsilon}' = \Psi[\mathbf{R}(t)] = \Psi[\exp(-t\mathbf{B})]. \tag{3.1.7b}$$

The ***Probability Distribution Function*** (PDF) is

$$B(t) = 1 - R(t) = 1 - \Psi[\exp(-t\mathbf{B})], \tag{3.1.7c}$$

and the probability density function (pdf) is

$$b(t) = \frac{dB(t)}{dt} = \Psi\left[\frac{d}{dt}[\mathbf{I} - \exp(-t\mathbf{B})]\right] = \Psi[\mathbf{B}\exp(-t\mathbf{B})]. \tag{3.1.7d}$$

To prove that

$$\frac{d\,\mathbf{r}(t)}{dt} = -\mathbf{r}(t)\mathbf{B},$$

replace $\exp(-t\mathbf{B})$ with its Maclaurin series expansion, differentiate each term with respect to t, while treating all matrices as constants (they are, because they do not depend upon t), factor out $\mathbf{B}$, and put everything back together again.

3.1.3 Properties of B and V

Equation (3.1.7d) can be used to extract many desired properties of S. For instance, $b(0) = \Psi[\mathbf{B}]$. In fact, all derivatives can be simply computed. Let $b^{(k)}(t)$ be the k-th derivative of $b(t)$ with respect to t; then

$$b^{(k)}(t) = -R^{(k+1)}(t) = (-1)^k \Psi\left[\mathbf{B}^{k+1}\exp(-t\mathbf{B})\right], \tag{3.1.8a}$$

and for $t = 0$,

$$b^{(k)}(0) = -R^{(k+1)}(0) = (-1)^k \Psi\left[\mathbf{B}^{k+1}\right]. \tag{3.1.8b}$$

The moments of the distribution are also easy to get. The formal procedure of integrating matrix expressions as though they were scalars turns out to give the correct results, although the proof is a bit cumbersome. Remember that a matrix commutes with every power of itself, including its inverse, and even sums of scalars times powers of itself. Also recall that $\mathbf{V} = \mathbf{B}^{-1}$, so

$$\mathbb{E}\left[T^k\right] = \int_0^\infty t^k\, b(t)\, dt = \int_0^\infty t^k \Psi[\mathbf{B}\exp(-t\mathbf{B})]\, dt$$

$$= \Psi\left[\int_0^\infty t^k \mathbf{B}\exp(-t\mathbf{B})dt\right] = \Psi\left[\mathbf{V}^k\left(\int_0^\infty (t\mathbf{B})^k \exp(-t\mathbf{B})d(t\mathbf{B})\right)\right].$$

The expression inside the large round brackets (which is a square matrix) actually turns out to be $k!\mathbf{I}$, so

$$\mathbb{E}\left[T^k\right] = k!\Psi\left[\mathbf{V}^k\right]. \tag{3.1.9}$$

The mean service time of S, as given in (3.1.4b) is a special case of (3.1.9) for $k = 1$.

The ***Laplace transform*** of $b(t)$ can be found in a similar fashion. By definition,

$$B^*(s) = \int_0^\infty e^{-st} b(t)\, dt,$$

so [using (3.1.7d)],

$$\begin{aligned} B^*(s) &= \Psi\left[\int_0^\infty \mathbf{B} e^{-st} \exp(-t\mathbf{B}) dt\right] = \Psi\left[\int_0^\infty \mathbf{B} \exp[-t(s\mathbf{I} + \mathbf{B})] dt\right] \\ &= \Psi\left[\mathbf{B}(s\mathbf{I} + \mathbf{B})^{-1} \left(\int_0^\infty \exp[-t(s\mathbf{I} + \mathbf{B})] d[t(s\mathbf{I} + \mathbf{B})]\right)\right]. \end{aligned}$$

Again, the expression inside the large round brackets is $\mathbf{I}$, so

$$B^*(s) = \Psi\left[\mathbf{B}(s\mathbf{I} + \mathbf{B})^{-1}\right] = \Psi\left[(\mathbf{I} + s\mathbf{V})^{-1}\right]. \tag{3.1.10}$$

Equations (3.1.7d), (3.1.8b), (3.1.9), and (3.1.10) are all equivalent in that each can be derived from the others, assuming that $b(t)$ is not too badly behaved. These results are important enough to summarize in a theorem.

Theorem 3.1.1: If a vector-matrix pair $\langle \mathbf{p}, \mathbf{B} \rangle$ (or equivalently, $\langle \mathbf{p}, \mathbf{V} \rangle$ with $\mathbf{V} = \mathbf{B}^{-1}$) satisfies any one of the following properties of a probability distribution [(3.1.7b), (3.1.7d), (3.1.8b), (3.1.9), and (3.1.10) respectively]:

$$R(t) = 1 - B(t) = \Psi\left[\exp(-t\mathbf{B})\right], \tag{3.1.7b}$$

$$b(t) = \frac{dB(t)}{dt} = \Psi\left[\mathbf{B} \exp(-t\mathbf{B})\right], \tag{3.1.7d}$$

$$b^{(k)}(0) = -R^{(k+1)}(0) = (-1)^k \Psi\left[\mathbf{B}^{k+1}\right], \tag{3.1.8b}$$

$$\mathbb{E}\left[T^k\right] = k!\Psi\left[\mathbf{V}^k\right], \tag{3.1.9}$$

$$\begin{aligned} B^*(s) &= \int_0^\infty e^{-st} b(t) dt \\ &= \Psi\left[\mathbf{B}(s\mathbf{I} + \mathbf{B})^{-1}\right] = \Psi\left[(\mathbf{I} + s\mathbf{V})^{-1}\right], \end{aligned} \tag{3.1.10}$$

then the other four relations must also be true (i.e., each equation can be used to prove the other four). The pair $\langle \mathbf{p}, \mathbf{V} \rangle$ (or $\langle \mathbf{p}, \mathbf{B} \rangle$), is said to be a ***generator***, or ***representation***, of the process whose probability distribution is $B(t)$ [and therefore of $b(t)$ and $R(t)$]. The matrix, $(\mathbf{I} + s\mathbf{V})^{-1}$, appears often, and is sometimes called the ***resolvent matrix***. ■

The Laplace transform has an interesting interpretation. Suppose that new customers are arriving at S with exponential interarrival times with parameter s. Then $B^*(s)$ is the probability that the customer in service will finish before the next customer arrives, given that service has just begun. [See (2.1.1b).]

We have occasion to describe processes other than the time a customer spends in S. Therefore we provide the following generic definition.

Definition 3.1.3

Let X be the random variable for some process (e.g., *system time*, or *interdeparture time*) whose pdf is $b_X(t)$. Then $\langle\, \mathbf{p_x}\,,\, \mathbf{B_x}\,\rangle$ is a generator of process X if the equations of Theorem 3.1.1 are satisfied. $\mathbf{p_x}$ is the ***startup vector*** or ***initial vector*** for the process (or ***startup process vector***), and $\mathbf{B_x}$ is the ***process rate matrix***, or the ***rate matrix*** for the process X. Only when we are dealing with the service time distribution of S do we use the terms *entrance vector* and *service rate matrix.* □

What If Phases are Nonexponential?

In deriving Theorem 3.1.1 we have assumed that each of the phases in S is exponential. One might ask what happens if this constraint is relaxed. Given that the customer wanders sequentially from phase to phase until he leaves, it would be expected that $\mathbb{E}[T]$ would depend only on the mean time for each of the phases. (Recall that for sequential processes, the sum of the means is equal to the mean of the sum.) In Section 9.3 we prove that this is so. But the higher moments and the overall distribution are different. In particular, the variance for a network of nonexponential servers is given by:

$$\sigma^2 = \sigma_e^2 + \Psi\,[\mathbf{V}\,\mathbf{T}\,\boldsymbol{\Gamma}]\,, \tag{3.1.11}$$

where $\mathbf{T} = \mathbf{M}^{-1}$ and $\boldsymbol{\Gamma}$ is a diagonal matrix with $[\boldsymbol{\Gamma}]_{ii} = (C_i^2 - 1)$. For exponential distributions, $C_i^2 = 1$, so $\boldsymbol{\Gamma} = \mathbf{0}$ and thus the second term on the right is 0, as it should be. If all the distributions are deterministic, then $C_i^2 = 0$, and

$$\sigma_D^2 = \sigma_e^2 - \Psi\,[\mathbf{VT}]\,.$$

For more information the reader is referred to Section 9.3.

3.1.4 Numerical Algorithm for Evaluating $b(x)$ and $R(x)$

The formulas given in Theorem 3.1.1 are not merely formal connections between functions and matrices. They can actually be used to calculate, efficiently and accurately, the values of $b(x)$, $R(x)$, and therefore $B(x)$, over a set of equally spaced values of x. First note that because of Theorem 1.3.2, and Equation (3.1.6b),

$$\mathbf{R}(x+y) = \exp[-(x+y)\mathbf{B}] = \mathbf{R}(x)\,\mathbf{R}(y),$$

for any x and y. This is often called the ***semigroup property***, and is part of all Markov processes. This equation reduces to (1.2.6c) for 1-dimensional matrices. However, in general the semigroup property does not hold for the reliability functions themselves. That is,

$$R(x+y) = \mathbf{p}\exp(-(x+y)\mathbf{B})\boldsymbol{\epsilon}' = \mathbf{p}\exp(-x\mathbf{B})\exp(-y\mathbf{B})\boldsymbol{\epsilon}' = \mathbf{p}\mathbf{R}(x)\mathbf{R}(y)\boldsymbol{\epsilon}',$$

but

$$R(x)R(y) = \mathbf{p}\exp(-x\mathbf{B})\,\boldsymbol{\epsilon}'\mathbf{p}\exp(-y\mathbf{B})\boldsymbol{\epsilon}' = \mathbf{p}\mathbf{R}(x)\mathbf{Q}\,\mathbf{R}(y)\boldsymbol{\epsilon}'.$$

The $\boldsymbol{\epsilon}'\mathbf{p} = \mathbf{Q}$ in the middle prevents $R(x)R(y)$ from being equal to $R(x+y)$ unless $\mathbf{Q} = 1$, which can only occur if $m = 1$, that is, only if $R(x)$ is an exponential function.

Now pick some small, positive δ and some positive integer k (bigger than 1, but not too big - more about this later), and evaluate

$$\mathbf{R}(\delta) \approx \mathbf{I} - \delta\mathbf{B} + \frac{1}{2}\delta^2\mathbf{B}^2 - \frac{1}{6}\delta^3\mathbf{B}^3 + \cdots + \frac{1}{k!}(-\delta)^k\mathbf{B}^k. \tag{3.1.12}$$

If this expression is sufficiently accurate (it certainly can be if δ and k have been chosen wisely), then we have for $x = n\delta$:

$$\mathbf{R}(x+\delta) = [\mathbf{R}(\delta)]^{n+1} = \mathbf{R}(x)\mathbf{R}(\delta),$$

where n can be as large as one needs to get sufficiently large $x = n\delta$.

If it is desired that $\mathbf{R}(x)$ be evaluated on N equally spaced points then, using ***Horner's rule*** [CONTE-DEBOER80] (a nested multiplication algorithm), to evaluate (3.1.12), $N + k$ matrix-matrix multiplications and k matrix additions are required. The computational complexity is linear in the number of points (one multiplication for each successive point) and of order m^3 in the dimension of the matrix. That is, the computational complexity is of order

$$\mathrm{O}\left((N+k)m^3\right).$$

We can do much better if we are interested only in the vector $\mathbf{r}(x)$ and the scalars $b(x)$, $R(x)$, and $B(x)$. We can compute them in the following way. Given a matrix representation, $\langle\, \mathbf{p}\,,\, \mathbf{B}\,\rangle$:

1. Calculate $\mathbf{b}' := \mathbf{B}\boldsymbol{\epsilon}'$; $b(0) = \mathbf{p}\mathbf{b}'$; $R(0) = 1$.
2. Calculate $\mathbf{R}(\delta)$ from (3.1.12) using Horner's rule.
3. Set $\mathbf{r}(0) = \mathbf{p}$.
4. Then (where $x_n = n\delta$),

   BEGIN FOR $n = 1$ to $n = N$, calculate

   $$\mathbf{r}(x_n) = \mathbf{r}(x_{n-1})\mathbf{R}(\delta)$$
   $$R(x_n) = \mathbf{r}(x_n)\boldsymbol{\epsilon}'$$
   $$b(x_n) = \mathbf{r}(x_n)\mathbf{b}'.$$

   END FOR

This involves only k matrix multiplications and additions, N matrix on vector multiplications, and $2N$ vector on vector multiplications (dot products). This means, then, that the computational complexity is of order

$$\mathrm{O}\left(Nm^2\right) + \mathrm{O}\left(km^3\right).$$

The term with N is sure to be the larger by far, therefore we see that this algorithm saves a factor of m in computational time over the brute-force procedure with which we started. Throughout this book, judicious selection of procedures can make many computations feasible that were previously impossible by other methods.

We point out from numerical analysis that the problem of selecting appropriate δ and k is the same as the problem one has in trying to solve (3.1.6a) as m coupled differential equations, using k-th order *Ordinary Differential Equation* (ODE) methods. In fact, the method we gave above is related to a method gaining favor in some quarters for more general ODEs, namely the *Taylor series expansion method*. We can even claim that our method is very stable, because all the eigenvalues of $\mathbf{B}$ have positive real parts (so there is no exponential blowup, the primary cause of instability). There may be a *stiffness* problem if the smallest eigenvalue is very small compared to the desired distance between points; we must make δ small enough to accommodate this.

Our last point has to do with accuracy. From Taylor's remainder theorem, we know that the error in $\mathbf{R}(\delta)$ is of order

$$\mathrm{O}\left(\delta^{k+1}\right).$$

Because the method is stable, the roundoff error accumulates linearly with n; therefore, the roundoff error at x is

$$\mathrm{Err}(x) = n\,\mathrm{O}\left(\delta^{k+1}\right) = x\,\mathrm{O}\left(\delta^{k}\right).$$

This expression can actually be used to estimate the error by evaluating for two different δ's, and performing an *extrapolation* procedure. See, for example, [CONTE-DEBOER80], or any standard text on numerical analysis for more insight.

Exercise 3.1.3: Evaluate $R(x)$, $B(x)$, $b(x)$, $b^{(\ell)}(0)$, $\mathbf{E}[T^\ell]$, and $B^*(s)$ for an Erlangian-2 distribution, using the formulas of this section. Let $0 \le x \le 10\mathbf{E}[T]$, $\delta = 0.1\mathbf{E}[T]$, and $k = 6$ in evaluating $R(x)$, $B(x)$, and $b(x)$. Compare with the exact answers.

Exercise 3.1.4: Repeat Exercise 3.1.3 for a 2-phase hyperexponential distribution.

3.2 Matrix Exponential Distributions

Up to now we have been vague about the constraints for $\mathbf{p}$ and $\mathbf{P}$, and so on. As long as $M_{ii} > 0$, $\mathbf{P}_{ij} \ge 0$, $(\mathbf{P}\boldsymbol{\epsilon}')_i \le 1$ for all i, j, and $(\mathbf{I} - \mathbf{P})^{-1}$ exists, proofs abound that guarantee good behavior. Such distributions are called ***PHase (PH) distributions*** * by Marcel F. Neuts [NEUTS75], [NEUTS81],

*In order to distinguish between PHase distributions and the phase components that are used to build ME distributions we always use the double capital PH to refer to PHase distributions only.

who has studied them extensively. On the other hand, there is a larger class of pdfs for which the conditions may not hold, yet still have a matrix representation. In fact, any pdf that has a rational Laplace transform (RLT) also has a matrix representation [LIPSKY-RAM85]. Such functions are sometimes called ***Kendall distributions*** [KENDALL64], with symbol, K_m (m is the number of phases), and their representations are often referred as ***Coxian servers*** [COX55], [LIPSKY-FANG86], with symbol C_m. We will not use those notations further.

An interesting and mathematically important point of view is to start with a representation and see if it corresponds to a true pdf. This and related questions are discussed in great detail in the literature, so we only summarize here. By a ***matrix representation*** of some distribution function, we mean a vector-matrix pair $\langle \mathbf{p}, \mathbf{B} \rangle$ (or equivalently, $\langle \mathbf{p}, \mathbf{V} \rangle$, because $\mathbf{B} = \mathbf{V}^{-1}$) which can be used in (3.1.7) to (3.1.10), and thus generates that function. This much we know. As long as $\mathbf{B}$ is finite-dimensional (as is always the case here unless we say otherwise), $B^*(s)$ as defined in (3.1.10) will always be a ratio of two polynomials, and $b(t)$, from(3.1.7d), will always be a sum of terms of the form $[f_n(x)e^{-\mu x}]$, where f_n is a polynomial of degree n, and $\Re(\mu) > 0$. Furthermore, if all the eigenvalues of $\mathbf{B}$ have positive real parts, then $b(t)$ is integrable and integrates to 1. The critical question remains as to whether $b(t)$ is a pdf [i.e., is it true that $b(t) \geq 0$ for all real $t > 0$?]. At present, there is no way one can look at $\langle \mathbf{p}, \mathbf{B} \rangle$, or $B^*(s)$ to answer this. The only sure way that it can be done is to examine $b(t)$ for all relevant t.

We first describe the simple and well-known Erlangian [ERLANG17] and hyperexponential distributions. We then introduce several useful and interesting distributions, including one with phases having complex service rates. We then introduce a ***canonical*** form for representations, namely Erlangians in parallel, sometimes with complex parameters. It turns out (see Section 3.4) that every representation is equivalent to one of these. Furthermore, the canonical representation is of minimal dimension.

3.2.1 Commonly Used Distributions

Before we look at the general classes of ME distributions, we discuss the two most commonly used, overused, and abused types. The reader was already introduced to their simplest nontrivial representatives in the exercises, but it pays to discuss them in some depth.

3.2.1.1 Erlangian Distributions

The Erlangian-m distribution [for which we use the symbol $E_m(t; \mu)$] describes the time it takes for a customer to be served by m identical exponential servers, one at a time (or one server exactly m times). Formally, let X_i be the random variable representing the time it takes for a customer to be served by the i-th server, with pdf, $\mu e^{-\mu t}$ (same μ for each server). Let Y_i be the total time it takes for the customer to be served by i servers (i.e., $Y_i = X_1 + X_2 + \cdots + X_i$). Obviously $Y_1 = X_1$, so its pdf is also $E_1(t; \mu) := \mu e^{-\mu t}$. The pdf for Y_2 is the

convolution of X_1 with X_2. That is,

$$E_2(t;\mu) := \int_0^t b_{X_1}(s)\, b_{X_2}(t-s)\, ds = \int_0^t \mu e^{-\mu s} \mu e^{-\mu(t-s)} ds$$

$$= \mu^2 e^{-\mu t} \int_0^t ds = \mu(\mu t) e^{-\mu t}.$$

We deliberately introduced the notation $b_{X_i}(t)$ to represent the pdfs of the X_i, even though in this case they are the same exponential function. Then by the definition of the Erlangians, we can say that $b_{Y_i}(t) = E_i(t;\mu)$. It is well known in general that

$$b_{Y_m}(t) = \int_0^t b_{Y_{m-1}}(s) b_{X_m}(t-s) ds,$$

which gives us, for exponentials (provable by induction),

$$E_m(t;\mu) := \int_0^t E_{m-1}(s;\mu)\mu e^{-\mu(t-s)} ds = \mu \frac{(\mu t)^{m-1}}{(m-1)!} e^{-\mu t}. \tag{3.2.1a}$$

The n-th moment for the Erlangian-m† is known from elementary calculus to be

$$\mathbf{E}\left[Y_m^n\right] = \int_0^\infty t^n\, E_m(t;\mu)\, dt = \frac{(n+m-1)!}{\mu^n (m-1)!}. \tag{3.2.1b}$$

In particular, the first two moments are

$$\mathbf{E}[Y_m] = \frac{m}{\mu}, \quad \text{and} \quad \mathbf{E}[Y_m^2] = \frac{m^2+m}{\mu^2},$$

with a variance of

$$\sigma_m^2 := \mathbf{E}[Y_m^2] - (\mathbf{E}[Y_m])^2 = \frac{m}{\mu^2},$$

giving a squared coefficient of variation of

$$C_m^2 = \frac{\sigma_m^2}{(\mathbf{E}[Y_m])^2} = \frac{1}{m}. \tag{3.2.1c}$$

For completeness and for future reference we also evaluate the Laplace transform for the Erlangian-m distribution. It is well known that the Laplace transform distribution of the sum of two random variables is the product of the Laplace transforms of the two distributions. That is, if $Z = X + Y$, then

$$B_Z^*(s) = B_X^*(s)\, B_Y^*(s).$$

The Laplace transform for the exponential distribution is simply:

$$B_{Y_1}^*(s) = \int_0^\infty E_1(t;\,\mu) e^{-st}\, dt = \int_0^\infty \mu e^{-\mu t}\, e^{-st}\, dt = \frac{\mu}{s+\mu}.$$

†Observe that we use the *italic* E for the "*E*rlangian" pdf and a fancy $\mathbf{E}$ for the "**E**xpected value" symbol.

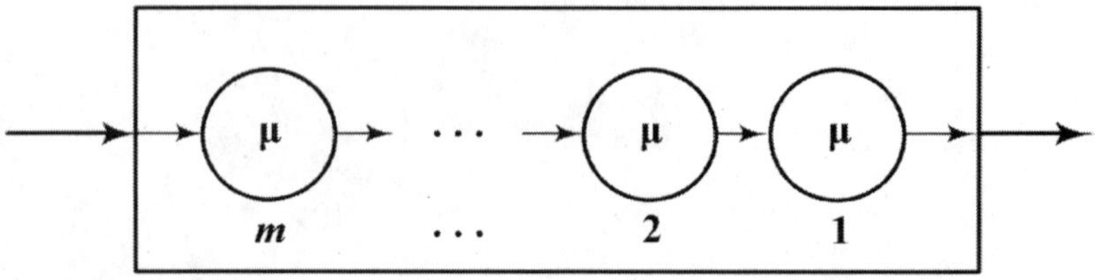

Figure 3.2.1: Subsystem containing m phases arranged into a string. Each phase has completion rate μ. A customer, upon entering, always goes to phase m. When finished there he goes to phase $m-1$, and so on until phase 1, after which he leaves. The density function for this excursion is the Erlangian-m, $E_m(t;\mu)$, as given in (3.2.1a). Note that the phase numbers are in reverse order.)

It then follows, either by direct integration, or by use of the above product theorem, that

$$B^*_{Y_m}(s) = \int_0^\infty E_m(t,\,\mu)e^{-st}\,dt = \left(\frac{\mu}{s+\mu}\right)^m. \tag{3.2.1d}$$

We make three trivial observations before moving on. The Erlangian-1 is an exponential distribution; only two parameters (μ and m) need be specified, and; all other Erlangians have $C_v^2 < 1$.

There is a natural extension of this distribution, the ***gamma distribution***, where m can take on noninteger as well as integer values. The ***gamma density function*** is defined in [AbramowitzStegun64] as

$$g(x|\alpha;\mu) := \mu\frac{(\mu x)^{\alpha-1}}{\Gamma(\alpha)}e^{-\mu x}, \tag{3.2.2a}$$

where $\Gamma(\alpha)$ is the ***gamma function***, defined by

$$\Gamma(\alpha+1) := \int_0^\infty x^\alpha\, e^{-x}\,dx. \tag{3.2.2b}$$

By integrating by parts, it is easy to see that $\Gamma(\alpha+1) = \alpha\Gamma(\alpha)$. Also,

$$\mathbf{E}[X^\ell] = \frac{\Gamma(\ell+\alpha)}{\mu^\ell\,\Gamma(\alpha)} \tag{3.2.2c}$$

Furthermore, if $\alpha = m$, a positive integer, then $\Gamma(m+1) = m!$, and from (3.2.1a)

$$g(x|m;\mu) = E_m(x;\mu).$$

Although the nonintegral gamma distributions have awkward mathematical properties at $t = 0$ (try to find their derivatives there), they are used by many researchers because any coefficient of variation less than 1 can be fit by these. We do not use them, because they cannot be represented by finite-dimensional matrices. Besides, we have other ways to fit any C_v^2.

From our own description, Erlangian distributions should be generated by the subsystem that looks like Figure 3.2.1. Since this is merely a representation of a distribution, we change our terminology for each component from *server* to *phase*. Remember, a phase is always has an exponential distribution, with a completion rate that may be a complex number, but its real part is always positive. For Erlangian-m distributions, all the phases have the same μ, so the completion rate matrix is the m-dimensional matrix satisfying $\mathbf{M} = \mu\mathbf{I}$. The transition matrix is given by the following.

$$\mathbf{P} = \left.\begin{bmatrix} 0 & 1 & 0 & \cdots & 0 & 0 \\ 0 & 0 & 1 & \cdots & 0 & 0 \\ \vdots & \vdots & \vdots & \cdots & \vdots & \vdots \\ 0 & 0 & 0 & \cdots & 0 & 1 \\ 0 & 0 & 0 & \cdots & 0 & 0 \end{bmatrix}\right\} \quad m \text{ rows and columns.} \tag{3.2.3a}$$

Note that, as in the figure, the matrix elements are in reverse order from the formulas. That is, the 1 in the second column of the first row corresponds to the customer going from phase m to $m-1$. This convention is adhered to whenever we deal with Erlangians.

Next define the auxiliary matrix

$$\mathbf{L} := \mathbf{I} - \mathbf{P} = \begin{bmatrix} 1 & -1 & 0 & \cdots & 0 & 0 \\ 0 & 1 & -1 & \cdots & 0 & 0 \\ \vdots & \vdots & \vdots & \cdots & \vdots & \vdots \\ 0 & 0 & 0 & \cdots & 1 & -1 \\ 0 & 0 & 0 & \cdots & 0 & 1 \end{bmatrix}. \tag{3.2.3b}$$

The completion rate matrix for the process is

$$\mathbf{B} = \mathbf{M}(\mathbf{I} - \mathbf{P}) = \mu\mathbf{I}\,\mathbf{L} = \mu\mathbf{L},$$

with service time matrix

$$\mathbf{V} = \mathbf{B}^{-1} = \frac{1}{\mu}\mathbf{L}^{-1}$$

and m-dimensional entrance vector

$$\mathbf{p} = [1\ 0\ 0\ \cdots\ 0].$$

One can verify directly that the inverse of $\mathbf{L}$ is given by

$$\mathbf{L}^{-1} = \begin{bmatrix} 1 & 1 & 1 & \cdots & 1 & 1 \\ 0 & 1 & 1 & \cdots & 1 & 1 \\ \vdots & \vdots & \vdots & \cdots & \vdots & \vdots \\ 0 & 0 & 0 & \cdots & 1 & 1 \\ 0 & 0 & 0 & \cdots & 0 & 1 \end{bmatrix}. \tag{3.2.3c}$$

From the well-known summation rule of binomial coefficients,

$$\binom{n+m+1}{m} = \sum_{j=0}^{m} \binom{n+j}{j}, \tag{3.2.4a}$$

it follows that

$$\left[\mathbf{L}^{-n}\right]_{ij} = \binom{n+j-i-1}{j-i} \quad \text{for} \quad i \le j. \tag{3.2.4b}$$

For instance (if you are concerned, just try a few matrix multiplications),

$$\mathbf{L}^{-3} = \begin{bmatrix} 1 & 3 & 6 & 10 & 15 & \cdots \\ 0 & 1 & 3 & 6 & 10 & \cdots \\ 0 & 0 & 1 & 3 & 6 & \cdots \\ 0 & 0 & 0 & 1 & 3 & \cdots \\ 0 & 0 & 0 & 0 & 1 & \cdots \\ \vdots & \vdots & \vdots & \vdots & \vdots & \vdots \end{bmatrix}.$$

Note that all these matrices are triangular, in that every element below the diagonal is 0 (e.g., $L_{ij} = 0$ if $i > j$). If $\mathbf{P}$ (or $\mathbf{B}$ or $\mathbf{V}$) is of this form, this is referred to as a ***feedforward network***. In any case, it can be shown that these matrices reproduce Equations (3.2.1) by purely algebraic manipulation of the equations in Theorem 3.1.1. Indeed, $\langle \mathbf{p}, \mathbf{B} \rangle$ as given here is a faithful representation of the Erlangian-m pdf.

Example 3.2.1: The values of Erlangians for several values of m have

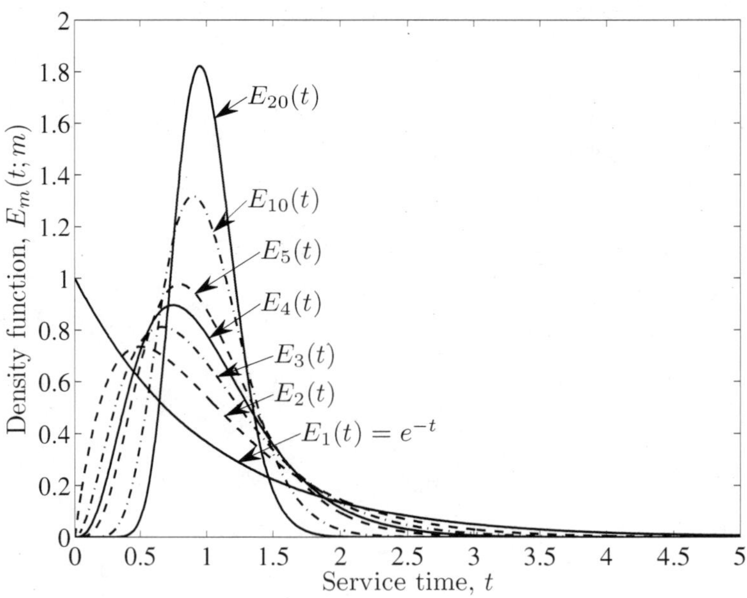

Figure 3.2.2: The pdfs for the Erlangian distributions $E_m(x; m)$ [see (3.2.1a)], with parameter $m = 1$, 2, 3, 4, 5, 10, and 20. All have a mean of 1. They all peak at a value less than their means, namely $1 - 1/m$, and get narrower with increasing m, agreeing with the fact that $C_v^2 = 1/m$ also gets smaller.

been calculated and plotted in Figure 3.2.2. These all have a mean of 1 (we set $\mu = m$) and, except for the exponential, are 0 at $t = 0$. Consistent with their values for C_v^2, these functions get narrower and narrower with increasing m ($\sigma_m = 1/\sqrt{m}$). In fact, the ***Dirac delta function*** $\delta(x)$ [see (5.1.12a) and following] can be defined by the limit

$$\delta(t - T) := \lim_{m\to\infty} E_m(t; m/T) \tag{3.2.5a}$$

and is a representation of the ***deterministic distribution***, the one that always gives a service time of T. In fact one can use the same matrices to represent the ***Uniform distribution*** (with r.v. $\boldsymbol{U}$) with pdf

$$b_U(x) = \begin{cases} 1/2 & \text{for } 0 < x < 2T \\ 0 & \text{otherwise} \end{cases}, \tag{3.2.5b}$$

having $\mathbb{E}[U] = T$. This is done by replacing $\mathbf{p} = [1 \ \ 0 \ \ 0 \ \ \cdots \ \ 0]$ with $\mathbf{p} = [1 \ \ 1 \ \ 1 \ \ \cdots \ \ 1]/m$. This is discussed further below, and in Exercise 3.5.8.▲

The representation as given in Figure 3.2.1 always has the customer starting at phase m. Suppose instead, that he starts at phase j with probability p_j, where $\sum_{j=i}^{m} p_j = 1$. In other words, the entrance vector is $\mathbf{p} = [p_m, p_{m-1}, \ldots, p_1]$, where $\mathbf{p}\boldsymbol{\epsilon}' = 1$. Then the pdf for such a process is:

$$b(t) = \sum_{j=1}^{m} p_j\, E_j(t;\, \mu) = \mu\, e^{-\mu t} \left[\sum_{j=1}^{m} p_j \frac{(\mu\, t)^j}{(j-1)!} \right] = f(t)\, e^{-\mu t}. \tag{3.2.6a}$$

This then, tells us that any polynomial multiplying an exponential function $e^{-\mu t}$ can be written as a sum of E_j pdfs with parameter μ. The constraint that $\mathbf{p}\boldsymbol{\epsilon}' = 1$ is equivalent to

$$\int_0^\infty b(t)\, dt = 1.$$

The condition that $p_i \geq 0$ guarantees that $b(t) \geq 0 \quad \forall \quad t \geq 0$.

It easily follows from (3.2.1d) that the Laplace transform is

$$B^*(s) = \int_0^\infty b(t)\, e^{-st}\, dt = \sum_{j=1}^{m} p_j \left(\frac{\mu}{s+\mu} \right)^j = \frac{q_1(s)}{(s+\mu)^m}. \tag{3.2.6b}$$

The rightmost term comes from combining fractions, and $q_1(s)$ is a polynomial of degree less than m.

We know from Equations (3.2.1) that $E_m(t;\, \mu)$ gives $C_m^2 = 1/m$. But we can get other values of C_v^2 between $1/m$ and 1 by varying the p_js in (3.2.6a). In particular, the reliability function,

$$R(t) = (1 + p\mu t)e^{-\mu t}$$

can give any value for C_v^2 between 1/2 and 1 by varying $0 \leq p \leq 1$. Obviously, for $p = 1$, $C_v^2 = 1/2$, whereas for $p = 0$, $C_v^2 = 1$. This is considered further in the following exercise.

Exercise 3.2.1: Give algebraic expressions for $\Psi[\mathbf{V}]$ and $\Psi[\mathbf{V}^2]$ in terms of p and μ, where

$$\mathbf{p} = [p \ \ (1-p)], \qquad \mathbf{M} = \mu \mathbf{I},$$

and $\mathbf{P}$ is given in (3.2.3a) for $m = 2$. Show that this produces the reliability function given by the equation just before this exercise. Express p and μ in terms of $\mathbb{E}[X]$ and C_v^2. In particular, show that

$$p = \frac{1 - C_v^2 + \sqrt{2(1 - C_v^2)}}{1 + C_v^2}.$$

Show by direct substitution that this gives the correct values for p when $C_v^2 = 1/2$ and 1.

We have one last comment concerning Erlangians. The matrix $\mathbf{L}$ from (3.2.3b) as well as all its powers, including its inverse, is tridiagonal, with all its diagonal elements being equal ($L_{ii} = 1$). Therefore, all m of its eigenvalues are equal to 1, but interestingly enough, it only has one left- and one right-eigenvector. Thus, $\mathbf{L}$ is called a ***defective matrix***. In general, if the number of pairs of eigenvectors is less than the dimension of a matrix, then the matrix is defective. This can only happen if at least one eigenvalue is multiple valued (as is the case here), because every eigenvalue must have at least one pair of eigenvectors.

3.2.1.2 Hyperexponential Distributions

The other widely used class of functions is the family of hyperexponential distributions with density functions of the form

$$h_m(t) := p_1[\mu_1 e^{-\mu_1 t}] + p_2[\mu_2 e^{-\mu_2 t}] + \cdots + p_m[\mu_m e^{-\mu_m t}]$$

$$= \sum_{j=1}^{m} p_j[\mu_j\, e^{-\mu_j t}], \tag{3.2.7a}$$

and reliability function,

$$R_m(t) := \sum_{j=1}^{m} p_j\, e^{-\mu_j t}, \tag{3.2.7b}$$

where μ_j and $p_j > 0$ are real, and $\sum_{j=1}^{m} p_j = 1$. We can assume without loss of generality that the exponents $[\mu_j]$ are all distinct. Otherwise, we could combine two equal ones together. Also, we can assume that $p_j \neq 0 \forall j$. Otherwise we could just throw that term away. In both cases, we just make m smaller. With these conditions we can say that for $m \geq 1$, it follows that $C_v^2 \geq 1$. $C_v^2 = 1$ only when all the μs become equal, reducing to $h_1(t)$, the exponential distribution. Let Z_m be the random variable described by the distribution $h_m(t)$; then its moments are

$$\mathbf{E}[\, Z_m^n \,] = n! \sum_{j=1}^{m} \frac{p_j}{\mu_j^n}, \tag{3.2.7c}$$

and its Laplace transform is

$$B^*_{Z_m}(s) = \sum_{j=1}^{m} p_j \frac{\mu_j}{\mu_j + s} = \frac{q_1(s)}{q_2(s)}, \tag{3.2.7d}$$

where

$$q_2(s) = (\mu_1 + s)(\mu_2 + s) \cdots (\mu_j + s) \cdots (\mu_m + s)$$

is a polynomial of degree m, and $q_1(s)$ is a polynomial of degree $m-1$. When a function has a Laplace transform that is a ratio of polynomials we say it has a ***Rational Laplace Transform*** (RLT). Note that (3.2.6b) is of the same form. In fact, all ME distributions are RLT, and all RLT functions have an ME representation.

The H_m distributions have an obvious representation. A customer enters a subsystem, and with probability p_j goes to phase j, which has a completion rate of μ_j. When finished, he leaves. Then $M_{jj} = \mu_j$, $\mathbf{P} = \mathbf{O}$, and $\mathbf{p}$ is the entrance vector whose j-th component is p_j. From this it follows that $\mathbf{B} = \mathbf{M}$ (pretty simple). It is trivial to show that this is a faithful representation of the h_ms. Also, $q_2(-s)$ is the characteristic function for $\mathbf{B}$. That is,

$$q_2(s) = \mathrm{Det}[\mathbf{B} + s\mathbf{I}].$$

We show later that this is true for the minimal representation of all ME distributions.

Hyperexponential Distributions with Two States

The family of hyperexponentials is so rich in parameters that one is usually left in a quandary as to what values to give them. Even the h_2 function has three free parameters (e.g., p_1, μ_1, and μ_2), with the following representation:

$$\mathbf{p} = [p_1\ p_2\,], \quad \mathbf{B} = \begin{bmatrix} \mu_1 & 0 \\ 0 & \mu_2 \end{bmatrix}, \quad \text{and} \quad \mathbf{V} = \begin{bmatrix} T_1 & 0 \\ 0 & T_2 \end{bmatrix} \tag{3.2.8a}$$

where $T_i := 1/\mu_i$. After a specific $\mathbf{E}[Z_2]$ and σ_2^2 have been chosen, one more condition is still needed. One should try to fix the third parameter based on the physical system being examined. One possibility is to use the third moment. Assuming that the first three moments are known, one can find T_1, T_2, and p_1 by solving the simultaneous equations:

$$\begin{aligned} \bar{x} = \mathbf{E}[Z_2] &= p_1 T_1 + p_2 T_2 \\ \mathbf{E}[Z_2^2] &= 2(p_1 T_1^2 + p_2 T_2^2) \\ \mathbf{E}[Z_2^3] &= 6(p_1 T_1^3 + p_2 T_2^3), \end{aligned} \tag{3.2.8b}$$

remembering that $p_1 + p_2 = 1$. An alternative to using $\mathbb{E}[Z_2^3]$ could be to fit the value of the density function at 0. That is, use

$$b(0) = p_1\mu_1 + p_2\mu_2. \tag{3.2.8c}$$

In any case, recalling that $\sigma^2 = \mathbb{E}[Z_2^2] - (\mathbb{E}[Z_2])^2$, and manipulating the first two of the above equations, it follows that

$$C_v^2 = \frac{\sigma^2}{\bar{x}^2} = 1 + 2\,p_1\,p_2\left(\frac{T_1 - T_2}{\bar{x}}\right)^2. \tag{3.2.8d}$$

Clearly, $C_v^2 \geq 1$ as long as $p_1,\ p_2 \geq 0$. $C_v^2 = 1$ only if $p_1 = 0$, or $p_2 = 0$, or $T_1 = T_2$. In all such cases, h_2 reduces to the exponential distribution.

Another popular choice for parametric studies is to express T_1 and T_2 in terms of the first two moments and p_1. Under certain conditions there are two choices. First let

$$\gamma := \frac{C_v^2 - 1}{2}.$$

Then $(p_1 + p_2 = 1)$

$$\text{for } T_2 < T_1 \quad \left\{ \begin{array}{lcl} T_1 & = & \bar{x}\left[1 + \sqrt{p_2\,\gamma\,/\,p_1}\right] \\ T_2 & = & \bar{x}\left[1 - \sqrt{p_1\,\gamma\,/\,p_2}\right] \end{array} \right\} \tag{3.2.8e}$$

but only if $p_1\,\gamma < p_2$; that is,$p_1 < 2/(C_v^2 + 1)$ Violation of this inequality yields unphysical parameters (if $p_1\gamma > p_2$ then $T_2 < 0$). Alternatively,

$$\text{for } T_1 < T_2 \quad \left\{ \begin{array}{lcl} T_1 & = & \bar{x}\left[1 - \sqrt{p_2\,\gamma\,/\,p_1}\right] \\ T_2 & = & \bar{x}\left[1 + \sqrt{p_1\,\gamma\,/\,p_2}\right] \end{array} \right\} \tag{3.2.8f}$$

but only if $p_2\,\gamma < p_1$; that is, $p_1 > (C_v^2 - 1)/(C_v^2 + 1)$. Only for $1 < C_v^2 < 3$ (or equivalently, $0 < \gamma < 1$) do both sets of equations apply.

One interesting way to pick p_1 is to make the two phases contribute equally to the mean. That is, let $p_1\,T_1 = p_2\,T_2 = \bar{x}/2$. It then follows that

$$p_{1|2} = \frac{1}{2}\left(1 \pm \sqrt{\frac{\gamma}{(1+\gamma)}}\right),$$

and

$$T_{1|2} = \bar{x}\left[1 + \gamma \mp \sqrt{\gamma(1+\gamma)}\right].$$

Obviously, $\mathbb{E}[Z_2^2] = \bar{x}^2(1 + C_v^2)$, and

$$\mathbb{E}[Z_2^3] = 3\bar{x}^3\,C_v^2(C_v^2 + 1).$$

One advantage of this choice for parameterization is that it is valid for all $1 \leq C_v^2 < \infty$.

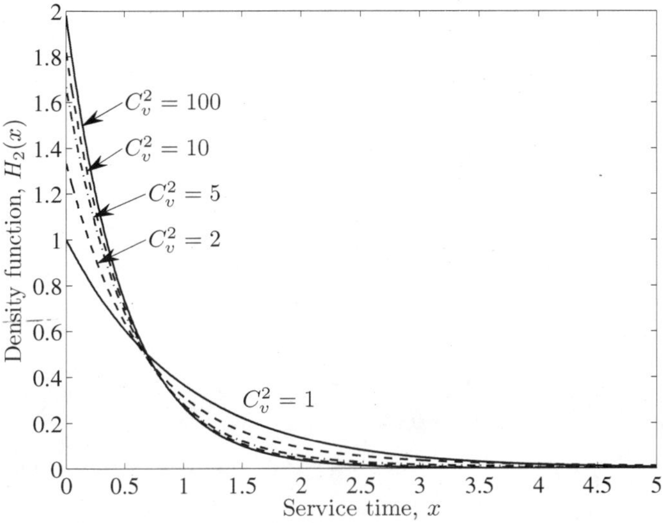

Figure 3.2.3: The density functions for a family of hyperexponential distributions with two phases, all with a mean value of 1, with $C_v^2 = 1, 2, 5, 10,$ and 100, respectively. The curve for $C_v^2 = 1$ is the exponential distribution. The third condition chosen for this three-parameter family was $2\alpha C_v^2 = 1 + \alpha^2$ ($\alpha = \mu_2/\mu_1$) for no good reason, except that we had to do something. Although the graph does not show it, all the curves cross twice, so they asymptotically are in the same sequence as they were at $x = 0$, ordered according to their value of C_v^2.

Example 3.2.2: The hyperexponential distribution $h_2(x)$, with mean of 1, has been calculated and plotted in Figure 3.2.3 for several different values for C_v^2. For mathematical convenience we have let $\alpha^2 - 2\alpha C_v^2 + 1 = 0$, where $\alpha = \mu_2/\mu_1$. This yielded third moments $\mathbb{E}[X^3]$, with values of 6.0, 18.0, 90.0, 330.0, and 30300.0, respectively. The pdfs themselves are as innocent looking as their representations, but as we show in Chapters 4 and 5, because they can have any value for the coefficient of variation (as long as it is greater than 1), they can disastrously affect mean system times. All true hyperexponentials are strictly greater than 0 at $x = 0$ and decay smoothly thereafter. Note that with this family, the larger C_v^2, the bigger $h(0)$ is. But as t gets larger, they all cross (not necessarily at the same place), and in the intermediate region they are in reverse order. An important aspect of these curves, which is shown clearly in Figure 3.2.4, is that they cross over once more, so for very large t they are in the same order in which they began.

The curves in Figure 3.2.4 display $\log[h_2(x)]$ versus x, and it is not hard to show that

$$\lim_{x\to\infty} \log[h_2(x)] = \log(p_2\mu_2) - \mu_2 x,$$

so each curve approaches a straight line with slope $-\mu_2$. The higher moments of these distributions are completely dominated by this tail behavior. ▲

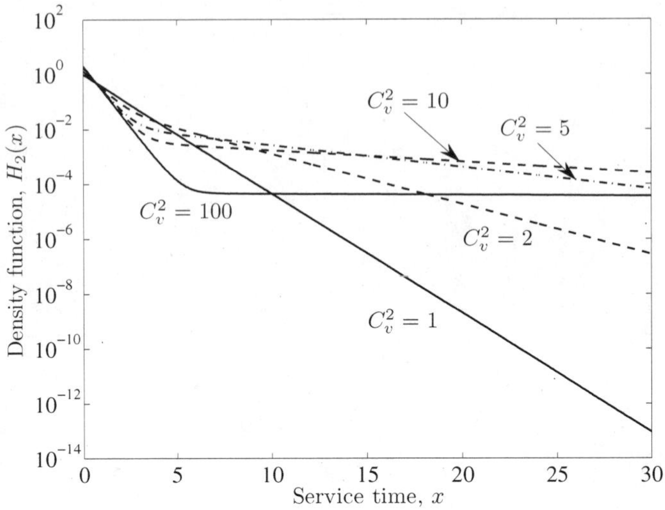

Figure 3.2.4: The same curves as Figure 3.2.3 but now the dependent variable is $\log[h_2(x|\, C_v^2)]$, thus showing some of the second crossings. The exponential function is a straight line on this graph. Also notice that the curves for $C_v^2 > 1$ change from one straight line to another. That is because $\mu_1 \gg \mu_2$, and $p_1 \gg p_2$, so they all start off (small x) with slope $-\mu_1$. The second term doesn't contribute until $\mu_1 x \gg 1$. The asymptotic slopes of all the curves are $-\mu_2$.

We are reluctant to make general claims about the behavior of functions beyond the significance of their second moments.

Distributions Coming from Singular B or V

An interesting special case of h_2 functions occurs when $p_1\gamma = 1 - p_1$, for then $T_1 = \bar{x}/p_1$ and $T_2 = 0$. For $x > 0$

$$\lim_{T_2 \to 0} e^{-x/T_2}/T_2 = \lim_{\mu_2 \to \infty} \mu_2\, e^{-\mu_2\, x} = 0.$$

In which case, the density function reduces to

$$b(x) = \frac{p_1}{T_1} e^{-x/T_1} \quad \text{for } x > 0$$

and $C_v^2 = (2 - p_1)/p_1$. So, depending on what is picked for p_1, C_v^2 can range anywhere from 1 to ∞. Because of the simple form for $b(x)$, this is sometimes called a ***generalized exponential function***. Gupta et.al [GUPTAETAL07] refer to it as a ***degenerate hyperexponential***. But it really is an exponential with an ***initial impulse***, because

$$R(x) = \int_x^\infty b(t)\, dt = p_1\, e^{-x/T_1}.$$

Therefore, $R(0_+) = p_1 < 1$. In other words, there is a finite probability that the event will take 0 time. That is, the pdf is more appropriately written as

$$b(x) = p_2\,\delta(x) + \frac{p_1}{T_1} e^{-x/T_1},$$

where $\delta(x)$ is the Dirac δ function introduced in Example 3.2.1. From (3.2.8a), the service rate matrix **B**, no longer exists (because $\mu_2 \to \infty$). Even so, matrix methods can still be used as long as all measurable quantities can be expressed in terms of the service time matrix,

$$\mathbf{V} = \begin{bmatrix} T_1 & 0 \\ 0 & 0 \end{bmatrix}.$$

Clearly, **V** no longer has an inverse, but (3.1.9) and the rightmost term in (3.1.10) are still valid. This generalizes to any distribution. That is, if **V** is not invertible, it must have a 0 eigenvalue with corresponding state with 0 service time (multiple 0 eigenvalues can be collapsed to 1 state). The probability of going to this state is the size of the initial impulse.

We have seen that **V** has a meaning even when it has no inverse. The case where **B** has no inverse also has a meaning. In this case we have what Feller [FELLER71] calls a ***defective distribution***, in that

$$\lim_{x\to\infty} R(x) = \lim_{x\to\infty} \mathbf{Pr}(X > x) > 0.$$

That is, there is a finite probability that the process will never end, so it has a ***defective probability measure***. (Note that defective distributions and ***defective matrices*** are unrelated concepts. Defective distributions may have nondefective representations, and nondefective distributions may have defective representations.) In this case,

$$R(x) = p + (1-p)R_d(x),$$

where $R_d(x)$ has all the properties of a reliability function; that is, it is monotonic, nonincreasing, $R_d(0) = 1$ and $R_d(\infty) = 0$. In this case, (3.1.7d), (3.1.8b), and (3.1.10) (the expression with **B** in it) are still valid. Only the moments are meaningless.

Exercise 3.2.2: Show by direct integration and use of (3.1.9) and (3.1.10) that $b(x)$ and **V** produce the same moments and Laplace transform.

Distribution functions with impulse at $x = 0$ are used in Section 4.5.4, and fully discussed in Section 5.1.3. Researchers who use this function as a simple way to get a large variance are introducing a highly singular behavior that may not be reflected in the actual system being investigated.

Often, abuse comes in when the functional form is picked for mathematical convenience, which may badly distort physical reality. We may be guilty of that in the various examples given in this chapter, but we are not looking at any particular system at present, so there should be no harm.

3.2.2 Sums of Erlangian Functions

We now generalize the Erlangian functions and hyperexponential functions to yield a class of functions that is equivalent to all possible ME functions, and are in fact the matrices of smallest dimension. This is proven in Section 3.4, but for now, consider functions of the form

$$b(t) = \sum_{k=1}^{K} f_k(t) e^{-\mu_k t} \quad \text{with} \quad \Re(\mu_k) > 0, \tag{3.2.9a}$$

where $f_k(t)$ is a polynomial of degree $m_k - 1$, and m_k can be any positive integer. That is, $b(t)$ is a sum of polynomials times exponentials, where

$$f_k(t) = \sum_{j=0}^{m_k-1} a_{jk}\, t^j.$$

We give a different look to the equation by introducing the Erlangian functions of order j as given in (3.2.1a). Then the expression for $b(t)$ can be rewritten in the form

$$b(t) = \sum_{k=1}^{K} a_k \left(\sum_{j=1}^{m_k} p_j^{(k)} E_j(t; \mu_k) \right). \tag{3.2.9b}$$

We have split a_{jk} into two terms such that

$$\sum_{j=1}^{m_k} p_j^{(k)} = 1 \quad \text{for } 1 \le k \le K.$$

Furthermore, because

$$\int_0^\infty b(t) dt = 1,$$

we must also have $\sum_{k=1}^{K} a_k = 1$. The number of terms all told is $m = \sum_{k=1}^{K} m_k$. As you might expect, m turns out to be the dimension of the representation we are constructing. In general, from (3.2.1b) we can write down the moments of $b(t)$ in terms of the binomial coefficients. If T is the random variable described by this process, we can write, with the aid of (3.2.1b) and (3.2.8b),

$$\mathbf{E}[T^n] := \int_0^\infty t^n\, b(t)\, dt = n! \sum_{k=1}^{K} \frac{a_k}{\mu_k^n} \left[\sum_{j=1}^{m_k} \binom{n+j-1}{j-1} p_j^{(k)} \right]. \tag{3.2.10}$$

The only requirement for these integrals to exist is that the real part of each μ_k be positive, which we have already assumed. We can even let the a_k and $p_n^{(k)}$ be complex (negative or positive) numbers, as long as they appear in complex conjugate pairs to guarantee that $b(t)$ and its moments are real (this is a subsidiary requirement, which we assume here).

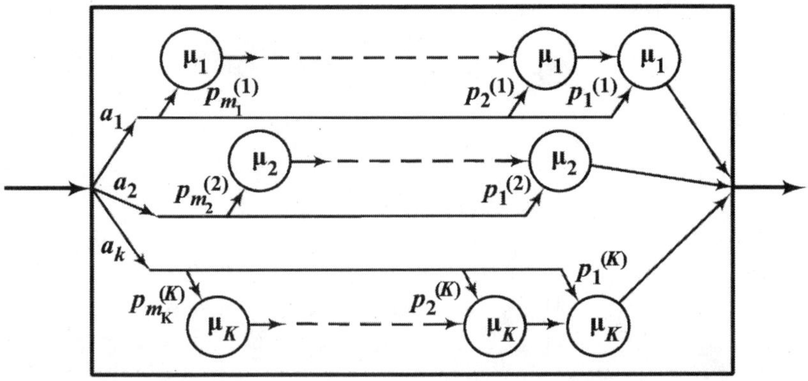

Figure 3.2.5: Subsystem containing m exponential phases. The phases are arranged into K strings, where string k has m_k identical phases in tandem, each with completion rate μ_k. A customer can go to any phase (with probability $a_k p_j^{(k)}$), but then must proceed along that string until the end, and then leave. Note that phase 1 for each string is the last one before leaving. The probability density function for this excursion is $b(t)$ as given in (3.2.9b). a_k and $p_{m_k}^{(k)}$ are assumed to be nonzero, otherwise the corresponding phases can be eliminated, yielding a smaller representation. Every representation is equivalent to one and only one of these, wherea_k, μ_k, and p_k are allowed to be complex, if necessary. No equivalent representation can have fewer dimensions.

Next we give a pseudophysical interpretation to $b(t)$. Look at Figure 3.2.5. This exactly describes the expression for $b(t)$. A customer enters a subsystem and goes to string k (made up of m_k identical phases with completion rate μ_k) with probability a_k. He then goes directly to phase j (counting from the departing end) of that string with probability $p_j^{(k)}$, and proceeds to the end, being served en route by each of the j phases. The customer then leaves. We now construct a matrix representation for this process. The transition matrix for a single line $\mathbf{P}_k$, is an m_k−dimensional matrix of form given in (3.2.3a): The completion rate matrix for the k-th string is also of dimension m_k, and because all the completion rates for that string are equal, it is simply $\mathbf{M_k} := \mu_k \mathbf{I_k}$. Next let $\mathbf{L_k}$ be the square matrix of dimension m_k of the form in (3.2.3b). The m-dimensional completion and transition matrices for the entire process can be written as

$$\mathbf{P} := \begin{bmatrix} \mathbf{P_1} & 0 & 0 & \cdots & 0 \\ 0 & \mathbf{P_2} & 0 & \cdots & 0 \\ \vdots & \vdots & \vdots & \cdots & \vdots \\ 0 & 0 & 0 & \cdots & 0 \\ 0 & 0 & 0 & \cdots & \mathbf{P_K} \end{bmatrix}; \quad \mathbf{M} := \begin{bmatrix} \mathbf{M_1} & 0 & 0 & \cdots & 0 \\ 0 & \mathbf{M_2} & 0 & \cdots & 0 \\ \vdots & \vdots & \vdots & \cdots & \vdots \\ 0 & 0 & 0 & \cdots & 0 \\ 0 & 0 & 0 & \cdots & \mathbf{M_K} \end{bmatrix},$$

where each entry is an appropriately sized and valued matrix (e.g., $\mathbf{0}$ is a matrix of all 0's). The *entrance* or *initial vector* for the process is given by the ***direct sum*** (the components of the vectors are concatenated to produce a single vector with as many components as all the others put together):

$$\mathbf{p} := a_1\mathbf{p^{(1)}} \oplus a_2\mathbf{p^{(2)}} \oplus \cdots \oplus a_K\mathbf{p^{(K)}}, \tag{3.2.11a}$$

where $\mathbf{p^{(k)}} = [p^{(k)}_{m_k} \; p^{(k)}_{m_k-1} \; \cdots \; p^{(k)}_2 \; p^{(k)}_1]$, and $p^{(k)}_{m_k} \neq 0$. See the comments after (3.2.3a) concerning the reverse order of the components.

We next construct the m-dimensional *service rate matrix* for this subsystem:

$$\mathbf{B} := \mathbf{M}(\mathbf{I}-\mathbf{P}) = \begin{bmatrix} \mu_1\mathbf{L_1} & \mathbf{0} & \mathbf{0} & \cdots & \mathbf{0} \\ \mathbf{0} & \mu_2\mathbf{L_2} & \mathbf{0} & \cdots & \mathbf{0} \\ \vdots & \vdots & \vdots & \cdots & \vdots \\ \mathbf{0} & \mathbf{0} & \mathbf{0} & \cdots & \mathbf{0} \\ \mathbf{0} & \mathbf{0} & \mathbf{0} & \cdots & \mu_K\mathbf{L_K} \end{bmatrix}. \tag{3.2.11b}$$

Because all the elements below the diagonal are zero (remember, the $\mathbf{L}$ matrices are triangular), we see that μ_k is an eigenvalue of $\mathbf{B}$, with multiplicity m_k. We know this because there is an obvious theorem in matrix theory which states that the eigenvalues of a triangular matrix are its diagonal elements.

If none of the μ's is equal to 0, we can let

$$\mathbf{V} = \mathbf{B}^{-1}, \tag{3.2.11c}$$

where $\mathbf{V}$ looks just like $\mathbf{B}$ with each $\mu_k\mathbf{L_k}$ replaced by $(1/\mu_k)\mathbf{L_k}^{-1}$.

Our purpose now is to show that the important properties of matrix representations are valid for purely algebraic reasons. To do this, first recall (3.2.4). Then look at the scalar reduction of the matrices by multiplying both sides of $\mathbf{L_k}^{-n}$ with the vectors $\mathbf{p^{(k)}}$ and $\boldsymbol{\epsilon}'_\mathbf{k}$ to get

$$\mathbf{p^{(k)}}\mathbf{L_k}^{-n}\boldsymbol{\epsilon}'_\mathbf{k} = \sum_{j=1}^{m_k} p_j^{(k)} \begin{pmatrix} n+j-1 \\ j-1 \end{pmatrix}. \tag{3.2.12}$$

This expression is identical to the term in the brackets in (3.2.10).

Now when we put (3.2.10) to (3.2.12) together and recall the definition of $\Psi[\,\cdot\,]$, we get

$$\mathbb{E}[T^n] = n!\Psi[\mathbf{V}^n].$$

Note that this relation is valid even if $b(t)$ is not a pdf. It only requires that the moments exist (i.e., the moments must be finite). Because we are dealing with finite sums of terms, the moments exist if and only if $\Re(\mu_k) > 0$. No probability assumptions are required for the component parts.

By algebraic manipulations and arguments similar to the preceding paragraph, noting that $(\mathbf{I}+\mathbf{sV})^{-1}$ is a block diagonal and triangular matrix, we can show that the Laplace transform of $b(t)$ satisfies the following.

$$B^*(s) := \int_0^\infty e^{-st}\, b(t)\, dt = \Psi\left[(\mathbf{I}+s\mathbf{V})^{-1}\right] = \frac{q_2(s)}{q_1(s)}.$$

But from (3.2.6b) and (3.2.7d) we have (after combining fractions)

$$B^*(s) = \sum_{k=1}^{K} a_k \sum_{j=1}^{m_k} p_j^{(k)} \left(\frac{\mu_k}{s+\mu_k}\right)^j = \frac{q_2(s)}{q_1(s)}. \tag{3.2.13a}$$

Clearly, $q_1(s)$ and $q_2(s)$ have no common roots, $q_1(s)$ is a polynomial of degree m, and $q_2(s)$ is of degree $m_2 < m$. In fact, from (3.2.13a) it must follow that

$$q_1(s) = (s+\mu_1)^{m_1} (s+\mu_2)^{m_2} \cdots (s+\mu_K)^{m_K}. \tag{3.2.13b}$$

The relation between $\Psi\left[(\mathbf{I}+s\mathbf{V})^{-1}\right]$ and $q_2(s)/q_1(s)$ is valid even if $\Re(\mu_k) < 0$ for some k. In other words, this equation is an algebraic relation among $\mathbf{V}$, $\mathbf{p}$, and the polynomials, $q_i(s)$. It reduces to the Laplace transform when all the μ_ks have positive real parts.

Let $\phi(y)$ be the characteristic polynomial of $\mathbf{B}$. Then from (3.2.11b), $\phi(y)$ has K distinct roots, each with multiplicity m_k $(1 \le k \le K \le m)$, that is,

$$\phi(y) = \text{Det}[y\mathbf{I} - \mathbf{B}] = (y-\mu_1)^{m_1}(y-\mu_2)^{m_2} \cdots (y-\mu_K)^{m_K}, \tag{3.2.13c}$$

where $1 \le m_k \le m$ and $\sum_{k=1}^{K} m_k = m$. Comparing (3.2.13b) and (3.2.13c), we get the important relation:

$$q_1(s) = (-1)^m \phi(-s). \tag{3.2.13d}$$

If $K = m$ the distribution is a pure hyperexponential, but if $K < m$, or equivalently, if $m_k > 1$ for at least one k, then $\mathbf{B}$ is a ***defective matrix***. We elaborate on this further in Section 3.4.

The third relationship that can be proven by direct algebraic manipulation is the following:

$$b(t) = \Psi[\mathbf{B}\exp(-t\mathbf{B})] := \sum_{n=0}^{\infty} \frac{(-t)^n}{n!} \Psi\left[\mathbf{B}^{n+1}\right]. \tag{3.2.13e}$$

Whereas $(\mathbf{I}+s\mathbf{V})^{-1}$ has a direct matrix meaning, $\exp(-t\mathbf{B})$ is only defined in terms of its Maclaurin series expansion (as given in the rightmost expression of the equation above). However, the exponential function has an infinite radius of convergence, therefore this formula is also valid for all $\mathbf{B}$. That is why it is so tempting to call this class of functions *matrix exponential*. We have now shown that for functions of the form of Figure 3.2.5 our wonderful formulas from Theorem 3.1.1, namely,

$$b(t) = \Psi[\exp(-t\mathbf{B})], \tag{3.2.14a}$$

$$B^*(s) := \Psi\left[(\mathbf{I}+s\mathbf{V})^{-1}\right] = \frac{q_2(s)}{q_1(s)}, \tag{3.2.14b}$$

where

$$q_1(s) = (-1)^m \phi(-s) \tag{3.2.14c}$$

and (if the moments exist)

$$\mathbb{E}[T^n] = n!\Psi[\mathbf{V}^n] \tag{3.2.14d}$$

are purely matrix identities, having no dependence on probability laws. We define the vector-matrix pair $\langle \mathbf{p}, \mathbf{B} \rangle$ (or $\langle \mathbf{p}, \mathbf{V} \rangle$) to be a ***faithful representation*** of $b(t)$ if these equations hold.

So, in summary, every distribution of the form in Figure 3.2.5 has a faithful matrix exponential representation as given by Equations (3.2.11). Later we show that this is true for all $\langle \mathbf{p}, \mathbf{B} \rangle$.

3.2.3 Other Examples of ME Functions

The class of ME functions described in the previous section are as general as one can get, even if complex probabilities and service rates are allowed. But before proving this assertion we discuss several specific representations. These will be used in succeeding chapters to examine the dependence of performance on variation of distributions. First we provide a definition for describing functions that "look alike".

Definition 3.2.1

Two random variables T_1 and T_2 have distributions with the ***same shape***, or of the ***same type*** if $T_1 = cT_2$, or equivalently, if their PDFs satisfy:

$$F_1(t) = F_2(ct), \quad \text{where } c > 0. \tag{3.2.15a}$$

We also say that "$F_1(t)$ and $F_2(t)$ are ***similar distributions*** if they have the same shape." It follows that $f_1(t) = c\, f_2(ct)$, and

$$\mathbb{E}[T_2^\ell] = c^\ell \mathbb{E}[T_1^\ell] \quad \forall\ \ell \geq 0. \tag{3.2.15b}$$

In Definition 3.4.1 of Section 3.4.2 we introduce the idea of ***equivalent representations***. Anticipating that, we can say the following. Let $F_i(t)$, $i = 1, 2$ be ME distributions that have the same shape; that is, they satisfy (3.2.15a). Then their representations satisfy:

$$\langle \mathbf{p_1}, \mathbf{B_1} \rangle \equiv \langle \mathbf{p_2}, c\mathbf{B_2} \rangle. \tag{3.2.15c}$$

In other words, $\langle \mathbf{p_2}, c\mathbf{B_2} \rangle$ is a faithful representation of $F_1(t)$, and $\langle \mathbf{p_1}, c^{-1}\mathbf{B_1} \rangle$ is a faithful representation of $F_2(t)$.

If T_1 and T_2 are ME, then (3.2.15a), (3.2.15b), and (3.2.15c) are equivalent in that each can be used to prove the others. Even in cases where moments and representations do not exist (we show a few in what follows), (3.2.15a) still is meaningful.

Functions that have the *same shape* form an equivalence class. We can write

$$F_1(\cdot) \sim F_2(\cdot)$$

if F_1 and F_2 have the same shape, and '$\sim$' is an equivalence relation in that it is symmetric, transitive, and reflexive.

[Note: Feller [FELLER71] says that "two distributions F_1 and F_2, are of the ***same type*** if

$$F_1(x) = F_2(ax + b),$$

or equivalently, if their random variables satisfy

$$X_1 = aX_2 + b.$$

He was concerned with distributions that could be greater than 0 for all values of $-\infty < x < \infty$. In such cases, b allows the two functions to align their origins, often to let $\mathbb{E}[X_1] = 0$. We, however, are only concerned with distributions over the range $0 \leq x < \infty$; that is, $F_i(x) = 0$ for $x < 0$. In other words, we are willing to *scale* the means, but not shift them. For example, we would not consider the uniform distribution for $x \in [0, 1]$ to be similar to the uniform distribution for $x \in [1, 2]$, whereas Feller, by setting $b = 1$ would say they are the same type. In any case, the two ideas are the same as long as $b = 0$.] □

From this definition then, all exponential distributions have the same shape. Also, all Erlangians of the same degree have the same shape. But not all hyperexponential distributions have the same shape, even if they have the same degree.

3.2.3.1 A 4-State Hyper-Erlangian

In various modeling applications, the class of Erlangian distributions is used when studying systems where it is expected that $C_v^2 < 1$, whereas hyperexponentials are used when it is expected that $C_v^2 > 1$. But both classes have properties that may be unrealistic in certain applications. For instance, we show in Chapter 5 that the behavior of a G/M/1 queue depends heavily on the behavior of $b(x)$ near $x = 0$. But all Erlangians have the property that $E_m(0) = 0$ for all $m \geq 2$. On the other hand, all true hyperexponentials have the property that $h_m(0) > 0$. What does one do if the true $b(x)$ has high variance but is still 0 at $x = 0$? What if the reverse is true? We show how to get large variance and still have $b(0) = 0$ in examining a 4-state representation made up of two Erlangian-2 distributions in parallel.

Consider the following representation (where as before, $T_i = 1/\mu_i$),

$$\mathbf{p} = [p_1 \;\; 0 \;\; p_2 \;\; 0], \tag{3.2.16a}$$

and

$$\mathbf{B} = \begin{bmatrix} \mu_1 & -\mu_1 & 0 & 0 \\ 0 & \mu_1 & 0 & 0 \\ 0 & 0 & \mu_2 & -\mu_2 \\ 0 & 0 & 0 & \mu_2 \end{bmatrix}, \quad \mathbf{V} = \begin{bmatrix} T_1 & T_1 & 0 & 0 \\ 0 & T_1 & 0 & 0 \\ 0 & 0 & T_2 & T_2 \\ 0 & 0 & 0 & T_2 \end{bmatrix}. \tag{3.2.16b}$$

This represents two Erlangian-2 functions in parallel (as in Figure 3.2.5), namely,

$$b(x) = p_1 \left[\mu_1(\mu_1 x)e^{-\mu_1 x}\right] + p_2 \left[\mu_2(\mu_2 x)e^{-\mu_2 x}\right], \tag{3.2.16c}$$

with the properties, $b(0) = 0$, and, as we now show, $0.5 \le C_v^2 < \infty$. In direct analogy with Equations (3.2.8b) we can write:

$$\begin{aligned} \bar{x} = \mathbb{E}[Z_2] &= 2(p_1 T_1 + p_2 T_2) \\ \mathbb{E}[Z_2^2] &= 6(p_1 T_1^2 + p_2 T_2^2) \\ \mathbb{E}[Z_2^3] &= 24(p_1 T_1^3 + p_2 T_2^3), \end{aligned} \tag{3.2.16d}$$

which we manipulate to get:

$$C_v^2 = \frac{\sigma^2}{\bar{x}^2} = \frac{1}{2} + 6\, p_1\, p_2 \left(\frac{T_1 - T_2}{\bar{x}}\right)^2. \tag{3.2.16e}$$

Clearly, when $T_1 = T_2$, $C_v^2 = 1/2$. Also, the difference between T_1 and T_2 can be made as large as desired, so C_v^2 is unbounded from above.

Next, we express T_i in terms of the parameters $\bar{x}$, C_v^2, and p_1. First let

$$\gamma = \frac{2C_v^2 - 1}{3}.$$

Then

$$\text{for } T_2 < T_1 \quad \left\{ \begin{aligned} 2T_1 &= \bar{x}\left[1 + \sqrt{p_2\,\gamma\,/\,p_1}\right] \\ 2T_2 &= \bar{x}\left[1 - \sqrt{p_1\,\gamma\,/\,p_2}\right] \end{aligned} \right\} \tag{3.2.16f}$$

but only if $p_1\,\gamma < p_2$; that is, $p_1 < 3/2(C_v^2 + 1)$. Alternatively,

$$\text{for } T_1 < T_2 \quad \left\{ \begin{aligned} 2T_1 &= \bar{x}\left[1 - \sqrt{p_2\,\gamma\,/\,p_1}\right] \\ 2T_2 &= \bar{x}\left[1 + \sqrt{p_1\,\gamma\,/\,p_2}\right] \end{aligned} \right\} \tag{3.2.16g}$$

but only if $p_2\,\gamma < p_1$; that is, $p_1 > (2C_v^2 - 1)/[2(C_v^2 + 1)]$. Only for $1/2 < C_v^2 < 2$ (or equivalently, $0 < \gamma < 1$) do both sets of equations apply.

As with the hyperexponential distribution, p_1 can be chosen so that the two Erlangians contribute the same to the mean. That is,

$$p_1\, T_1 = p_2\, T_2 = \bar{x}/4$$

$$p_{1|2} = \frac{1}{2}\left(1 \pm \sqrt{\frac{\gamma}{1+\gamma}}\right),$$

$$T_{1|2} = \frac{\bar{x}}{2}\left[1 + \gamma \mp \sqrt{\gamma(1+\gamma)}\right],$$

$$\mathbb{E}[Z_2^2] = \bar{x}^2(1 + C_v^2),$$

and

$$\mathbb{E}[Z_2^3] = \frac{2}{3}\bar{x}^3(C_v^2 + 1)(4\,C_v^2 + 1).$$

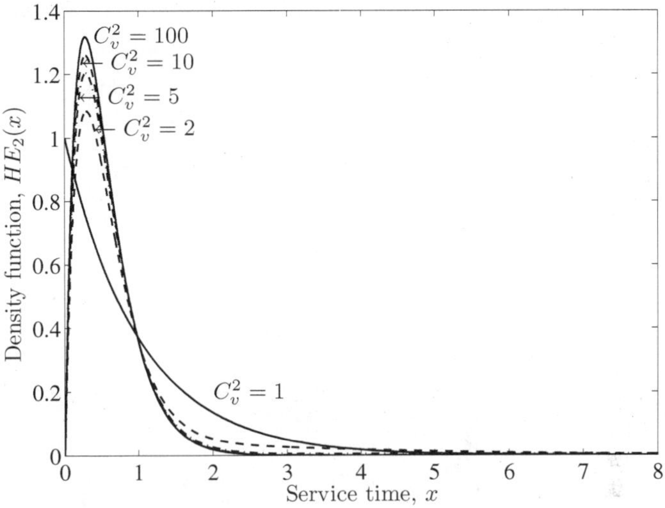

Figure 3.2.6: Density functions for a family of hyper-Erlangian-2 distributions with four phases, as defined by Equations (3.2.16). All have a mean value of 1, with $C_v^2 = 1$, 2, 5, 10, and 100, respectively. The curve corresponding to $C_v^2 = 1$ is the exponential distribution. The third condition was chosen to have the same $\mathbb{E}[X^3]$ as the hyperexponentials in Figure 3.2.3.

Note that these formulas are valid for all $1/2 \le C_v^2 < \infty$, but the third moments are somewhat different from those of the hyperexponential distributions.

Example 3.2.3: The density function in (3.2.16c) with $\bar{x} = 1$ has been plotted in Figure 3.2.6 for the same values of C_v^2 and $\mathbb{E}[X^3]$ as for the hyperexponential in Figure 3.2.3. There are several differences between the two sets of curves despite the fact that they have the same first three moments. In addition to having $b(0) = 0$ (except for the exponential curve, which is included here for comparison), most of these curves are bimodal. That is, they have two relative maxima. This cannot be seen on the regular graphs, but are clear in Figure 3.2.7 in the region $T_2 \gg T_1$.

Clearly, looks can be deceiving. Although these curves look very much like the Erlangian-2 (but with $\mathbb{E}[X] \approx 0.5$ in Figure 3.2.2), these all have $C_v^2 > 1$, whereas the Erlangian-2 has $C_v^2 = 1/2$. These functions do not even have tails similar to the corresponding ones for the $h_2(x)$ functions. They don't look alike for small x, and they don't look alike for large x (different slopes on the semilog plots), even though they have the same first three moments. ▲

In studying various queues in Chapters 4 and 5, we use this class of functions together with the hyperexponentials in order to study how different pdfs with the same first three moments can affect performance.

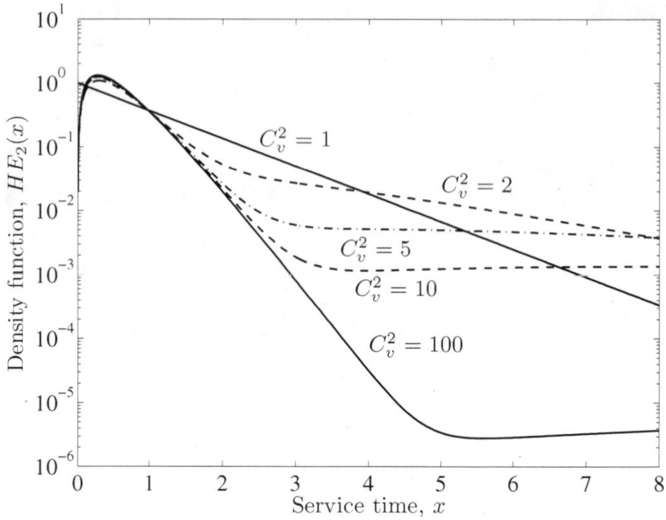

Figure 3.2.7: The same curves as in Figure 3.2.6 except that the dependent variable is $\log[HE_2(x|C_v^2)]$**.** In this form it is seen that for functions with large C_v^2, the curves reach a relative minimum and then rise again before finally going to 0 as $x \to \infty$. In other words, these functions are bimodal.

3.2.3.2 A Non PHase Distribution

We now present an interesting function, first presented by O'Cinneide [O'CINNEIDE91], whose usefulness in queueing theory has not as yet been demonstrated, but it nonetheless shows that non-PHase distributions exist.

Consider the function:

$$b(x) = c\,[1 + a\,\cos(\omega\, x + \delta)]\; e^{-\mu\, x}. \tag{3.2.17a}$$

Assume that all the constants (c, a, ω, δ, and μ) are real. Then, as long as $\mu > 0$, the function is integrable over the interval $[\,0,\, \infty\,)$. Furthermore, if $|\,a\,| \leq 1$ it follows that $b(x) \geq 0$ for all $x \geq 0$. Under these conditions, $b(x)$ is a perfect candidate to be a pdf. Subject to the constraints mentioned above, the parameters ω, δ, and μ are arbitrary, but c must be picked to satisfy:

$$\int_0^\infty b(x)\, dx = 1.$$

Note that if $a = \pm 1$ then $b(x) = 0$ for an infinite number of values of x. Neuts [NEUTS89] has shown that if a function has n roots, it must have a PH (all states are real) representation of dimension of at least n. Therefore there exists no (finite) PHase representation of this $b(x)$. But we now find an ME (complex) representation with only three states.

If one recalls the calculus, and has a table of integrals available, it is straightforward, but rather tedious, to perform the integration needed to determine c. However, with the aid of complex analysis, it is possible to rewrite

(3.2.17a) so it has the simple form of a hyperexponential distribution with three terms. First let $i = \sqrt{-1}$, and recall that:

$$e^{\pm i\,t} = \cos(t) \pm i\,\sin(t),$$

or equivalently,

$$\cos(t) = \frac{e^{i\,t} + e^{-i\,t}}{2}, \quad \text{and} \quad \sin(t) = \frac{e^{i\,t} - e^{-i\,t}}{2\,i}.$$

Then let $t = \omega\,x + \delta$ and insert the expression for $\cos(t)$ into (3.2.17a) to get

$$b(x) = c\left[1 + \frac{a}{2}\left(e^{i(\omega\,x+\delta)} + e^{-i(\omega\,x+\delta)}\right)\right]e^{-\mu\,x}.$$

Multiplying out and regrouping, we get a sum of three terms:

$$b(x) = p_1\left[\mu\,e^{-\mu\,x}\right] + p_2\left[(\mu - i\omega)e^{-(\mu-i\omega)x}\right] + p_3\left[(\mu + i\omega)e^{-(\mu+i\omega)x}\right],$$

where

$$\mathbf{p} := [\,p_1\ p_2\ p_3\,] = c\begin{bmatrix} \frac{1}{\mu} & \frac{a\,e^{i\delta}}{2(\mu - i\omega)} & \frac{a\,e^{-i\delta}}{2(\mu + i\omega)} \end{bmatrix}. \tag{3.2.17b}$$

This is exactly in the form of (3.2.7a), with the faithful ME representation, $\langle\,\mathbf{p},\,\mathbf{B}\,\rangle$, where

$$\mathbf{B} = \begin{bmatrix} \mu & 0 & 0 \\ 0 & \mu - i\omega & 0 \\ 0 & 0 & \mu + i\omega \end{bmatrix}. \tag{3.2.17c}$$

We still must find c, but that is simple enough, because $\mathbf{p}\,\boldsymbol{\epsilon}' = 1$. Evaluating this expression yields:

$$\frac{1}{c} = \frac{1}{\mu} + a\,\frac{\mu\,\cos(\delta) - \omega\,\sin(\delta)}{\mu^2 + \omega^2} = \frac{1}{\mu} + \frac{a\cos(\delta + \theta)}{\sqrt{\mu^2 + \omega^2}}, \tag{3.2.17d}$$

where $\cos\theta = \mu/\sqrt{\mu^2 + \omega^2}$. Because $\mathbf{B}$ is diagonal, it follows that

$$\mathbf{R}(x) := \exp(-x\mathbf{B}) = e^{-\mu\,x}\begin{bmatrix} 1 & 0 & 0 \\ 0 & e^{i\omega\,x} & 0 \\ 0 & 0 & e^{-i\omega\,x} \end{bmatrix}.$$

From this we can get the reliability function:

$$R(x) = \Psi[\,\mathbf{R}(x)\,]$$

$$= ce^{-\mu\,x}\left[\frac{1}{\mu} + \frac{a}{\mu^2 + \omega^2}[\mu\cos(\omega x + \delta) - \omega\sin(\omega\,x + \delta)]\right]. \tag{3.2.17e}$$

As is required, this equation satisfies $R(0) = 1$. One, of course, could get the same expression by evaluating $\int_x^\infty b(x)\,dx$. Try it.

The ***service time matrix*** **V**, is obvious, and after some work, one can write down the mean, namely:

$$\mathbb{E}[X] = \Psi[\,\mathbf{V}\,] = \int_0^\infty x\, b(x)\, dx$$

$$= c\left[\frac{1}{\mu^2} + \frac{a}{(\mu^2+\omega^2)^2}[2(\mu^2-\omega^2)\cos(\delta) + 4\,\mu\,\omega\,\sin(\delta)]\right]. \qquad (3.2.17f)$$

It's easy enough to write down the general expression for the n-th moment using (3.2.7c), but it takes some effort to express it as a manifestly real number. We leave special cases to the following example and exercise.

Example 3.2.4: In examining this function we have selected two extreme cases. Let $a = \pm 1$, $\delta = 0$, and $\omega = \mu = 1$. Then

$$b_\pm(x) := \frac{2}{2\pm 1}[1 \pm \cos(x)]e^{-x},$$

and

$$R_\pm(x) = \frac{1}{2\pm 1}\left(2 \pm [\cos(x) - \sin(x)]\right) e^{-x}.$$

Both sets of functions are plotted in Figure 3.2.8 together with e^{-x} for comparison. On Figure 3.2.9 the y-axis is presented on a log scale. In this mode, the exponential function shows up as a straight line, and the zeros of $b_\pm$ show up as downward spikes at $x = n\pi$, even n for b_+, and odd n for b_-. After some manipulation, and using $(1\pm i) = \sqrt{2}\, e^{\pm i\pi/4}$, we get the moments:

$$\mathbb{E}[X_\pm^n] = \frac{2\,n!}{2\pm 1}\left[1 \pm \frac{1+i}{4}\left(\frac{1+i}{2}\right)^n \pm \frac{1-i}{4}\left(\frac{1-i}{2}\right)^n\right]$$

$$= \frac{2\,n!}{2\pm 1}\left[1 \pm \left(\frac{1}{\sqrt{2}}\right)^{n+1} \cos[(n+1)\pi/4]\right].$$

In particular, for $n = 0$, this expression is 1. Other parameters are

$$\mathbb{E}[X_+] = \frac{2}{3}; \qquad \mathbb{E}[X_+^2] = 1; \qquad \sigma_+^2 = \frac{5}{9} \quad \text{and} \quad C_+^2 = \frac{5}{4},$$

and

$$\mathbb{E}[X_-] = 2; \qquad \mathbb{E}[X_-^2] = 5; \qquad \sigma_-^2 = 1 \quad \text{and} \quad C_-^2 = \frac{1}{4}.$$

Obviously, this class of functions can yield C_v^2 both greater than and less than 1. ▲

Exercise 3.2.3: Put in all the missing steps in deriving Equations (3.2.17). Also, redo all of Example 3.2.4, but with $\delta = \pi/2$. That is, replace $\cos(x)$ with $\sin(x)$ in $b_\pm(x)$.

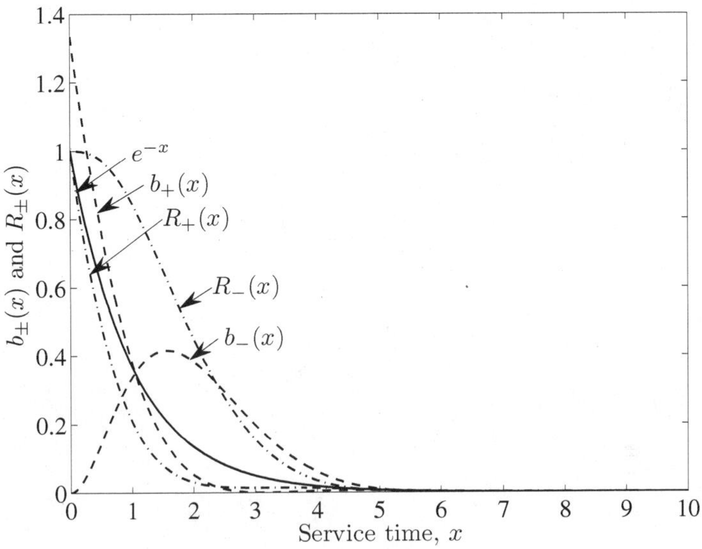

Figure 3.2.8: Density and reliability functions $b_\pm(x)$ and $R_\pm(x)$ of Equations (3.2.17), where $a = \pm 1$, $\delta = 0$, and $\mu = \omega = 1$. Although $b_\pm(x)$ increase and decrease an infinite number of times (not visible on this scale), the $R_\pm(x)$ are monotonically nonincreasing functions of x, as they must be. The exponential function, e^{-x}, is included for comparison.

3.3 Distributions With Heavy Tails

As might be presumed, and is shown in Section 3.4.2.2, all ME distributions have ***exponential tails***. The ***tail*** refers to the behavior of $R(x)$ when x is very large. That is, for ME distributions, when x is very large,

$$R(x) \rightarrow c\, x^n\, e^{-ax}.$$

In recent years there has been an increasing interest in distributions that are "not well behaved". That is, they go to 0 more slowly than ME functions. Some common terms used are *subexponential, heavy-, fat-, or long-tailed* distributions. Loosely they have the property

$$\lim_{x \to \infty} \frac{x^n\, e^{-\alpha\, x}}{R(x)} = 0, \qquad ; \forall\ \alpha > 0, \quad \text{and } \forall\ n. \tag{3.3.1a}$$

Equivalently, such functions satisfy the property:

$$\int_0^\infty e^{ax}\, R(x)\, dx = \infty \qquad \forall\ \ a > 0. \tag{3.3.1b}$$

Hence the term *subexponential.*

3.3.1 Subexponential Distributions

The expressions above are good enough for most applications, but some researchers (see e.g. [ASMUSSEN03]) have need for a tighter definition. Consider

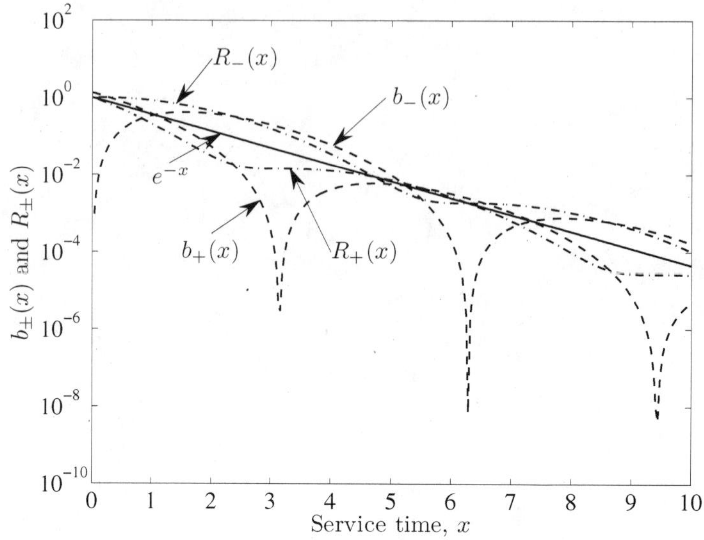

Figure 3.2.9: $\log[b_\pm(x)]$ and $\log[R_\pm(x)]$, as defined in Figure 3.2.8, as functions of x. The exponential function e^{-x} shows up as a straight line. The rapid dips of $b_\pm(x)$ actually extend infinitely downward, because $b_\pm(x) = 0$ at $x = 2n\pi$ for b_+, and $x = (2n+1)\pi$ for b_-. The corresponding $R_\pm$ has zero slope at those points.

one whose reliability function $R(x) = \mathbf{Pr}(X > x)$ satisfies the following.

$$\lim_{x\to\infty} \frac{R(x+t)}{R(x)} = 1, \qquad \forall\ t \geq 0. \tag{3.3.1c}$$

It says that if a process has been going on for a very long time $[x]$, then it is likely to last for an unboundedly longer time $[t]$.

A stronger condition, useful for studying waiting time tails is given by Asmussen [ASMUSSEN03] as

$$\lim_{x\to\infty} \frac{\mathbf{Pr}[X_1 + X_2 > x]}{\mathbf{Pr}[X_1 > x]} = 2, \tag{3.3.1d}$$

where X_1 and X_2 are independent and identically distributed.

Every function that satisfies (3.3.1c) also satisfies (3.3.1a) or (3.3.1b), but there are functions satisfying (3.3.1b) that do not satisfy (3.3.1c), so (3.3.1c) defines a class of functions that is a proper subset of the class of functions defined by (3.3.1b). The same is true for the classes defined by (3.3.1d) and (3.3.1c).

Some researchers use the term *long-tailed distribution* for functions satisfying (3.3.1c), and *subexponential* for those satisfying (3.3.1d). Others use *heavy-tailed* for functions satisfying (3.3.1a) or (3.3.1b). This can be confusing, because (3.3.1b) should be the natural owner of *subexponential.* Following [ASMUSSEN03] we summarize these terms in the following. Other definitions are also in use. See, for instance, Trivedi [TRIVEDI02] and the discussion following Definition 3.3.3 below.

Definition 3.3.1

Let L_1 be the set of functions that satisfy (3.3.1a) or (3.3.1b). That is,

$$L_1 := \{R(x) \mid (3.3.1b) \text{ is satisfied}\}.$$

Then L_1 is the set of ***heavy-tailed distributions***. Next let

$$L_2 := \{R(x) \mid (3.3.1c) \text{ is satisfied}\}.$$

Then L_2 is the set of ***long-tailed distributions***. Finally, let

$$L_3 := \{R(x) \mid (3.3.1d) \text{ is satisfied}\}$$

Members of L_3 are called ***subexponential distributions***. It can be shown [EMBR-KLUP-MIK07] that

$$L_3 \subset L_2 \subset L_1.$$

We use all the terms interchangably here, since we will never have a need to make a distinction. We also say that such functions are ***ill-behaved functions***, or ***not well behaved***. All other functions are ***well behaved***. □

Subexponential distributions can be divided into two classes: those for which $\mathbf{E}[X^\ell] < \infty$ for all ℓ, and those that have infinite moments for $\ell > \alpha > 0$. An example of the former is given here.

Example 3.3.1: An example of a function that can be heavy-tailed and has all finite moments is the ***Weibull distribution*** (see, e.g., [TRIVEDI02]). Its reliability function is given by

$$R(x) = e^{-\lambda x^a}, \quad \text{for} \quad \lambda,\ a > 0, \tag{3.3.2a}$$

with pdf

$$f(x) = -\frac{d}{dx} R(x) = \lambda\, a\, x^{a-1}\, e^{-\lambda x^a}. \tag{3.3.2b}$$

We use (3.3.1c) to get

$$\phi(t;x) := \frac{R(x+t)}{R(x)} = e^{-\lambda[(x+t)^a - x^a]} = e^{-\lambda x^a[(1+t/x)^a - 1]} \longrightarrow e^{-a\lambda t\, x^{a-1}},$$

where we have replaced $(1+t/x)^a$ with $1+at/x$, its linear Taylor approximation for large x. It is not hard to see that

$$\lim_{x\to\infty} \phi(t,x) = \begin{cases} 0 & \text{for } a > 1 \\ e^{-\lambda t} & \text{for } a = 1 \\ 1 & \text{for } a < 1 \end{cases}$$

We see then, that for $a < 1$ the Weibull distribution is subexponential (actually, heavy-tailed); for $a = 1$ it has an ***exponential tail***; and for $a > 1$ it is, shall we say, ***superexponential***. Equations (3.3.1a) and (3.3.1b) can easily be applied to yield the same conclusions, and thus, that the Weibull distributions are heavy-tailed for $a < 1$. However (3.3.1d) requires more effort.

The moments can be found by direct integration:

$$\mathbf{E}[X^\ell] = \int_0^\infty x^\ell \lambda\, a\, x^{a-1}\, e^{-\lambda x^a} = \lambda\, a \int_0^\infty x^{\ell+a+1}\, e^{-\lambda x^a}\, dx$$

$$= \left(\frac{1}{\lambda}\right)^{\ell/\alpha} \int_0^\infty u^{\ell/a} e^{-u}\, du = \left(\frac{1}{\lambda}\right)^{\ell/\alpha} \Gamma(1 + \ell/a),$$

where we made the substitution $x^a \to u$. $\Gamma(x)$ is the gamma function given by (3.2.2b). ▲

We do not dwell further on this class of functions, except to say that they can be quite troublesome in trying to solve queueing systems using matrix methods, because they need ME representations of large dimension to be approximated adequately. But they do have all their moments about them.

3.3.2 Power-Tailed (PT) Distributions

For the rest of this section we focus on distributions for which $\mathbf{E}[X^\ell] = \infty$ for ℓ greater than some $\alpha > 0$, the very troublesome, but very interesting, class of ***Power-Tailed* (PT) *distributions***. Suppose a random variable, X, has a reliability function $R(x)$ satisfying

$$R(x) \Longrightarrow \frac{c}{x^\alpha}. \tag{3.3.3a}$$

Obviously, its tail goes to 0 as some power of x, hence the term *power-tail.* Then it must have infinite moments. Its pdf satisfies

$$f(x) = -\frac{dR(x)}{dx} \Longrightarrow \frac{c\alpha}{x^{\alpha+1}},$$

implying, therefore:

$$\mathbf{E}[X^\ell] = \int_0^\infty x^\ell\, f(x)\, dx$$

$$= A(z) + c\alpha \int_z^\infty x^{\ell-1-\alpha}\, dx = \infty, \quad \text{for } \ell > \alpha, \tag{3.3.3b}$$

where z is a value for x above which the asymptotic behavior in (3.3.3a) is satisfied, and $A(z)$ is the value of the integral from 0 to z. But (3.3.3a) doesn't have to be precisely true for (3.3.3b) to be true. The more general formula,

$$\lim_{x\to\infty} x^\ell\, R(x) = \begin{cases} 0 & \text{for } \ell < \alpha \\ \infty & \text{for } \ell > \alpha \end{cases} \tag{3.3.3c}$$

is more useful (see Figure 3.3.10 below). However, a definition that reflects the property of interest is best. By integrating by parts we can show that for $\ell > 0$,

$$\mathbb{E}[X^\ell] = \int_0^\infty x^\ell \, f(x)\, dx = \ell \int_0^\infty x^{\ell-1}\, R(x)\, dx.$$

Definition 3.3.2

A random variable X is ***power-tailed with parameter***, $\boldsymbol{\alpha}$, if its reliability function $R(x)$ satisfies the following:

$$\mathbb{E}[X^\ell] = \ell \int_0^\infty x^{\ell-1}\, R(x)\, dx = \infty \quad \text{for } \ell > \alpha,$$

$$\mathbb{E}[X^\ell] = \ell \int_0^\infty x^{\ell-1}\, R(x)\, dx < \infty \quad \text{for } \ell < \alpha, \tag{3.3.3d}$$

These functions are often called ***Pareto distributions*** after the 19th-century economist, Vilfredo Pareto, who used densities of the form $cx^{\mu-1}/(1+x)^{\alpha+\mu}$ to describe the distribution of wealth in the industrialized world. They are also known as ***Lévy distributions***, or ***Lévy-Pareto distributions***, because P. Lévy defined and found the class of ***stable distributions*** that have these power-tails (but only $0 < \alpha < 2$ give non-Gaussian results). □

Feller defines a ***slowly varying function*** as one which satisfies

$$\lim_{t\to\infty} \frac{L(tx)}{L(t)} = 1.$$

He then says that $R(x)$ is ***regularly varying*** with exponent $-\alpha$ if

$$R(x) = \frac{L(x)}{x^\alpha}$$

and $L(x)$ is slowly varying. Although this is an interesting property in its own right, it is too restrictive and doesn't explain the vast number of phenomena that have PT behavior. Therefore we do not rely on this property in our presentation. See for example, [FELLER71] for a general discussion, [SAM-TAQQU94] for details about stable distributions, and [GREIN-JOB-LIP99] and [KLINGER97] for full details of material covered here.

The conclusion that a process can have infinite moments requires some discussion. If $\alpha < 2$ then X has an infinite variance, and if $\alpha < 1$ then X has an infinite mean! What does an infinite moment indicate? Or, it might be asked, why should we consider them at all? Such questions would normally be outside the scope of this book, but in recent years processes that are important in areas where queueing theory is applied seem to show this kind of behavior. Therefore we must provide some insight to PT behavior so that we can make sense of the solutions to various queues we solve in the next chapters. The rest of this section can be skipped over on first reading.

This subject has been of interest to statisticians for many years, and in recent years it has shown up in many places. It appears that the size of earthquakes, avalanches (see [BAK96]), solar flares, and white noise are power-tailed. Health insurance claims also are PT ([LOWRIE-LIP93]). Although it is considered controversial, it appears that the distribution of wealth is also power-tailed. After all, it is a fact that 1% of the population owns 40% of everything in this country, just as it did in the 19th century when Pareto did his studies. (This percentage was at its lowest in the mid 1970's when it dipped to 28% [PHILLIPS02].) In subjects closer to queueing applications, in particular computer science and telecommunications, Leland and Ott [LELAND-OTT86] found that the distribution of CPU times at BELLCORE satisfied the PT properties we discuss in this section. (The longest job took over 1,200,000 seconds, 2 weeks, whereas the mean time for the 6 million jobs measured was about 1 second.) Garg et al. [LIPGARGROBBERT92], Hatem [HATEM97], Crovella and Bestavros [CROVELLABESTAVROS96], and others have found that file sizes stored on disks, and even Web page sizes are PT for many orders of magnitude beyond the mean. In a related phenonemon, Leland et al., [LELANDETAL94], followed by many others, found that Ethernet, and telecomunications traffic generally, are ***self-similar***. If these observations are correct, then system performance prediction must be able to include power-tail behavior, or some truncated version of it.

3.3.3 What Do PT Distributions Look Like?

How can we tell that a process is PT, and why is it only recently being observed? The first question is easy enough to show, but part of the second is answered in Chapter 4. The most characteristic feature of PT distributions is masked when one looks at a plot of $R(x)$ or $B(x)$ versus x, since they are both monotonic, approaching a horizontal limit. But if one plots $\log(R(x))$ versus $\log(x)$ then one gets a straight line with slope $-\alpha$, because, from (3.3.3a),

$$\log(R(x)) \Longrightarrow \log(c) - \alpha \log(x)$$

This characteristic is unmistakable, as we now show with a simple example.

Example 3.3.2: Consider the r.v., X_a, with reliability function

$$R_a(x) = a \cdot e^{-x} + \frac{1-a}{(1+x)^2} \quad \text{for } 0 \le a \le 1. \tag{3.3.5}$$

It is easy to show that $\mathbb{E}(X_a] = 1$ for all a. But for $a < 1$, it has a power tail with $\alpha = 2$, and thus has infinite variance. Figure 3.3.1 shows this function for $a \in \{0.0, 0.5, 0.8, 1.0\}$. For $a = 1$ we have the pure exponential function, but on a normal scale (left-hand figure) the other three curves look very similar to the first, so one would expect no surprises, even though they actually have infinite variance. However, in the log-log plot (right-hand figure) the different behavior of the tails becomes visible: all three PT functions show the straight-line behavior described above, with negative slope $\alpha = 2$. ▲

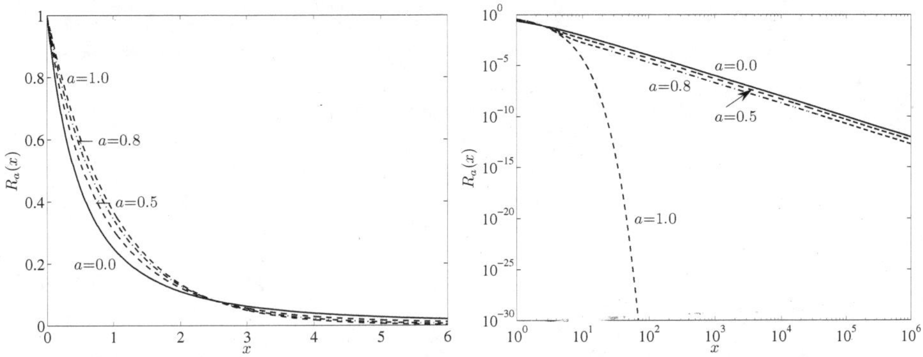

Figure 3.3.1: Four reliability functions, three with power-tails and infinite variance (plotted on both linear and log-log scale). These are all taken from Equation (3.3.5), for $a \in \{0.0, 0.5, 0.8, 1.0\}$. All the curves are equal at $\exp(x/2) = (1 + x)$, but this is just an artifact of the functional form chosen.

This characteristic can be duplicated with real data if enough data are available. Let $\{y_i \,|\, 0 \le i \le N,\, y_i \ge 0\}$, with $y_o := 0$, be a set of experimental data points of, say CPU times. Let $\{x_i\}$ be the same set of data points, reordered in size place. That is, $x_o = y_o = 0 \le x_1 \cdots \le x_n \le \cdots x_N$. Then the function

$$R_e(x \,|N) := \frac{N-n}{N}, \quad \text{for } x_n < x \le x_{n+1} \tag{3.3.4a}$$

should approach the underlying reliability function for the process being measured. That is,

$$\lim_{N\to\infty} R_e(x \,|N) = R(x) \tag{3.3.4b}$$

in the sense that $|R(x) - R_e(x \,|N)| = \mathrm{O}(1/N)$. Note that $R_e(x)$ is a monotonic non-increasing function of x, $R_e(0 \,|N) = 1$, and $R_e(x > x_N \,|N) = 0$.

As an example of the statistical behavior of (3.3.4), we have done the following simulation.

Example 3.3.3: We have simulated two sets of 1,000,000 random samples from (3.3.5) for $a = 0$. $R_o(x)$ and the two sets are plotted together in Figure 3.3.2 using the expression for $R_e(x \,|10^6)$ from (3.3.4a). The three sets of curves are very close. On a normal plot there would be little else to say, but on the log-log plot shown, the match is precise up to 100 times the mean, and we see, for both $R_e(x)$ curves, a more or less straight line stretching out for three orders of magnitude beyond the mean. The largest dozen or so points cover most of that range. This is typical of PT distributions. We discuss these data in more detail in the next few sections. ▲

3.3.4 Statistical Behavior of Large Samples

The behavior shown in the above example, together with some insight as to the significance of infinite moments, may be understood in the following way.

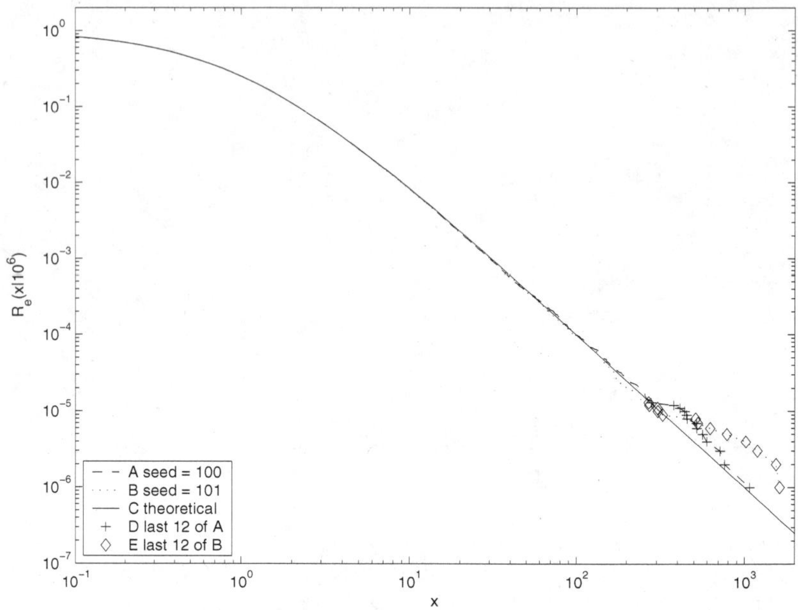

Figure 3.3.2: Comparison of $R_o(x) = 1/(1+x)^2$ and two sets of 1,000,000 randomly generated samples taken from that distribution, and presented as $R_e(x)$. On a standard (linear) plot, we would see no difference whatsoever, but even on a log-log plot the three curves are virtually indistinguishable except for the last dozen or so points. The largest 12 samples for each set are shown with +s and ◇s. There are not enough data at the end of the curve to give a smooth fit, but those last points still track the straight line. If we had sampled 10,000,000 points instead, the fit would have extended out farther.

First we discuss residual time behavior, that is, time remaining after some time has already elapsed. Trivedi [TRIVEDI02] calls this the ***conditional mean exceedance*** (CME_x).

Definition 3.3.3

Let $X_>(x)$ be the r.v. denoting the time for a task, given that it is greater than x. It is not hard to show that the mean remaining time is

$$CME_x := \mathbf{E}[X_>(x)] - x = \frac{\int_x^\infty y f(y)\,dy}{R(x)} = \frac{\int_x^\infty R(y)\,dy}{R(x)}, \qquad (3.3.6a)$$

where the last expression comes from the previous one by integrating by parts. □

Obviously, $\mathbf{E}[X_>(x)] > x$, but how much greater? If $R(x) = 0$ for $x > C$, as is the case for the uniform distribution, then $\mathbf{E}[X_>(x)]$ can never exceed C, so

$$\lim_{x \to C} \{\mathbf{E}[X_>(x)] - x\} = \lim_{x \to C} CME_x = 0. \qquad (3.3.6b)$$

One way to interpret this is to observe that as a task progresses (x increases) the expected time remaining goes to zero. This would seem to be trivially obvious, but consider the following. If $R(x)$ is exponentially distributed, say $R(x) = e^{-\mu x}$, then

$$\mathbf{E}[X_>(x)] = x + \frac{\int_x^\infty e^{-\mu y}\,dy}{e^{-\mu x}} = x + \frac{1}{\mu}.$$

In this case then,

$$\mathbf{E}[X_>(x)] - x = CME_x = \frac{1}{\mu}.$$

In other words, no matter how long a task has been running, if the task hasn't finished yet it still has time $1/\mu$ remaining. This is no more than another example of the memoryless property of the exponential distribution.

It can be shown that all ME distributions satisfy

$$\lim_{x\to\infty} CME_x = \frac{1}{\mu_K}, \tag{3.3.6c}$$

where $1/\mu_K$ is the largest eigenvalue of $\mathbf{V}$. [We might mention that μ_K must be real and positive in order for $\langle\, \mathbf{p},\, \mathbf{B}\,\rangle$ to generate a (real, positive) PDF.] In other words, the mean time remaining will approach a constant. This may be larger or smaller than the mean. For Erlangians, this is smaller, whereas for hyperexponentials it will be larger than the mean. But it is not easy to say in general which way it will go.

As implied by Definition 3.3.1, subexponential distributions have the property that

$$\lim_{x\to\infty} \{\mathbf{E}[X_>(x)] - x\} \to \infty. \tag{3.3.6d}$$

In other words, the longer a task has already taken, the longer it has yet to go. According to Trivedi [TRIVEDI02], distributions satisfying (3.3.6d) are ***heavy-tailed***. Distributions satisfying (3.3.6c) are ***medium-tailed***, and (3.3.6b) he calls ***light-tailed***. We prefer to call distributions that satisfy (3.3.6c) ***exponential-tailed distributions***.

We now look at CME_x for PT distributions. Consider (3.3.6a) and suppose that x is large enough so that (3.3.3a) is valid. Then for $\alpha > 1$

$$\begin{aligned}\mathbf{E}[X_>(x)] - x = CME_x &\approx \frac{\int_x^\infty c/y^\alpha\,dy}{c/x^\alpha}\\ &= x^\alpha \int_x^\infty \frac{dy}{y^\alpha} = \frac{x^\alpha}{\alpha-1}\frac{1}{x^{\alpha-1}} = \frac{x}{\alpha-1}.\end{aligned} \tag{3.3.7a}$$

This tells us that if a task has already lasted a time x, it's likely to last a comparable amount of time longer, and the longer it has run, the longer it is likely to run. In fact, if $1 < \alpha < 2$ the task will last an additional time longer than it has already run. Of course, if $\alpha \le 1$ the mean time is itself infinite.

The random variable $X_>(x)$ can be interpreted in a somewhat different way in examining a set of independent samples. Let us suppose that a set of N samples, $s_N := \{x_n \mid 1 \le n \le N\}$, has already been picked from $R(x)$. Then we would hope that if N is large enough, the average satisfies

$$\bar{x}(N) = \frac{1}{N}\sum_{n=1}^{N} x_n \approx \mathbf{E}[X]. \tag{3.3.7b}$$

Let

$$y_1 := \max_{x_n \in s_N} \{x_n\};$$

then we continue to pick more samples. Let Y_2 be the r.v. denoting the value of the first sample subsequently chosen that is bigger than y_1. Then $y_2 := \mathbf{E}[Y_2] = \mathbf{E}[X_>(y_1)]$, and $1/R(y_1)$ is an estimate of the number of samples chosen before the bigger sample came. Let M_1 be the actual number of new samples taken. All the other samples are less than y_1, so they collectively should not change the average very much. Let $N_2 = N + M_1 - 1$; then,

$$\bar{x}(N_2) = \frac{1}{N_2}\sum_{n=1}^{N_2} x_n$$

will probably not be much different from $\bar{x}(N)$. Only y_2 can appreciably affect the running average. But for well behaved distributions, when N is large enough y_2 is only, on average, $1/\mu_K$ bigger than y_1, whereas, N_2 is usually more than twice as big as N_1. Its contribution to the average, $R(y_1) \times y_2$ is small and goes to 0 as the number of samples increases. That is, as y_1 gets bigger, $R(y_1)$ goes to 0 faster than Y_2 goes to ∞. Put another way, when the sample size is large, out-of-range events are so rare that they have little effect on the running average.

The above statement holds true for the estimate of any moment of X, because $R(y_1)y_2^\ell \approx (y_1 + 1/\mu_K)^\ell / e^{y_1\mu_k}$ goes to zero for any ℓ. However, the number of samples must be larger with increasing ℓ for the running average to settle down.

What we have just said applies only to ***well-behaved functions***. From (3.3.7) we see that for PT functions

$$R(y_1)\mathbf{E}[X_>(y_1)]^\ell \approx \frac{c}{y_1^\alpha}\left[\frac{y_1}{\alpha-1}\right]^\ell = \frac{c}{(\alpha-1)^\ell}\, y_1^{\ell-\alpha}.$$

We see here that for $\ell > \alpha$ the contribution of y_2 to the running average is likely to grow with increasing number of samples. That is, x_N may appear to stabilize for a while [$1/R(y_1)$ new samples], but then y_2 arrives, and is so much bigger than y_1 that it causes the running average of $\{x_n^\ell\}$ to be even bigger than its previous maximum. A formal statement of this is the following. Let

$$\overline{x^\ell}(N) := \frac{1}{N}\sum_{n=1}^{N} x_n^\ell.$$

Then for $\ell < \alpha$, and for any z,

$$\mathbf{Pr}\left(\overline{x^\ell}(N) > z\right) = 1 \quad \text{for some } N \text{ large enough.}$$

This is another way of saying that if one selects enough samples, one will (almost surely) get a running average bigger than any previously chosen number, or $\lim_{N\to\infty} \overline{x^\ell}(N) = \infty$. That's the statistical meaning of $\mathbb{E}[X^\ell] = \infty$.

3.3.5 The Central Limit Theorem and Stable Distributions

In the previous section we loosely discussed the "closeness of $\bar{x}(N)$ to $\mathbb{E}[X]$." Here we give it some quantitative meaning. We invoke the ***Central Limit Theorem*** (CLT) and describe what is meant by a *stable distribution*. In particular, we show by example that distributions with finite means, but infinite variance, do not satisfy the CLT as usually applied, and thus cause problems with statistical convergence. For a fuller understanding, the books by Feller [FELLER71], and Samorodnitsky and Taqqu [SAM-TAQQU94] are necessary. We restrict ourselves to the range $1 < \alpha \le 2$.

3.3.5.1 Distributions with Finite Variance

The concept of a ***stable distribution*** is of some use in understanding the advanced literature concerning PT distributions and self-similar traffic. We follow Feller (with a slight modification) [FELLER71], in defining it now. First let $X_1, X_2, X_3, \ldots, X_n, \ldots$ be independent random variables with the same distribution $F(\cdot)$. Define the random variable corresponding to their statistical average

$$A_n := \frac{1}{n}\sum_{j=1}^{n} X_j. \tag{3.3.8}$$

Definition 3.3.4

The distribution, $F(\cdot)$***, with random variable X is Stable*** if for each n there exist constants $c_n > 0$ and γ_n such that

$$A_n \stackrel{d}{=} c_n X + \gamma_n \tag{3.3.9a}$$

and $F(\cdot)$ is not concentrated at one point. The symbol $\stackrel{d}{=}$ indicates that the r.v. on the left has the same distribution as the r.v. on the right. It can be shown that

$$c_n = \frac{1}{n^\kappa}, \quad \text{where} \quad \kappa = \begin{cases} 1 - 1/\alpha & \text{for } \alpha < 2 \\ 1/2 & \text{otherwise} \end{cases}.$$

This is the same α as the power-tail exponent if $\alpha < 2$. For all functions with finite variance, including well-behaved functions, $\kappa = 1/2$. Also, if $\alpha > 1$,

$$\gamma_n = \mathbb{E}[X].$$

What does all this mean? Well, we hope it becomes clear as we go through the rest of this section. □

If the mean and variance of $F(\cdot)$ exist, call them $\bar{x} = \mathbb{E}[X]$ and σ^2, respectively, and define the random variable

$$Z_n := n^{1/2}(A_n - \bar{x}). \tag{3.3.9b}$$

Next define the r.v.,

$$Z := \lim_{n\to\infty} Z_n.$$

The ***central limit theorem*** states that Z is ***normally distributed*** with mean of 0 and variance σ^2. Let $\phi(w) = \exp(-w^2/2)/\sqrt{2\pi}$ be the pdf of the standard normal distribution ($\bar{x} = 0$ and $\sigma = 1$), and $\Phi(w)$ be its PDF. Then for n "large enough", A_n is normally distributed with mean $\bar{x}$ and variance σ^2/n. From a measurement viewpoint, we can state that the probability that A_n will be within w standard deviations of its mean is given by

$$\mathbb{P}\mathbf{r}\left(\bar{x} - w\frac{\sigma}{\sqrt{n}} < A_n < \bar{x} + w\frac{\sigma}{\sqrt{n}}\right) = \Phi(w) - \Phi(-w) = 2\Phi(w) - 1. \tag{3.3.10a}$$

[We have used the fact that ϕ is symmetric, so $\Phi(w) = 1 - \Phi(-w)$.] Equivalently,

$$\mathbb{P}\mathbf{r}\left(\left|\frac{A_n - \bar{x}}{\bar{x}}\right| > \epsilon\right) = 2[1 - \Phi(w)] = 2\Phi(-w), \tag{3.3.10b}$$

where $\epsilon = w\sigma/(\bar{x}\sqrt{n})$ is the relative error. In other words, for a fixed probability (or fixed w), the range of $A_n - \bar{x}$ contracts as $1/\sqrt{n}$. Thus one can be 95% sure $[2\Phi(2) - 1 = .9545]$ that the average of 10,000 samples taken from a normal distribution with $\sigma = 1$ [or any other well-behaved distribution] will agree with its expectation value to within two parts in 100, (I.e., $w\sigma/\bar{x}\sqrt{n} = 2/\sqrt{10,000} = 0.02$).

Loosely speaking, we can say that

$$|A_n - \bar{x}| = \mathrm{O}\left(\frac{1}{\sqrt{n}}\right). \tag{3.3.10c}$$

This tells us that if one wants to double the accuracy (reduce ϵ to $\epsilon/2$), one must sample four times as many points.

Example 3.3.4: For demonstrative purposes, we have simulated 100,000 realizations of A_n for each of $n = 10$, 100, 1000, and 10,000. Each random number was taken from the exponential distribution with $\bar{x} = 1$. That is, $F(x) = 1 - e^{-x}$. In Figure 3.3.3, we have plotted the number of realizations of A_n that fall in each 0.1 interval. It is seen how the distribution for A_n narrows as n increases, according to (3.3.10a). The number of realizations of Z_n from (3.3.9b) (where $\mathbb{E}[Z_n] = 0$) in each 0.1 interval, is plotted in Figure 3.3.4, where it is seen that the distributions approach $\phi(x)$ (the normal distribution with 0 mean and unit variance) as n increases. The different curves visually have approximately the same width and shape, verifying that the original distributions do narrow according to $1/\sqrt{n}$. Note that even though the exponential distribution is highly unsymmetric, Z_n looks

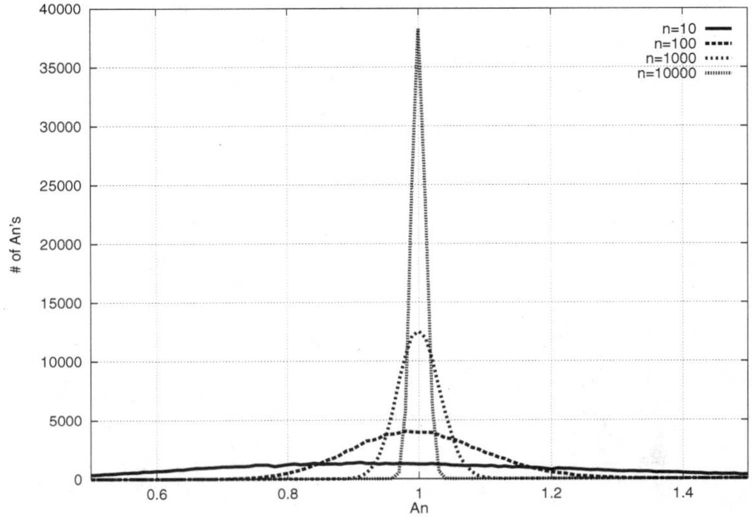

Figure 3.3.3: The measured average interarrival time for a Poisson distribution. The figure shows 100,000 samples of A_n as defined by (3.3.8), with a mean of 1.0, for $n = 10$, 100, 1000 and 10000. The curves get narrower with n, showing how the measured average approaches its mean as the number of samples increases.

symmetric, even for $n = 10$. ▲

Now let us go back to our definition of stable distributions. We see that Z is normally distributed with a mean of 0, and $\sigma^2 = 1$. Suppose we added two such normal random variables together. We know from elementary calculus that the distribution of their sum is also normal, with variance $1/2$, and a mean of 0. That is, the convolution of the normal distribution with itself is a normal distribution with one half the variance. Now look at (3.3.9a) ($c_2 = 1/\sqrt{2}$ and $\gamma_2 = 0$).

$$Z + Z \stackrel{d}{=} \frac{1}{\sqrt{2}} Z.$$

This equation says exactly the same thing. In other words, the normal distribution is stable. In fact, it is the only distribution with finite variance that is stable. As supported in Figure 3.3.4, all well-behaved functions tend toward the normal, and thus can be considered to be *asymptotically stable*, in that if n is large enough, the distribution of the sum approaches a fixed function (the ***normal distribution***).

We next see that for functions with infinite variance, an entire 4-parameter family of stable distributions must be considered.

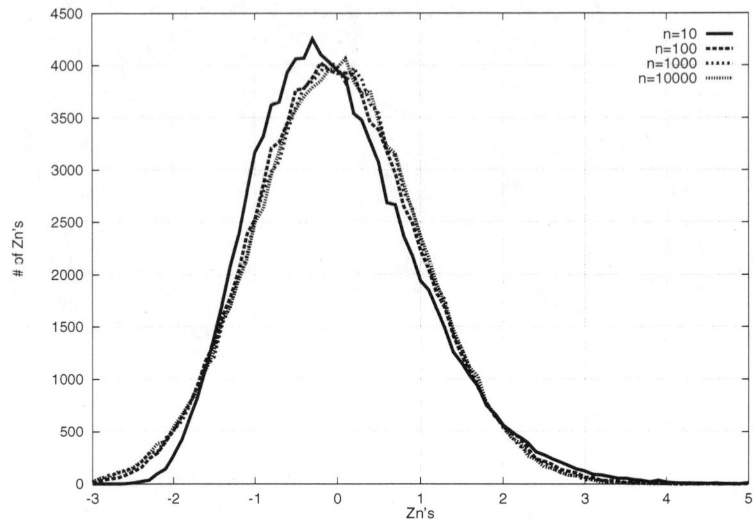

Figure 3.3.4: This figure shows curves for 100,000 samples of Z_n, matching those for A_n in Figure 3.3.3. Z_n is defined in (3.3.9b). The shapes tend toward the normal distribution with 0 mean and unit variance as n increases (see [KLINGER97])

3.3.5.2 Distributions with Infinite Variance

The problem becomes much more complex if $F(\cdot)$ has infinite variance. Various researchers have shown (see Feller [FELLER71] or Samorodnitsky and Taqqu [SAM-TAQQU94] for details) that if X is power-tailed with $1 < \alpha \leq 2$, Z_n must be modified to

$$Z_n := n^{\kappa}(A_n - \bar{x}), \quad \text{where } \kappa = 1 - 1/\alpha. \tag{3.3.11}$$

As n grows larger, Z_n approaches Z, a random variable from a 4-parameter family of distributions, the ***α-stable distributions*** described in [SAM-TAQQU94]. They label them as $S_\alpha(\sigma, \beta, \mu)$, where for $1 < \alpha < 2$, σ is a ***generalized width*** (or ***scale parameter***), μ is the mean, and β is a generalized *skewness parameter*. From its definition, Z has zero mean, and because we are here dealing only with one-sided distributions [$F(x) = 0$ for $x < 0$], it turns out that $\beta = 1$. Thus, for distributions of interest in this chapter, Z_n approaches the α-stable random variable $S_\alpha(\sigma, 1, 0)$, and thus Z has the same distribution as $S_\alpha(\sigma, 1, 0)$. That is,

$$Z = \lim_{n\to\infty} Z_n \stackrel{d}{=} S_\alpha(\sigma, 1, 0).$$

Let $\phi_\alpha(x|\,\sigma, 1, 0)$ be the pdf for $S_\alpha(\sigma, 1, 0)$, and $\Phi_\alpha(x|\,\sigma, 1, 0)$ be its PDF, satisfying

$$\Phi_\alpha(x|\,\sigma, 1, 0) := \int_{-\infty}^{x} \phi_\alpha(x'|\,\sigma, 1, 0)\, dx'.$$

For convenience, we also define the reliability function

$$R_\alpha(x|\,\sigma,1,0) := 1 - \Phi_\alpha(x|\,\sigma,1,0).$$

That σ is a scale parameter is verified by the following property.

$$\phi_\alpha(x|\,\sigma,1,0) = \frac{1}{\sigma}\phi_\alpha(x/\sigma|\,1,1,0),$$

or equivalently,

$$\begin{aligned}\Phi_\alpha(x|\,\sigma,1,0) &= \Phi_\alpha(x/\sigma|\,1,1,0) \quad \text{and}\\ R_\alpha(x|\,\sigma,1,0) &= R_\alpha(x/\sigma|\,1,1,0).\end{aligned}$$

From [SAM-TAQQU94], $S_\alpha(\sigma,1,0)$ has the following behavior for large x,

$$\lim_{x\to\infty} R_\alpha(x|\,\sigma,1,0) = C_\alpha\left(\frac{\sigma}{x}\right)^\alpha, \tag{3.3.12a}$$

where

$$C_\alpha = \frac{\alpha-1}{\Gamma(2-\alpha)|\cos(\pi\alpha/2)|}. \tag{3.3.12b}$$

As x goes to $-\infty$, $\Phi_\alpha(x)$ has the property (drops very rapidly to 0)

$$\lim_{x\to-\infty}[\Phi_\alpha(x|\,1,1,0)] = \mathrm{O}\left(\frac{\exp\left[-c_2(\alpha)|x|^\varphi\right]}{|x|^{\varphi/2}}\right), \tag{3.3.12c}$$

where $\varphi := \alpha/(\alpha-1)$. The equations in V. M. Zolotarev [ZOLOTAREV86] imply that

$$\Phi_\alpha(0|1,1,0) = \frac{1}{\alpha} \quad \text{for } 1<\alpha<2. \tag{3.3.12d}$$

That is, the probability that a given sample will be below the mean is $1/\alpha$, which is greater than 1/2. This seems to agree with our simulations and with the tables in [DUMOUCHEL71]. This formula also shows that for $\alpha = 2$, $\Phi_2(0|\,1,1,0) = 1/2$, agreeing with our knowledge that $\Phi_2(x|\,1,\beta,0)$ is symmetric for all β. However, as $\alpha \Rightarrow 1_+$, the probability that a single sample will be less than the mean approaches 1. In other words, very few samples will be greater than the mean, but, boy will they be big. Of course, for $\alpha \le 1$ there is no mean, so for such cases, the formula is meaningless.

The generalization of (3.3.10a) is given by

$$\mathbf{Pr}\left(\bar{x} - w\frac{\sigma}{n^\kappa} < A_n < \bar{x} + \frac{\sigma}{n^\kappa}\right) = \Phi_\alpha(w|\,1,1,0) - \Phi_\alpha(-w|\,1,1,0) \tag{3.3.13a}$$

for n large enough. To demonstrate this, Klinger [KLINGER97] performed calculations similar to those used for Figures 3.3.3 and 3.3.4, but for the power-tail function given in Section 3.3.6.2 below. He set $\bar{x} = 1$ and $\alpha = 1.4$. The results are displayed in Figures 3.3.5 and 3.3.6. He was also able to calculate the generalized width to be $\sigma = 0.581259\ldots$. The partial curve in Figure 3.3.6 is for $S_{1.4}(0.581259,1,0)$, as given by [DUMOUCHEL71]. For full details, see [KLINGERETAL97].

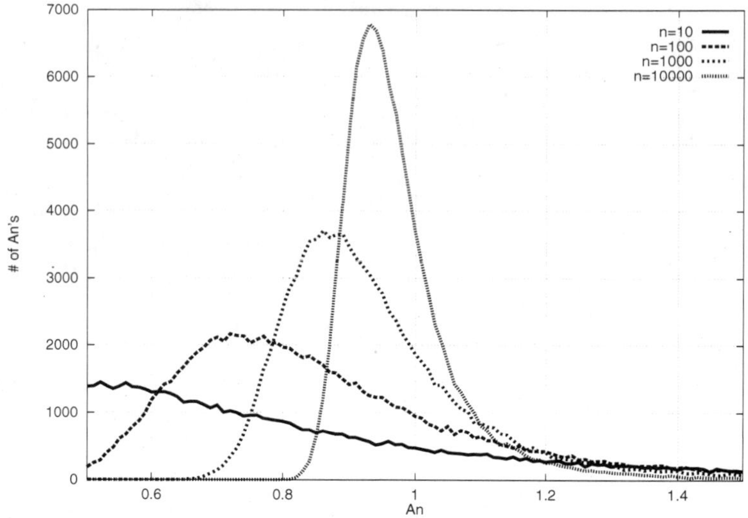

Figure 3.3.5: 100,000 samples of the average of n power-tail samples of A_n, for $n = 10$, 100, 1000, and 10,000. The PT distribution function is taken from Section 3.3.6.2, with $\bar{x} = 1$, $\alpha = 1.4$, and $\theta = 0.5$. The scale parameter σ was measured to be ≈ 0.58126 (this is not the standard deviation, which is infinite because $\alpha < 2$; see text and [KLINGERETAL97]). Note how broad the curves are, even for the average of 10,000 samples.

There are several interesting features displayed in Figure 3.3.5. First observe how broad the distributions are, even for $n = 10,000$. Next note that the peaks occur well below the mean, indicating that most measurements (realizations of A_n) will underestimate the mean. Third, observe that the distributions do not tend to become symmetric, a consequence of the one-sidedness of $R_Y(x)$ [$R_Y(x) = 0$ for $x < 0$]. Next, it can be seen from Figure 3.3.6 that the Z_n for different n have more or less the same width, with peaks at about the same position, albeit of different heights. They clearly are approaching the α-stable distribution for $S_\alpha(\sigma, 1, 0)$, but more slowly than well-behaved functions approach the normal distribution. This also demonstrates that the distributions become narrower as n increases, according to $1/n^\kappa$. Last, it appears that convergence to the α-stable distribution starts at the tail (very large x) and gradually converges below the mean [$\mathbb{E}[Z_n] = 0$].

There is further discussion of convergence in the next section. But before going on, observe that if $(X - \bar{x}) \stackrel{d}{=} S_\alpha(\sigma, 1, 0)$ [i.e., if X is itself an α-stable variable, which strictly speaking, can't be if $F(\cdot)$ is one-sided, see below], then $Z_n \stackrel{d}{=} S_\alpha(\sigma, 1, 0)$ for all n, or

$$(A_n - \bar{x}) \stackrel{d}{=} S_\alpha(\sigma/n^\kappa, 1, 0). \tag{3.3.13b}$$

Therefore the random variables, $A_1, A_2, A_3, \ldots, A_n, \ldots$ have distributions that are similar in that they have the same shape, differing only by the scale σ/n^κ

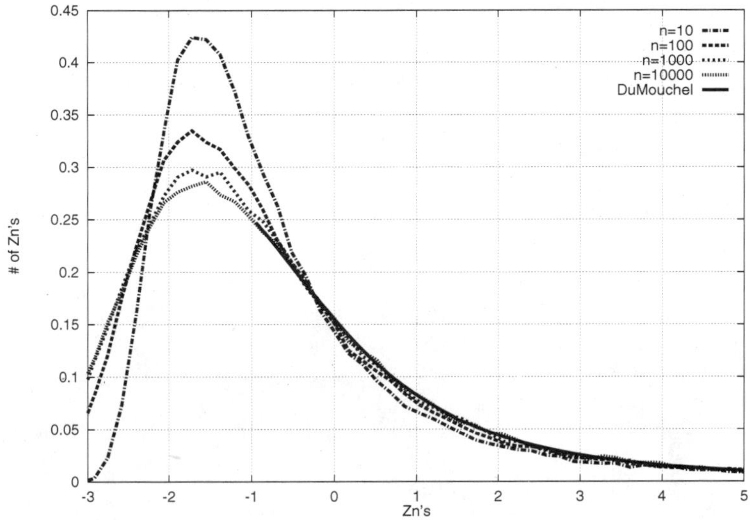

Figure 3.3.6: The sample sets of Figure 3.3.5 were modified by (3.3.11) to get samples of Z_n, where $\mathbb{E}[Z_n] = 0$. The most salient features are: the curves do not approach a symmetric limit; the peaks occur at $\approx -\alpha$; the power-tail behavior is still there. The $\alpha-$stable distribution, taken from [DUMOUCHEL71], is also plotted, but only for $Z \geq -1$.

(see Definition 3.2.1). In this sense, $A_n - \bar{x}$ is ***self-similar*** (S-S). But because $Z = \lim Z_n$ for any distribution $F(\cdot)$, one can say that every distribution is *asymptotically self-similar.* This is again a generalization of the CLT which states that all sums of random variables with finite variance approach the normal distribution (Compare Figures 3.3.4 and 3.3.6). However, the term, ***self-similar***, is reserved for distributions with infinite variance, the α-stable distributions $S_\alpha(\sigma, \beta, \mu)$.

Admittedly, this material may be difficult to absorb, and one should read [SAM-TAQQU94] and [FELLER71] for greater insight to this subject. However, for our purposes, we can summarize all this by the generalization of (3.3.10c). Thus, the deviation of a measured average from its mean satisfies

$$|A_n - \bar{x}| = \mathrm{O}\left(\frac{1}{n^\kappa}\right), \tag{3.3.13c}$$

where κ is given in Definition 3.3.4. Equation (3.3.10c) told us that if a distribution is well behaved (and $\kappa = 1/2$), then a factor of two increase in accuracy requires four times as many data points. But if $\alpha < 2$, the number of samples needed is much bigger. A typical value for α as seen in data-file sizes or CPU times is $\alpha \approx 1.4$. In this instance, $\kappa = 1 - 1/1.4 = 2/7 = .2857$. In order for $|A_{n_2} - \bar{x}|$ to be half as large as $|A_{n_1} - \bar{x}|$, according to (3.3.13c) it is required that

$$\frac{n_2^\kappa}{n_1^\kappa} = 2,$$

or for $\kappa = 1 - 1/\alpha = 1 - 1/1.4 = .4/1.4 = 2/7$,

$$\left(\frac{n_2}{n_1}\right) = 2^{1/\kappa} = 2^{3.5} = 11.3137.$$

That is, one would need over 11 times as many samples to increase accuracy by a factor of 2. We pursue this further in the next section.

3.3.5.3 Stable Distributions and Measured Averages

From (3.3.13a) and Figure 3.3.5, it can be seen that as with *normal* distributions, for fixed w, as n is increased the range of $(A_n - \bar{x})$ contracts for PT distributions, but now as $1/n^\kappa$. Because $\kappa < 1/2$ the contraction iwith increasing n is much slower than for distributions with finite variance. Furthermore, because $R_\alpha(x|\,\sigma, 1, 0)$ drops off as $1/x^\alpha$, there will always be a nonnegligible probability that the deviation will be large. In other words, no matter how large w is chosen to be, there will always be a non-negligible (i.e., power-tail law) probability that the error bound will be exceeded, but on the high side only. To give some practical meaning to this, consider the following hypothetical situation.

Suppose that responses to requests over the Internet are sent in some orderly fashion (e.g., a burst of packets with exponential interarrival times - Poisson arrivals), but that the amount of data (in packet units) in each burst-response is distributed according to a PT distribution $F(\cdot)$, with mean $\bar{x}$ and parameter α. A potential design criterion could be to create a host node that can handle a given traffic rate λ (in packets/sec), for some specified time interval, with the understanding that it will sometimes be exceeded by more than fraction δ. p is the probability that it will be exceeded. Let A_n be the r.v. denoting the average number of packets contained in each of n successive bursts (i.e., $A_n \times n$ is the total number of packets). Then,

$$\mathbf{Pr}(A_n > \bar{x} + w\sigma/n^\kappa) = R_\alpha(w|\,1, 1, 0),$$

where σ is the generalized width of $F(\cdot)$. We have assumed that n is large enough so that the difference between the distributions for Z_n and Z is negligible, an assumption that must still be investigated. Based on their definitions, p and δ must satisfy

$$p = R_\alpha(w|\,1, 1, 0), \quad \text{and} \quad \delta = w\sigma/(\bar{x}\, n^\kappa). \tag{3.3.14}$$

The equation for p allows us to find w, and then the equation for δ allows us to solve for n, the number of burst-responses needed to have the specified stability. n/λ is the mean time interval one must wait for the n bursts to arrive.

To see how this works, we set $p \in \{0.1,\ 0.05,\ 0.01\}$; $\delta = 0.1$, $\bar{x} = \sigma = 1.0$, and solved for $T = n/\lambda$ for various values of α. The following table gives the values of w, as a function of p and α. The entries for $\alpha = \infty$ are for the normal distribution.

Table 3.3.1 : w as a Function of p and α.
(w is the Number of "Standard Deviations" One Must Go Above The Mean to Get a Reliability of p.)

α	$1/\kappa$	$p = 0.10$	$p = 0.05$	$p = 0.01$
∞	2.0	1.281	1.644	2.32
2.0	2.0	1.812	2.326	3.29
1.5	3.0	2.146	3.824	11.65
1.4	3.5	2.209	4.343	15.08
1.1	11.0	−0.521	4.355	36.81

Note that for $\alpha = 1.1$, the entry for $p = 0.1$ is negative. This is a consequence of (3.3.12d), where it is seen that Z_n falls below 0 over 90% of the time $(1/\alpha = 1/1.1 = 0.90909 \cdots > 1 - p)$.

The next table shows T in seconds, as a function of p and α. For convenience, $\lambda = 328.48$ bursts, or requests/second was chosen.

Table 3.3.2 : Time (in Seconds) Needed for a System to Stabilize to a Given Probability, p.

α	$p = 0.10$	$p = 0.05$	$p = 0.01$
∞	0.500	0.823	1.639
2.0	1.000	1.647	3.295
1.5	30.087	170.233	4,813.587
1.4	154.233	1,643.446	128,202.284
1.1	–	1.03×10^8 years	5×10^{20} years

We see that under normal operations (Poisson arrivals) for intervals of 0.5 seconds, only one interval in ten will have an arrival rate greater than $(1 + \delta)\lambda = 1.1 \times \lambda$. If the measurement interval is increased to 1.639 seconds, then only one such interval in a hundred will see an arrival rate greater than $1.1 \times \lambda$. The story is entirely different for PT processes. For $\alpha = 1.5$ an interval of 30.087 seconds must be taken for overloads to occur in only one interval in 10. To reduce that to one interval in one hundred, intervals of over one hour in duration are required. If $\alpha = 1.4$, then the situation worsens by an order of magnitude, and for $\alpha = 1.1$, the concept of stability no longer exists!

3.3.6 Truncated Power-Tailed (TPT) Distributions

Many researchers have argued that PT distributions cannot actually exist. After all, we live in a finite world, and there must be a biggest member of any set. In principle, this may be true for items such as file sizes that are presently in existence, but it certainly cannot apply to such items as program execution time, if one replaces the concept of ∞ with ***unboundedness***. Yes it's true that only a finite number of programs have run since computers were invented, and therefore there must be one that ran for the longest time (not counting the ones that are still running, a nontrivial complication). But that does not guarantee that a future program will not run even longer. In fact we can be sure that ultimately many will. In other words, the size of execution times to come is unbounded. (That's also true of files to come, but we are usually interested in files that presently exist.)

3.3.6.1 Truncation and Range of a Distribution

What we are really interested in is finding a function that represents well the behavior of a given process that produces a large number of samples. If that process is well behaved, then it doesn't make any difference whether the domain of $F(\cdot)$ is allowed to be finite or infinite. (See Section 3.3.4 for further discussion.) If for instance, $F(x) = 1 - e^{-x}$, then the probability that we will ever get a sample more than 50 times greater than the mean is $e^{-50} = 1.93 \times 10^{-22}$. If we selected a sample from this distribution every nanosecond, it would take over 160,000 years before even one such sample is likely to occur. Therefore, the debate between finite and infinite extent is meaningless. Thus the practical people let us theoreticians integrate from 0 to ∞ without any worries.

The problem is quite different when we are dealing with PT functions, because, as shown in Section 3.3.4, very big samples occur often enough to affect system averages. For $R(x) = 1/(1+x)^2$, a sample greater than 50 times the mean would occur once every 2500 times, or 400 times in a million samples. In fact, a sample more than 1000 times the mean would very likely occur in a million samples, as occurred more than once in Figure 3.3.2. We are really dealing with two issues that are interrelated.

(1) Is the distribution limited in range (or at least does it have an exponentially decaying tail; i.e., is it well behaved)?

(2) Will the system of interest be measured long enough to produce a number of samples N sufficient to produce a stable average, as in (3.3.7b)?

If both are true, then we can say that the ***system is in its steady state.*** If (2) is false, then the system is still in its ***transient region***. If (1) is not true, then (2) may never be true, no matter what N is.

The trouble is, unless there are good theoretical reasons, we can never really know if either of (1) and (2) is true. After all, it would take an infinite number of samples (and an infinite amount of time) to test the entire tail. The best that can be done is to collect data, and do some statistical analysis. One direct way is to plot the data according to (3.3.4a) on a log-log scale, as was done in Figure 3.3.2. If the process is well behaved, *and* enough samples have been taken, then the curve will drop rapidly above some value of $x = x_r$, which we might call the ***Range of the distribution***. In Figure 3.3.1 we see that the exponential curve ($a = 1$) drops rapidly for $x > 2$, whereas, the other curves never drop below a straight line. Figure 3.3.2 shows that the two $R_e(x|10^6)$ curves don't drop rapidly, they just stop at about $x = 1074.47$ and $x = 1624.53$, respectively. (Remember that $\bar{x} = 1$, we're seeing events that are over 1000 times the mean.) Does this mean that:

(1) 1624.53 is the largest value that will ever be seen (rigid cutoff); or

(2) Only somewhat larger values will be seen (exponential drop in the curve); or

(3) Much larger values will occur as the number of samples increases (the curve continues in a straight line); or

(4) The curve will take some other unknown path?

Of course, without taking any further measurements, we can't tell which of the four will happen. But surely the third option is most likely, at least for one more unit to the right. Since this is a logarithmic scale, multiple samples bigger than 5000 would be expected in the course of selecting another 10,000,000 samples.

Suppose that there are about 10^6 events in the course of the busy part of any given day. Then the two sets of samples of Figure 3.3.2 could be considered typical days. But one day in ten (a total of 10^7 events) there will be one or more events that are over 5000 time units. So if we used either of these data sets as the model for a typical day, one day in ten would be very much *out of the ordinary*.

The example we have chosen has $\alpha = 2$, so although it (just barely) has an infinite variance, it has a finite mean that can be measured with the same accuracy as well-behaved functions. That is, given that $\kappa = 1 - 1/\alpha = 1 - 1/2 = 1/2$, (3.3.10c) applies. For instance, the measured parameters for the two sample sets have averages of $\bar{x}_1 = 0.998606$ and $\bar{x}_2 = 0.996596$, respectively. Both are within a few parts per thousand of each other and of the true mean, satisfying $O(1/\sqrt{10^6}) = 1/1000$. However, the variances of the two sets are, respectively, $\text{Var}_1 = 11.7748$ and $\text{Var}_2 = 16.3986$. Clearly, these give no reasonable estimate of anything. If we had chosen a function that has $\alpha < 2$, then $\bar{x}_1$ and $\bar{x}_2$ would not be so close to each other or the theoretical mean, and Var_1 and Var_2 would both most likely be much bigger (depending on α) and much further apart. In choosing $\alpha = 2$ we demonstrated the best of the worst.

Let us construct a truncated test function version of $R(x) = 1/(1+x)^2$, with random variable $X_T(x_r)$, that satisfies (2) above as follows.

$$R_T(x|x_r) = \begin{cases} 1/(1+x)^2 & \text{for} \quad x < x_r \\ e^{(1-x/x_r)}/(1+x_r)^2 & \text{for} \quad x > x_r \end{cases}, \tag{3.3.15}$$

where x_r is the range of $R_T(x|x_r)$. It can be shown that

$$\mathbf{E}[X_T] = 1 - \frac{1}{(1+x_r)^2}$$

and

$$\mathbf{E}[X_T^2] = 2\,\log(x_r + 1) + \frac{2x_r(1+3x_r)}{(1+x_r)^2}.$$

If we let $x_r = 1624.53$, then this function very well represents the second set of data, but it may be a little too extended for the first set. Plugging into the above equations, we get:

$$\mathbf{E}[X_T(1624.53)] = 0.999,999,620, \quad \mathbf{E}[X_T(1074.45)] = 0.999,999,135,$$

and

$$\sigma^2(1624.53) = 19.781, \qquad \sigma^2(1074.45) = 18.952.$$

Obviously, any value picked for x_r that's in this range or bigger will have a negligible affect on the measured mean, but the variance grows as $\log(x_r)$, and any performance parameters that depend on the variance will be affected strongly by what is selected for x_r. If we had chosen a function with $1 < \alpha < 2$ then even the mean, although it exists, would be unstable to numerical measurement, and the variance would grow linearly with x_r. In the following chapters we give numerous examples of various performance parameters that depend heavily on the variance (and higher moments), and even other factors such as the value of the pdf near $x = 0$.

So the big question for this section is: "What value for x_r should be chosen for a given application?" This has not been studied significantly until now, but it is worthy of serious research. In any case, based on what has been discussed here, we summarize what can be said at present about TPT distributions with respect to x_r.

First determine how many events $[N]$ are likely to occur during the time period of interest. If the distribution is truly truncated, and:

(1) the number of events is large enough for samples comparable to or bigger than x_r to occur $[N > 1/R(x_r)]$, then standard steady-state analytic techniques or simulations will give acceptable results for describing performance during a typical time period; or

(2) the number of events is too small for events as big as x_r to occur even once with significant probability, then for more accurate results, methods designed for transient systems should be used if possible. As a first approximation, reduce x_r to match the sample size and apply standard steady-state techniques. The results should be interpreted as good "most of the time," with the expectation that once in a while performance will be much worse. How often? About once in every $1/(1 - (F(\hat{x}_r))^N)$ time periods, where $\hat{x}_r$ is the range that matches the sample size. How bad the extreme periods are likely to be depends upon x_r. The bigger x_r is, the worse the extreme periods are likely to be.

Note that if $x_r \gg \hat{x}_r$, then it is not possible to tell the difference between a truncated tail and an infinite one. The extreme periods will occur equally often, and will be very different from the "usual" periods. To put this into everyday perspective, consider the occurence of earthquakes (the size of earthquakes have been measured to be PT over at least 10 orders of magnitude of energy released). On most days the subterranean earth moves very little, and no quakes, or quakes that measure less than 3.0 on the Richter scale occur. Thus no public action is needed. But every few years an earthquake of > 7.0 occurs, causing serious damage. In terms of planning, it is of no interest to be told that quakes of size > 12.0 can never occur.

3.3.6.2 An ME Representation of a TPT Distribution

In the previous section we examined reasons why we should look at truncated versions of PT distributions, and showed in (3.3.15) that truncation was easy enough to implement if an appropriate choice could be made for the range $[x_r]$ of the process. However, when one takes integrals involving such functional forms (i.e., functions that explicitly have terms such as $1/x^\alpha$), numerical techniques often must be used. Furthermore, they are ill-suited for use in Markov-type modeling. In particular, they are not ME distributions.

In this section we present a model that mimics in a simple way what could be causing PT behavior. It thus gives some insight as to why power-tails occur. At the same time it provides us with a functional form (first introduced in [LIPSKY86]) that has a power-tail, can be truncated, and, depending on the base function used, can be matrix-exponential, and thus can be used for analytic Markov modeling. The contents of this section are taken from [GREIN-JOB-LIP99].

First consider the following scenario, a variant of which was known in the eighteenth century as Bernoulli's ***St. Petersberg paradox*** [JENSEN67]. Suppose a typical computer user chooses to run a program whose CPU time is best described by a distribution function $F_o(x)$, with a mean of 1.0 seconds. After receiving the result, he decides, with probability 1/2, to run the program again, but with modifications that increase its CPU time by a factor of 2. After receiving the second result, he decides (again with probability 1/2) whether to run the program yet again, with more modifications which increase its CPU time by another factor of 2. Even if this looping continued indefinitely, only 1/2 the users would run their programs more than once, only 1 in 4 users would run their programs more than twice, and less than 1 in a thousand $(1/2^{10})$ would run their programs more than 10 times. Call each run a *job*. On average, each user will only run two jobs. So, the frequent user is not common, yet the ***mean CPU time*** per job grows unboundedly. If all the jobs executed are taken collectively, then 1/2 of them will be first runs, 1/4 will be second runs, and so on. The mean time per job is given by:

$$\bar{x} = \frac{1}{2} \cdot 1 + \frac{1}{4} \cdot 2 + \frac{1}{8} \cdot 4 + \frac{1}{16} \cdot 8 + \cdots + = \frac{1}{2} + \frac{1}{2} + \frac{1}{2} + \frac{1}{2} + \cdots = \infty.$$

Of course, it would take an infinite amount of time and an infinite number of users for this sum to be complete. But what would be seen over time is a user behavior that seems to stabilize (an average of two runs per user), but with the infrequent arrival of very big jobs, that get bigger, and cause the mean CPU time per use to grow ever bigger as well. This is a reasonable qualitative description of power-tail behavior generally, where "ℓ-th moment" $(\ell \geq \alpha)$ replaces "mean CPU time."

A formal mathematical description of the above process is as follows. Let $X_o, X_1, \ldots X_n, \ldots$ be random variables representing the time for the n-th rerun of a program, given that it will run at least that many times (X_o is the initial run, X_1 is the first rerun, etc.). Let $F_n(x)$ be the distribution function for X_n, with reliability function $R_n(x)$, and density function $f_n(x)$. Next, let

$0 < \theta_n \le 1$ be the conditional probability that a program will be run at least one more time, given that it ran n times. Now define

$$\gamma_n := \mathbf{E}[X_n]/\mathbf{E}[X_{n-1}].$$

For the example just given, we have for $n > 0$, $\theta_n = 1/2$, $\gamma_n = 2$, and $\mathbf{E}[X_o] = 1$.

For notational convenience, we define

$$\theta(n) := \theta_1\theta_2 \cdots \theta_n$$

starting with $\theta_o := 1$, $\theta(0) := 1$, and

$$\gamma(n) := \gamma_1\gamma_2 \cdots \gamma_n = \mathbf{E}[X_n]/\mathbf{E}[X_o].$$

Then

$$\Theta_T := \sum_{n=0}^{T-1} \theta(n), \tag{3.3.16a}$$

where Θ_T is the expected number of times a user will run a program (original or modified), with up to $T-1$ modifications. The random variable Y_T given by

$$Y_T := \frac{1}{\Theta_T} \sum_{n=0}^{T-1} \theta(n) X_n \tag{3.3.16b}$$

represents the CPU time of a program, among all those that have not run more than N jobs. The distribution function for Y_T is given by

$$F_{Y_T}(x) = \frac{1}{\Theta_T} \sum_{n=0}^{T-1} \theta(n) F_n(x), \tag{3.3.16c}$$

with mean

$$\mathbf{E}[Y_T] = \frac{\mathbf{E}[X_o]}{\Theta_T} \sum_{n=0}^{T-1} \theta(n)\gamma(n). \tag{3.3.16d}$$

These formulas are far too rich in parameters for our expository purposes, so we now make some simplifying assumptions. We point out, however, that the power-tail behavior we demonstrate is valid for this general expression as long as $\theta(n) \to 0$ and $\gamma(n) \to \infty$, with $1 \ge \theta_n \ge a > 0$ and $\gamma_n \ge b > 1$, for some infinite subset of the positive integers, and for some a and b.

Assume that

$$\theta_n = \theta \quad \text{and} \quad \gamma_n = \gamma \qquad \text{for all } n > 0. \tag{3.3.17a}$$

Then $\theta(n) = \theta^n$, and $\gamma(n) = \gamma^n$. Consequently,

$$\Theta_T = \sum_{n=0}^{T-1} \theta^n = \frac{1-\theta^T}{1-\theta}. \tag{3.3.17b}$$

For demonstrative purposes let us make the simplifying assumption that all the $F_n(x)$s have the same shape as $F_o(x)$, and that $F_o(x)$ is well behaved. That is,

$$F_n(x) = F_o(x/\gamma^n), \quad \text{and thus } \mathbf{E}(X_n] = \gamma^n \mathbf{E}[X_o] \quad \forall \quad n. \tag{3.3.18a}$$

The corresponding formula for $R_n(x)$ is obvious, but

$$f_n(x) = \gamma^{-n} f_o(x/\gamma^n). \tag{3.3.18b}$$

The density function for Y_T becomes

$$f_{Y_T}(x) = \frac{1-\theta}{1-\theta^T} \sum_{n=0}^{T-1} \left(\frac{\theta}{\gamma}\right)^n f_o(x/\gamma^n), \tag{3.3.19a}$$

with reliability function

$$R_{Y_T}(x) = \frac{1-\theta}{1-\theta^T} \sum_{n=0}^{T-1} \theta^n R_o(x/\gamma^n). \tag{3.3.19b}$$

We presently show that these are TPT distributions. They are well behaved if $R_o(x)$ is, and converge to

$$f(x|\theta, \gamma) := \lim_{T\to\infty} f_{Y_T}(x) = (1-\theta) \sum_{n=0}^{\infty} \left(\frac{\theta}{\gamma}\right)^n f_o(x/\gamma^n), \tag{3.3.20a}$$

and

$$R(x|\theta, \gamma) := \lim_{T\to\infty} R_{Y_T}(x) = (1-\theta) \sum_{n=0}^{\infty} \theta^n R_o(x/\gamma^n). \tag{3.3.20b}$$

Although $R_{Y_T}(\cdot)$ is well behaved for all T, the limit function $R(x)$ is not (see Definition 3.3.1). The moments of $F_{Y_T}(\cdot)$ are easy to find. From the definition,

$$\mathbf{E}[Y_T^\ell] = \frac{1-\theta}{1-\theta^T} \sum_{n=0}^{T-1} \left(\frac{\theta}{\gamma}\right)^n \int_o^\infty x^\ell f_o(x/\gamma^n)\, dx.$$

We make the substitution, $x = u\gamma^n$, and get

$$\begin{aligned} \mathbf{E}[Y_T^\ell] &= \frac{1-\theta}{1-\theta^T} \sum_{n=0}^{T-1} \left(\frac{\theta}{\gamma}\right)^n \gamma^{n(\ell+1)} \int_o^\infty u^\ell f_o(u)\, du \\ &= \frac{1-\theta}{1-\theta^T} \sum_{n=0}^{T-1} (\theta\gamma^\ell)^n \, \mathbf{E}[X_o^\ell], \end{aligned}$$

and finally,

$$\mathbf{E}[Y_T^\ell] = \frac{1-\theta}{1-\theta^T} \cdot \frac{1-(\theta\gamma^\ell)^T}{1-\theta\gamma^\ell} \cdot \mathbf{E}[X_o^\ell]. \tag{3.3.21}$$

As long as $\theta\,\gamma^{\ell} < 1$, the limit can be taken to get (where $Y := \lim Y_T$)

$$\mathbb{E}[Y^{\ell}] := \lim_{T\to\infty} \mathbb{E}[Y_T^{\ell}] = \frac{1-\theta}{1-\theta\,\gamma^{\ell}} \cdot \mathbb{E}[X_{\rm o}^{\ell}]. \tag{3.3.22a}$$

But if $\theta\,\gamma^{\ell} \geq 1$ the limit diverges (infinite moments). We identify α by the relation

$$\theta\,\gamma^{\alpha} = 1 \quad \text{or} \quad \alpha := -\frac{\log(\theta)}{\log(\gamma)}. \tag{3.3.22b}$$

This is the same α as in Definition 3.3.2, leading to the typical power-tail relation for moments:

$$\mathbb{E}[Y^{\ell}] < \infty \quad \Longleftrightarrow \quad \ell < \alpha. \tag{3.3.22c}$$

Therefore, for any well-behaved $f(x)$, Y is power-tailed.

Example 3.3.5: We now give a specific example of (3.3.19b). Let

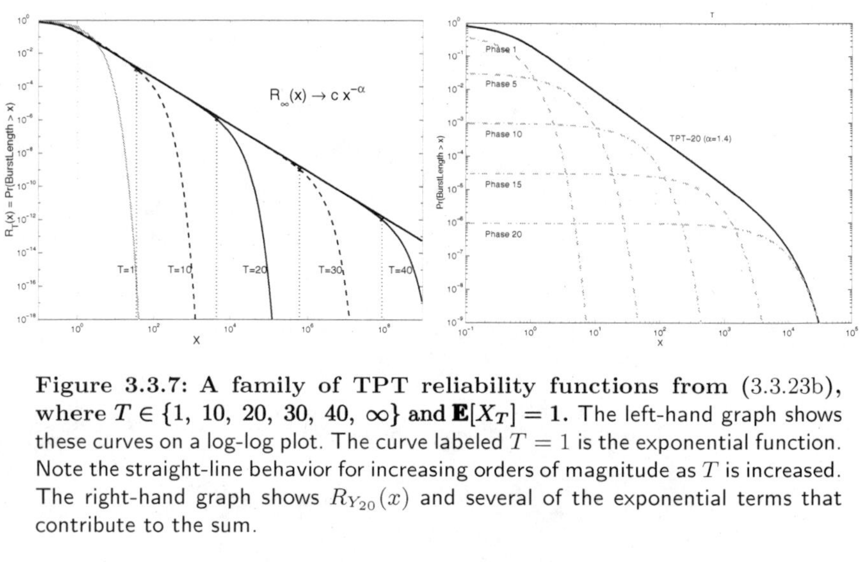

Figure 3.3.7: A family of TPT reliability functions from (3.3.23b), where $T \in \{1,\ 10,\ 20,\ 30,\ 40,\ \infty\}$ and $\mathbb{E}[X_T] = 1$. The left-hand graph shows these curves on a log-log plot. The curve labeled $T = 1$ is the exponential function. Note the straight-line behavior for increasing orders of magnitude as T is increased. The right-hand graph shows $R_{Y_{20}}(x)$ and several of the exponential terms that contribute to the sum.

$$R_{\rm o}(x) = e^{-\mu(T)x}, \quad \text{where} \quad \mu(T) = \frac{1-\theta}{1-\gamma\,\theta} \cdot \frac{1-(\theta\,\gamma)^T}{1-\theta^T}. \tag{3.3.23a}$$

This choice for $\mu(T)$, from (3.3.21), guarantees that $\mathbb{E}[Y_T] = 1$ for all T. Also, we have

$$R_{Y_T}(x) = \sum_{n=0}^{T-1} p_n(T) e^{-x\,\mu(T)/\gamma^n}. \tag{3.3.23b}$$

and

$$p_n(T) = \frac{\theta^n(1-\theta)}{1-\theta^T}, \quad \text{for } 0 \leq n \leq (T-1). \tag{3.3.23c}$$

In general, from (3.3.21), all the moments are given by

$$\mathbb{E}[Y_T^\ell] = \frac{1-\theta}{1-\theta^T} \cdot \frac{1-(\theta\,\gamma^\ell)^T}{1-\theta\,\gamma^\ell} \cdot \frac{\ell!}{[\mu(T)^\ell]}. \tag{3.3.23d}$$

Obviously, the additional assumptions (3.3.17a), (3.3.18a), and (3.3.23a) cause Y_T to be hyperexponentially distributed, as shown in Figure 3.3.8, with the ME represention $\langle\, \mathbf{p}(T),\, \mathbf{B}(T)\,\rangle$:

$$\mathbf{p}(T) = \frac{1-\theta}{1-\theta^T}[1,\ \theta,\ \theta^2,\ \ldots,\ \theta^{(T-1)}\,],$$

and

$$\mathbf{B}(T) = \mu(T) \begin{bmatrix} 1 & 0 & 0 & \cdots & 0 \\ 0 & 1/\gamma & 0 & \cdots & 0 \\ 0 & 0 & 1/\gamma^2 & \cdots & 0 \\ \cdots & \cdots & \cdots & \cdots & \cdots \\ 0 & 0 & 0 & \cdots & 1/\gamma^{T-1} \end{bmatrix}. \tag{3.3.24}$$

The individual phases are exponentially distributed with parameter $\mu(T)/\gamma^\ell$ and $\mathbf{p}(T)\boldsymbol{\epsilon}' = \sum_{j=0}^{T-1} p_j(T) = 1$. Figure 3.3.8 is a diagram of this representation.

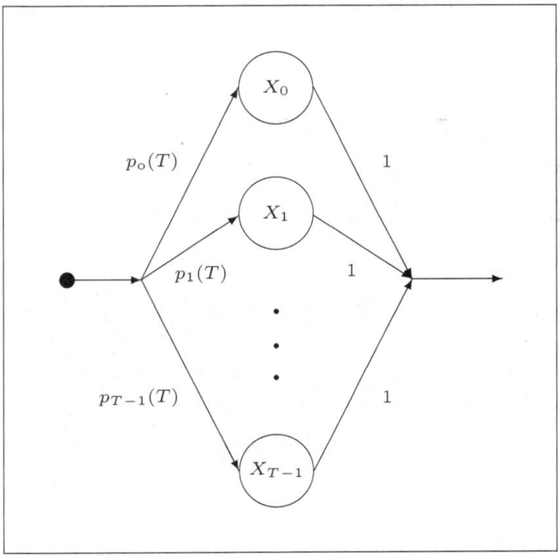

Figure 3.3.8: Canonical representation of f_{Y_T}. The X_js are exponentially distributed with rates $\mu(T)/\gamma^j$, the diagonal elements of $\mathbf{B}(T)$ in (3.3.24). $p_j(T)$ is the j-th component of $\mathbf{p}(T)$.

We have made some specific calculations of (3.3.23b) with parameters $\alpha = 1.4$, $\theta = 0.5$, $\gamma = 1/\theta^{1/\alpha} = 1.64067$, $\mathbb{E}[Y_T] = 1.0$, and $T \in \{1,\ 10,\ 20,\ 30,\ 40,\ \infty\,\}$, and have presented them as log-log graphs in Figure 3.3.7. The left-hand graph shows all six functions, and the ever-increasing extension of the straight line ($T = \infty$). The right-hand graph shows $R_{Y_{20}}(x)$ and the contributions of the terms for $n+1 = 1, 5, 10, 15,$ and 20. For instance, the curve labeled "Phase 1" is $0.5e^{-\mu(20)x}$, where $\mu(20) = 2.729958$ from (3.3.23a). Here we see how the tail "fills in" for increasing T. In some sense, this mimics the way data points accumulate for real systems. For a given set of data, there is a largest member, and very few other elements of comparable size. As more samples are added, a few will be much larger than all previous ones, and the tail fills in. Thus we can map, at least qualitatively, the increase in number of samples (N) with increase in T.

We explore the structure of (3.3.23b) further by evaluating $R_Y(x)$ ($T = \infty$) for various values of α, with $\mathbf{E}[X_\alpha] = 1$. The results are plotted in Figure 3.3.9, both on linear scale and log-log scale. The unlabeled curve is the exponential ($\alpha = \infty$). All start at $R_\alpha(0) = 1$. The smaller α is, the faster the curve drops initially, but eventually the curves cross, with smaller α ending up on top. This is a manifestation of the property described earlier for PT distributions, namely that an individual event is likely to be well below average, but when an above average event occurs, it will likely be well above the mean. This statement becomes more extreme with decreasing α [see (3.3.12d) and surrounding discussion]. The log-log graph shows the crossings and the straight-line behavior.

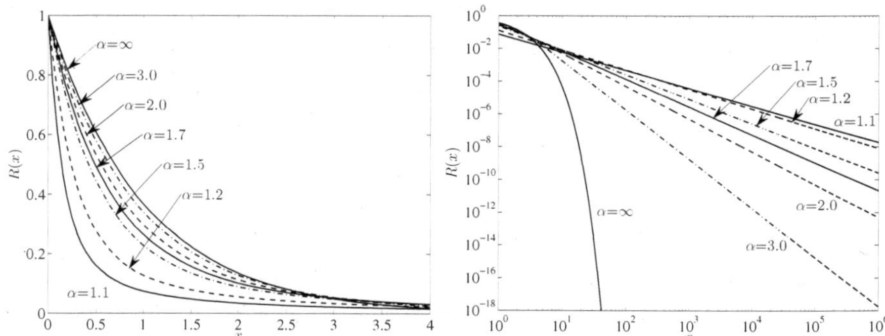

Figure 3.3.9: $R(x|\theta, \gamma)$ as a function of x (plotted on both linear and log-log scale) for $\alpha = -\log(\theta)/\log(\gamma) \in \{1.1, 1.2, 1.5, 1.7, 2.0, 3.0, \infty\}$ and $\theta = 0.5$ [See (3.3.20b)]. At $x \approx 3$ the curves start to cross until finally for $x \approx 216$ the curves for $\alpha = 1.1$ and $\alpha = 1.2$ cross and complete the reordering of the curves. As α approaches ∞, $R(x)$ approaches e^{-x} for finite x.

The class of functions given by (3.3.23b) is clearly of the hyperexponential type, as in (3.2.7b). But, as seen in Figure 3.3.7, depending on the size of T, $R_{Y_T}(x)$ looks very much like a PT distribution for several orders of magnitude. The concept of ***range*** was discussed in the previous section, and can be taken here to be (see [SCHWEFEL00] for a detailed discussion):

$$x_r(T) = \frac{\gamma^T}{\mu(T)}.$$

From this formula we see that an increase of T by 1 increases the range of Y_T

by a factor of γ. On a log-log scale, this would appear as equal spacing, as it is in Figure 3.3.7. Note that $\gamma = 1/\theta^{1/\alpha}$, so for a fixed α, the bigger θ is, the smaller γ is. That means that bigger θ (smaller γ) requires a bigger T to get the same range x_r.

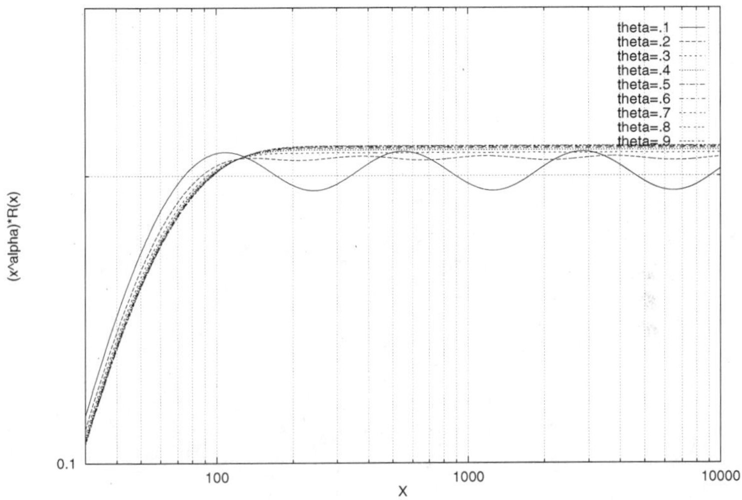

Figure 3.3.10: The PT function of (3.3.23b) ($T = \infty$) multiplied by x^α, for $\alpha = 1.4$ and various values of θ. If $R(x)$ were a true power-tail function, all these curves would be asymptotic straight lines. Although the vertical axis has no scale marked on it, the horizontal line is at $c \approx .214$, and the relative fluctuations are all less than 2%. In any case, (3.3.3a) is still valid, and $R(x)$ is bounded from above and below by true PT functions.

As a final example, we display in Figure 3.3.10 the function $c(x) := x^\alpha R(x)$ [from (3.3.23b) with $T = \infty$] for various values of θ. We see that the "straight lines" are not as straight as we might think from Figures 3.3.7 and 3.3.9. However, the relative fluctuations are never more than 2%. We also see that $c(x)$ is very stable to changes in θ (same 2% variation for $0.1 \le \theta \le 0.9$). Note that the period of the oscillation on the log scale is $\log(\gamma)$. That is, $c(\log(x)) = c(\log(x\gamma))$. This is proven below for any $R_o(x)$. ▲

We next show that $R(x)$ given in (3.3.20b) is asymptotically bounded by c/x^α for any well-behaved (and continuous) $R_o(x)$. Consider (3.3.20b), evaluated at $x = \gamma t$,

$$R(\gamma t) = (1-\theta)\sum_{n=0}^{\infty} \theta^n R_o(t/\gamma^{n-1}) = (1-\theta)\sum_{n=-1}^{\infty} \theta^{n+1} R_o(t/\gamma^n)$$

$$= \theta(1-\theta)\sum_{n=0}^{\infty} \theta^n R_o(t/\gamma^n) + (1-\theta)R_o(\gamma t) = \theta R(t) + (1-\theta)R_o(\gamma t).$$

But $R_o(t)$ is well behaved, and drops off at least as fast as some negative exponential, so for t large enough, $R_o(\gamma t)$ must be small compared to the sum, therefore,

$$R(\gamma t) \longrightarrow \theta R(t) \quad \text{as} \quad t \longrightarrow \infty.$$

This can be done any number of times, so we have, for large t

$$R(\gamma^k t) = \theta^k R(t).$$

Let $u = \gamma^k$, solve for k $[k = \log(u)/\log(\gamma)]$, and substitute for it to get

$$\theta^k = e^{k\log(\theta)} = e^{\log(\theta)\log(u)/\log(\gamma)}.$$

But from (3.3.22b), $\alpha = -\log(\theta)/\log(\gamma)$, so

$$\theta^k = e^{-\alpha\log(u)} = e^{\log(u^{-\alpha})} = u^{-\alpha}.$$

Therefore

$$R(\gamma^k t) = R(ut) = R(t)/u^{\alpha}.$$

Let t be large enough, but fixed, and let $x = ut$; then finally

$$R(x) = R(t)/(x/t)^{\alpha} = \frac{R(t)t^{\alpha}}{x^{\alpha}} = \frac{c}{x^{\alpha}}.$$

Figure 3.3.10 already showed that c is not really constant, but is a periodic function of $\log(x)$. What we have proven is that $c(x) := x^{\alpha} R(x)$ satisfies $c(x) = c(\gamma x) = c(\gamma^2 x) = \cdots = c(\gamma^n x) = \cdots$ for x large enough. But $R(x)$ still satisfies the most critical property of PT functions, namely Equation (3.3.22c), or (3.3.3b).

Now it is clear why we called Y_T *truncated power-tailed*: Y_T is well-behaved for finite T, but exhibits the characteristic power-tail properties and therefore behaves as a power-tailed random variable in the limit $T \to \infty$. In the following chapters, we use the family of functions in Example 3.3.5 to study the behavior of various queues.

3.3.6.3 A TPT Distribution Where $f(0) = 0$

In general, the distribution of Y_T [as defined in (3.3.16b)] has a matrix exponential representation if each X_k does. If every X_k satisfies (3.3.18a), then Y_T is ME if X_o is. The example we presented is quite specific. It was presented to show how one can build a power-tail distribution in the first place. The behavior of the distribution for small x may also be important for specific applications, so the first few terms can be modified to accomodate those properties, without affecting the properties of the tail. One can also use a different base function for $R_o(x)$. Alternatively, our $R_T(x)$ can be mixed with, or convoluted with, any other reliability function to get additional desired properties. For instance, $\langle \mathbf{p}(T), \mathbf{B}(T) \rangle$ of (3.3.24) represents a true hyperexponential, therefore it follows that $f_T(0) > 0$ (see Section 3.2.1.2). If it were necessary to have a function for which $f(0) = 0$, then one could replace the exponential terms with say, Erlangian distributions, as was done in Section 3.2.3.1. However this would double the dimension of the representation from T to $2T$. Another way to achieve the same effect is to convolute (3.3.24) with a single exponential function, that is, have an exponential of the form $\nu\, e^{-\nu x}$ follow the TPT function. Then the new PDF, call it $G(x)$ with pdf $g(x)$, has a representation of the form:

$$\mathbf{p} = \frac{1-\theta}{1-\theta^T}[1,\ \theta,\ \theta^2,\ \ldots,\ \theta^{(T-1)},\ 0],$$

and

$$\mathbf{B} = \mu \begin{bmatrix} 1 & 0 & 0 & \cdots & 0 & -1 \\ 0 & 1/\gamma & 0 & \cdots & 0 & -1/\gamma \\ 0 & 0 & 1/\gamma^2 & \cdots & 0 & -1/\gamma^2 \\ \cdots & \cdots & \cdots & \cdots & \cdots & \cdots \\ 0 & 0 & 0 & \cdots & 1/\gamma^{T-1} & -1/\gamma^{T-1} \\ 0 & 0 & 0 & \cdots & \cdots & \nu/\mu \end{bmatrix}. \tag{3.3.25}$$

This only increases the dimension by one, from T to $T+1$. An alternate representation that is equivalent to $G(x)$ puts the extra exponential in front of the TPT function. This is left as an exercise.

Exercise 3.3.1: Find $\mathbf{V}$ from (3.3.25) for arbitrary μ, T, and ν, and evaluate the first three moments of $g(x)$ using Theorem 3.1.1. Show, using (3.1.8b), that $g(0) = 0$. Why must this be true?

Exercise 3.3.2: Construct a representation of $G(x)$ where the exponential with parameter ν is in front of the TPT distribution. Find $\mathbf{V}$, and evaluate the first three moments. These should be identical to those in the previous example. Why do the two representations yield the same $G(x)$?

As a final comment, TPT distributions are clearly characterized by their very large C_v^2. A common belief about distributions with very large coefficient of variation is that most tasks are small to reasonable in magnitude, but every once in a while a big one comes along. This allows for the interpretation that the big ones are exceptional and can be ignored as outliers (lightning struck again). For TPT's this is clearly untrue, for there is no clear boundary between *big* and *small*. Consider, for instance, the α-th moment over scaled intervals. We can say that any TPT density function has asymptotic form $f(x) \Rightarrow c/x^{\alpha+1}$ up until x approaches its range x_r, when it then drops off more rapidly. Let γ be any number greater than 1, and consider all k such that $\gamma^k < x_r$. Then the partial integrals given by

$$\mathbb{E}_k(X^\alpha) := \int_{\gamma^k}^{\gamma^{k+1}} x^\alpha\, f(x)\, dx \approx \int_{\gamma^k}^{\gamma^{k+1}} \frac{cx^\alpha}{x^{\alpha+1}} dx$$

$$= \int_{\gamma^k}^{\gamma^{k+1}} \frac{c\,dx}{x} = c[\log(\gamma^{k+1} - \log(\gamma^k)] = c\log\gamma$$

are all the same size. That is, each interval in the power-tail region $[\gamma^k, \gamma^{k+1}]$ contributes exactly the same amount to $\mathbb{E}[X^\alpha]$. Tasks of all sizes (up to x_r) contribute significantly to the α-th moment. There are no boundaries between large and small.

The TPT introduced in this section shows the same behavior, component by component. That is, each term in the sum of (3.3.19a) contributes exactly the same amount to $\mathbb{E}[X^\alpha]$. We show this in the following equation.

$$\mathbb{E}[X_T^\alpha] = \int_o^\infty x^\alpha f_{Y_T}(x)\,dx = \frac{1-\theta}{1-\theta^T}\sum_{n=o}^{T-1}\left(\frac{\theta}{\gamma}\right)^n \int_o^\infty x^\alpha f_o(x/\gamma^n)\,dx$$

$$= \frac{1-\theta}{1-\theta^T}\sum_{n=o}^{T-1}\left(\frac{\theta}{\gamma}\right)^n (\gamma^n)^{\alpha+1}\int_o^\infty u^\alpha f_o(u)\,du = \frac{1-\theta}{1-\theta^T}\sum_{n=o}^{T-1}(\theta\gamma^\alpha)^n \mathbb{E}[X_o^\alpha].$$

But from (3.3.22b), $\theta\gamma^\alpha = 1$, so every term contributes the amount $(1-\theta/(1-\theta^T)\mathbb{E}[X_o^\alpha]$ to $\mathbb{E}[X_T^\alpha]$.

Of course, for $\mathbb{E}[X^\ell]$, $\ell < \alpha$, the smaller tasks collectively contribute more, but for $\ell > \alpha$ the larger tasks contribute ever more. Only the finite range of $f(\cdot)$ keeps these moments finite. For $1 < \alpha < 2$, the range of greatest interest, the larger tasks are not sufficient to overly affect the mean, but they cause havoc for the variance. As we show in later chapters, second-order performance measures such as the waiting, and residual times are highly dependent on the variance, and the stability of the queue length depends on the third moment, so PT distributionss, even the truncated variety, cannot be ignored.

3.4 Equivalent Representations

One might ask if there are more general representations than those discussed in Section 3.2, namely those of Figure 3.2.5. The answer is no!. First we prove that by using Laplace transforms, we introduce a type of similarity transformation which preserves all the structure of all the matrix equations, and gives some insight into why Figure 3.2.5 is minimal. These transformations are used in later chapters for more general applications.

3.4.1 The Canonical Minimal Representation

Consider the expression $B^*(s) = \Psi\left[(\mathbf{I} + s\mathbf{V})^{-1}\right]$ built from the vector-matrix pair, $\langle \mathbf{p}, \mathbf{B} \rangle$ both of dimension m. Let $\{\mu_j \,|\, 1 \le j \le m\}$ be the set of eigenvalues (not necessarily all distinct) of $\mathbf{B}$. We know from Theorem 3.1.1 that if $B^*(s)$ is the Laplace transform of some ME distribution, namely $b(x) = \Psi[\exp(-x\mathbf{B})\mathbf{B}]$, then $\Re(\mu_j) > 0$ for all μ_j. Furthermore, $\min|\mu_j|$ must be real (and positive). We also know that when $s = -\mu_j$ $(\mathbf{I}+s\mathbf{V})$ has no inverse. One would therefore expect that $B^*(-\mu_j) = \infty$ for all j, but this is not necessarily the case, although it is true that if $B^*(s) = \infty$, then $s = -\mu_j$

for some j. We discuss the reason why this can happen in the next section, but for now observe that $(\mathbf{I} + s\mathbf{V})^{-1}$ must be proportional to $1/\phi(s)$, where $\phi(s) = (\text{Det}[\mathbf{I}+s\mathbf{V}])$. Then $\Psi\left[(\mathbf{I} + s\mathbf{V})^{-1}\right]$ must yield a ratio of polynomials, say $q_2(s)/q_1(s)$, where common factors between $q_1(s)$ and $q_2(s)$ have been removed. Let the degree of q_1 be m_1 (the dimension of $\mathbf{V}$ is m). Then $m_1 \le m$. All the roots of q_1 must be elements of the set $\{-\mu_j\}$, but if $m_1 < m$ then not all members of that set are roots of q_1.

We are now ready to state and prove the theorem for the unique minimal representations.

Theorem 3.4.1: Every vector-matrix pair, $\langle\, \mathbf{p},\, \mathbf{B}\, \rangle$ (or $\langle\, \mathbf{p},\, \mathbf{V}\, \rangle$) with dimension m, and its generated distribution as given in Theorem 3.1.1, is equivalent to a vector-matrix pair (call it $\langle\, \mathbf{p_c},\, \mathbf{B_c}\, \rangle$, with dimension m_c) of the form surrounding Figure 3.2.5. That is, $\langle\, \mathbf{p_c},\, \mathbf{B_c}\, \rangle$ generates the same moments and $b(x)$ as $\langle\, \mathbf{p},\, \mathbf{B}\, \rangle$, and $m_c \le m$. Furthermore there are no other representations whose dimensions are smaller than m_c. This representation is unique to within a reordering of the μ_js. Therefore, we call it the ***canonical representation*** of $b(x)$. ■

Proof: First recall that $\langle\, \mathbf{p},\, \mathbf{B}\, \rangle$ generates a Laplace transform by (3.2.14b) that is RLT. Next note that every ratio of polynomials can be written as partial fractions [sums of terms whose denominators are of the form $(s - \mu_i)^{m_i}$], which can then be manipulated into the form given in (3.2.13a). The parameters in (3.2.13a) then map directly into Figure 3.2.5 and the minimal representation $\langle\, \mathbf{p_c},\, \mathbf{B_c}\, \rangle$. The Laplace transform of every well-behaved function is unique (to within a set of measure 0), and because $\langle\, \mathbf{p_c},\, \mathbf{B_c}\, \rangle$ and $\langle\, \mathbf{p},\, \mathbf{B}\, \rangle$ have the same Laplace transform, they must represent the same $b(x)$. **QED**

3.4.2 Isometric Transformations

We now present a purely linear algebraic approach that yields Theorem 3.4.1. It is also more general because it does not rely on a specific entrance vector $\mathbf{p}$. This can be useful in analyzing compound processes and semi-Markov processes. First consider the following definition.

Definition 3.4.1

Let $\langle\, \mathbf{p_1}\,,\, \mathbf{B_1} \rangle$ and $\langle\, \mathbf{p_2}\,,\, \mathbf{B_2} \rangle$ *be two vector-matrix pairs. Then they are* ***equivalent*** *if and only if they have the same moments according to* (3.2.14c), *or have the same Laplace transform according to* (3.2.14b), *or represent the same function according to* (3.2.14a). Any one of the three can prove the other two if the $\mathbf{B}$ matrices are invertible. If they are equivalent, we write

$$\langle\, \mathbf{p_1}\,,\, \mathbf{B_1} \rangle \equiv \langle\, \mathbf{p_2}\,,\, \mathbf{B_2} \rangle.$$

They do not have to be of the same dimension to be equivalent. □

Next consider any vector matrix pair $\langle\, \mathbf{p},\, \mathbf{B}\, \rangle$, where $\mathbf{B}$ has inverse $\mathbf{V}$, and $\mathbf{p}\,\boldsymbol{\epsilon}' = 1$. We now apply a particular ***similarity transformation*** to this pair, yielding another pair that is equivalent. We then have the following theorem.

Theorem 3.4.2: Take any nonsingular, ***isometric matrix*** $\mathbf{S}$ (i.e., $\mathbf{S}\boldsymbol{\epsilon}' = \boldsymbol{\epsilon}'$, and $\mathbf{S}^{-1}\boldsymbol{\epsilon}' = \boldsymbol{\epsilon}'$). Apply the following ***isometric transformation***.

$$\tilde{\mathbf{p}} := \mathbf{p}\mathbf{S}^{-1} \quad \text{and} \quad \tilde{\mathbf{B}} := \mathbf{S}\mathbf{B}\mathbf{S}^{-1}. \tag{3.4.1}$$

Then $\langle\, \tilde{\mathbf{p}},\, \tilde{\mathbf{B}}\, \rangle = \langle\, \mathbf{p},\, \mathbf{B}\, \rangle$ in the following sense.

$$b(t) := \tilde{\Psi}\left[\exp(-t\tilde{\mathbf{B}})\tilde{\mathbf{B}}\right] = \Psi\left[\exp(-t\mathbf{B})\mathbf{B}\right],$$

$$\tilde{\Psi}\left[\tilde{\mathbf{V}}^{\ell}\right] = \Psi\left[\mathbf{V}^{\ell}\right], \quad \forall\ \ell \geq 0,$$

and

$$B^*(s) := \tilde{\Psi}\left[(\mathbf{I} + s\tilde{\mathbf{V}})^{-1}\right] = \Psi\left[(\mathbf{I} + s\mathbf{V})^{-1}\right]$$

where $\tilde{\Psi}\left[\mathbf{X}\right] := \tilde{\mathbf{p}}\,\mathbf{X}\,\boldsymbol{\epsilon}'$ for any square matrix $\mathbf{X}$. This is true for every invertible isometric matrix, therefore there are an infinite number of equivalent representations of every ME function. Put differently, all the equations in Theorem 3.1.1 are ***invariant in form*** with respect to isometric transformations. ■

Proof: First note that

$$\tilde{\mathbf{p}}\,\boldsymbol{\epsilon}' = (\mathbf{p}\,\mathbf{S}^{-1})\,\boldsymbol{\epsilon}' = \mathbf{p}(\mathbf{S}^{-1}\,\boldsymbol{\epsilon}') = \mathbf{p}\,\boldsymbol{\epsilon}' = 1.$$

It is well known that $\mathbf{S}\mathbf{B}^n\mathbf{S}^{-1} = (\mathbf{S}\mathbf{B}\mathbf{S}^{-1})^n$ for all n. For instance,

$$\mathbf{S}\mathbf{B}^2\mathbf{S}^{-1} = \mathbf{S}\mathbf{B}\mathbf{S}^{-1}\mathbf{S}\mathbf{B}\mathbf{S}^{-1} = (\mathbf{S}\mathbf{B}\mathbf{S}^{-1})^2.$$

Therefore,

$$\begin{aligned}\mathbf{S}\exp(-t\mathbf{B})\mathbf{S}^{-1} &= \mathbf{S}\left(\sum_{n=0}^{\infty}\frac{(-t)^n}{n!}\mathbf{B}^n\right)\mathbf{S}^{-1} = \sum_{n=0}^{\infty}\frac{(-t)^n}{n!}\mathbf{S}\mathbf{B}^n\mathbf{S}^{-1}\\ &= \sum_{n=0}^{\infty}\frac{(-t)^n}{n!}(\mathbf{S}\mathbf{B}\mathbf{S}^{-1})^n = \exp(-t\mathbf{S}\mathbf{B}\mathbf{S}^{-1}).\end{aligned}$$

Thus we can write:

$$\begin{aligned}b(t) &= \Psi\left[\exp(-t\mathbf{B})\mathbf{B}\right] = \Psi\left[\mathbf{S}^{-1}\mathbf{S}\exp(-t\mathbf{B})\mathbf{S}^{-1}\mathbf{S}\,\mathbf{B}\,\mathbf{S}^{-1}\,\mathbf{S}\right]\\ &= (\mathbf{p}\mathbf{S}^{-1})\exp(-t\mathbf{S}\mathbf{B}\mathbf{S}^{-1})\mathbf{S}\mathbf{B}\mathbf{S}^{-1}\boldsymbol{\epsilon}' = \tilde{\mathbf{p}}\exp(-t\tilde{\mathbf{B}})\tilde{\mathbf{B}}\,\boldsymbol{\epsilon}'\\ &= \tilde{\Psi}\left[\exp(-t\tilde{\mathbf{B}})\tilde{\mathbf{B}}\right].\end{aligned}$$

The other relations can be proven in similar fashion. **QED**

This theorem is true even if one of the eigenvalues of $\mathbf{B}$, call it μ, satisfies $\Re(\mu) < 0$ [i.e., $b(t)$ is not a density function]. Then,

1. $\lim_{t\to\infty} b(t) = \infty$
2. The integral definition of $B^*(s)$ only exists for $\Re(s) > -\Re(\mu)$
3. The moments, $\mathbf{E}[X^\ell]$, do not exist.

The term ***isometric transformation*** was chosen for the following reason. If we consider the sum of the components of a vector $\mathbf{r}$ to be its (pseudo)"***length***," then an isometric transformation preserves the length of every row vector; that is, $\mathbf{r}\,\boldsymbol{\epsilon}'$ is invariant. However, we must be careful, because the sum can be negative and thus cannot be used as a "metric" in the mathematical metric space sense. In any case, a transformation which does not change that length is *iso-metric* (*iso* means "same", and *metric* means "length").

We now show that any matrix that preserves length in this sense must be isometric. Let $\mathbf{r}$ be any row vector, and $\mathbf{S}$ be an invertible matrix. Then $\tilde{\mathbf{r}} = \mathbf{r}\,\mathbf{S}^{-1}$ is the transformed vector, and

$$\left[\tilde{\mathbf{r}}\,\boldsymbol{\epsilon}' = \mathbf{r}\,\mathbf{S}^{-1}\boldsymbol{\epsilon}' = \mathbf{r}\,\boldsymbol{\epsilon}' \quad \forall \quad \mathbf{r}\right] \iff \left[\mathbf{S}^{-1}\,\boldsymbol{\epsilon}' = \boldsymbol{\epsilon}'\right].$$

The proof follows from the fact that the only column vector which is orthogonal ($\mathbf{u}\,\mathbf{v}' = 0$) to every row vector is the one with all zeros, therefore, $\mathbf{v}' := \mathbf{S}^{-1}\boldsymbol{\epsilon}' - \boldsymbol{\epsilon}' = \mathbf{o}'$, because $\mathbf{r}\mathbf{v}' = 0$ for all $\mathbf{r}$. See [LIPSKY-RAM85] for details.

Example 3.4.1: A straightforward example of the invariance of isometric transformations is permuting the labels of the phases of any $\langle\, \mathbf{p},\, \mathbf{B}\,\rangle$. Changing the labels requires interchanging the components of $\mathbf{p}$ and interchanging the rows and columns of $\mathbf{B}$. It is well known that this can be done formally with the use of ***permutation matrices***. These are $0-1$ matrices with exactly one '1' in each row and column. In all cases, then, their row-sums are 1, so they are automatically isometric. For instance, for a two-dimensional representation, in order to interchange phases 1 and 2, one uses the matrix:

$$\mathbf{S} = \begin{bmatrix} 0 & 1 \\ 1 & 0 \end{bmatrix}.$$

In this case, $\mathbf{S}^{-1} = \mathbf{S}$, so

$$\tilde{\mathbf{p}} = \mathbf{p}\mathbf{S}^{-1} = [p_1,\, p_2] \begin{bmatrix} 0 & 1 \\ 1 & 0 \end{bmatrix} = [p_2,\, p_1],$$

and

$$\tilde{\mathbf{B}} = \begin{bmatrix} 0 & 1 \\ 1 & 0 \end{bmatrix} \begin{bmatrix} B_{11} & B_{12} \\ B_{21} & B_{22} \end{bmatrix} \begin{bmatrix} 0 & 1 \\ 1 & 0 \end{bmatrix} = \begin{bmatrix} B_{22} & B_{21} \\ B_{12} & B_{11} \end{bmatrix}.$$

Thus by Theorem 3.4.2, we have proven what most people would consider obvious, namely that changing the numbering on the phases leaves all properties of the representation unchanged. ▲

We now discuss the issue as to why two representations can be equivalent and yet have different dimension. The following observation was first made by Neuts in [NEUTS81].

Example 3.4.2: Let $\mathbf{B}$ be any matrix such that:

$$\mathbf{B}\boldsymbol{\epsilon}' = \mu\boldsymbol{\epsilon}'$$

(i.e., $\boldsymbol{\epsilon}'$ is a right-eigenvector of $\mathbf{B}$ with eigenvalue, μ). Then for every $\mathbf{p}$, $\langle\, \mathbf{p},\, \mathbf{B}\,\rangle$ represents the (one-dimensional) exponential function. That is,

$$b(x) = \Psi\left[\exp(-x\mathbf{B})\mathbf{B}\right] = \mu\, e^{-\mu x}.$$

Because $\mathbf{B}\boldsymbol{\epsilon}' = \mu\boldsymbol{\epsilon}'$ it follows that $\mathbf{B}^{\ell}\boldsymbol{\epsilon}' = \mu^{\ell}\boldsymbol{\epsilon}' \quad \forall \quad \ell$. Then, $\Psi\left[\mathbf{B}^{\ell}\right] = \mathbf{p}\mathbf{B}^{\ell}\boldsymbol{\epsilon}' = \mu^{\ell}$. The proof follows directly by substituting this into (3.2.13e). Thus, a representation with dimension $m = \text{Dim}[\mathbf{B}]$ is equivalent to a representation whose dimension is 1. A specific example of this is given in Section 3.4.3. ▲

The above example is a special case of the following. After reviewing Section 1.3.3.1, consider the set of column vectors:

$$\boldsymbol{\epsilon}',\ \mathbf{B}\boldsymbol{\epsilon}',\ \mathbf{B}^2\boldsymbol{\epsilon}',\ \cdots,\ \mathbf{B}^{m-1}\boldsymbol{\epsilon}',$$

where $m = \text{Dim}[\mathbf{B}]$. There exists a smallest integer, n, such that $\mathbf{B}^n\boldsymbol{\epsilon}'$ can be written as a linear combination of the vectors with a lower power of $\mathbf{B}$. That is

$$\mathbf{B}^n\,\boldsymbol{\epsilon}' = a_o\,\boldsymbol{\epsilon}' + a_1\mathbf{B}\boldsymbol{\epsilon}' + \cdots + a_{n-1}\,\mathbf{B}^{n-1}\boldsymbol{\epsilon}'$$

or

$$(\mathbf{B}^n - a_o\,\mathbf{I} - a_1\mathbf{B} - \cdots - a_{n-1}\,\mathbf{B}^{n-1})\boldsymbol{\epsilon}' = f_n(\mathbf{B})\boldsymbol{\epsilon}' = \mathbf{o}'.$$

We know that $n \le m$, because it is well known that the characteristic polynomial (a polynomial of degree m) always allows us to write $\mathbf{B}^m\boldsymbol{\epsilon}'$ in terms of the others. In fact, $f_n(y)$ can be written as

$$f_n(y) = (y-\mu_1)^{n_1}(y-\mu_2)^{n_2}\cdots(y-\mu_K)^{n_K}, \tag{3.4.2a}$$

with the same set of μ's as $\phi(y)$, the characteristic polynomial of $\mathbf{B}$ (3.2.13c). In this case,

$$0 \le n_k \le m_k \quad \text{and} \quad \sum_{k=1}^{K} n_k = n. \tag{3.4.2b}$$

If n is strictly less than m, we can actually find a representation of lesser dimension that is equivalent to the one given. In Example 3.4.2, $n = 1$. The underlying cause of this drop in dimensionality is the fact that one or more left-eigenvectors of $\mathbf{B}$ are orthogonal to $\boldsymbol{\epsilon}'$. The different possibilities for reduction are sketched here.

1. $m_k = 1$ and $n_k = 0$; then $\mathbf{u_k}\,\boldsymbol{\epsilon}' = 0$,

2. $m_k > 1$ but there is only one left eigenvector; then either $n_k = m_k$ or $n_k = 0$. In the latter case, $\mathbf{u_k}\,\boldsymbol{\epsilon}' = 0$,

3. $m_k > 1$ and there are several left eigenvectors; then $n_k \leq m_k$. If $n_k = 0$, then all the eigenvectors are orthogonal to $\boldsymbol{\epsilon}'$. If $n_k > 0$ then a linear combination of the eigenvectors can be found such that all but one (at most) are orthogonal to $\boldsymbol{\epsilon}'$.

In other words, every eigenvalue that appears in $f_n(y)$ has exactly one left eigenvector that is not orthogonal to $\boldsymbol{\epsilon}'$. The number of such eigenvectors is κ. We next show how the others can be thrown away.

Consider the ***Jordan canonical form*** (see, e.g., [HORN-JOHNSON85]) for matrices, For each finite-dimensional square matrix), call it $\mathbf{B}$, there always exists a nonsingular matrix $\mathbf{R}$ such that

$$\mathbf{RBR}^{-1} = \begin{bmatrix} \mu_1\mathbf{X_1} & \mathbf{0} & \mathbf{0} & \cdots & \mathbf{0} \\ \mathbf{0} & \mu_2\mathbf{X_2} & \mathbf{0} & \cdots & \mathbf{0} \\ \vdots & \vdots & \vdots & \cdots & \vdots \\ \mathbf{0} & \mathbf{0} & \mathbf{0} & \cdots & \mu_{K_B}\mathbf{X_{K_B}} \end{bmatrix}, \tag{3.4.3a}$$

where K_B is the number of (independent) left eigenvectors and the μ's are the eigenvalues of $\mathbf{B}$. The μ's are not necessarily distinct (i.e., there may be two or more eigenvectors with the same eigenvalue). The reader should compare this with (3.2.11b) before going on. Each matrix $\mathbf{X_k}$ is of the form

$$\mathbf{X_k} = \begin{bmatrix} \mu_k & \alpha_k & 0 & \cdots & 0 & 0 \\ 0 & \mu_k & \alpha_k & \cdots & 0 & 0 \\ \vdots & \vdots & \vdots & \cdots & \vdots & \vdots \\ 0 & 0 & 0 & \cdots & \mu_k & \alpha_k \\ 0 & 0 & 0 & \cdots & 0 & \mu_k \end{bmatrix}, \tag{3.4.3b}$$

where $\alpha_k \neq 0$, and is otherwise not specified. The usual Jordan normal form sets $\alpha_k = \pm 1$, but we ultimately set it to $\alpha_k = -\mu_k$ so that $\mathbf{X_k} = \mu_k\,\mathbf{L_k}$, where $\mathbf{L_k}$ is given by (3.2.3b). As an example, consider the 2-dimensional similarity transformation equation showing that α can be given any value, and furthermore, there are enough free constants available to do more.

$$\mathbf{R\,L\,R}^{-1} := \begin{bmatrix} \alpha/a & \alpha b/a^2 \\ 0 & -1/a \end{bmatrix} \begin{bmatrix} 1 & -1 \\ 0 & 1 \end{bmatrix} \begin{bmatrix} a/\alpha & b \\ 0 & -a \end{bmatrix} = \begin{bmatrix} 1 & \alpha \\ 0 & 1 \end{bmatrix} = \mathbf{X},$$

where a, b, $\alpha \neq 0$ but are otherwise anything. This can easily be made into an isometric transformation by making $b = 1 + 1/\alpha$ and $a = -1$, for then

$$\mathbf{R} \Longrightarrow \mathbf{S} = \begin{bmatrix} -\alpha & 1+\alpha \\ 0 & 1 \end{bmatrix}, \quad \mathbf{S}^{-1} = \begin{bmatrix} -1/\alpha & 1+1/\alpha \\ 0 & 1 \end{bmatrix},$$

and $\mathbf{S}\,\boldsymbol{\epsilon}' = \mathbf{S}^{-1}\,\boldsymbol{\epsilon}' = \boldsymbol{\epsilon}'$. After picking α, there were still two free parameters (a and b) available to make the transformation an isometric one. The reader should check out these equations.

We now discuss what to do with those left eigenvectors that sum to 0. When such vectors occur, the rows in $\mathbf{S}$ corresponding to that block also sum to 0. Let us assume then, that the blocks in (3.4.3a) are already ordered so that all those corresponding to 0-sum eigenvectors are placed at the end. Let us also assume that all the rows that do not sum to zero are normalized so that they sum to 1. One other consideration must be made. If there are two or more eigenvectors with the same eigenvalue, then there will be a block for each. It is not hard to show that the eigenvectors can be recombined to produce one that sums to 1 (the one that goes with the biggest block), with all the others summing to 0. Yes, all this can be done by successive isometric transformations. Then we end up with

$$\tilde{\mathbf{B}} = \mathbf{S}\mathbf{B}\mathbf{S}^{-1} = \begin{bmatrix} \mu_1\mathbf{L_1} & \mathbf{0} & \mathbf{0} & \cdots & \mathbf{0} & \mathbf{E_1} \\ \mathbf{0} & \mu_2\mathbf{L_2} & \mathbf{0} & \cdots & \mathbf{0} & \mathbf{E_2} \\ \vdots & \vdots & \vdots & \cdots & \vdots & \vdots \\ \mathbf{0} & \mathbf{0} & \mathbf{0} & \cdots & \mu_\kappa\mathbf{L}_\kappa & \mathbf{E}_\kappa \\ \mathbf{0} & \mathbf{0} & \mathbf{0} & \cdots & \mathbf{0} & \mathbf{E} \end{bmatrix},$$

where $\mathbf{S}$ satisfies

$$\mathbf{S}\,\boldsymbol{\epsilon}'_{\mathbf{m}} = \mathbf{S}\begin{bmatrix} 1 \\ \vdots \\ 1 \\ 1 \\ \vdots \\ 1 \end{bmatrix} = \begin{bmatrix} 1 \\ \vdots \\ 1 \\ 0 \\ \vdots \\ 0 \end{bmatrix} \quad \text{and} \quad \mathbf{S}^{-1}\begin{bmatrix} 1 \\ \vdots \\ 1 \\ 0 \\ \vdots \\ 0 \end{bmatrix} \doteq \boldsymbol{\epsilon}'_{\mathbf{m}}.$$

The new column vector has n ones and $m_e = m - n$ zeroes, where n comes from (3.4.2b). $\mathbf{E_k}$ is of dimension $n_k \times m_e$ and $\mathbf{E}$ is of dimension $m_e \times m_e$. $\kappa \leq K_B$ is the number of left eigenvectors for which $\mathbf{u_k}\boldsymbol{\epsilon}'_{\mathbf{k}} \neq 0$. It is also the minimum number of blocks for a representation that is valid for all entrance vectors $\mathbf{p}$.

Following the notation of (3.2.11a), observe that:

$$\Psi\,[\mathbf{B}] = \mathbf{p}\,\mathbf{B}\boldsymbol{\epsilon}' = \mathbf{p}\,\mathbf{S}^{-1}\mathbf{S}\,\mathbf{B}\,\mathbf{S}^{-1}\,\mathbf{S}\,\boldsymbol{\epsilon}'_{\mathbf{m}} = \tilde{\mathbf{p}}\,\tilde{\mathbf{B}}\,\mathbf{S}\boldsymbol{\epsilon}'_{\mathbf{m}}$$

$$= \begin{bmatrix} a_1\tilde{\mathbf{p}}^{(1)} \; a_2\tilde{\mathbf{p}}^{(2)} \; \cdots \; a_\kappa\tilde{\mathbf{p}}^{(\kappa)} \end{bmatrix} \begin{bmatrix} \mu_1\mathbf{L_1} & \mathbf{0} & \mathbf{0} & \cdots & \mathbf{0} & \mathbf{E_1} \\ \mathbf{0} & \mu_2\mathbf{L_2} & \mathbf{0} & \cdots & \mathbf{0} & \mathbf{E_2} \\ \vdots & \vdots & \vdots & \cdots & \vdots & \vdots \\ \mathbf{0} & \mathbf{0} & \mathbf{0} & \cdots & \mu_\kappa\mathbf{L}_\kappa & \mathbf{E}_\kappa \\ \mathbf{0} & \mathbf{0} & \mathbf{0} & \cdots & \mathbf{0} & \mathbf{E} \end{bmatrix} \begin{bmatrix} \boldsymbol{\epsilon}'_{\mathbf{1}} \\ \boldsymbol{\epsilon}'_{\mathbf{2}} \\ \vdots \\ \boldsymbol{\epsilon}'_{\boldsymbol{\kappa}} \\ \mathbf{o}' \end{bmatrix}.$$

$\boldsymbol{\epsilon}'_{\mathbf{k}}$ is the m_k-dimensional column vector of all 1's, and $\mathbf{o}'$ is the m_e dimensional column vector of all 0's. Clearly, whatever the $\mathbf{E}$ matrices are, they do not contribute to $\Psi\,[\mathbf{B}]$, because the number of zeroes in the column vector exactly matches the row dimension of the $\mathbf{E}$ matrices. The same is true of all powers of $\mathbf{B}$, including $\mathbf{V}$ and its powers. Therefore, we can throw away all last m_e

rows and columns and end up with a new vector-matrix pair, which we also call $\langle\, \tilde{\mathbf{p}}, \tilde{\mathbf{B}}\,\rangle$.

Hereafter we include the dimension reduction, if appropriate, whenever we make an isometric transformation. $\tilde{\mathbf{B}}$ is the smallest matrix that is equivalent to $\mathbf{B}$ for all possible $\mathbf{p}$. However, it can be reduced further, depending on the specific $\mathbf{p}$ chosen. The pair $\langle\, \tilde{\mathbf{p}}, \tilde{\mathbf{B}}\,\rangle$ is in the form given by Equations (3.2.11), but they are not necessarily equal. It may happen that some n_k are actually larger than those found by the Laplace transform. Note that in (3.2.11) it was required that $p^{(k)}_{m_k} \neq 0$, but here, it is possible that $p^{(k)}_{n_k} = 0$. If so, we throw it away, together with the corresponding row and column of $\tilde{\mathbf{B}}$. When all this trimming is done, we *do* end up with the same vector-matrix pair as in Theorem 3.4.1.

Yes, it was a long way to get there, and you might have preferred to stick with the Laplace transform view, but here we found a minimal representation of $\mathbf{B}$ that is good for all entrance vectors, and we did it with only matrix arguments. The only step remaining, if appropriate, is to examine the particular $\tilde{\mathbf{p}} = \mathbf{p}\,\mathbf{S}^{-1}$, and do the final trimming then.

3.4.2.1 Summary

We have now seen that all functions of exponential type [i.e., of the form given in Equations (3.2.8)] have rational Laplace transforms (RLTs) and can be represented by a vector-matrix pair $\langle \mathbf{p}\,,\, \mathbf{B}\rangle$ of the form (3.2.11a) and (3.2.11b). Conversely, for every $\langle \mathbf{p}\,,\, \mathbf{B}\rangle$ there exists an equivalent vector-matrix pair $\langle \tilde{\mathbf{p}}\,,\, \tilde{\mathbf{B}}\rangle$ of equal or lesser dimension that is of the form (3.2.11b) and represents the same function as given by Equations (3.2.14). There is no representation that has a smaller dimension. In general, one can say that if $\langle \mathbf{p}\,,\, \mathbf{B}\rangle$ is a representation of $b(t)$, so is $\langle\, \mathbf{pS}^{-1}\,,\, \mathbf{SBS}^{-1}\,\rangle$, where $\mathbf{S}$ is any nonsingular isometric matrix of appropriate dimension. Clearly, there are an infinite number of equivalent representations of every pdf (including, interestingly enough, the exponential distribution, which has an infinite number of equivalent representations, but of dimension >1). Thus it would seem useless to try to give real physical meaning to the individual components of $\mathbf{p}$ or $\mathbf{B}$.

It is important to note that if the a_is, $p_i^{(k)}$s, and μ_is are real and positive, we are dealing with a ***PHase distribution*** [NEUTS81], but they do not have to be for $b(t)$ to be a proper pdf. Neuts has defined a PHase distribution to be a distribution for which there exists a representation where $\mathbf{p}$, $\mathbf{P}$, and $\mathbf{M}$ have only real, non-negative components. Such a representation said to be of ***PHase type***. (See the footnote at the beginning of Section 3.2.) We give several examples where the original representation is of PHase type, but the canonical one is not (e.g., Erlangian distributions with feedback). A detailed classification of matrix exponential functions is given in [LIPSKY-FANG86].

Now we state the ***representation theorem.***

Theorem 3.4.3: Consider any finite vector-matrix pair $\langle \mathbf{p}\,,\, \mathbf{B}\rangle$ with the following properties. $\mathbf{p}$ is isometric; $\mathbf{B}$ is invertible and has no eigenvalues with nonpositive real part. Then:

1. The three equations in Theorem 3.1.1 [or (3.2.14)] are algebraically correct.
2. Let $\mathbf{S}$ be any isometric invertible matrix. Then
$$\langle\, \mathbf{p}\,,\, \mathbf{B}\,\rangle \equiv \langle\, \mathbf{pS}^{-1}\,,\, \mathbf{SBS}^{-1}\,\rangle.$$
3. There exists a special $\mathbf{S}$ such that $\mathbf{SBS}^{-1}$ is of the form (3.4.3), with K_B blocks. If the last m_e rows and columns are discarded, the resulting matrix has $\kappa \le K_B$ blocks. This is the smallest $\mathbf{B}$ matrix that is valid for all $\mathbf{p}$.
4. For a specific $\mathbf{p}$, if for each k, those rows and columns corresponding to $p^{(k)}_{m_k} = 0$ are discarded, then the reduced vector-matrix pair $\langle\, \tilde{\mathbf{p}}\,,\, \tilde{\mathbf{B}}\,\rangle$ is the ***canonical representation*** with the following properties.
    (a) It is unique to within an exchange of blocks.
    (b) It is equivalent to $\langle\, \mathbf{p}\,,\, \mathbf{B}\,\rangle$.
    (c) It has $K \le \kappa \le K_B$ blocks.
    (d) No other representation is of smaller dimension.
    (e) The characteristic equation for $\tilde{\mathbf{B}}$ satisfies (3.2.13b).

The various components may not be physically realizable even if the components of the original representation are, but diagrammatically it looks like Figure 3.2.5. If the reduced m_k is greater than 1 for any k, then the canonical representation is ***defective***. It follows then, that if the canonical representation is defective ($\mathbf{B}$ is a defective matrix), no diagonal representation of $b(x)$ exists. ■

Remember, even if individual components of $\mathbf{p}$ or $\mathbf{B}$ are complex, $b(x)$ is unchanged by an isometric transformation, so the physical consequences are unchanged. D. R. Cox was the first one to consider complex probabilities [Cox55] in this context, but made little use of it. In the next chapters we derive numerous equations, all of which are invariant to this class of isometric transformations.

3.4.2.2 Hierachy of ME Functions

In the following set of definitions, when we talk about $R(x)$ we will, by implication, include $B(x) = 1 - R(x)$ and $b(x) = (d/dx)B(x)$.

We wish to define and classify five sets of ME functions that are mutually inclusive (nested subsets).

Definition 3.4.2

Let $\langle\, \mathbf{p},\, \mathbf{B}\,\rangle$ be any finite-dimensional vector-matrix pair with possibly complex components, and $\mathbf{p}\boldsymbol{\epsilon}' = 1$. Then:

$$R(x) = \Psi[\exp(-x\mathbf{B})], \quad \text{with} \ \ R(0) = 1$$

and RLT

$$B^*(s) = \Psi[\,\mathbf{B}(s\mathbf{I} + s\mathbf{B})^{-1}] = \Psi[\,(\mathbf{I} + s\mathbf{V})^{-1}] = \frac{q_2(s)}{q_1(s)},$$

where $\mathbf{V} = \mathbf{B}^{-1}$, if it exists. Let $\{\mu_i\}$ be the set of roots of $q_1(s)$, and let $\sigma = \min[\Re(\mu_i)]$. We define five sets of functions where each one is a superset of the one below it.

1. ***ME functions*** [$R(x)$ is complex].
2. ***Real ME functions*** [$R(x)$ is real].
3. ***Integrable (real) ME functions*** [$\lim_{x\to\infty} R(x) = 0$].
4. ***ME distributions*** [$b(x) \geq 0 \;\forall\; x \geq 0$].
5. ***PHase representations.***

(There are some interesting subsets between (3) and (4), and after (5), and others, no doubt.)

There are three domains in which these functions can be defined/tested: matrix domain, function domain, and Laplace transform domain. These sets of functions have the following properties in each of the domains:

Table 3.4.1. Properties of ME Functions in Three Domains

	$\langle \mathbf{p}, \mathbf{B} \rangle$	$R(x),\ b(x),\ F(x)$	$B^*(x)$
(1)	Finite (complex)	$\sum f_i(x) e^{-\mu_i x}$	$q_2(s)/q_1(s)$
(2)	$\Phi(\mu) = \text{Det}\lvert\mathbf{B} - \mu\mathbf{I}\rvert$ is real; $\Phi(\mu_i) = 0$	If μ is complex, then μ^* is also a term; $f_{\mu_i}(s) = f^*_{\mu^*_i}(s)$	$q_1(s)$ and $q_2(s)$ are real; $q_1(s)$ divides $\Phi(s)$
(3)	$\sigma > 0$	$\sigma > 0$	$\sigma > 0$
(4)	Not known	$b(x) \geq 0$	Not known
(5)	$B_{ii} > 0,\ \ B_{ij} \leq 0$ $p_i \geq 0,\ \ (\mathbf{B}\epsilon')_i \geq 0$ $\mathbf{V} = \mathbf{B}^{-1}$ exists	Not known	Not known

Classes (1) to (3) are not appropriate for use in queueing theory (except, perhaps as approximations to probability functions), but they have some interesting properties as seen below. □

For instance, the LT matrix as defined in (3.1.10) exists irrespective of whether the integral definition of B*(s) exists (even if $\mathbf{V}$ doesn't exist). The integral definition for the Laplace transform,

$$B^*(s) = \int_0^\infty e^{-sx}\, b(x)\, dx$$

exists on the positive real line only for $s > -\sigma$.

If $q_1(s)$ and $q_2(s)$ are real (i.e., they are both polynomials with real coefficients), then $R(x)$ is real for all real x [class (2)]. That is, the $\mu_i's$ and the polynomials, $f_i(x)$, occur in complex conjugate pairs.

If $\sigma > 0$, then all the moments of $b(x)$ exist, and satisfy [class (3)]:

$$\mathbb{E}[X^\ell] = \int_0^\infty x^\ell \, b(x)\, dx = \ell!\Psi[\mathbf{V}^\ell].$$

Furthermore, if σ is an eigenvalue of $\mathbf{B}$ (i.e., it has no imaginary component) then $R(x)$ has an exponential tail. That is,

$$R(x) \longrightarrow c\, x^m \, e^{-\sigma x}$$

for x large enough. m is the multiplicity of σ.

But $B(x)$ may not be a PDF. For this to be true, we must have [class (4)]

$$b(x) \geq 0 \quad \forall \;\; x \geq 0,$$

or equivalently, $R(x)$ must be a monotonically nonincreasing function of x. After 40 years of research we still don't know how (or if) this can be shown directly from the matrix or LT domains, but if the above inequality is true, $\langle\, \mathbf{p}, \mathbf{B}\, \rangle$ represents a ***matrix exponential distribution***. This is the class of functions of interest to us here.

An important subclass of ME distributions in great use today, and first defined by [NEUTS75] is the class of PHase distributions. This class is defined in the matrix domain as given in the table above [class (5)]. The inequalities are equivalent to having a representation that is truly physical. That is, $\mathbf{B} = \mathbf{M}(\mathbf{I} - \mathbf{P})$ with $M_{ii} > 0$, $1 \geq P_{ij} \geq 0$, $(\mathbf{P}\boldsymbol{\epsilon}')_i \leq 1$, and $(\mathbf{I} - \mathbf{P})$ has an inverse. As is shown by, for instance, Example 3.4.3 below, a given PHase distribution may have representations that are not PHase (in fact, it will have an infinite number of them). So we say that:

A distribution is a ***PHase distribution*** if it has at least one ***PHase represention***.

3.4.3 Examples of Equivalent Representations

Despite the powerful theorem we stated in the preceding section about minimal and unique representations, a feeling persists that somehow one can construct a set of phases that can do better (sort of like looking for a perpetual motion machine). A common example, which some people have called a ***generalized Erlangian***, has the historically older name of ***hypoexponential distribution***. The simplest example is given by the following.

Example 3.4.3: Consider a server with two phases in tandem that do not have equal completion rates. The straightforward representation of this is

$$\mathbf{p} = [1 \;\; 0]; \quad \mathbf{M} = \begin{bmatrix} \mu_1 & 0 \\ 0 & \mu_2 \end{bmatrix}; \quad \mathbf{P} = \begin{bmatrix} 0 & 1 \\ 0 & 0 \end{bmatrix},$$

and thus,

$$\mathbf{B} = \begin{bmatrix} \mu_1 & -\mu_1 \\ 0 & \mu_2 \end{bmatrix}.$$

This is a triangular matrix, therefore the eigenvalues of $\mathbf{B}$ are equal to μ_1 and μ_2. If the μ's are not equal, $\mathbf{B}$ can be diagonalized by the matrix made up of its eigenvectors. Look at

$$\mathbf{S}^{-1} = \frac{1}{\mu_2 - \mu_1}\begin{bmatrix} \mu_2 & -\mu_1 \\ 0 & \mu_2 - \mu_1 \end{bmatrix}, \quad \mathbf{S} = \frac{1}{\mu_2}\begin{bmatrix} \mu_2 - \mu_1 & \mu_1 \\ 0 & \mu_2 \end{bmatrix}.$$

First note that $\mathbf{S}\,\boldsymbol{\epsilon}' = \boldsymbol{\epsilon}'$. Then

$$\tilde{\mathbf{p}} = \mathbf{p}\mathbf{S}^{-1} = \begin{bmatrix} \dfrac{\mu_2}{\mu_2 - \mu_1} & \dfrac{\mu_1}{\mu_1 - \mu_2} \end{bmatrix}, \quad \tilde{\mathbf{B}} = \mathbf{S}\mathbf{B}\mathbf{S}^{-1} = \begin{bmatrix} \mu_1 & 0 \\ 0 & \mu_2 \end{bmatrix},$$

and $\langle\, \mathbf{p}\,,\, \mathbf{B}\,\rangle \equiv \langle\, \tilde{\mathbf{p}}\,,\, \tilde{\mathbf{B}}\,\rangle$. So a hypoexponential distribution is just another hyperexponential distribution, but with a difference. Suppose that $\mu_2 > \mu_1$. Then $(\tilde{\mathbf{p}})_2 < 0$ and $(\tilde{\mathbf{p}})_1 > 1$. This is not very physical, but it gives the right pdf, namely,

$$b(t) = \frac{\mu_2}{\mu_2 - \mu_1}\left(\mu_1 e^{-\mu_1 t}\right) + \frac{\mu_1}{\mu_1 - \mu_2}\left(\mu_2 e^{-\mu_2 t}\right) = \frac{\mu_1 \mu_2}{\mu_1 - \mu_2}\left(e^{-\mu_2 t} - e^{-\mu_1 t}\right),$$

and

$$R(t) = \frac{\mu_2}{\mu_2 - \mu_1}\left(e^{-\mu_1 t}\right) + \frac{\mu_1}{\mu_1 - \mu_2}\left(e^{-\mu_2 t}\right) = \frac{1}{\mu_1 - \mu_2}\left(\mu_1 e^{-\mu_2 t} - \mu_2 e^{-\mu_1 t}\right).$$

You can check these out by taking the direct convolution of two nonequivalent exponentials, and then evaluating $R(t) = \int_t^\infty b(y)\, dy$.

This equation, by the way, gives us a second difference. The value of $b(0)$ is 0, whereas every true hyperexponential must be greater than 0 at the origin. In any case, which representation would you want to use? Which is easier to handle? In either case there is a problem. If μ_1 and μ_2 get arbitrarily close to each other, then the formula becomes numerically unstable. But if they are exactly equal, we have an Erlangian-2 distribution. In fact, if we take the limit very carefully, we will get $E_2(t) = \mu(\mu t)e^{-\mu t}$.

There is (at least) one last observation to be made here. From Definition 3.4.2, $\langle\, \mathbf{p}\,,\, \mathbf{B}\,\rangle$ is clearly a PHase representation, but $\langle\, \tilde{\mathbf{p}}\,,\, \tilde{\mathbf{B}}\,\rangle$ is not. In any case, $R(t)$ is a PHase distribution. ▲

The problem is somewhat complicated algebraically. This is what happens in general. Take any two-dimensional representation. As long as the two eigenvalues are different, we have two pairs of eigenvectors, and the canonical representation looks like a hyperexponential. If we then let the two eigenvalues approach each other, suddenly the two left (and right) eigenvectors become equal to each other, and we are left with a degenerate eigenvalue with only one pair of eigenvectors. This means that there is no isometric (or any other) transformation that will diagonalize $\mathbf{B}$, so we are stuck with the E_2 representation (not so terrible). This demonstrates what happens when a matrix (in this case, $\mathbf{B}$) becomes defective.

An alternative possibility is for there to be two independent eigenvectors with the same eigenvalue (e.g., a true h_2 function where the two completion rates are the same). In this case we can throw away one of the phases and permit our customer to go to the other phase with the sum of the probabilities,[†] again yielding the exponential distribution.

Confusing enough? Well, let us try another example, a specific case of Example 3.4.2.

Example 3.4.4: Consider once again two phases in tandem, but now the customer can leave after finishing phase 1 with probability θ. Then the **P** matrix and entrance vector are

$$\mathbf{P} = \begin{bmatrix} 0 & 1-\theta \\ 0 & 0 \end{bmatrix} \quad \text{and} \quad \mathbf{p} = [\, p \;\; q \,],$$

where $p + q = 1$. This leads to a completion rate matrix of the form

$$\mathbf{B} = \begin{bmatrix} \mu_1 & -\mu_1(1-\theta) \\ 0 & \mu_2 \end{bmatrix}.$$

This too can be made to look like an h_2 function, but if $\mu_2 = \theta\mu_1$, then suddenly, $\boldsymbol{\epsilon}'$ is a right eigenvector of **B**, with eigenvalue μ_2. This means that this subsystem is only an exponential server, even though nothing special seems to have happened. From Example 3.4.2 this leads to $\Psi\left[\exp(-t\mathbf{B})\right] = \exp(-t\mu_2)$ for any entrance vector. Observe what has happened here. When $\mu_2 = \theta\mu_1$, one of the two left eigenvectors becomes orthogonal to $\boldsymbol{\epsilon}'$ and thus is discarded, together with the reduction of dimension. Here is the isometric transformation:

$$\mathbf{S}^{-1} = \frac{1}{\mu_2 - \mu_1} \begin{bmatrix} \mu_2 - \mu_1\theta & -\mu_1(1-\theta) \\ 0 & \mu_2 - \mu_1 \end{bmatrix},$$

and

$$\mathbf{S} = \frac{1}{\mu_2 - \mu_1\theta} \begin{bmatrix} \mu_2 - \mu_1 & \mu_1(1-\theta) \\ 0 & \mu_2 - \mu_1\theta \end{bmatrix}.$$

Again note that $\mathbf{S}\boldsymbol{\epsilon}' = \boldsymbol{\epsilon}'$, and

$$\tilde{\mathbf{p}} = \mathbf{p}\mathbf{S}^{-1} = \left[\frac{p(\mu_2 - \mu_1\theta}{\mu_2 - \mu_1} \quad \frac{p\mu_1\theta + q\mu_2 - \mu_1}{\mu_2 - \mu_1} \right], \qquad \tilde{\mathbf{B}} = \mathbf{S}\mathbf{B}\mathbf{S}^{-1} = \begin{bmatrix} \mu_1 & 0 \\ 0 & \mu_2 \end{bmatrix},$$

But when $\mu_2 = \theta\mu_1$ the equations fall apart. For this specific case,

$$\mathbf{S}^{-1} = \begin{bmatrix} 1/a & 1 \\ 0 & 1 \end{bmatrix}, \quad \mathbf{S} = \begin{bmatrix} a & -a \\ 0 & 1 \end{bmatrix}.$$

Any a will yield the same $\tilde{\mathbf{B}}$, but note that the first row of **S** sums to 0, and no value for a can change that. Also note that

$$\mathbf{S}\boldsymbol{\epsilon}' = \begin{bmatrix} 0 \\ 1 \end{bmatrix} \quad \text{and} \quad \mathbf{S}^{-1}\begin{bmatrix} 0 \\ 1 \end{bmatrix} = \boldsymbol{\epsilon}'.$$

[†]This property is quite different from the apparently similar situation in control theory. There, if a degenerate eigenvalue has two eigenvectors, that implies a feedback loop, which can cause instability.

Throwing away the first row and first column of every matrix, and the first component of every vector, yields the 1-dimensional representation of the exponential distribution. ▲

As a last example, consider the following defective 3-dimensional representations.

Example 3.4.5: The left half of Figure 3.4.1 is a diagram of a server with three phases where the customer, upon entering, goes to phase 1 ($\mathbf{p} = [1 \quad 0 \quad 0]$). After finishing at phase 1 he goes to phase 2 with probability p, and to phase 3 with probability $q = 1 - p$. After that he leaves. Phases 1 and 2 have service rate $\mu_1 = \mu_2 = 2$ and phase 3 has $\mu_3 = 1$. Then

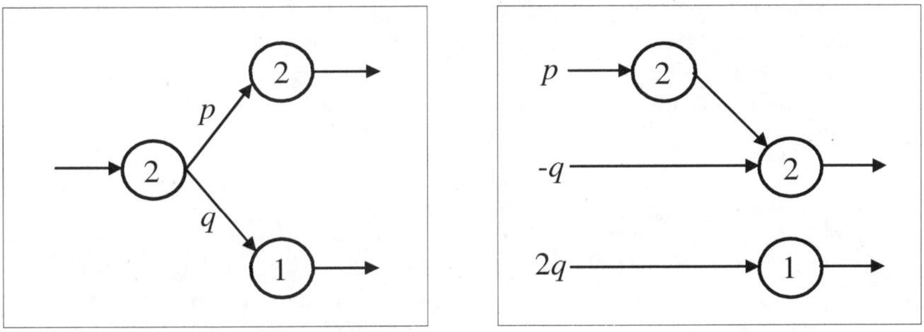

Figure 3.4.1: Two defective representations of the function given in equation (3.4.4). The left-hand figure is a PHase representation, whereas the right-hand one is not, but is in canonical form.

$$\mathbf{P} = \begin{bmatrix} 0 & p & q \\ 0 & 0 & 0 \\ 0 & 0 & 0 \end{bmatrix} \quad \mathbf{M} = \begin{bmatrix} 2 & 0 & 0 \\ 0 & 2 & 0 \\ 0 & 0 & 1 \end{bmatrix} \quad \text{and} \quad \mathbf{B} = \begin{bmatrix} 2 & -2p & -2q \\ 0 & 2 & 0 \\ 0 & 0 & 1 \end{bmatrix}.$$

Given that $\mathbf{B}$ is triangular, its three eigenvalues are its diagonal elements, 2, 2 and 1. But it only has two sets of eigenvectors, one for eigenvalue 1 and one for 2. Thus it is defective. The canonical form for $\tilde{\mathbf{B}}$ must be:

$$\tilde{\mathbf{B}} = \begin{bmatrix} 2 & -2 & 0 \\ 0 & 2 & 0 \\ 0 & 0 & 1 \end{bmatrix}.$$

An easy way to find the ***isometric transformation*** that yields $\tilde{\mathbf{B}}$ is to solve the set of homogeneous equations implied by

$$\mathbf{S}\,\mathbf{B} = \tilde{\mathbf{B}}\,\mathbf{S},$$

and selecting the undetermined constants so as to satisfy $\mathbf{S}\boldsymbol{\epsilon}' = \boldsymbol{\epsilon}'$. They turn out to be

$$\mathbf{S} = \frac{1}{p}\begin{bmatrix} 1 & q & -2q \\ 0 & p & 0 \\ 0 & 0 & p \end{bmatrix} \qquad \mathbf{S}^{-1} = \begin{bmatrix} p & -q & 2q \\ 0 & 1 & 0 \\ 0 & 0 & 1 \end{bmatrix},$$

and $\tilde{\mathbf{p}} = \mathbf{p}\,\mathbf{S}^{-1} = [\,p \quad -q \quad 2q\,]$. The diagram of the canonical representation is shown on the right diagram of Figure 3.4.1. Here we have an E_2 component and a hypoexponential part with a negative probability of going to phase 2. The density function can be written down directly as

$$b(x) = (2p\,x - q)\left(2\,e^{-2x}\right) + 2q\,e^{-x}. \tag{3.4.4}$$

Note that, as with all distributions where the customer must go through at least two phases before exiting, $b(0) = 0$.

It is easy to check that rows 2 and 3 of $\mathbf{S}$ are left eigenvectors of $\mathbf{B}$, and columns 1 and 3 of $\mathbf{S}^{-1}$ are right eigenvectors, but the other row and column are not. ▲

Perhaps we have tried to say too much in too little space. Rest assured that there are an infinity of examples that can force us into confusing interpretations of the various components. Therefore, we reiterate that it is the matrix as a whole that describes any subsystem, or nonexponential server, not its components.

3.4.4 On the Completeness of ME Distributions

Despite the richness of possibilities we have just seen, not every pdf has an exact representation. On the other hand, it is well known that the set of polynomials times exponentials forms a complete set in that (almost?) every integrable function can be approximated arbitrarily closely by a sum of members of that set. This approximation concept is discussed in detail elsewhere and is becoming an increasingly important area of research, with few clear answers at present.

By ***completeness*** we mean that for every pdf of interest there exists a sequence of finite-dimensional vector-matrix pairs (perhaps of ever-increasing dimension) whose properties converge to those of that pdf. Suppose that $\{\langle\, \mathbf{p_m}\,,\, \mathbf{B_m}\,\rangle \mid m = 1, 2, \ldots\}$ is such a sequence; then in some meaningful sense,

$$\lim_{m\to\infty} \Psi_m\left[\exp(-t\mathbf{B_m})\right] = R(t) \tag{3.4.5a}$$

and

$$\lim_{m\to\infty} \Psi_m\left[\mathbf{V}^{\ell}_{\mathbf{m}}\right] = \int_0^{\infty} t^{\ell} b(t)dt, \qquad \ell \ge 0, \tag{3.4.5b}$$

with equivalent limits for other properties of $b(t)$. We have discussed three such sequences up to now; the TPT distributions of Section 3.3.6.2, the deterministic distribution of (3.2.5a), and the uniform distribution (to be discussed further in Exercise 3.5.8). All three involve an ever-increasing sequence of representations whose properties approach ever closely those of the function they approximate, so Equations (3.4.5) are satisfied. But what about

$$\lim_{m\to\infty} \langle\, \mathbf{p_m}\,,\, \mathbf{B_m}\,\rangle?$$

The TPT representation in (3.3.24) does indeed have a limit, but the representation of (3.2.5a) does not. Recall that the Erlangian-m functions have a mean of m/μ, so to maintain a mean of 1, we let $\mu = m$. Then, in the limit as $m \to \infty$ we also have $\mu \to \infty$, so $\lim_{m\to\infty} \mathbf{B_m}$ does not exist. The uniform distribution is even worse. The sequence of approximate representations has the same $\mathbf{B_m}$s, whereas the entrance vectors are

$$\mathbf{p_m} = \frac{1}{m}[1\ 1\ \cdots\ 1\ 1],$$

so $\lim\ \mathbf{p_m} = \mathbf{o}$. These examples tell us we must be careful when we let the dimensions of a representation become unboundedly large, and we cannot necessarily deal directly with infinite-dimensional matrices and vectors. But we can (in principle) deal with matrices of whatever size is needed to yield accurate enough approximations to any desired PDF.

Before moving on, we discuss the meaning of a representation for which $\mathbf{B}$ or $\mathbf{V}$ is singular (i.e., either matrix has no inverse). First we consider finite representations. If $\mathbf{B}$ is singular, exactly one of the parallel paths of its minimal representation (Figure 3.2.5) has a single phase with a 0 completion rate, or equivalently, an infinite completion time (multiple phases in tandem with infinite completion times would be redundant). This corresponds to one of two possibilities. Either (at least) one of the phases in the original representation is broken, or there is a possibility that a customer can be trapped in an infinite loop. In either case, there is a greater than zero probability that a customer can take an infinite time to complete service. In other words, the mean service time for this distribution is infinite. This is consistent with (3.2.14c) because $\mathbf{V}$ does not exist if $\mathbf{B}$ is singular. Next, suppose that $\mathbf{V}$ exists and is singular. Then it has at least one 0 eigenvalue, and exactly one parallel path of its minimal representation has a single phase with zero completion time. This is physically equivalent to the possibility that a customer may bypass service altogether. In other words, there is a probability greater than 0 that a customer will have 0 service time, or the PDF, $B(t)$ at $t = 0$, is greater than 0. Because

$$B(t) = \int_0^t b(x)dx,$$

$b(x)$ must be singular at $x = 0$. This is consistent with (3.1.8b) and the fact that $\mathbf{B}$ does not exist. We get around this without much difficulty later.

Infinite matrices have a much greater variety of singularities, thus making them more difficult to analyze mathematically (aside from the technical problem of dealing with an infinite set of numbers). A detailed discussion of this must wait for further research. It is sufficient for our purposes to deal only with finite matrices, and to represent distribution functions that have special properties (e.g., functions with nonexponential tails and have infinite moments) by a sequence of finite representations of ever-increasing dimension, as described above in our definition of ME functions.

3.4.5 Setting Up Matrix Representations

It is one thing to talk abstractly about a pdf that describes the behavior of a server or process. It is another thing to say explicitly what the pdf is, based on real-world examination. "What is the pdf?" is definitely not a trivial question to answer nor is, "What is its matrix representation?" We discuss the two questions briefly here. There are various ways in which the behavior of subsystems shows up in the course of examining queueing systems. Several of them, together with how they can be represented in LAQT, follow.

1. If a Markov chain, or transition graph description is given, $\mathbf{p}$, $\mathbf{P}$, and $\mathbf{M}$ are included as part of the description. In effect, this gives us Figure 3.1.1.
2. If a density function is given, and one of the following is true;
   (a) $b(t)$ only has terms that are exponentials times powers of t, then it can be rewritten in the form of (3.2.1), from which the appropriate parameters corresponding to Figure 3.2.1 can be found,
   (b) $b(t)$ is not as in part (a), then an approximation must be found that obeys (a).
3. If the Laplace transform for the pdf of the subsystem is given, and
   (a) $B^*(s)$ is RLT, then expand it in terms of its partial fractions. This entails finding the roots of its denominator polynomial. Each term will be of the form $[a_i p_j^{(i)}]/(1 + s\mu_i)^j$, from which Figure 3.2.1 can be drawn, or
   (b) $B^*(s)$ is not RLT, then an approximation must be found that is RLT.
4. Only a finite set of data is available that reflects the performance of the subsystem. Then a suitable function must be constructed that reflects this performance (i.e., another approximation).

It is not at all clear what a 'good' approximation might mean in a queueing theory context. Its goodness depends very much on what use will be made of the function and in what context. Even if two functions seem to look alike, they may yield radically different results in any given application. The commonly accepted procedure of picking approximate functions that have the correct first two (or more) moments (i.e., $\mathbb{E}[T]$ and σ^2, etc.) has been shown to be inadequate and even very misleading in solving various problems. The value of $b(t)$ and its derivatives at 0 may be more important at times. This is discussed in Chapter 5. Until then, we assume in all topics we cover here that a representation, or a series of approximate representations converging to $b(t)$, has already been selected.

3.5 Renewal Processes and Residual Times

Consider a sequence of positive random variables (e.g., service times), $\{X_1, X_2, \ldots X_k, \ldots\}$ where all the X_ks are independent and, except perhaps X_1, are identically distributed. Its relationship with the material in this chapter is straightforward. Let our subsystem S start with an infinite number of customers waiting to enter while C_1 is being served. Call them $C_2, C_3, C_4, \ldots$. When C_1 is finished, he leaves, and C_2 immediately enters, and so on (see Figure 3.5.1). The time C_k spends in S is X_k. It is clear that the X_ks have the same pdf. There is one possible exception, namely if C_1 had entered S at some indeterminate time before our observer started her clock. Then X_1

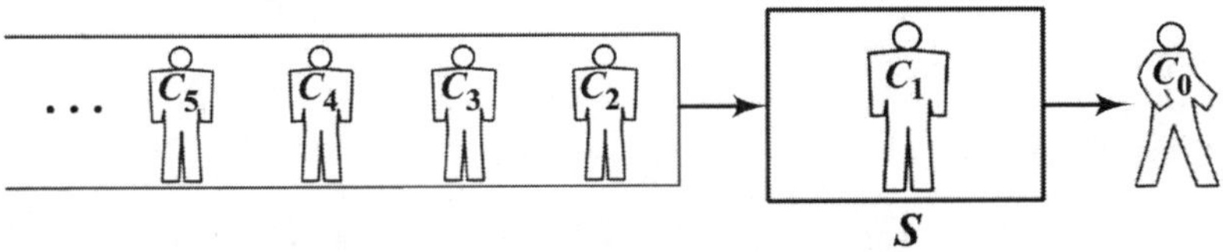

Figure 3.5.1: Renewal process viewed as a sequence of departures from a single subsystem S, able to serve one customer at a time. There is an infinite queue of customers waiting to enter S, and at time = 0, C_1 is already being served. He leaves at time Y_1 (= X_1), after which C_2 immediately enters. At time Y_2 (= $Y_1 + X_2$) he leaves and C_3 enters. This goes on indefinitely, generating the renewal epochs, Y_1, Y_2, Y_3, Y_4, ... , Y_k ....

would come from the PDF [see (3.1.7c)]

$$\mathbb{P}\mathbf{r}(X_1 < x) := B_1(x) = 1 - \boldsymbol{\pi}\,[\exp(-x\mathbf{B})]\boldsymbol{\epsilon}',$$

where π_i is the probability that C_1 was at phase i when she started looking, and x is the time elapsed thereafter. This subtle change of $\boldsymbol{\pi}$ for $\mathbf{p}$ in (3.1.7a) is quite a powerful technique in analyzing a sequence of events. In general, one can take the vector that describes what happened up to the present $[\boldsymbol{\pi}]$ and premultiply it to the vector of probabilities of future events (recall from Definition 3.1.1 that $[\exp(-x\mathbf{B})\boldsymbol{\epsilon}']_i$ is the probability that C_1 will still be in S at time x, given that it was in state i at time 0) to get the total probability for any given event to occur. If observation began at the moment C_1 entered S, then $\boldsymbol{\pi} = \mathbf{p}$, and X_1 has the same distribution as the other X_ks.

An interesting event to examine is the time for the n-th customer to complete service. That time is the random variable Y_n, called a ***renewal epoch***, and defined by the obvious relation

$$Y_n := \sum_{k=1}^{n} X_k = Y_{n-1} + X_n, \quad n > 1, \tag{3.5.1a}$$

where $Y_1 = X_1$. In our picture, the Y_ns are the ***departure times***, and the X_n's are the ***interdeparture times***. If one thinks of these customers as having already departed from S and then arrive at some point downstream then the X_ns become the ***interarrival times*** and the Y_n's become the ***arrival times***. We remind the reader that in this book we use ***epoch*** to mean not only the time Y_n, but the entire interval from Y_{n-1} up to and including Y_n.

A formal definition of a *renewal process* as given by Feller [FELLER71] follows.

Definition 3.5.1

Let X_1, X_2, ..., X_n, ... be a sequence of independent random variables having the same distribution as X (i.e., $X_n = X$). Furthermore, let Y_n be defined by (3.5.1a). Then the sequence of Y_ns constitute a ***renewal process***. Alternatively, the sequence of X_ns can be called a renewal process. Furthermore, if $X_1 \neq X$ Feller calls it a ***delayed renewal process***. It has also been referred to as a ***generalized renewal process***.

An associated process can be defined as follows. Let $N_j(\Delta)$ be the non-negative integer random variable denoting the number of customers that have departed (or arrived) in the time interval $((j-1)\Delta, j\Delta]$, where $\Delta > 0$. Then the sequence $\{N_j(\Delta)\}$, is the ***counting process*** associated with the renewal process $\{X_n\}$. Even though the X_n's are iid, the N_j's (except for Poisson) in general, are not independent. □

We already know quite a bit about these variables from elementary probability theory [TRIVEDI02]. The classic survey is given in [COX62].

3.5.1 Matrix Representations for the pdf of Y_n

We know that the mean time for C_n to finish is the sum of the mean service times for all customers up to and including n. Because all customers, except perhaps C_1, share the same distribution, we have

$$\mathbf{E}[\,X_k^j\,] := \mathbf{E}[\,X^j\,], \quad k > 1,\ j \geq 0.$$

The variance of X_k $(k > 1)$ is

$$\mathrm{Var}(X_k) := \sigma^2 := \mathbf{E}[\,X^2] - \bar{x}^2.$$

Then [where only $\mathbf{E}[X_1^j]$ and σ_1^2 are different]

$$\mathbf{E}[Y_n] = \mathbf{E}[X_1] + (n-1)\mathbf{E}[X] \quad \text{and} \quad \mathrm{Var}(Y_n) = \sigma_1^2 + (n-1)\sigma^2.$$

These properties follow from the fact that the pdf for Y_n [call it $b_n(x)$] is the convolution of the pdfs of the X_ks. For instance,

$$b_2(x) = \int_0^x b_1(s)b(x-s)ds,$$

and generally,

$$b_{k+1}(x) = \int_0^x b_k(s)b(x-s)ds, \quad k > 1, \tag{3.5.1b}$$

where $b(x)$ comes from (3.1.7d), and $b_1(x)$ is similar, with $\boldsymbol{\pi}$ replacing $\mathbf{p}$. Similarly, the PDFs, $B_k(x)$, satisfy

$$B_{k+1}(x) = \int_0^x B_k(s)b(x-s)ds. \tag{3.5.1c}$$

Note that $b_1(x)$ is the pdf for both X_1 and Y_1, and $b(x)$ is the pdf for every other X_k.

Equations (3.5.1) are not in a form conducive to producing a useful matrix representation, but let us try anyway. After all, it is often as important to know what cannot be done as it is to know what can. For $k = 2$,

$$\begin{aligned} b_2(x) &= \int_0^x \boldsymbol{\pi}\,\mathbf{B}\exp(-s\mathbf{B})\boldsymbol{\epsilon}'\mathbf{p}\,\exp[-(x-s)\mathbf{B}]\mathbf{B}\boldsymbol{\epsilon}'\,ds \\ &= \boldsymbol{\pi}\,\mathbf{B}\left[\int_0^x \exp[-s\mathbf{B}]\mathbf{Q}\exp[-(x-s)\mathbf{B}]ds\right]\mathbf{B}\,\boldsymbol{\epsilon}', \end{aligned}$$

where[†] $\mathbf{Q} := \boldsymbol{\epsilon}'\mathbf{p}$ is an idempotent matrix (see Exercise 1.3.5) and does not commute with $\mathbf{B}$ or $\mathbf{V}$. This matrix appears over and over and has many useful properties, some of which we summarize here as a lemma.

Lemma 3.5.1: Let $\mathbf{Q} = \boldsymbol{\epsilon}'\mathbf{p}$; then $\mathbf{Q}$ has one eigenvalue equal to 1, and $m-1$ eigenvalues equal to 0, where m is the dimension of $\mathbf{Q}$. In other words, $\mathbf{Q}$ is of rank 1. $\boldsymbol{\epsilon}'$ and $\mathbf{p}$ are its right and left eigenvectors belonging to eigenvalue 1. That is, they satisfy

$$\mathbf{Q}\,\boldsymbol{\epsilon}' = \boldsymbol{\epsilon}' \quad \text{and} \quad \mathbf{pQ} = \mathbf{p}.$$

$\mathbf{Q}$ is ***idempotent***, because $\mathbf{Q} = \mathbf{Q}^2$. Also, for any square matrix $\mathbf{D}$, the following are true.

$$\mathbf{QDQ} = \Psi[\mathbf{D}]\,\mathbf{Q}, \quad \mathbf{QD}\,\boldsymbol{\epsilon}' = \Psi[\mathbf{D}]\,\boldsymbol{\epsilon}', \quad \mathbf{pDQ} = \Psi[\mathbf{D}]\,\mathbf{p}.$$

The proofs are straightforward by substituting for $\mathbf{Q}$. Recall that $\Psi[\mathbf{D}] = \mathbf{pD}\boldsymbol{\epsilon}'$ is a scalar and can be brought outside any matrix algebraic expression. For instance, for some arbitrary multiplication string of matrices with at least two appearances of $\mathbf{Q}$, we can write

$$\mathbf{AQBQC} = \mathbf{A}\;\mathbf{QBQ}\;\mathbf{C} = \Psi[\mathbf{B}]\,\mathbf{AQC}.$$

Therefore, every matrix string can be reduced to a scalar times a matrix string with at most one $\mathbf{Q}$ in it. ■

We return now to the last equation preceding Lemma 3.5.1. Because $\mathbf{Q}$ is in the middle of this expression, no simplification can be made in this form. Expanding both exponentials in power series will allow the integrals to be performed. There are two paths that one can take. We do both in turn. First,

$$\begin{aligned} b_2(x) &= \boldsymbol{\pi}\,\mathbf{B}\int_0^x \sum_{k=0}^{\infty}\frac{(-\mathbf{B})^k}{k!}\mathbf{Q}\sum_{j=0}^{\infty}\frac{(-\mathbf{B})^j}{j!}s^k(x-s)^j ds\mathbf{B}\boldsymbol{\epsilon}' \\ &= \boldsymbol{\pi}\,\mathbf{B}\sum_{k=0}^{\infty}\sum_{j=0}^{\infty}\frac{(-\mathbf{B})^k\mathbf{Q}(-\mathbf{B})^j}{k!j!}\left[\int_0^x s^k(x-s)^j ds\right]\mathbf{B}\boldsymbol{\epsilon}'. \end{aligned}$$

[†]We point out that this $\mathbf{Q}$ has nothing whatever to do with the transition rate matrix $\boldsymbol{Q}$ of Chapter 1.

The expression in brackets, as defined in [ABRAMOWITZSTEGUN64], is the ***beta function***, and is equal to

$$\beta(k+1, j+1) := \int_0^x s^k (x-s)^j ds = \frac{k!j!}{(k+j+1)!} x^{k+j+1}.$$

Therefore,

$$b_2(x) = x\boldsymbol{\pi}\,\mathbf{B}\left[\sum_{k=0}^{\infty}\sum_{j=0}^{\infty}\frac{(-x\mathbf{B})^k\mathbf{Q}(-x\mathbf{B})^j}{(k+j+1)!}\right]\mathbf{B}\boldsymbol{\epsilon}'. \tag{3.5.2a}$$

As far as we know, there is no closed-form expression for this. However, see Exercises 3.5.5 and 3.5.6 for a meaning of these terms.

Exercise 3.5.1: If S is one-dimensional (i.e., exponential), then $\mathbf{Q} = 1, \boldsymbol{\pi} = 1$, and $\mathbf{B} = \mu$. Show directly from the expression above that $b_2(x) = \mu^2 x e^{-\mu x}$.

Alternatively, we can write

$$\begin{aligned} b_2(x) &= \boldsymbol{\pi}\,\mathbf{B}\left[\int_0^x \exp(-s\mathbf{B})\mathbf{Q}\exp(+s\mathbf{B})ds\right]\exp(-x\mathbf{B})\mathbf{B}\boldsymbol{\epsilon}' \\ &= \boldsymbol{\pi}\,\mathbf{B}\sum_{k=0}^{\infty}\sum_{j=0}^{\infty}\frac{(-\mathbf{B})^k\mathbf{Q}(\mathbf{B})^j}{k!j!}\left[\int_0^x s^{k+j}ds\right]\exp(-x\mathbf{B})\mathbf{B}\boldsymbol{\epsilon}', \end{aligned}$$

and finally,

$$b_2(x) = x\boldsymbol{\pi}\,\mathbf{B}\left[\sum_{k=0}^{\infty}\sum_{j=0}^{\infty}\frac{(-x\mathbf{B})^k\mathbf{Q}(x\mathbf{B})^j}{k!j!(k+j+1)}\right]\exp(-x\mathbf{B})\mathbf{B}\boldsymbol{\epsilon}'. \tag{3.5.2b}$$

This does not seem to be much better, if at all, and we can expect $b_3(x)$ to yield even messier expressions for either form. Our purpose in going through this at all was to warn the reader that matrix functions are not always as easy to manipulate as their scalar counterparts. We must look elsewhere for useful expressions.

Exercise 3.5.2: Show that (3.5.2b) also reduces to $b_2(x) = \mu^2 x e^{-\mu x}$ when S is one-dimensional.

Rather than trying to convert a convolution into a matrix expression, let us instead look at Y_k as a single process. Consider Figure 3.5.2 where we have k identical subsystems in tandem, each described by the same pair $\langle \mathbf{p}, \mathbf{V}\rangle$, except for S_1, which has $\boldsymbol{\pi}$ instead of $\mathbf{p}$. A customer starts at the i-th phase

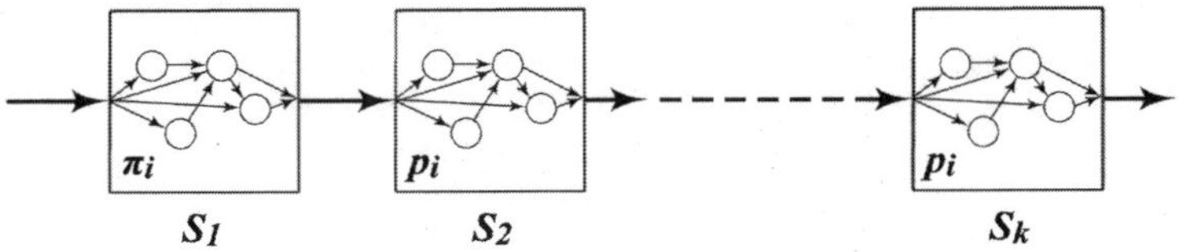

Figure 3.5.2: Representation of the distribution of Y_k, the k-th convolution of S with itself. All the S's are identical, except that the starting vector for S_1 may be different.

of S_1 with probability π_i. After meandering for a while $[\mathbf{P}]$, he leaves $[\mathbf{q}']$, and immediately goes to S_2, entering there and going to phase i with probability p_i. Instead of having a convolution of k m-dimensional objects, our process is described by the $(k \times m)$-dimensional arrays $\{\mathbf{p_k}, \boldsymbol{\epsilon}'_\mathbf{k}, \mathbf{P_k}, \mathbf{M_k}, \text{etc.}\}$. $\boldsymbol{\epsilon}'_\mathbf{k}$ is a $k \times m$ vector of all 1's. The process must start in one of the first m states, so

$$\mathbf{p_k} = [\boldsymbol{\pi}, \mathbf{o}, \mathbf{o}, \ldots, \mathbf{o}] \tag{3.5.3a}$$

(each $\mathbf{o}$ is an m-vector of all 0's) and will go from i to j in S_1 with probability P_{ij}, or go to the phase j in S_2 with probability $q_i p_j = (\mathbf{q}'\mathbf{p})_{ij}$. For $k = 3$, for instance,

$$\mathbf{P_3} = \begin{bmatrix} \mathbf{P} & \mathbf{q}'\mathbf{p} & \mathbf{O} \\ \mathbf{O} & \mathbf{P} & \mathbf{q}'\mathbf{p} \\ \mathbf{O} & \mathbf{O} & \mathbf{P} \end{bmatrix} \quad \text{and} \quad \mathbf{M_3} = \begin{bmatrix} \mathbf{M} & \mathbf{O} & \mathbf{O} \\ \mathbf{O} & \mathbf{M} & \mathbf{O} \\ \mathbf{O} & \mathbf{O} & \mathbf{M} \end{bmatrix}. \tag{3.5.3b}$$

The rate matrix for the process is (remember that $\mathbf{Bq}'\mathbf{p} = \mathbf{BQ}$)

$$\mathbf{B_3} = \mathbf{M_3}(\mathbf{I_3} - \mathbf{P_3}) = \begin{bmatrix} \mathbf{B} & -\mathbf{BQ} & \mathbf{O} \\ \mathbf{O} & \mathbf{B} & -\mathbf{BQ} \\ \mathbf{O} & \mathbf{O} & \mathbf{B} \end{bmatrix}$$

$$= \mathbf{B} \begin{bmatrix} \mathbf{I} & -\mathbf{Q} & \mathbf{O} \\ \mathbf{O} & \mathbf{I} & -\mathbf{Q} \\ \mathbf{O} & \mathbf{O} & \mathbf{I} \end{bmatrix} \tag{3.5.3c}$$

with process time matrix

$$\mathbf{V_3} = \mathbf{B_3}^{-1} = \begin{bmatrix} \mathbf{I} & \mathbf{Q} & \mathbf{Q} \\ \mathbf{O} & \mathbf{I} & \mathbf{Q} \\ \mathbf{O} & \mathbf{O} & \mathbf{I} \end{bmatrix} \mathbf{V}. \tag{3.5.3d}$$

The generalization to any k should be clear. We can now write down the pdf for this process:

$$b_k(x) = \mathbf{p_k}\left[\mathbf{B_k} \exp(-x\mathbf{B_k})\right] \boldsymbol{\epsilon}'_\mathbf{k} \quad \text{and} \quad \mathbb{E}[Y_k^\ell] = \frac{1}{\ell!} \mathbf{p_k} \left[\mathbf{V_k}^\ell\right] \boldsymbol{\epsilon}'_\mathbf{k}. \tag{3.5.3e}$$

Exercise 3.5.3: Prove by direct calculation that (3.5.3d) is the inverse of $\mathbf{B_3}$. Also, give the general expression for $\mathbf{V_k}$ and $\mathbf{B_k}$, and find the mean and variance of $b_k(x)$ using only these formulas.

3.5.2 Renewal Function and Transient Renewal Processes

If all that renewal theory had to offer was another view of convolutions, the topic would not have arisen at all. Its importance comes in studying the number of events that occur in a given interval of time. Suppose that we observe S for a time 0 to Δ. What is the probability that exactly n customers will depart in that time? Let that probability be P_n. Then

$$P_n(\Delta) = \mathbb{P}\mathbf{r}(Y_n \leq \Delta < Y_{n+1}). \tag{3.5.4a}$$

Now, the PDF corresponding to (3.5.3e), $B_n(T)$, is the probability that Y_n is less than Δ, but does not exclude the possibility that Y_m, for $m > n$ is also less than Δ. Therefore,

$$\begin{aligned} B_n(\Delta) &= P_n(\Delta) + P_{n+1}(\Delta) + P_{n+2}(\Delta) + \cdots \\ &= \sum_{m=n}^{\infty} P_m(\Delta) = P_n(\Delta) + B_{n+1}(\Delta). \end{aligned}$$

It then follows that

$$P_n(\Delta) = B_n(\Delta) - B_{n+1}(\Delta). \tag{3.5.4b}$$

We are already familiar with the well-known example for exponential distributions, namely the ***Poisson distribution***, for which

$$P_m(\Delta) = \frac{(\mu\Delta)^m}{m!} e^{-\mu\Delta}. \tag{3.5.4c}$$

We now derive this formula with the aid of (3.5.4b). The m-th convolution of an exponential with itself is the Erlangian density function, already defined in (3.2.1a) and satisfying (3.5.1a),

$$E_m(x) = \mu \frac{(\mu x)^{m-1}}{(m-1)!} e^{-\mu x},$$

whose PDF is

$$B_m(\Delta) = \int_o^{\Delta} E_m(x)dx = 1 - \left[\sum_{k=0}^{m-1} \frac{(\mu\Delta)^k}{k!}\right] e^{-\mu\Delta} = \sum_{k=n}^{\infty} \frac{(\mu\Delta)^k}{k!} e^{-\mu\Delta}.$$

The desired result follows directly.

A useful function in renewal theory is the average number of departures in the interval $(0, \Delta]$.† The initial time $t = 0$ is not included in the interval

†We follow standard mathematical practice, where $(a, b]$ stands for: "all the points between a and b, not including a, but including b." Put another way, $'('$ and $')'$ mean *open* (does not include), and $'['$ and $']'$ mean *closed* (does include).

because we do not wish to count the departure of C_o, if it existed. Define the ***renewal function*** to be the expected number of departures in this interval. Then

$$M(T) := \sum_{n=0}^{\infty} nP_n(T) = \sum_{n=0}^{\infty} nB_n(T) - \sum_{n=0}^{\infty} nB_{n+1}(T)$$
$$= \sum_{n=1}^{\infty} n\, B_n(T) - \sum_{n=1}^{\infty} (n-1)B_n(T).$$

Note that two terms cancel, leaving the well-known formula

$$M(\Delta) = \sum_{n=1}^{\infty} B_n(\Delta). \tag{3.5.5}$$

Following [TRIVEDI02], from (3.5.1b),

$$M(\Delta) = B_1(\Delta) + \int_o^{\Delta} B_1(s)b(\Delta - s)\, ds + \int_o^{\Delta} B_2(s)b(\Delta - s)\, ds + \cdots$$
$$= B_1(\Delta) + \int_o^{\Delta} [B_1(s) + B_2(s) + B_3(s) + \cdots]b(\Delta - s)\, ds,$$

yielding an integral equation (the ***renewal equation***) for the renewal function

$$M(\Delta) = B_1(\Delta) + \int_o^{\Delta} M(s)b(\Delta - s)ds$$
$$= B_1(\Delta) + \int_o^{\Delta} M(\Delta - s)b(s)ds. \tag{3.5.6}$$

Actually, it has been found to be easier to study the derivative of $M(\Delta)$, because $M(\Delta)$ goes to infinity as Δ goes to infinity, but its derivative does not. Therefore, define the ***renewal density***

$$m(x) := \frac{dM(x)}{dx} = \sum_{n=1}^{\infty} b_n(x) = b_1(x) + \int_o^{x} m(s)b(x - s)ds. \tag{3.5.7}$$

$m(x)$ can be interpreted as the instantaneous completion (or service, or arrival) rate of the renewal process. A solution of this equation is not easy to come by, although its Laplace transform is, giving us little insight into what is going on. It is known, however, that if $b(x)$ is exponential, then $m(\Delta) = \mu$ is constant for all Δ, which is what one would expect for all distributions. The expected number of completions in the interval $(0, \Delta]$ is $M(\Delta) = \mu\,\Delta$, no matter how big or small Δ is. It is somewhat surprising that this is not true for general servers. We find $m(x)$ by looking at a different problem that turns out to simultaneously solve (3.5.7).

Consider our same S with only one customer, who, after visiting S leaves, and with probability α immediately returns to S, as shown in Figure 3.5.3.

Feller calls this a ***transient renewal process***. This is also referred to as a ***feedback loop***. We use the symbol S_r for the subsystem that generates this. For the rest of this chapter, r is used as a subscript for objects that are properties of S_r, as distinct from the use of any other symbols, such as i, j, k, l, and n, which are numerical subscripts. So, for instance, S_k is the k-th subsystem in tandem in Figure 3.5.2. We can construct the pdf for S_r by the following argument. Our customer will visit S exactly k times with probability $\alpha^{k-1}(1-\alpha)$. Given that the pdf for visiting k times is $b_k(x)$, the pdf for S_r is

$$f(x;\alpha) := (1-\alpha)\sum_{k=1}^{\infty}\alpha^{k-1}b_k(x) := (1-\alpha)m(x;\alpha). \tag{3.5.8a}$$

From previous discussion, it follows that $m(x;\,\alpha)$ satisfies the integral equa-

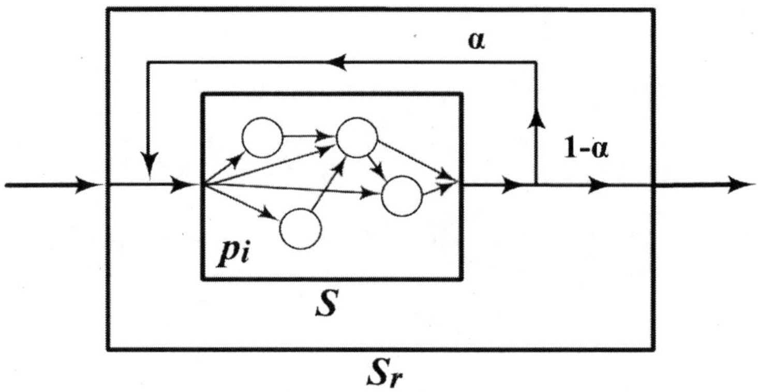

Figure 3.5.3: Representation of the pdf of $f(x;\,\alpha)$. After leaving S, a customer can either leave S_r or, with probability α, return to S. It has a representation given by $\langle \boldsymbol{\pi},\, \mathbf{B_r}(\alpha)\rangle$, as given in the text.

tion

$$m(x;\alpha) = b_1(x) + \alpha\int_0^x m(s;\alpha)b(x-s)\,ds, \tag{3.5.8b}$$

from which we get

$$m(x) = m(x;1) = \lim_{\alpha\to 1}\frac{f(x;\alpha)}{1-\alpha}. \tag{3.5.8c}$$

By integrating (3.5.8a) and (3.5.8b) one can also get a formal expression for $M(x;\alpha)$ with the following properties.

$$\begin{aligned} M(x;\alpha) :&= \int_0^x m(s;\alpha)\,ds = B_1(x) + \alpha\int_0^x M(s;\alpha)B(x-s)ds \\ &= \frac{F(x;\alpha)}{1-\alpha}. \end{aligned} \tag{3.5.8d}$$

Parallel with (3.5.8c), the renewal function satisfies

$$M(x) = M(x;1) = \lim_{\alpha \to 1} \frac{F(x;\alpha)}{1-\alpha}, \tag{3.5.8e}$$

where $F(x;\, \alpha)$ is the PDF of S_r. Its functional form is given below.

This process can be viewed directly as an m-dimensional subnetwork. Let $(\mathbf{P_r})_{ij}$ be the probability of going from i to j, either directly $[P_{ij}]$, or by leaving $[q_i]$, and then immediately returning $[\alpha]$, and going to $j[p_j]$. Then

$$\mathbf{P_r} = \mathbf{P} + \alpha\, \mathbf{q}'\, \mathbf{p}. \tag{3.5.9a}$$

$\mathbf{M_r}$ is the same as $\mathbf{M}$, so the service rate matrix for S_r is

$$\mathbf{B_r}(\alpha) = \mathbf{M_r}(\mathbf{I} - \mathbf{P_r}) = \mathbf{M}(\mathbf{I} - \mathbf{P} - \alpha \mathbf{q}'\, \mathbf{p}) = \mathbf{B} - \alpha \mathbf{M}\mathbf{q}'\mathbf{p}.$$

Recall that $\mathbf{M}\mathbf{q}' = \mathbf{B}\boldsymbol{\epsilon}'$. Therefore, we have

$$\mathbf{B_r}(\alpha) = \mathbf{B}\,(\mathbf{I} - \alpha\mathbf{Q}), \tag{3.5.9b}$$

and because $f(x;\alpha)$ is a density function, generated by $\langle \boldsymbol{\pi}\,,\, \mathbf{B_r}(\alpha) \rangle$, we can write

$$f(x;\alpha) = \boldsymbol{\pi} \exp[-x\mathbf{B_r}(\alpha)]\, \mathbf{B_r}(\alpha)\boldsymbol{\epsilon}' = \boldsymbol{\pi} \exp[-x\mathbf{B}(\mathbf{I} - \alpha\mathbf{Q})]\; \mathbf{B}(\mathbf{I} - \alpha\mathbf{Q})\boldsymbol{\epsilon}'$$

and

$$F(x;\, \alpha) = 1 - \boldsymbol{\pi}[\exp(-x\mathbf{B_r}(\alpha))]\boldsymbol{\epsilon}'. \tag{3.5.9c}$$

But $(\mathbf{I} - \alpha\mathbf{Q})\boldsymbol{\epsilon}' = (1-\alpha)\boldsymbol{\epsilon}'$, so

$$f(x;\alpha) = (1-\alpha)\boldsymbol{\pi} \exp[-x\mathbf{B}(\mathbf{I} - \alpha\mathbf{Q})]\, \mathbf{B}\, \boldsymbol{\epsilon}', \tag{3.5.9d}$$

and

$$m(x;\, \alpha) = \boldsymbol{\pi} \exp[-x\mathbf{B}(\mathbf{I} - \alpha\mathbf{Q})]\, \mathbf{B}\boldsymbol{\epsilon}'. \tag{3.5.9e}$$

A similar expression can be found for its integral,

$$M(x;\, \alpha) = \frac{1 - \boldsymbol{\pi}\, \exp[-x\mathbf{B_r}(\alpha)]\, \boldsymbol{\epsilon}'}{1-\alpha}. \tag{3.5.9f}$$

Let us digress for a moment to observe that $m(x;\alpha)$ is actually the generating function of the $b_k(x)$s. Thus $m(x;0) = b_1(x)$, and in general the k-th derivative of $m(x;\alpha)$ with respect to α evaluated at $\alpha = 0$ is $(k!)b_{k+1}(x)$, where $b_k(x)$ is the pdf of the k-th convolution of $b(x)$ with itself. That is,

$$b_k(x) = \frac{1}{(k-1)!} \left[\left(\frac{\partial}{\partial \alpha} \right)^{(k-1)} m(x;\alpha) \right]_{\alpha=0}. \tag{3.5.9g}$$

This must reduce to the familiar when S is a pure exponential, where as usual, $\mathbf{Q}, \mathbf{p}$, and $\boldsymbol{\epsilon}'$ all equal 1, and $\mathbf{B} = \mu$, so

$$m(x;\alpha) = \mu e^{-\mu x(1-\alpha)} = \mu e^{-\mu x} e^{\mu x \alpha}.$$

For $\alpha = 0$, we get as expected, $b_1(x) = \mu e^{-\mu x}$. There is more to be said about this result. As we pointed out previously in (3.5.8a), the density function of a subsystem with feedback $f(x;\alpha)$, is equal to $(1-\alpha)m(x;\alpha)$. So if S is exponential, with mean service rate μ, then $f(x;\alpha)$ is also exponentially distributed, with mean service rate $(1-\alpha)\mu$. But this is a special case of the following rather interesting lemma, which we state in two apparently unrelated ways.

Lemma 3.5.2: Let $b(x)$ be any pdf with m-dimensional representation $\langle \mathbf{p}, \mathbf{B} \rangle$.

(a) Then the representation of $b(x)$ with feedback [i.e., $\langle \mathbf{p}, \mathbf{B_r}(\alpha) \rangle \rightarrow f(x;\,\alpha)$] is also m-dimensional.

(b) The average of $b(x)$ with its convolutions of all orders, weighted over a geometric distribution $[(1-\alpha)\alpha^{k-1}]$, has a representation which has the same dimension as $b(x)$ itself [(3.5.8a)]. ■

What makes this interesting is the following. We know from the discussion in Section 3.4.5 that the representation of $b_k(x)$ is of dimension $m \times k$. Yet an appropriately weighted average of all these functions has a representation that is no more complicated than the one for $b(x)$. The example of an exponential distribution shows this clearly. The exponential distribution has a one-dimensional representation. Its k-th convolution, the Erlangian-k distribution, has a smallest representation that is of dimension k. Yet the weighted sum is again exponential (i.e., its representation is one-dimensional).

Exercise 3.5.4: Show, using (3.5.9g), that the expression above for $m(x;\alpha)$ does indeed generate the Erlangian-k distributions defined in (3.2.1).

It is not as easy to take the derivative of a matrix function as it would seem. First of all, $\mathbf{B}$ and $\mathbf{Q}$ do not commute (see Theorem 1.3.2), therefore we cannot write $[\exp(-x\mathbf{B})][\exp(x\alpha\mathbf{BQ}]$ for $\exp[-x\mathbf{B}(\mathbf{I}-\alpha\mathbf{Q})]$. Second, the function must be replaced by its Taylor series expansion, and then each term differentiated separately. For instance (here, $'$ stands for the derivative with respect to α),

$$\frac{d}{d\alpha}\mathbf{B_r}^3 = \frac{d}{d\alpha}(\mathbf{B_r}\mathbf{B_r}\mathbf{B_r}) = \mathbf{B_r'}\mathbf{B_r^2} + \mathbf{B_r}\mathbf{B_r'}\mathbf{B_r} + \mathbf{B_r^2}\mathbf{B_r'}.$$

Now from (3.5.9b), $\mathbf{B_r}(\alpha = 0) = \mathbf{B}$ and

$$\frac{d}{d\alpha}\mathbf{B}\,(\mathbf{I}-\alpha\mathbf{Q}) = -\mathbf{BQ},$$

so (suppressing $\mathbf{B_r}$'s dependence on α),

$$\left(\frac{d\mathbf{B_r}^3}{d\alpha}\right)_{\alpha=0} = -\left(\mathbf{BQB}^2 + \mathbf{B}^2\mathbf{QB} + \mathbf{B}^3\mathbf{Q}\right).$$

This expression clearly is not the same as $-3\mathbf{B}(\mathbf{BQ})^2$, and in fact is typical of the terms appearing in Equations (3.5.2).

Exercise 3.5.5: Show in general that

$$\left(\frac{d\mathbf{B_r}^n}{d\alpha}\right)_{\alpha=0} = -\mathbf{B}\left(\sum_{k=0}^{n-1} \mathbf{B}^k\mathbf{Q}\mathbf{B}^{n-k-1}\right).$$

Exercise 3.5.6: Use Exercise 3.5.5 to show that the expression for $b_2(x)$ in (3.5.2a) is actually

$$-\left(\frac{\partial}{\partial\alpha}\Psi\left[\exp(-x\mathbf{B_r})\right]\right)_{\alpha=0},$$

which is the derivative of $F_r(x;\,\alpha)$ for $\mathbf{p} = \boldsymbol{\pi}$, and then evaluated at $\alpha = 0$.

Returning to (3.5.9e), we can take the limit as α goes to 1 directly and get

$$m(x) = \boldsymbol{\pi}\exp[-x\mathbf{B}(\mathbf{I}-\mathbf{Q})]\mathbf{B}\,\boldsymbol{\epsilon}'. \tag{3.5.9h}$$

It is not so easy to find $M(x)$ from $M(x;\alpha)$ in (3.5.9f) because both numerator and denominator approach 0 as $\alpha \to 1$. For exponential distributions, $\mathbf{B} \Rightarrow \mu$, $\mathbf{Q} \Rightarrow 1$, and $\boldsymbol{\pi} \Rightarrow 1$, so $m(x) = \mu$. Clearly, for all other distributions $m(x)$ varies with x. However, we have the first of three versions of the ***renewal theorem***:

Theorem 3.5.3a: Let S represent an ME distribution generating a renewal process; then

$$\lim_{x\to\infty} m(x) = \frac{1}{\bar{x}}. \tag{3.5.10a}$$

∎

Proof: First observe that because $\mathbf{V} = \mathbf{B}^{-1}$, we can state that

$$\boldsymbol{\pi}_\mathbf{r} := \frac{\mathbf{pV}}{\Psi\left[\mathbf{V}\right]} \tag{3.5.10b}$$

is the left eigenvector of $\mathbf{B}(\mathbf{I}-\mathbf{Q})$ with eigenvalue 0, and corresponding right eigenvector $\boldsymbol{\epsilon}'$, with length $\boldsymbol{\pi}_\mathbf{r}\,\boldsymbol{\epsilon}' = 1$. (We take another look at the ***mean residual vector*** $\boldsymbol{\pi}_\mathbf{r}$, in the next section.) Then as we showed in Chapter 1 [Equations (1.3.3a) and (1.3.10a)], for large x,

$$\exp[-x\mathbf{B}(\mathbf{I}-\mathbf{Q})] \to \boldsymbol{\epsilon}'\,\boldsymbol{\pi}_\mathbf{r}.$$

Recall from (3.1.4b) that $\Psi[\mathbf{V}] = \bar{x}$ and that $\boldsymbol{\pi}\boldsymbol{\epsilon}' = 1$, so we have

$$\lim_{x\to\infty} m(x) = (\boldsymbol{\pi}\boldsymbol{\epsilon}')\boldsymbol{\pi}_{\mathbf{r}}\,\mathbf{B}\boldsymbol{\epsilon}' = \frac{\mathbf{pV}}{\bar{x}}\mathbf{B}\boldsymbol{\epsilon}' = \frac{\mathbf{pVB}\boldsymbol{\epsilon}'}{\bar{x}} = \frac{1}{\bar{x}}.$$

QED

This tells us that only if the interval is large enough will the mean number of customers departing approach $\Delta/\bar{x}$. This is true because the initial state of the system has to be "forgotten" before the steady-state average can be achieved. We show this more clearly in the next section.

3.5.3 Residual Times and Delayed Intervals

Numerous books have been written exclusively on renewal theory, so one should not expect to be able to cover too much in three sections. There are, however, two related points that we wish to discuss. First, how do we decide what the starting vector $\boldsymbol{\pi}$, is? Even if we have a concise answer for that, we only have formulas describing the first interval of time $(0, \Delta]$. What about later intervals $(\Delta, 2\Delta], (2\Delta, 3\Delta], \ldots, (k\Delta, (k+1)\Delta]$, and even more generally $(x, x+\Delta]$, for any $x > 0$?

3.5.3.1 Residual Vector

Let us consider the simplest case where our time begins at the moment C_1 enters S, or equivalently, just after C_o (if we had defined it) leaves. Then $\boldsymbol{\pi} = \mathbf{p}$, and we have a renewal process describing the number of customers who complete service in the interval $(0, \Delta]$, which we can (at least in principle) calculate using Equations (3.5.4) together with (3.5.9) or (3.5.3) (see the next section for another way). But suppose that we wanted to do the equivalent for a later interval $(x, x+\Delta]$. What would the starting vector $\boldsymbol{\pi}(x)$ be then? Well, if we knew that customer C_1 was still in service at time x, then $\boldsymbol{\pi}(x)$ would be proportional to $\mathbf{r}(x) = \mathbf{p}\exp(-x\mathbf{B})$, whose i-th component is the probability that C_1 is still in service and is at phase i (recall the discussion in Section 3.1.2). The proportionality constant is $\Psi[\exp(-x\mathbf{B})]$, which is $R_1(x)$. What is to be done if C_1 has already finished or we have not kept track of the number of completions until x? We consider the first alternative in the next section and consider the second one here.

Suppose that we do not know, or do not care, how many customers have been served in previous intervals. Can we say something about the probability state of the presently active customer? We can answer the question in a manner similar to that for the transient renewal process, as in Figure 3.5.3. The only difference is that the customer always returns to S (i.e., $\alpha = 1$). We are now describing a closed system, just as was done in Chapter 1. Our customer after leaving phase i can get to j either by going directly there $[P_{ij}]$, or by leaving $[q_i]$, and immediately re-entering and going to j, $[p_j]$. Thus we have an ***isometric matrix*** satisfying (1.3.1b):

$$\mathbf{P_r} := \mathbf{P} + \mathbf{q}'\mathbf{p}. \tag{3.5.11a}$$

But this is identical to (3.5.9a) with $\alpha = 1$, with matching transition rate matrix (1.3.2c), $\mathbf{B_r} := \mathbf{B}(\mathbf{I} - \mathbf{Q}) = \mathbf{B_r}(1)$, which is (3.5.9b) with $\alpha = 1$. We can now define the mean residual vector, or simply the ***residual vector***

$$\boldsymbol{\pi}_\mathbf{r}(x) := \mathbf{p}\exp(-x\mathbf{B_r}), \tag{3.5.11b}$$

whose i-th component is the probability that the trapped customer is at phase i at time x irrespective of how many times he has gone around the loop. From its definition in (3.5.11b) it follows that

$$\lim_{x\to\infty} \boldsymbol{\pi}_\mathbf{r}(x) = \frac{1}{\Psi[\mathbf{V}]}\mathbf{p}\mathbf{V} = \boldsymbol{\pi}_\mathbf{r}, \tag{3.5.12a}$$

where $\boldsymbol{\pi}_\mathbf{r}$ is the mean residual vector defined by (3.5.10b). Note that $m(x) = \boldsymbol{\pi}_\mathbf{r}(x)\mathbf{B}\boldsymbol{\epsilon}'$, but more important, we can evaluate a delayed renewal process starting at any time, x. For instance, suppose that it is desirable to find the renewal density for some interval starting at time x. Then, replacing $\boldsymbol{\pi}$ with $\boldsymbol{\pi}_\mathbf{r}(x)$ in (3.5.11b) yields

$$m_r(\Delta; x) := \boldsymbol{\pi}_\mathbf{r}(x)\exp(-\Delta\mathbf{B_r})\mathbf{B}\boldsymbol{\epsilon}'$$

$$= \mathbf{p}\exp(-x\mathbf{B_r})\exp(-\Delta\mathbf{B_r})\mathbf{B}\boldsymbol{\epsilon}' = \Psi\left[\exp[-(x+\Delta)\mathbf{B_r}]\mathbf{B}\right].$$

Now, because $\boldsymbol{\pi}_\mathbf{r}(x)$ goes to $\boldsymbol{\pi}_\mathbf{r}$ as x goes to infinity [from (3.5.12a)], we have what Feller calls the second form of the renewal theorem [FELLER71].

Theorem 3.5.3b: Let S represent an ME distribution generating a renewal process where measurement starts at time x after C_1 began service; then

$$\lim_{x\to\infty} m_r(\Delta; x) = \frac{1}{\bar{x}}.$$

In words, if measurement is delayed long enough so that the initial state of the system is forgotten, the mean number of customers being served in a time interval Δ is $\Delta/\bar{x}$. ■

This discussion leads us to yet another form of the renewal theorem. If the measuring interval begins at a time completely uncorrelated with the time a customer begins service, the best we can say is that he is at phase i with probability $(\boldsymbol{\pi}_\mathbf{r})_i$. Then we have a third form for the renewal theorem.

Theorem 3.5.3c: Let S represent an ME distribution generating a renewal process in which it is not known when the customer in service (call it C_1) first entered; then $m(\Delta)$ is the same for all Δ and is equal to $1/\bar{x}$, thus $M(\Delta) = \Delta/\bar{x}$. ■

This is what we felt all along. In any experiment of this type, one must decide ahead of time when to start counting and when to stop counting service completions, so that there will be no correlation between when the first customer starts service and when measurement begins. To do otherwise would yield a mean departure rate different from the long-term average.

Almost as an afterthought, we can derive the well-known expression for the ***mean residual time***, which is the mean time that a customer will remain in service, given that it was not known when he began. Let X_r be the r.v. for that remaining time. Then consistent with our notation, we use the symbol $\bar{x}_r := \mathbb{E}[X_r]$.[†] Recall that $\boldsymbol{\pi}_\mathbf{r}$ is the left eigenvector of $\mathbf{B}_\mathbf{r}$, which in turn is the transition rate matrix for our trapped customer of Figure 3.5.3, with $\alpha = 1$. Therefore, the component i of $\boldsymbol{\pi}_\mathbf{r}$ is the steady-state probability of finding him at phase i. Lacking any knowledge of where or when the process began originally, the best we can say at any given moment is that $\boldsymbol{\pi}_\mathbf{r}$ describes all we know about where our customer is. Let us imagine that as of now, we shall let him leave the system once he has finished his present trip through S, then

Theorem 3.5.4: Let X_r be the r.v. for the time remaining for a customer who has been in service for an indefinite period. Then

$$\bar{x}_r = \mathbb{E}[X_r] = \boldsymbol{\pi}_\mathbf{r}\mathbf{V}\boldsymbol{\epsilon}' = \frac{\mathbf{p}\,\mathbf{V}\mathbf{V}\,\boldsymbol{\epsilon}'}{\Psi\left[\mathbf{V}\right]} = \frac{\Psi\left[\mathbf{V}^2\right]}{\Psi\left[\mathbf{V}\right]} = \frac{\mathbb{E}[X^2]}{2\bar{x}}. \tag{3.5.12b}$$

In fact, one gets the rather unusual relationship between the moments of the residual distribution and the original one:

$$\mathbb{E}[X_r^n] = n!\,\boldsymbol{\pi}_\mathbf{r}\,\mathbf{V}^n\boldsymbol{\epsilon}' = \frac{n!}{\bar{x}}\mathbf{p}\mathbf{V}\mathbf{V}^n\boldsymbol{\epsilon}'$$

$$= \frac{n!}{\bar{x}}\Psi\left[\mathbf{V}^{n+1}\right] = \frac{\mathbb{E}[X^{n+1}]}{(n+1)\bar{x}}. \tag{3.5.12c}$$

The proof comes directly from (3.1.9). ■

Exercise 3.5.7: Evaluate $\bar{x}_r$ for an E_2 and an h_2 distribution (see Exercises 3.1.1 and 3.1.2). For the h_2 distribution, let $\alpha = 0.1$, and $\mu_2/\mu_1 = 10$. Note that for E_2, $\bar{x}_r$ is always less than $\bar{x}$, whereas for h_2, $\bar{x}_r$ is always greater than $\bar{x}$. In fact, show in general that $\bar{x}_r$ can be written in either of the two following ways.

$$\bar{x}_r = \bar{x}\,\frac{C_v^2 + 1}{2} = \bar{x} + \bar{x}\,\frac{C_v^2 - 1}{2}, \tag{3.5.12d}$$

so the mean residual time is bigger (smaller) than the mean time whenever the squared coefficient of variation C_v^2, is greater (less) than 1.

The concept of a mean residual vector is useful in succeeding chapters. Here we derive the known result that gives the pdf of X_r, the time remaining for a customer who has been in service for an indefinite period. We do this simply by replacing $\mathbf{p}$ with $\boldsymbol{\pi}_\mathbf{r}$ in (3.1.7d). Then

$$b_r(x) = \boldsymbol{\pi}_\mathbf{r}\,\mathbf{B}\exp(-x\mathbf{B})\boldsymbol{\epsilon}' = \frac{\mathbf{p}\mathbf{V}}{\Psi\left[\mathbf{V}\right]}\mathbf{B}\exp(-x\mathbf{B})\boldsymbol{\epsilon}' = \frac{\Psi\left[\exp(-x\mathbf{B})\right]}{\bar{x}}.$$

[†]So the secret is out; the subscript r stands for *residual*, not renewal, or reliability, or whatever.

But the numerator is $R(t)$, the reliability function of (3.1.7b), so

$$b_r(t) = \frac{R(t)}{\bar{x}}. \tag{3.5.13}$$

Exercise 3.5.8: You have to catch a train to Leipzig from the Hauptbahnhof Station in Munich, which you know leaves every hour. Therefore, the time between departures is exactly one hour, and its density function is given by $b(x) = \delta(x - 1)$ from (3.2.5a). x is measured from the time of the previous departure, but you don't know what that time is when you arrive at the station. You could have just missed it, so you may have to wait a whole hour for the next train, or you could be just on time and get on board right away. Or, it could be anywhere in between, all with equal probability. In other words, the time remaining is uniformly distributed with a mean of 1/2 hour. Find a representation of the uniform distribution using the residual vector in (3.5.10b) and the representation of the Dirac delta function of (3.2.5a) to create $b_r(x)$ as given by (3.5.13).

3.5.3.2 Renewal Processes

We now return to the question presented in the first paragraph of the preceding section. For definiteness, suppose that at time 0, C_1 began service, and that at time $x > 0$, n customers had already been served (i.e., $Y_n \leq x < Y_{n+1}$). What can be said of the events occurring in the interval $(x, x+\Delta]$? It turns out that the generalizations of (3.5.3) contain all the information needed. Define the vector $\mathbf{r}(x, n)$ with $m \times n$ components

$$\mathbf{r}(x, n) := \mathbf{p_n} \exp(-x\mathbf{B_n}), \tag{3.5.14}$$

where, from Exercise 3.5.3, we know that $\mathbf{B_n}$ is an $n \times n$ matrix whose components are $m \times m$ matrices. The matrices on the diagonal are all $\mathbf{B}$, and all the matrices on the super diagonal are $-\mathbf{BQ}$ as, for instance, (3.5.3c). $\mathbf{r}(x, n)$ is actually the reliability vector function already defined in (3.1.7a) for the process described by Figure 3.5.2. Component $(km+j)$ is the probability that our customer is at phase j in S_{k+1} at time x, for $0 \leq k < n$ and $1 \leq j < m$. This in turn means that he has already visited S_1 through S_k but is presently in S_{k+1}. We have already argued that a single customer passing successively through k identical subsystems is equivalent to a renewal epoch of k customers going through S one at a time. Therefore, the sum of probabilities of being somewhere in S_{k+1} must be the same as the $P_k(x)$ defined by (3.5.4a). That is,

$$P_k(x, n) = \sum_{j=km+1}^{(k+1)m} [\mathbf{r}(x, n)]_j$$

is the probability that exactly k customers have been served in the interval (0, x]. Strictly speaking, this is true only for $k \le n$. The complete analysis should only apply for $n = \infty$ or at least for n large enough so that $P_k(x)$ is negligible for all $k > n$. How large n must be to achieve this depends strongly on how large x is, because longer intervals of time permit more customers to be served.

The problem of choosing n for practical computation is not as serious as it would seem. $\mathbf{B_n}$ describes a system with no feedback (all the matrices below the diagonal are $\mathbf{0}$) and consistent with its definition,

$$P_k(x, n_1) = P_k(x, n_2) = P_k(x), \quad \forall\ k \le n_1 \le n_2.$$

This must be true, because whether a customer leaves after visiting n subsystems or moves on to S_{n+1} should have no effect on how much time was spent at each previous S. This must hold true for the components of $\mathbf{r}(x, n)$ as well. Therefore,

$$[\mathbf{r}(x, n)]_i = [\mathbf{r}(x, n+1)]_i \quad \forall\ i \le n \times m.$$

There are no convergence difficulties in talking about an infinite-dimensional $\mathbf{B}_\infty$, therefore we delete the argument, n, in $P_k(x, n)$ and $\mathbf{r}(x, n)$, and define the set of m-dimensional vectors $\boldsymbol{\pi}(x, k)$ as

$$\boldsymbol{\pi}(x, k) := \frac{1}{P_k(x)} \left[r_{km+1}(x), r_{km+2}(x), \ldots, r_{(k+1)m}(x)\right], \tag{3.5.15a}$$

where

$$\boldsymbol{\pi}(x, k)\boldsymbol{\epsilon}' = 1.$$

Put differently,

$$\mathbf{r}(x, \infty) = [P_o(x)\boldsymbol{\pi}(x, 0),\ P_1(x)\boldsymbol{\pi}(x, 1),\ P_2(x)\boldsymbol{\pi}(x, 2),\ \ldots] \tag{3.5.15b}$$

[P_k is a scalar and $\boldsymbol{\pi}(x, k)$ is an m-vector]. We are coming down the home stretch now.

It should be clear that $[\boldsymbol{\pi}(x, k)]_i$ is the conditional probability that C_{k+1} is at phase i at time x, given that C_k has finished. Therefore it can be used in the same way that the initial vector $\boldsymbol{\pi}$ is used, except that we now start measuring at time x. For instance, the renewal density for the interval $(x, x + \Delta]$, given that exactly k customers were served from 0 to x, is

$$m(\Delta; x, k) := \boldsymbol{\pi}(x, k) \exp(-\Delta \mathbf{B_r})\mathbf{B}\, \boldsymbol{\epsilon}'. \tag{3.5.15c}$$

Let $X_n(x)$ be the r.v. for the service time remaining for C_{n+1} given that it was in service at time x (a conditional residual time). Then

$$\bar{x}(x, n) = \mathbf{E}[X_n(x)] = \boldsymbol{\pi}(x, n)\mathbf{V}\, \boldsymbol{\epsilon}'. \tag{3.5.15d}$$

The number of sequences of events that can be analyzed in this way is unlimited. For instance, one can analyze the renewal process starting at some time x_2, given that k_1 customers were served in the interval before x_1, and k_2 customers were served in the interval $(x_1, x_2]$, and so on. Of course, the longer the sequence of conditions, the less interesting the results, for they must ultimately converge to the results using $\boldsymbol{\pi}_\mathbf{r}$. Well, maybe.

3.5.4 Two Illustrations of Renewal Processes

In discussing renewal theory, we have introduced three views, corresponding to Figures 3.5.1 to 3.5.3, none of which actually correspond to the standard description in terms of arrivals. There should be no problem of changing our view from arrivals to departures, but the formulas derived from the three distinct viewpoints given in the previous sections are bound to be at least somewhat confusing. In this subsection we illustrate the various formulas for two distributions. The first assumes that S has only one internal state, and thus represents an exponential server. This leads us to yet another derivation of the Poisson process. In the second example S represents the Erlangian-2 distribution.

3.5.4.1 The Poisson Process

As always, for exponential distributions, $\mathbf{B} \Rightarrow \mu$, and $\mathbf{p}, \mathbf{Q}$, and $\boldsymbol{\epsilon}'$ all equal 1. Many formulas have already been reduced to their exponential results (or have been left to the exercises). We finish the job here. First consider (3.5.9d). The pdf $f(x;\alpha)$ is the density function for a subsystem with external feedback, as shown in Figure 3.5.3. If S itself is exponential, so is S_r, for, as we showed for $m(x;\alpha)$ following (3.5.9g),

$$f(x;\,\alpha) = (1-\alpha)\mu\, e^{-(1-\alpha)\mu x}.$$

This is an exponential distribution with mean service rate $\mu' = (1-\alpha)\mu$. We discussed the underlying significance of this in Lemma 3.5.2. But this tells us something else as well, which we state as another lemma.

Lemma 3.5.5: If any diagonal element of a transition matrix is greater than 0, it can be replaced by 0, with a commensurate change in its service rate and the other elements of $\mathbf{P}$ in that row. That is, suppose that $P_{ii} > 0$. Then let $\alpha = P_{ii}$ and

$$\text{new } P_{ii} = 0; \qquad \text{new } P_{ij} = \frac{P_{ij}}{1-\alpha} \quad \text{for } j \neq i;$$

$$\text{new } M_{ii} = M_{ii}(1-\alpha).$$

The new $\mathbf{P}$ and new $\mathbf{M}$ will yield the same results as the original ones. Thus one can assume (if convenient) that the diagonal elements of a transition matrix are all 0, without loss of generality. ■

The discussion on residual and delayed times has no significance when applied to exponential servers, because $\boldsymbol{\pi}_{\mathbf{r}}(x)$ as defined in (3.5.11b) is always 1 because $\mathbf{B}_{\mathbf{r}} = \mathbf{0}$. Everything is memoryless, and remains the same as it was at the beginning, until the customer leaves.

We then go to (3.5.14), for $n = \infty$. Here [compare with (3.5.3c) and (3.2.3b)]

$$\mathbf{B}_\infty = \mu \begin{bmatrix} 1 & -1 & 0 & 0 & 0 & \cdots \\ 0 & 1 & -1 & 0 & 0 & \cdots \\ 0 & 0 & 1 & -1 & 0 & \cdots \\ 0 & 0 & 0 & 1 & -1 & \cdots \\ \vdots & \vdots & \vdots & \vdots & \vdots & \cdots \end{bmatrix}.$$

To evaluate $\exp(-x\mathbf{B}_\infty)$, one needs $(\mathbf{B}_\infty)^k$ for all k. It can be proven by induction that

$$(\mathbf{B}_\infty{}^k)_{ij} = \mu^k(-1)^{j-i}\binom{k}{j-i} \quad \text{for } j \geq i, \tag{3.5.16a}$$

and 0 otherwise. Therefore, without too much mathematical difficulty, we get the expression (using $y = \mu x$)

$$\exp(-x\mathbf{B}_\infty) = e^{-y} \begin{bmatrix} 1 & y & y^2/2! & y^3/3! & y^4/4! & \cdots \\ 0 & 1 & y & y^2/2! & y^3/3! & \cdots \\ 0 & 0 & 1 & y & y^2/2! & \cdots \\ 0 & 0 & 0 & 1 & y & \cdots \\ \vdots & \vdots & \vdots & \vdots & 1 & \cdots \\ \vdots & \vdots & \vdots & \vdots & \vdots & \cdots \end{bmatrix}.$$

From its definition in (3.5.3a),

$$\mathbf{p}_\infty = [1, 0, 0, 0, 0, \cdots],$$

so $\mathbf{r}(x, \infty)$ is the top row of $\exp(-x\mathbf{B}_\infty)$, or

$$\mathbf{r}(x, \infty) = \left[e^{-y}, ye^{-y}, \frac{y^2e^{-y}}{2!}, \frac{y^3e^{-y}}{3!}, \cdots\right].$$

We know that $m = 1$ from Section 3.5.3, so we get (as no surprise to anyone)

$$P_k(x) = \frac{(\mu x)^k e^{-\mu x}}{k!}, \tag{3.5.16b}$$

the Poisson probabilities of finding k departures in time interval x [compare with (2.1.15) and (3.5.4c)].

3.5.4.2 Renewal Process with E_2 Interdeparture Times

One of the advantages of the methods in this book is that the expressions can easily be directly numerically evaluated automatically by computer. However, it is not easy to get physical insight unless one carries out many parametric studies, presenting the results graphically. As it happens, if m (the dimensionality of S) is small enough, we can find explicit expressions from the matrix formulas. The smallest nontrivial case is then $m = 2$. We now consider one such example.

The Erlangian distribution was discussed in Section 3.2.1 and Equation (3.2.1a). Recall that $E_k(x)$ corresponds to k identical exponential phases in tandem, each with service rate μ. Then for $k = 2$,

$$\mathbf{B} = \mu \begin{bmatrix} 1 & -1 \\ 0 & 1 \end{bmatrix} \quad \text{and} \quad \mathbf{Q} = \begin{bmatrix} 1 & 0 \\ 1 & 0 \end{bmatrix}.$$

From (3.5.9b),

$$\mathbf{B_r}(\alpha) = \mathbf{B}(\mathbf{I} - \alpha\mathbf{Q}) = \mu \begin{bmatrix} 1 & -1 \\ -\alpha & 1 \end{bmatrix}.$$

To get explicit expressions for $f(x;\alpha)$, $m(x;\,\alpha)$, and whatever else might be interesting, we must first get an explicit form for $\exp[-x\mathbf{B_r}(\alpha)]$. It is not hard to show that the eigenvalues for $\mathbf{B_r}(\alpha)$ are $(1 \pm \sqrt{\alpha})$, with eigenvectors (for convenience let $\beta = \sqrt{\alpha}$):

$$\mathbf{u}_\pm = [-1, \pm\beta] \quad \text{and} \quad \mathbf{v}'_\pm = \frac{1}{2}\begin{pmatrix} -1 \\ \pm 1/\beta \end{pmatrix}.$$

Because the eigenvalues are distinct, we can use (1.3.8c) to get (where $y = \mu x \beta$)

$$\exp[-x\mathbf{B_r}(\alpha)] = e^{-\mu x} \begin{bmatrix} \cosh y & \sinh y/\beta \\ \beta \sinh y & \cosh y \end{bmatrix}. \tag{3.5.17}$$

We use this to find $f(x;\alpha)$ from (3.5.9d). Let $\boldsymbol{\pi}$ have components π_1 and π_2, whose sum is 1; then

$$f(x;\alpha) = (1-\alpha)\mu e^{-\mu x}\left(\pi_1 \frac{\sinh y}{\beta} + \pi_2 \cosh y\right).$$

This certainly is not a simple expression even if $\pi_2 = 0$, that is, when $\boldsymbol{\pi} = \mathbf{p}$. In this case

$$f(x;\,\alpha) = \frac{1-\alpha}{2\beta}\mu\left(e^{-\mu x(1-\beta)} - e^{-\mu x(1+\beta)}\right).$$

It is not clear what the generalization for Lemma 3.5.5 is when S is not exponential. We have already noted (Lemma 3.5.2) that a subsystem with external feedback, as in Figure 3.5.3, has the same dimensionality as the subsystem without feedback. The last equation shows that an Erlangian-2 with feedback is equivalent to a subsystem of two unequal phases in tandem, with *no* feedback. The service rates of the two phases are the eigenvalues of $\mathbf{B_r}(\alpha)$. But, of course, this should have been clear from Section 3.2.1. As might be expected, when $\alpha = 1$, $f(x;1)$ is identically 0, corresponding to the fact that our looping customer is forever imprisoned in S_r.

We know from (3.5.8a) that $m(x;\alpha) = f(x;\alpha)/(1-\alpha)$, therefore

$$m(x;\alpha) = \frac{\mu}{2}e^{-\mu x}\left(\pi_1\beta(e^{\mu\beta x} - e^{-\mu\beta x}) + \pi_2(e^{\mu\beta x} + e^{-\mu\beta x})\right).$$

Recall from (3.5.9g) that $m(x;\alpha)$ is the generator of the convolutions of $b(x)$. In this case

$$b(x) = b_1(x) = m(x;0) = \pi_1\, E_2(x;\mu) + \pi_2\, \mu\, e^{-\mu x}.$$

This makes sense. If our customer starts at the second phase (π_2), he will leave in exponential time. But if he starts at the first phase (π_1), he must go through both phases, taking Erlangian-2 time to leave.

Exercise 3.5.9: From (3.5.9g), find the k-th convolutions of $b(x)$. In particular, show that if $\pi_1 = 1$, then the k-th convolution is the Erlangian-$2k$, but if $\pi_2 = 1$, then the k-th convolution is the Erlangian of order $2k - 1$.

From (3.5.8c) the renewal density for our example is (recall that $\beta = \sqrt{\alpha}$)

$$m(x) = m(x; 1) = \frac{\mu}{2}\left[1 + (\pi_2 - \pi_1)e^{-2\mu x}\right]. \tag{3.5.18a}$$

Observe that as x goes to infinity $m(x)$ approaches $\mu/2$, which is $1/\bar{x}$, consistent with the first form of the renewal theorem (Theorem 3.5.3a). Also note that if $\pi_1 = \pi_2$, then $m(x)$ is always $1/\bar{x}$. This is consistent with the third form of the renewal theorem (Theorem 3.5.3c), because the mean residual vector [from (3.5.10b)] is $\boldsymbol{\pi}_\mathbf{r} = [0.5,\ 0.5]$. In words, given that both phases have equal service times and we do not know where our customer started, it will be at either one with equal probability.

The renewal function can be found from $m(x)$ by simple integration,

$$M(\Delta) = \int_0^\Delta m(x)dx = \frac{\Delta}{\bar{x}} + \frac{\pi_2 - \pi_1}{2\,\mu\,\bar{x}}\left(1 - e^{-2\mu\Delta}\right). \tag{3.5.18b}$$

Given that$M(\Delta)$ is the mean number of departures in interval Δ, $M(\Delta)/\Delta$ is the mean number of departures per unit time in that interval. This has a finite limit as Δ goes to infinity, and should be compared with $m(\Delta)$, which is the departure rate at the end of the interval. Note that

$$\frac{M(\Delta)}{\Delta} = \frac{1}{\bar{x}} + \frac{\pi_2 - \pi_1}{\bar{x}}\frac{1 - e^{-2\mu\Delta}}{2\,\mu\,\Delta}. \tag{3.5.18c}$$

We see that $M(\Delta)/\Delta$ approaches the same limit as $m(\Delta)$, but much more slowly. Even when $\exp(-\mu\Delta)$ is negligible, a term in $1/\Delta$ persists (unless the system started in the mean residual state). This is analogous to the average system behavior described in Chapter 1 [see (1.3.12b) and the discussion following it], and in fact, the dependence on Δ is identical. We next move on to the residual vector defined in (3.5.11b). Instead of starting with $\mathbf{p}$, we start with the more general $\boldsymbol{\pi}$, and get with the aid of (3.5.17) for $\alpha = \beta = 1$,

$$\begin{aligned}\boldsymbol{\pi}_\mathbf{r}(x) &= \boldsymbol{\pi}\exp(-x\mathbf{B}_\mathbf{r})\\ &= e^{-\mu x}[\pi_1\cosh(\mu\,x) + \pi_2\sinh(\mu\,x),\ \ \pi_1\sinh(\mu\,x) + \pi_2\cosh(\mu\,x)],\end{aligned}$$

which in this case rearranges to

$$\boldsymbol{\pi}_\mathbf{r}(x) = [0.5,\ 0.5] + \frac{\pi_2 - \pi_1}{2}e^{-2\mu\,x}[-1,\ 1]. \tag{3.5.19}$$

This can be used, for instance, to calculate $X_r(x)$, the time remaining for the trapped customer to complete his present service, given that he has been going in circles for time x. That is,

$$\bar{x}_r(x) := \mathbb{E}[X_r(x)] = \boldsymbol{\pi}_{\mathbf{r}}(x)\mathbf{V}\boldsymbol{\epsilon}' = \frac{1}{2\,\mu}[3 - (\pi_2 - \pi_1)e^{-2\mu x}].$$

As x goes to infinity, we get the mean residual time $\bar{x}_r$, which is $3/(2\mu)$, or $3\bar{x}/4$, irrespective of the initial state.

Exercise 3.5.10: Prove the formula above. Show that $\bar{x}_r(0) = \bar{x}$ for $\boldsymbol{\pi} = [1,\ \ 0]$.

We next evaluate the delayed renewal density, either using the material preceding Theorem 3.5.3b or by taking (3.5.19) as the starting vector for $m(x)$. In either case we get

$$m_r(\Delta; x) = \frac{\mu}{2}\left[1 + (\pi_2 - \pi_1)e^{-2\mu\,(x+\Delta)}\right]. \tag{3.5.20a}$$

For any finite Δ, as x grows large, $m_r(\Delta;\ x)$ approaches $1/\bar{x}$, as was described in the second form of Theorem 3.5.3.

The delayed renewal function also follows easily. As above,

$$M_r(\Delta; x) := \int_0^\Delta m_r(s;\ x)\,ds$$

$$= \frac{\mu\,\Delta}{2} + \frac{\pi_2 - \pi_1}{2}e^{-2\,\mu\,x}\left(1 - e^{-2\,\mu\,\Delta}\right). \tag{3.5.20b}$$

As with (3.5.18c) the behavior as x goes to infinity can be examined best by looking at M/Δ. Then for any Δ,

$$\frac{M(\Delta; x)}{\Delta} = \frac{1}{\bar{x}}\left[1 + (\pi_2 - \pi_1)e^{-2\,\mu\,x}\frac{1 - e^{-2\,\mu\,\Delta}}{2\,\mu\,\Delta}\right]. \tag{3.5.20c}$$

Note that $M(\Delta;\ x)$ approaches the expected limit $(1/\bar{x})$ much more rapidly than does $M(\Delta)$ [which is really $M(\Delta;\ 0)$]. Thus if one waits some time, x, before beginning measurements, successive intervals of Δ will yield the same average number of completions.

Exercise 3.5.11: Let $2\,\mu = 1$ and $\boldsymbol{\pi} = [0\ \ 1]$; then compare Equations (3.5.18) and (3.5.20c) for $\Delta = 2$ and increasing x.

In dealing with residual vectors, we have given the impression that all information about the internal state of the subsystem is gradually lost as time goes on. This is true only because observations concerning past behavior have not been included in estimating the future. In the discussion following (1.3.15b) it was pointed out that in a discrete Markov chain, time and the counting of events were synonymous, whereas a continuous chain soon loses track of the number of events. In the second part of Section 3.5.3 it was shown that knowledge of the number of past departures can be incorporated into estimations of future behavior. We will show presently that such information can affect appreciably what is likely to happen.

First we must determine $\mathbf{r}(x, \infty)$ from (3.5.14) for our present example. To do this, in addition to the matrices already evaluated at the beginning of this section, we need $\mathbf{BQ}$, which is easily shown to be

$$\mathbf{BQ} = \mu \begin{bmatrix} 1 & -1 \\ 0 & 1 \end{bmatrix} \begin{bmatrix} 1 & 0 \\ 1 & 0 \end{bmatrix} = \mu \begin{bmatrix} 0 & 0 \\ 1 & 0 \end{bmatrix}.$$

We must also have $\mathbf{p}_\infty$, which is the same as (3.5.3a), where each element is a two-vector, with $\boldsymbol{\pi} = [\pi_1, \ \pi_2]$.

We next set up $\mathbf{B}_\infty$ and find that it is identical with the $\mathbf{B}_\infty$ we had for the exponential distribution, except that all rows and columns are taken two at a time. Observe that each 2 by 2 block on the diagonal of $\mathbf{B}_\infty$ in the first part of Section 3.5.3.1 is precisely $\mathbf{B}$, and the 2 by 2 blocks above and to the right of the diagonal blocks are all $-\mathbf{BQ}$. We are indeed fortunate, because $\exp(-x\mathbf{B}_\infty)$ is the same as that in the preceding section. Equations (3.5.15) imply that (again $y = \mu\, x$)

$$\boldsymbol{\pi}(x,\, k) = \left[\pi_1 \frac{y^{2k}}{(2k)!} + \pi_2 \frac{\delta_{k0} y^{2k-1}}{(2k-1)!},\ \ \pi_1 \frac{y^{2k+1}}{(2k+1)!} + \pi_2 \frac{y^{2k}}{(2k)!}\right] \frac{e^{-y}}{P_k(x)}$$

and

$$P_k(x) = \frac{y^{2k-1} e^{-y}}{(2k+1)!}[(2k+1)y + \pi_1\, y^2 + \pi_2\,(2k)\,(2k+1)]. \tag{3.5.21a}$$

Therefore,

$$\boldsymbol{\pi}(x, k) = \frac{[\pi_1\,(2k+1)\,y + \pi_2\,(2k)(2k+1),\ \ \pi_1\, y^2 + \pi_2\,(2k+1)\,y]}{(2k+1)y + \pi_1\, y^2 + \pi_2\,(2k)(2k+1)}. \tag{3.5.21b}$$

Observe that $\boldsymbol{\pi}(0_+,\, 0) = [\pi_1, \ \pi_2]$, and for $k > 0$, $\boldsymbol{\pi}(0_+,\, k) = [1, \ 0]$.

Ordinarily, not too much credence should be placed in physical interpretations of the components of the internal states of a subsystem, because there may be many equivalent representations of S. In this case, however, there is some insight to be gained. When x is very small, one should expect C_1 to still be in S, and in his starting state. This is exactly the case, because $P_k(0_+)$ is essentially 0 except for $k = 0$. Given the highly unlikely event that $k-1$ customers have already left in 0_+ time, C_k would almost surely have not progressed much beyond just entering. This is indeed the case, because $\boldsymbol{\pi}(0_+, k) = \mathbf{p}$, the entrance vector.

As y increases, the second component of $\boldsymbol{\pi}(x, k)$ also increases, and when y is approximately equal to $2k$, the two components are comparable. As y

increases further, the second component becomes much larger than the first, and approaches 1. This has a direct physical interpretation. One would expect approximately k customers to be served in time $2k/\mu$, so if x is much larger than that, C_k has surely been in service a long time and must be at the second phase by now. Again the reader is warned that such interpretations are risky, and is referred to the discussion in Section 3.4. The important point to note is that depending on k and x, the internal state of S could be vastly different from $\mathbf{p}$ or $\boldsymbol{\pi}_{\mathbf{r}}$, the mean residual vector (which in this case is $[0.5,\ \ 0.5]$).

There is a useful statement that can be said in general. If many more customers have actually been served than one would expect in the time interval under measurement, the internal state vector of S will be close to the entrance vector. If the number that have been served is comparable to the expected number, the internal state will be closer to $\boldsymbol{\pi}_{\mathbf{r}}$. Finally, if far fewer customers have been served than might be expected, S will be described by a completely different state vector. In any case, the initial vector (in this case, $\boldsymbol{\pi} = [\pi_1,\ \ \pi_2]$) will be washed out.

Whatever might or might not be said about the internal state of S, many different predictions can be made. First, we can calculate the mean time to the next departure, given the number that have already departed, from Equations (3.5.21).

Exercise 3.5.12: Let $\mu = 2$ per minute, and suppose that measurement began at the moment a customer began service. In the interval $(0, 2]$, $0 \le k \le 10$ customers have been served. What is the mean time for the next customer to depart $[\bar{x}(2, k)]$? Make a table for k versus $\bar{x}$. Suppose the interval is $(0, 4]$. What are the $\bar{x}$s now?

Exercise 3.5.13: Do the same as in Exercise 3.5.12, except that now you have no idea when the first customer you counted began service. Compare and discuss the two pairs of results.

Another interesting number to look at is the renewal function conditioned on k departures in the previous interval of time. Equations (3.5.18) can be used for this purpose. But instead of using the initial vector $\boldsymbol{\pi}$, we use $\boldsymbol{\pi}(x, k)$, which is, after all, the initial vector starting at x.

Exercise 3.5.14: Suppose that $0 \le k \le 10$ customers have finished in the first 2 minutes, as in Exercise 3.5.12. What is the expected number of departures in the next 2 minutes? In the next 4 minutes? Summarize your answers in a table. Also calculate the number you would have expected in the first 2 minutes.

The marginal probabilities of having n departures in the interval $(x, x+\Delta]$, conditioned on having had k completions up to then can be calculated using (3.5.21a) (where n replaces k and Δ replaces x), again using the appropriate components from (3.5.21b) instead of the initial vector $\boldsymbol{\pi}$. The number of necessary parameters is growing steadily now; we have $n \times k \times x \times \Delta$ possibilities. A formal presentation of even more complex formulas becomes increasingly difficult, because one loses track of everything that is going on. But still, let us have one more exercise.

Exercise 3.5.15: Compare the $P_n(x)$ as defined in (3.5.4a) for a Poisson process, and a renewal process where the interdeparture times are distributed according to an Erlangian-2 distribution. Assume that measurement begins when C_1 enters S, and that the mean interdeparture time in all cases is 1 minute. Calculate the E_2 process for four different conditions.

1. The interval for counting the number of arrivals is $(0, 2]$ [Equation (3.5.21a)].
2. The interval for counting arrivals is $(2, 4]$, and no customer completed service previously [(3.5.21a) conditioned by (3.5.21b)].
3. The same as condition 2 except that two customers had completed service in the interval $(0, 2]$.
4. The same as condition 3, but for four customers.

Construct a single table of numbers that has the Poisson and all four Erlangian cases for $0 \le n \le 10$, and discuss their similarities and differences.

We have one more extension to discuss before giving up on this chapter. This is done by example, although it should be clear how one can generalize to any subsystem. Although it may be difficult (and often impossible) to know what is going on inside S, it is easy to keep track of the number of customers departing in successive intervals. In a different approach related to the technique of ***embedded Markov chains***, one waits until a customer begins service before taking measurements. In that case, the period always begins with $\boldsymbol{\pi} = \mathbf{p}$. When the interval is over, one waits for the next completion before measuring again. But then the mean number of departures is not $\Delta/\bar{x}$, even for large time, because we are always starting over. In Chapter 6, S is generalized so that several customers can be served at once. In that case, when a customer leaves, the internal state of the residual subsystem is not known, so one cannot start over until S is completely empty. Such behavior is called a *semi-Markov process*, and is discussed fully in Chapter 8. The technique described herein does generalize to multiple customer service without any conceptual complications.

Example 3.5.1: Consider an example such as Exercise 3.5.14. Initially, S is in state $a[1,0]$. Suppose that in the first minute C_1 and C_2 have both finished, but C_3 is still in S. At that moment, C_3 will be at phase 1 with probability $[\boldsymbol{\pi}(1,2)]_1$. Using (3.5.21b) (with $\pi_1 = 1$), this probability is 0.7143. Now suppose that C_3 is still busy by the end of the second minute; then at that moment it is at phase 1 with probability 0.2941. One gets this by using (3.5.21b) again, but this time $\pi_1 = 0.7143$, and of course, $\pi_2 = 0.2857$. If one measures the number of completions in the interval $(0,2]$ without noting how many finished in the first minute, the probability that C_3 will be at phase 1 is 0.5556.

Interestingly enough, if no customers finish in the first minute, and two finish in the second minute, the sequence for phase 1 to be busy is $1.0000 \to 0.3333 \to 0.6757$, but if one customer finishes in each of the two minutes, the sequence is $1.0000 \to 0.6000 \to 0.5556$. This happens to be the same as when going to 2 without considering the number at 1, but this is not always the case. Anyway, we see that the three different ways of having two completions in 2 minutes, keeping track of how many completed in the first minute, yield different results. Now, for instance, in calculating the mean time for C_3 to finish using the data above and (3.5.15d), we get three different answers, 0.837838, 0.777778, and 0.647059 minute, respectively, for 2, then 0; 1, then 1; and 0, then 2. ▲

Exercise 3.5.16: Extend the discussion above to three 1-minute intervals where a total of three customers finished service. What is the mean time until C_4 finishes in each case?

It is hoped that the reader can now extend this procedure to any example. Any information that one has concerning past behavior of a system should be usable in calculating conditional events in the future.

with Rational Laplace transform

Chapter 4

M/G/1 QUEUE

The shortest path between two truths in the real domain passes through the complex domain.
J. Hadamard

A mathematician may say anything he pleases, but a scientist must be at least partially sane.
Willard Gibbs

We are finally ready to look at nonexponential queues in earnest. In Chapter 2 we looked at closed loops in which both subsystems were single servers with exponential service time distributions. We showed how to transform a closed system into an open one, and how certain types of non steady-state behavior should be analyzed. In Chapter 3, we showed how a large class of nonexponential servers (ME distributions) can be treated exactly, using a matrix representation, and applied it to examining various aspects of renewal processes, as well as the specific behavior of a single general server, including residual times. We now combine those two chapters in studying the M/ME/1 queue, first looking at steady-state closed systems, then "opening" them, and finally, extending the transient results of Chapter 2. In those cases where a particular result does not depend on the specific properties of a matrix, the result becomes applicable to M/G/1 queues as well. Much of this material is an outgrowth of the Ph.D. thesis by John L. Carroll [CARROLL79], and the associated papers, [CARROLLLIPVDL82], and [TEHRANIPOURVDLLIP89]. Equivalent results were also obtained by Marcel Neuts [NEUTS82].

4.1 S.S. M/ME/1// N (and M/ME/1/ N) Loop

We start, as always, by making some new definitions. In Chapter 2 each state could be described uniquely by n, the number at S_1, whereas in Chapter 3 the states were described by identifying the phase in S_1 where the active customer was. Here both must be specified to describe uniquely a state of the system shown in Figure 4.1.1. This figure is itself a combination of Figures 2.1.1 and 3.1.1, where the single server, S_1 of Figure 2.1.1 is replaced by the m-phase subsystem, S, of Figure 3.1.1.

All the objects in the following list are the same as defined in Chapter 3: $\mathbf{p}$, $\mathbf{P}$, $\mathbf{q}'$, $\boldsymbol{\epsilon}'$, $\mathbf{M}$, $\mathbf{B}$, $\mathbf{V}$, $\mathbf{Q} = \boldsymbol{\epsilon}'\mathbf{p}$, and the linear operator, $\Psi[\,\cdot\,]$. For a closed

L. Lipsky, *Queueing Theory*, DOI 10.1007/978-0-387-49706-8_4,

system with N customers, define the following.

Definition 4.1.1

$[\boldsymbol{\pi}(n;N)]_i$:= *steady-state probability that there are n customers in the queue at* S_1, *and the one being served is at phase i.* n includes the customer being served, and $\boldsymbol{\pi}(n;N)$ is a row vector with m components. The associated scalar probability, $r(n;N)$ is the same as Definition 2.1.1. □

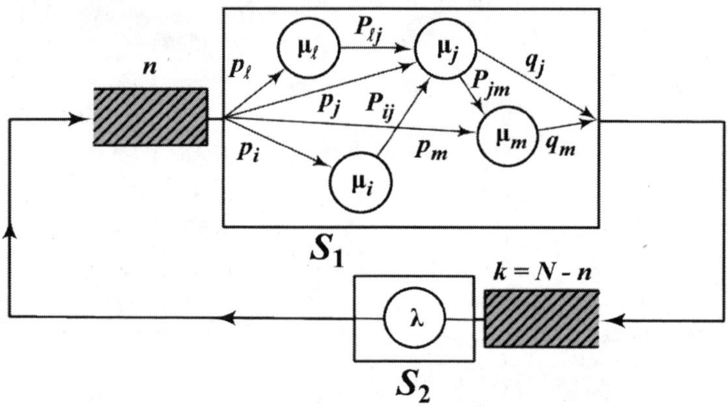

Figure 4.1.1: Closed loop made up of two subsystems. S_2 is purely exponential, with service rate λ, whereas S_1 is of the type described in Figure 3.1.1 and thus represents a matrix exponential distribution. There are n customers at S_1, with the active customer being at phase i (or in ***internal state*** i), and the other k $(= N - n)$ customers are at S_2.

Although $\boldsymbol{\pi}_i(0;N)$ has no meaning (if no customers are at S_1, no phase can be busy), it is useful to define the vector

$$\boldsymbol{\pi}(0;N) := r(0;N)\mathbf{p}. \tag{4.1.1}$$

Then for all n, $0 \le n \le N$,

$$r(n;\ N) = \sum_{i=1}^{m} \pi_i(n;N) = \boldsymbol{\pi}(n;N)\boldsymbol{\epsilon}'. \tag{4.1.2}$$

From these definitions, we see that there are $m\,N + 1$ states describing the closed system [or $m\,(N+1)$ states if we make believe that $\pi_i(0;N)$ has meaning], but they are grouped together as $(N+1)$ m-vectors. This way of grouping is the basis of LAQT and was first used to advantage by Victor Wallace [WALLACE69] in formalizing ***Quasi Birth-Death*** (**QBD**) ***processes***. He recognized that for many systems, the transition rate matrices $\boldsymbol{Q}$, as defined in Chapter 1, are block tridiagonal. That is, the $\mathbf{Q}$ of Chapter 1 can be considered as a matrix whose elements are themselves matrices. Only the diagonal, superdiagonal, and subdiagonal elements are nonzero matrices. He chose the term QBD because birth-death processes are also tridiagonal, but with scalar components. He also speculated about an algebraic theory for Markovian networks [WALLACE72]. All queueing systems considered here are special cases of QBD processes, but we do not look at them in that context.

4.1.1 Balance Equations

Let us first introduce some new notation.

Definition 4.1.2

$\{j; n; N\}$ *is an integer triplet that corresponds to one possible state of an M/ME/1//N loop.* N is the total number of customers in the system, n is the number of customers at S_1, including the one in service, and j is the phase in S_1 that is busy. We can say that the system is in state $\{j\,; n;\, N\}$. If we are dealing with an open system ($N = \infty$), we use the notation $\{j;\, n\}$.

$\boldsymbol{\Xi := \{j\,|1 \le j \le m,\ j \textit{ is a phase in } S_1\}}$. Only one customer can be active at a time in S_1, thus Ξ is the set of all *internal states* of S_1. We can say that the system is in internal state $j \in \Xi$, or that the active customer is at phase j in S_1. □

Remember, too, we are assuming that S_1 and S_2 operate independently. This means that only one thing happens at a time. The term "one thing" means whatever we wish. Thus a customer leaving S_i and being replaced immediately by the next customer in the queue is "one thing." Also, the process whereby a customer leaves one subsystem (and is replaced by a successor), goes to the other, and finding it empty immediately enters into service is "one thing." However, if two customers are active at the same time (e.g., one in each subsystem), only one at a time can change state. In general, those processes that take 0 time (moving from one subsystem to the other, entering S_i, moving from one phase to another) are considered to be part of the previous process.

Recall from Theorem 1.3.3 that balance equations are valid because they are the same as $\boldsymbol{\pi Q} = 0$, the steady-state ***Chapman-Kolmogorov equation***. As a direct generalization of Section 2.1.2. and (2.1.4a), [and as a special case of Equation (1.3.9a)] in order for the system to be in a steady state, the probability rate of leaving state $\{i;\, n;\, N\}$ must be equal to the probability rate of entering that state. Thus for state $\{\cdot;\, 0;\, N\}$ we have

$$\lambda r(0; N) = \sum_j \pi_j(1; N) M_{jj} q_j = \boldsymbol{\pi}(1; N)\mathbf{M}\mathbf{q}'.$$

In words, the probability rate of leaving the state where no one is at S_1 is equal to the probability of there being no one there $[r(0; N)]$ times the probability rate of a customer finishing at S_2 $[\lambda]$. The middle term of the equation above is the probability rate of entering state $\{\cdot;\, 0;\, N\}$. This is equal to the sum of probability rates of having the customer in S_1 being served by j $[\pi_j(1; N)]$, who then finishes there $[\mu_j = M_{jj}]$, and leaves $[q_j]$. The rightmost expression of the equation is the matrix equivalent of the middle expression. From (3.1.1b) and (3.1.3) it follows directly that

$$\mathbf{M}\mathbf{q}' = \mathbf{B}\boldsymbol{\epsilon}'. \tag{4.1.3a}$$

Thus if both sides of the preceding equation are multiplied on the right by $\mathbf{p}$, and we use (4.1.1), we get the vector balance equation:

$$\lambda\,\boldsymbol{\pi}(0;N) = \boldsymbol{\pi}(1;N)\mathbf{M}\mathbf{q}'\,\mathbf{p} = \boldsymbol{\pi}(1;N)\mathbf{B}\mathbf{Q}, \tag{4.1.3b}$$

where $\mathbf{Q} = \boldsymbol{\epsilon}'\mathbf{p}$ is the idempotent matrix defined in Section 3.5.1 and has nothing to do with the transition rate matrix $\boldsymbol{Q}$. Except when direct reference is made to Chapter 1, $\mathbf{Q}$ always has this meaning.

The balance equation for state $\{i;\ N;\ N\}$ is derived as follows. In this case there is no one at S_2, therefore there can be no arrivals to S_1, but instead, the customer who is active in S_1 can complete service at i $[\pi_i(N;N)M_{ii}]$, thereby causing the system to leave that state. The probability rate of entering state $\{i;\ N;\ N\}$ is made up of two parts. Either the system could be in state $\{i;\ N-1;\ N\}$, $[\pi_i(N-1;\ N)]$, and have the lone customer at S_2 finish $[\lambda]$, or all N customers could already be at S_1, but the active customer is at some other phase j, $[\pi_j(N;N)]$, finishes there $[M_{jj}]$, and goes to $i[P_{ji}]$. Note that a completion at S_2 changes the ***external state*** of the system (n goes from $N-1$ to N) but not the internal state (the active customer at S_1 does not move merely because a new customer has arrived at the queue, hence i in unchanged). So this equation is

$$\pi_i(N;N)M_{ii} = \lambda\,\pi_i(N-1;N) + \sum_j \pi_j(N;N)\,M_{jj}\,P_{ji}$$

or in matrix form,

$$\boldsymbol{\pi}(N;N)\mathbf{M} = \lambda\boldsymbol{\pi}(N-1;N) + \boldsymbol{\pi}(N;N)\mathbf{M}\mathbf{P}.$$

Remembering that $\mathbf{B} = \mathbf{M}(\mathbf{I}-\mathbf{P})$, the equation above can be rearranged to

$$\boldsymbol{\pi}(N;N)\mathbf{B} = \lambda\boldsymbol{\pi}(N-1;N),$$

or, using $\mathbf{B}^{-1} = \mathbf{V}$,

$$\boldsymbol{\pi}(N;N) = \boldsymbol{\pi}(N-1;N)\mathbf{V}\lambda. \tag{4.1.3c}$$

The balance equations for states where n is greater than 0 but less than N combine all the features of (4.1.3b) and (4.1.3c). It is useful to describe what happens in these cases with the help of the state transition diagram in Figure 4.1.2. As usual, the sum of the weights of the arrows going to $\{i;\ n;\ N\}$ equals the sum of those leaving. So for $i \in \Xi$, we have

$$\pi_i(n;N)(M_{ii}+\lambda)$$
$$= \sum_j \pi_j(n;N)M_{jj}P_{ji} + \sum_j \pi_j(n+1;N)M_{jj}q_j\,p_i + \pi_i(n-1;N)\lambda.$$

These m equations can be summarized by the vector equation

$$\boldsymbol{\pi}(n;\,N)(\mathbf{M}+\lambda\mathbf{I}) = \boldsymbol{\pi}(n;N)\mathbf{M}\,\mathbf{P} + \boldsymbol{\pi}(n+1;N)\mathbf{M}\,\mathbf{q}'\,\mathbf{p} + \boldsymbol{\pi}(n-1;N)\lambda\mathbf{I}.$$

This, in turn, can be rearranged, as with the previous equations, to yield the rest of the balance equations. For $0 < n < N$,

$$\boldsymbol{\pi}(n;N)(\mathbf{B}+\lambda\mathbf{I}) = \boldsymbol{\pi}(n+1;N)\mathbf{B}\,\mathbf{Q} + \boldsymbol{\pi}(n-1;N)\lambda\mathbf{I} \tag{4.1.3d}$$

We mention here that (4.1.3d) is valid for $n = 1$ by virtue of (4.1.1).

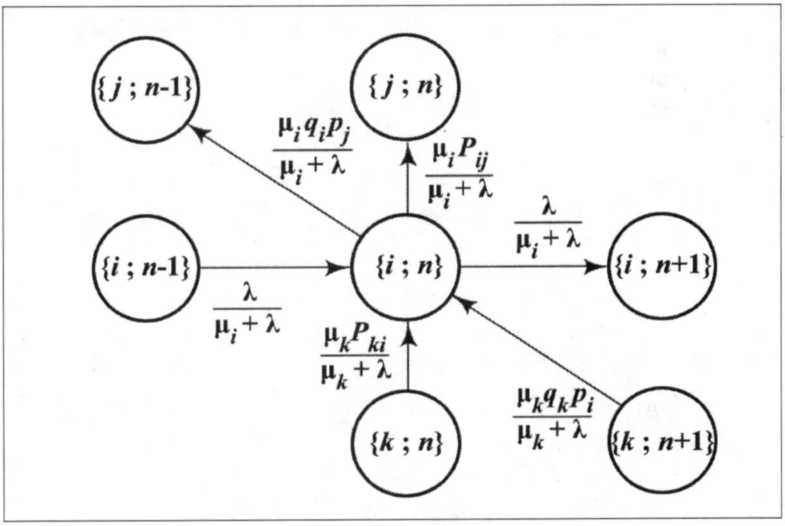

Figure 4.1.2: Steady-state transition diagram for state $\{i;\, n;\, N\}$ of an M/ME/1//N closed loop. An arrow pointing to the left represents a customer finishing at phase i, $\left[\{(\mathbf{M}+\lambda\mathbf{I})^{-1}\mathbf{M}\}_{ii}\right]$, and leaving S_1, $[\{\mathbf{q}\}_i]$, followed by another customer entering and going to j, $[\{\mathbf{p}\}_j]$. There is also implicitly an arrow pointing horizontally to the left to cover the possibility that the entering customer goes to the same phase left behind by the departing customer $[p_i]$. A vertical arrow corresponds to a customer finishing at phase i, $[(\mathbf{M}+\lambda\mathbf{I})^{-1}\mathbf{M}]$, and going to phase j, $[\{\mathbf{P}\}_{ij}]$. An arrow to the right (no diagonal arrows allowed) corresponds to a customer finishing at S_2, $[(\mathbf{M}+\lambda\mathbf{I})^{-1}\lambda]$, and immediately going to S_1, without changing the internal state.

The set of Equations (4.1.3) falls in the class of "second-order finite-difference vector equations," not a particularly informative name for our purposes. They are similar in appearance to the balance equations for the M/M/1 queue (2.1.4a) and reduce to them when S_1 is exponential. In the next section we prove that they reduce to first-order equations and then give an explicit expression for the general solution.

4.1.2 Steady-State Solution

First consider (4.1.3d) for $n = N - 1$:

$$\boldsymbol{\pi}(N-1;N)(\mathbf{B}+\lambda\mathbf{I}) = \boldsymbol{\pi}(N;N)\mathbf{B}\,\mathbf{Q} + \lambda\boldsymbol{\pi}(N-2;N).$$

Next replace $\boldsymbol{\pi}(N;N)$ with (4.1.3c), divide by λ, and regroup terms to get (recalling that $\mathbf{V}\,\mathbf{B} = \mathbf{I}$)

$$\boldsymbol{\pi}(N-1;N)\left(\mathbf{I} + \frac{1}{\lambda}\mathbf{B} - \mathbf{Q}\right) = \boldsymbol{\pi}(N-2;N).$$

Now define the important pair of matrices

$$\mathbf{A} := \mathbf{I} + \frac{1}{\lambda}\mathbf{B} - \mathbf{Q} \tag{4.1.4a}$$

and (assuming that it exists)

$$\mathbf{U} := \mathbf{A}^{-1}. \tag{4.1.4b}$$

It then follows that

$$\boldsymbol{\pi}(N-1;N) = \boldsymbol{\pi}(N-2;N)\mathbf{U}. \tag{4.1.5a}$$

Before proving by induction that this equation is true for all $n < N$, we enumerate a collection of simple relations (stated in the form of the following lemma) that prove useful throughout the rest of the book.

Lemma 4.1.1: For $\mathbf{A}$ and $\mathbf{U}$, defined by Equations (4.1.4), the following are matrix identities.

$$\lambda\mathbf{A}\boldsymbol{\epsilon}' = \mathbf{B}\,\boldsymbol{\epsilon}', \qquad \lambda\mathbf{V}\mathbf{A}\,\boldsymbol{\epsilon}' = \boldsymbol{\epsilon}', \qquad \mathbf{U}\,\mathbf{B}\,\boldsymbol{\epsilon}' = \lambda\boldsymbol{\epsilon}',$$

and since $\mathbf{Q} = \boldsymbol{\epsilon}'\mathbf{p}$,

$$\mathbf{UBQ} = \lambda\mathbf{Q} \quad \text{and} \quad \lambda\mathbf{AQ} = \mathbf{BQ}.$$

Similarly,

$$\lambda\mathbf{pA} = \mathbf{pB}, \qquad \lambda\mathbf{pAV} = \mathbf{p}, \qquad \mathbf{pBU} = \lambda\mathbf{p}.$$

Also,

$$\lambda\mathbf{QA} = \mathbf{QB} \quad \text{and} \quad \lambda\mathbf{QAV} = \mathbf{Q}.$$

There are several other variations. ■

Proof: By using $\mathbf{I}\boldsymbol{\epsilon}' = \mathbf{Q}\boldsymbol{\epsilon}' = \boldsymbol{\epsilon}'$ it follows that

$$\mathbf{A}\boldsymbol{\epsilon}' = \left(\mathbf{I} + \frac{1}{\lambda}\mathbf{B} - \mathbf{Q}\right)\boldsymbol{\epsilon}' = \boldsymbol{\epsilon}' + \frac{1}{\lambda}\mathbf{B}\boldsymbol{\epsilon}' - \boldsymbol{\epsilon}' = \frac{1}{\lambda}\mathbf{B}\boldsymbol{\epsilon}'.$$

All else follows trivially. **QED**

Now assume that for all k from $N-2$ down to n [by virtue of (4.1.5a) it is true for $k = N-2$],

$$\boldsymbol{\pi}(k+1; N) = \boldsymbol{\pi}(k; N)\mathbf{U}.$$

Insert this (with $k = n$) into (4.1.3d) and get

$$\boldsymbol{\pi}(n; N)(\mathbf{B} + \lambda\mathbf{I}) = \boldsymbol{\pi}(n; N)\mathbf{UBQ} + \lambda\boldsymbol{\pi}(n-1; N).$$

After using Lemma 4.1.1, and rearranging somewhat, we get what is needed for the proof by induction, namely the following first-order matrix difference equation promised previously:

$$\boldsymbol{\pi}(n; N) = \boldsymbol{\pi}(n-1; N)\mathbf{U}. \tag{4.1.5b}$$

Now (4.1.3d) is true for all n from 1 to $N-1$, so (4.1.5b) must be true also. In particular,

$$\boldsymbol{\pi}(1; N) = \boldsymbol{\pi}(0; N)\mathbf{U}$$

(note that this equation satisfies (4.1.3b)), because $\mathbf{UBQ} = \lambda\mathbf{Q}$, and

$$\boldsymbol{\pi}(2; N) = \boldsymbol{\pi}(1; N)\mathbf{U} = \boldsymbol{\pi}(0; N)\mathbf{U}^2.$$

In general, we have [using (4.1.1)]

$$\boldsymbol{\pi}(n; N) = \boldsymbol{\pi}(0; N)\mathbf{U}^n = r(0; N)\mathbf{p}\,\mathbf{U}^n \quad \text{for} \quad 0 \le n < N, \tag{4.1.6a}$$

and with the help of (4.1.3c),

$$\boldsymbol{\pi}(N; N) = \lambda r(0; N)\mathbf{p}\mathbf{U}^{N-1}\mathbf{V}. \tag{4.1.6b}$$

Every $\boldsymbol{\pi}$ is conveniently expressed in terms of $\boldsymbol{\pi}(0; N)$, which by virtue of (4.1.1) depends on only one scalar parameter, $r(0; N)$. This, in turn, can be evaluated by the usual requirement that the probabilities add up to 1:

$$\sum_{n=0}^{N} r(n; N) = \sum_{n=0}^{N} \boldsymbol{\pi}(n; N)\boldsymbol{\epsilon}'$$

$$= r(0; N)\mathbf{p}\left(\sum_{n=0}^{N-1} \mathbf{U}^n + \lambda\mathbf{U}^{N-1}\mathbf{V}\right)\boldsymbol{\epsilon}' = 1. \tag{4.1.6c}$$

This equation can be simplified both visually and computationally by defining the matrix in the large brackets to be the ***normalization matrix*** $\mathbf{K}(N)$, and observing that $\mathbf{K}(N)$ satisfies:

$$\mathbf{K}(N) := \mathbf{I} + \mathbf{U} + \mathbf{U}^2 + \cdots + \mathbf{U}^{N-1} + \lambda\mathbf{U}^{N-1}\mathbf{V}$$

$$= \mathbf{I} + \mathbf{U}(\mathbf{I} + \mathbf{U} + \mathbf{U}^2 + \cdots + \mathbf{U}^{N-2} + \lambda\mathbf{U}^{N-2}\mathbf{V}). \tag{4.1.6d}$$

The expression inside the parentheses is $\mathbf{K}(N-1)$, so, for $N > 1$ we have the recursive formula:

$$\mathbf{K}(N) = \mathbf{I} + \mathbf{UK}(N-1), \quad \text{where} \quad \mathbf{K}(1) = \mathbf{I} + \lambda\mathbf{V}. \tag{4.1.6e}$$

By virtue of the fact that for any $\mathbf{F}$ that has no unit eigenvalues,

$$\sum_{n=0}^{N-1} \mathbf{F}^n = [\mathbf{I} - \mathbf{F}^N][\mathbf{I} - \mathbf{F}]^{-1},$$

(4.1.6d) can also be written as

$$\mathbf{K}(N) = [\mathbf{I} - \mathbf{U}^N][\mathbf{I} - \mathbf{U}]^{-1} + \lambda \mathbf{U}^{N-1}\mathbf{V}. \tag{4.1.6f}$$

Finally recall that $\Psi[\cdot] = \mathbf{p}[\cdot]\boldsymbol{\epsilon}'$, so (4.1.6c) leads to

$$r(0; N) = \frac{1}{\Psi[\mathbf{K}(N)]}. \tag{4.1.6g}$$

Equations (4.1.6) are very interesting in that they give us an explicit closed-form expression for the M/ME/1 queue which retains the simple form the solution of the M/M/1 queue has, as given in (2.1.4) and (2.1.5). In particular, compare $\mathbf{K}(N)$ with $K(N)$ in (2.1.4c) and (2.1.4d). Furthermore, these equations are ideally suited for numerical computation, as well as algebraic manipulation. Efficient computational algorithms can be written to compute the steady-state and other properties. It should become apparent to the reader just how to do this, but these formulas are important enough to be summarized by the folowing.

Theorem 4.1.2: For any closed loop made of one exponential server with service rate λ, and one general server that has a matrix exponential representation $\langle \mathbf{p}, \mathbf{B} \rangle$, the steady-state queue-length probabilities are given by

$$r(n; N) = r(0; N)\Psi[\mathbf{U}^n] \quad \text{for} \quad 0 \le n < N, \tag{4.1.7a}$$

$$r(N; N) = \lambda r(0; N)\Psi\left[\mathbf{U}^{N-1}\mathbf{V}\right]. \tag{4.1.7b}$$

The matrix $\mathbf{U}$ is given by (4.1.4b), and $r(0; N)$ is given by (4.1.6e) or (4.1.6f), and (4.1.6g). The vector probabilities are given by (4.1.6a) and (4.1.6b):

$$\boldsymbol{\pi}(n; N) = r(0; N)\mathbf{p}\mathbf{U}^n \quad \text{for} \quad 0 \le n < N, \tag{4.1.7c}$$

$$\boldsymbol{\pi}(N; N) = \lambda r(0; N)\mathbf{p}\mathbf{U}^{N-1}\mathbf{V}. \tag{4.1.7d}$$

These equations give us a ***matrix geometric solution*** of the M/ME/1/ /N queue analogous to the geometric solution for the M/M/1/ /N queue given by Equations (2.1.4). ■

The term *geometric* refers to any series where the ratio of successive terms is a constant factor. Thus $1 + x + x^2 + x^3 + \cdots$ is the *geometric series*, where x is the ratio of terms. In our theorem, $\mathbf{U}$ is the ratio of successive terms, and since it is a matrix, we call this *matrix geometric*.

Example 4.1.1: Figure 4.1.3 shows the steady-state queue-length probabilities of an M/E_2/1/ /20 loop, for various values of $\rho = \lambda\Psi[\mathbf{V}] = \lambda\mathbf{E}[X]$. At first glance, this figure looks similar to Figure 2.1.3 for the M/M/1 queue, but there are several significant differences. First note that $r(N; N)$ comes from a different formula than $r(n < N; N)$ [Equations (4.1.7)], therefore we can expect the curve to deviate in going from 19 to 20. This does indeed show itself for $\rho = 1$, but it is not so clear for other values of ρ, either because the curve is growing too big (as with $\rho = 2$), or the values are too small to be seen ($\rho \leq 0.9$). A second feature is that the two curves corresponding to $\rho = 2$ and $\rho = 0.5$ are not mirror images of each other. For $\rho = 0.5$, $N = 20$ is sufficiently large so that S_2 is saturated, so $r(n; 20) \approx r(n)$ (i.e., the M/E_2/1 queue). On the other hand, the curve corresponding to $\rho = 2.0$ is very close to the E_2/M/1 queue, because now S_1 is saturated. As we show in detail in Chapter 5, the two queues are distinctly different in their performance. ▲

What we just described might be expected, but for the third distinctive feature observe that unlike the M/M/1 queue, $r(n; 20)$ is not a monotonically decreasing function of n, even when $\rho < 1$. Note that for $\rho = 0.9$ and 1, we have $r(1; N)/r(0; N) > 1$. But from (4.1.7a), as long as $N \geq 2$, the ratio of those two probabilities is $\Psi[\mathbf{U}]$ which for the M/E_2/1/ /N loop can be shown to be (also see the end of Section 4.4.4)

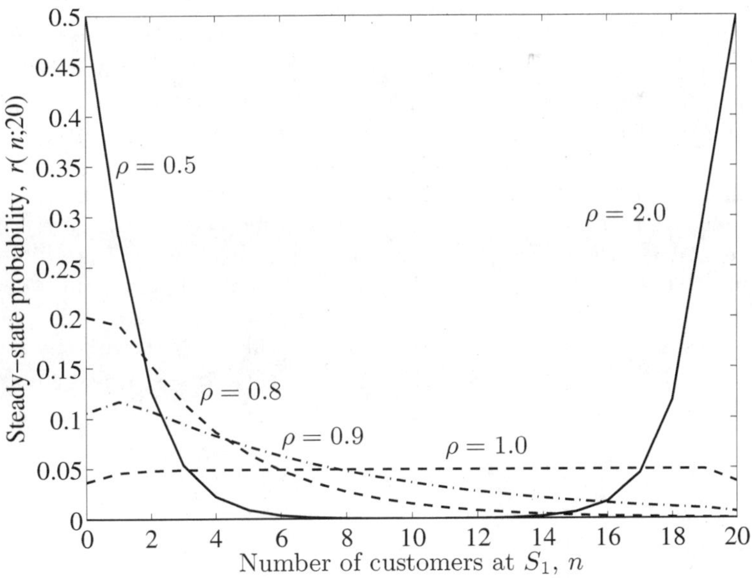

Figure 4.1.3: Steady-state queue-length probabilities for an M/E_2/1/ /20 loop, for $\rho = 0.5, 0.8, 0.9, 1.0$, and 2.0. For $\rho < 1$, the curves tend to decrease with n, but not universally so. Note that the curves for $\rho = 0.5$ and $\rho = 2.0$ are not mirror images of each other, nor is the curve for $\rho = 1$ horizontal (see Figure 2.1.3).

$$\Psi[\mathbf{U}] = \frac{\rho}{2}\left(2 + \frac{\rho}{2}\right).$$

This expression is greater than 1 as long as $\rho > 2\sqrt{2} - 2 \approx 0.8284$. Therefore, $r(n;N)$ will first rise and then decrease to zero with increasing n when $0.8284 < \rho \le 1$.

Exercise 4.1.1: Calculate the steady-state queue-length probabilities of an $M/E_2/1//N$ loop for $N = 20$ and $\rho = 0.5$, and 0.9. Compare your answers with those for an M/M/1//N queue by plotting both sets on the same graph, $r(n;N)$ versus n. By what percent do the two sets of numbers differ? Under what conditions could $r(3;N)$ be greater than $r(2;N)$?

Exercise 4.1.2: Do the same calculations as in Exercise 4.1.1, except here let S_1 be equivalent to an H_2 distribution (see Exercise 3.1.2). Let $pT_1 = (1-p)T_2 = 1/2$, and $C_v^2 = 10.0$. Are there values of ρ for which $\Psi[\mathbf{U}] > 1$ and $r(n;N)$ is not a monotonic function of n? Do the same calculations for the hyper-Erlangian function of Equations (3.2.14).

The queue-length probabilities are not often used in practice to analyze the performance of closed systems, partly because there is too much to measure. One important performance parameter that *is* measured is the rate at which customers make a full circuit of the loop. Aside from a multiplicative constant, we called this the ***system throughput*** in Definition 2.1.2. The number of customers who leave a single server per unit time is equal to the fraction of time that server is busy (or the probability that the server is busy), divided by the time it takes to service one customer. One can look at this in a different way. S_i releases customers at a constant rate $(1/\bar{x}_i)$ as long as it is busy, but does nothing when it is idle (i.e., when no customers are there). Any way one looks at it [see Equations (2.1.5)], the system throughput is (remember that $\lambda\bar{x}_1 = \rho$)

$$\Lambda(N) = \frac{1 - r(0;N)}{\bar{x}_1} = \frac{\Psi[\mathbf{K}(N)] - 1}{\bar{x}_1 \Psi[\mathbf{K}(N)]} = \frac{\lambda}{\rho}\frac{\Psi[\mathbf{UK}(N-1)]}{\Psi[\mathbf{K}(N)]}. \tag{4.1.8a}$$

The last form for $\Lambda(N)$ is interesting for comparing with (2.1.5b), but computationally, the first two forms are probably better. According to the discussion, and to (2.1.5d), one should be able to calculate the throughput based on the flow through any server. Therefore ($\bar{x}_2 = 1/\lambda$),

$$\Lambda(N) = \frac{1 - r(N;N)}{\bar{x}_2} = \lambda \frac{\Psi[\mathbf{K}(N)] - \Psi\left[\mathbf{U}^{N-1}\lambda\mathbf{V}\right]}{\Psi[\mathbf{K}(N)]}. \tag{4.1.8b}$$

Although the two equations for $\Lambda(N)$ must be equal, it takes some effort to prove that they are the same algebraically, which we leave for the following exercise.

Exercise 4.1.3: Prove by direct algebraic manipulation that

$$r(0; N) - \rho r(N; N) = 1 - \rho,$$

or equivalently,

$$(1-\rho)\Psi\left[\mathbf{K}(N)\right] = 1 - \rho\Psi\left[\mathbf{U}^{N-1}\lambda\mathbf{V}\right].$$

Exercise 4.1.4: Calculate $\Lambda(N)$ for the closed $M/E_2/1//N$ loop, where $\bar{x} + 1/\lambda = 1$ [i.e., $\lambda = 1 + \rho$, and $\bar{x} = \rho/(1+\rho)$] and $\rho = 0.5$ for $N = 1$ through 20. Repeat the calculations for $\rho = 0.9$, 1.0, and 2.0. Draw the four curves on the same graph and compare with the graphs in Exercise 2.1.3.

Exercise 4.1.5: Do the same as in Exercise 4.1.4, but now S_1 is the hyperexponential described in Exercise 4.1.2.

4.1.3 Departure and Arrival Queue-Length Probabilities

In the preceding section we derived the steady-state probabilities of what a ***random observer*** would see over a long period of time. There are two special sets of moments in time that deserve separate treatment. These time points are referred to as ***embedding points***. ***Embedded Markov chains*** are used to consider the following questions.

1. What will a customer see upon arriving at S_1?
2. What will a customer leave behind upon exiting S_1?

Given that it takes no time for a customer to go from one server to another, these questions are the same as asking the equivalent questions of S_2. In the case of the M/G/1 queue, the two questions turn out to have the same answer, and almost the same as $r(n; N)$, but this is not the case for other systems. We prove the equality here and at the same time demonstrate the method that can be used in the other cases.

First we define a set of steady-state vectors.

Definition 4.1.3

$[\mathbf{w}(n;N)]_i$:= *probability that between events, n customers are at* S_1 *and phase i is busy (or, the system is in internal state,* $i \in \Xi$*).* As with $\boldsymbol{\pi}(0;N)$, $\mathbf{w}(0;N)$ is defined to be proportional to $\mathbf{p}$. □

Nothing happens between events, so we can argue that this is the same as the probability of being in state $\{i;\ n;\ N\}$ just before, or just after, an event. How then, you may ask, does this differ from $[\boldsymbol{\pi}(n;N)]_i$? If the time interval between events was always the same (or is taken from some distribution that is independent of the state the system was in), the two would be identical (e.g., $\mathbf{M} = \mu\mathbf{I}$). However, a random observer is less likely to find the system in a state that is relatively short-lived than one that has a long mean time, $[(\lambda\mathbf{I} + \mathbf{M})^{-1}]$. On the other hand, internal and external transitions mark the moments of events and take no notice of the time between them, so you can say (in fact, we do say) that $\boldsymbol{\pi}(n;N)$ is related to $\mathbf{w}(n;N)$ by time-weighting (not waiting).

The $\mathbf{w}(n;N)$ vectors satisfy the following balance equations, which are similar to those for the $\boldsymbol{\pi}(n;N)$ vectors, except that the elapsed times between events are ignored. So we have the equivalent of a discrete Markov chain. For $n = 0$,

$$\mathbf{w}(0;N)\boldsymbol{\epsilon}' = \sum_{i=1}^{m} w_i(1;N)\mu_i(\lambda + \mu_i)^{-1}q_i.$$

In words, if there are no customers at S_1, $[\mathbf{w}(0;N)\boldsymbol{\epsilon}']$, then at the next event the system will certainly leave that state. On the other hand, the system can enter that state by first being in some internal state with one customer at S_1, $[w_i(1;N)]$, have the next event occur in S_1, $[\mu_i/(\mu_i + \lambda)]$, and have that event be a departure $[q_i]$. The probability that the next event will occur in S_1, $[\mu_i/(\mu_i + \lambda)]$, comes from Equation (2.1.1b). In vector form,

$$\mathbf{w}(0;\ N) = \mathbf{w}(1;\ N)(\lambda\mathbf{I} + \mathbf{M})^{-1}\mathbf{M}\mathbf{q}'\mathbf{p}.$$

The procedure should be sufficiently clear so that we can write the vector equations for $n > 0$ directly. Note that if S_1 and S_2 each have at least one customer, the probability that an event, when it occurs, will be in S_2 is $\lambda[(\lambda\mathbf{I} + \mathbf{M})^{-1}]_{ii}$, whereas if either is empty, the event will certainly occur in the other. Therefore,

$$\mathbf{w}(n;N) = \mathbf{w}(n;N)(\lambda\mathbf{I} + \mathbf{M})^{-1}\mathbf{M}\mathbf{P} + \mathbf{w}(n-1;N)(\lambda\mathbf{I} + \mathbf{M})^{-1}\lambda\mathbf{I}$$

$$+\mathbf{w}(n+1;N)(\lambda\mathbf{I} + \mathbf{M})^{-1}\mathbf{M}\mathbf{q}'\mathbf{p} \quad \text{for } 0 < n < N,$$

and

$$\mathbf{w}(N;N) = \mathbf{w}(N;N)\mathbf{P} + \mathbf{w}(N-1;N)(\lambda\mathbf{I} + \mathbf{M})^{-1}\lambda\mathbf{I}.$$

We next regroup terms, recall that $\mathbf{B} = \mathbf{M}(\mathbf{I} - \mathbf{P})$ and that $\mathbf{M}\mathbf{q}' = \mathbf{B}\boldsymbol{\epsilon}'$, to get

$$\mathbf{w}(0;N) = \mathbf{w}(1;N)(\lambda\mathbf{I} + \mathbf{M})^{-1}\mathbf{B}\mathbf{Q}, \tag{4.1.9a}$$

$$\mathbf{w}(n;N)(\lambda\mathbf{I} + \mathbf{M})^{-1}(\lambda\mathbf{I} + \mathbf{B})$$

$$= \lambda \mathbf{w}(n-1;N)(\lambda \mathbf{I}+\mathbf{M})^{-1} + \mathbf{w}(n+1;N)(\lambda \mathbf{I}+\mathbf{M})^{-1}\mathbf{BQ}, \qquad (4.1.9b)$$

and

$$\mathbf{w}(N;N)\mathbf{M}^{-1}\mathbf{B} = \lambda \mathbf{w}(N-1;N)(\lambda \mathbf{I}+\mathbf{M})^{-1}. \qquad (4.1.9c)$$

These equations look similar to (4.1.3). In fact, we can guess at their solution in the following.

Theorem 4.1.3: The steady-state vector probabilities of finding n customers at S_1 and $N-n$ customers at S_2 between events are

$$\mathbf{w}(0;N) = \lambda C(N)\boldsymbol{\pi}(0;N), \qquad (4.1.10a)$$
$$\mathbf{w}(n;N) = C(N)\boldsymbol{\pi}(n;N)(\lambda \mathbf{I}+\mathbf{M}), \qquad (4.1.10b)$$
$$\mathbf{w}(N;N) = C(N)\boldsymbol{\pi}(N;N)\mathbf{M}. \qquad (4.1.10c)$$

The $\boldsymbol{\pi}$s were defined by (4.1.6), and $C(N)$ is the normalizing constant chosen so that the sum of the w's is 1,

$$\frac{1}{C(N)} = \lambda[1 - r(N;N)] + \sum_{n=1}^{N} \boldsymbol{\pi}(n;N)\mathbf{M}\boldsymbol{\epsilon}'. \qquad (4.1.10d)$$

■

Proof: Substitute (4.1.10) into (4.1.9) and get (4.1.3). Proof of (4.1.10d) is left as an exercise. **QED**

Notice that the $\mathbf{w}$s are indeed related to the $\boldsymbol{\pi}$s by the state-dependent time it takes for an event to occur $[(\lambda \mathbf{I}+\mathbf{M})^{-1}]$.

Exercise 4.1.6: Prove that Equation (4.1.10d) is correct.

Having found expressions for the $\mathbf{w}$s, we are now prepared to define and then find the following vector probabilities.

Definition 4.1.4

$\mathbf{a}(n;N)$:= *probability vector that a customer arriving at* S_1 *will find* n *customers there already.* $[\mathbf{a}(n;N)]_i$ *is the probability that the active customer is at phase* $i \in \Xi$. *The associated scalar probability is* $a(n;N) = \mathbf{a}(n;N)\boldsymbol{\epsilon}'$. Note that there are $n+1$ customers at S_1 *after* the arrival. □

Definition 4.1.5

$\mathbf{d}(n;N)$:= *probability vector, whose component* $d_i(n;N)$, *is the probability that a customer departing* S_1 *will leave* n *customers behind, with the system in* $i \in \Xi$ *(immediately after the next customer enters). The associated scalar probability is* $d(n;N) = \mathbf{d}(n;N)\boldsymbol{\epsilon}'$. Note that there were $n+1$ customers at S_1 before the departure. □

Of course, $a(n; N)$ is also the probability that the customer will leave $N - n - 1$ customers behind at S_2, and $d(n; N)$ is the probability that the customer will find $N - n - 1$ other customers already waiting or being served at S_2. We look at our loop from this point of view in Chapter 5. It is not hard to see that $a(N; N) = d(N; N) = 0$, because the arriving or departing customer cannot count himself. The other probabilities can be evaluated using the following argument.

We know the steady-state vector probabilities $[\mathbf{w}(n; N)]$ of the system's state between events. There are two types of events. Either something happens in S_1, or something happens in S_2. The probability that the event will occur in S_1 is $(\lambda\mathbf{I} + \mathbf{M})^{-1}\mathbf{M}$ if n is not 0 or N, whereas it is 0 for $n = 0$, and 1 if $n = N$. If the event is in S_2, it will result in an arrival to S_1, and if the event is in S_1, one of two things can happen. Either the active customer will leave $[\mathbf{q}']$, with another (if available) taking his place $[\mathbf{p}]$, or he will just go to another phase $[\mathbf{P}]$. All together, there are six different kinds of terms, which we now list with their probabilities. In the following set of equations we use the notation "$\mathbb{P}\mathbf{r}[X \to Y]$" to mean "the probability that the system will go to state Y at the next event, AND that it is in state X at present."

$$
\begin{array}{llcll}
(1) & \mathbb{P}\mathbf{r}[\{\cdot;\, 0;\, N\} & \to & \{i;\, 1;\, N\}] & = [\mathbf{w}(0;\, N)]_i; \\
(2) & \mathbb{P}\mathbf{r}[\{i;\, n;\, N\} & \to & \{i;\, n+1;\, N\}] & = [\mathbf{w}(n;\, N)]_i\, [(\lambda\mathbf{I} + \mathbf{M})^{-1}\lambda\mathbf{I}]_{ii}; \\
(3) & \mathbb{P}\mathbf{r}[\{j;\, n;\, N\} & \to & \{i;\, n;\, N\}] & = [\mathbf{w}(n;\, N)]_j\, [(\lambda\mathbf{I} + \mathbf{M})^{-1}\mathbf{M}\mathbf{P}]_{ji}; \\
(4) & \mathbb{P}\mathbf{r}[\{j;\, n;\, N\} & \to & \{i;\, n-1;\, N\}] & = [\mathbf{w}(n;\, N)]_j\, [(\lambda\mathbf{I} + \mathbf{M})^{-1}\mathbf{M}\,\mathbf{q}'\mathbf{p}]_{ji}; \\
(5) & \mathbb{P}\mathbf{r}[\{j;\, N;\, N\} & \to & \{i;\, N;\, N\}] & = [\mathbf{w}(N;\, N)]_j\, [\mathbf{P}]_{ji}; \\
(6) & \mathbb{P}\mathbf{r}[\{j;\, N;\, N\} & \to & \{i;\, N-1;\, N\}] & = [\mathbf{w}(N;\, N)]_j\, [\mathbf{q}'\mathbf{p}]_{ji}.
\end{array}
\tag{4.1.11}
$$

Of course, the sum of these terms is 1, and if rearranged would yield the balance equations we just used to get the **w**s in the first place. We have enumerated them with a different purpose in mind. First, consider only those transactions that result in an arrival to S_1: namely, (1) and (2). Their sum is the probability of an arrival to S_1 irrespective of n. The sum of the two terms in (4.1.11), whose reciprocal we call $G_a(N)$, is [use Equations (4.1.10)]

$$
\begin{aligned}
\frac{1}{G_a(N)} &:= \mathbf{w}(0; N)\boldsymbol{\epsilon}' + \lambda \sum_{n=1}^{N-1} \mathbf{w}(n; N)(\lambda\mathbf{I} + \mathbf{M})^{-1}\boldsymbol{\epsilon}' \\
&= \lambda\, C(N) \left[r(0; N) + \sum_{n=1}^{N-1} r(n; N) \right].
\end{aligned}
$$

The sum of the r's must be 1, and the expression in brackets has all but one of them, therefore we get the following.

$$
\frac{1}{G_a(N)} = \lambda C(N)[1 - r(N; N)]. \tag{4.1.12a}
$$

By the rule of conditional probabilities $[P(B \mid A) = P(B \cap A)/P(A)]$, the marginal arrival probabilities are $G_a(N)$ times the appropriate terms above, so after some substitutions and cancellations, the following emerges. For $0 \leq n < N$,

$$\mathbf{a}(n;N) = \lambda G_a(N)\mathbf{w}(n;N)(\lambda\mathbf{I}+\mathbf{M})^{-1} = \frac{1}{1-r(N;N)}\boldsymbol{\pi}(n;N)$$

and

$$a(n;N) = \frac{r(n;N)}{1-r(N;N)}.$$

A similar argument holds for $\mathbf{d}(n;N)$. But now we must start in state $\{n+1;\, N\}$, so that the departing customer leaves n others behind; thus

$$\mathbf{d}(n;N) = G_d(N)\mathbf{w}(n+1;N)(\lambda\mathbf{I}+\mathbf{M})^{-1}\mathbf{BQ}.$$

As before, we get the probability of a departure from S_1 irrespective of n by adding the contributions from processes (4) and (6).

$$\frac{1}{G_d(N)} = \sum_{n=1}^{N-1} \mathbf{w}(n;N)(\lambda\mathbf{I}+\mathbf{M})^{-1}\mathbf{Mq}'\mathbf{p}\boldsymbol{\epsilon}' + \mathbf{w}(N;N)\mathbf{q}'\mathbf{p}\boldsymbol{\epsilon}'$$

$$= C(N)\sum_{n=1}^{N-1} \boldsymbol{\pi}(n;N)(\lambda\mathbf{I}+\mathbf{M})(\lambda\mathbf{I}+\mathbf{M})^{-1}\mathbf{B}\boldsymbol{\epsilon}' + C(N)\boldsymbol{\pi}(N;N)\mathbf{B}\boldsymbol{\epsilon}',$$

where we have used $\mathbf{p}\boldsymbol{\epsilon}' = 1$ and $\mathbf{Mq}' = \mathbf{B}\boldsymbol{\epsilon}'$. Next, recall from Lemma 4.1.1 that $\mathbf{B}\boldsymbol{\epsilon}' = \lambda\mathbf{A}\boldsymbol{\epsilon}'$, use Theorem 4.1.2, and get

$$\frac{1}{G_d(N)} = \lambda C(N)r(0;N)\left(\sum_{n=1}^{N-1} \mathbf{pU}^n\mathbf{A}\boldsymbol{\epsilon}' + \mathbf{pU}^{N-1}\mathbf{VB}\boldsymbol{\epsilon}'\right)$$

$$= \lambda C(N)r(0;N)\left(\sum_{n=1}^{N} \mathbf{pU}^{n-1}\boldsymbol{\epsilon}'\right),$$

which finally yields what we might have expected,

$$\frac{1}{G_d(N)} = \lambda C(N)[1-r(N;N)], \tag{4.1.12b}$$

the same as we got for sum of the arrivals. The fact that $G_a(N) = G_d(N)$ tells us that the steady-state probability of an arrival to a subsystem is equal to the steady-state probability of a departure from that subsystem. We would expect no less. The process of getting the $\mathbf{d}(n;N)$s and $d(n;N)$s is the same as that for evaluating $G_d(N)$, and gives the same results for $d(n;N)$ as for $a(n;N)$. These are summarized by the following theorem.

Theorem 4.1.4: The steady-state vector and scalar probabilities of finding n customers in an M/ME/1/ /N queue $[\boldsymbol{\pi}(n;N), r(n;N)]$, of an arriving customer finding n already in the queue $[\mathbf{a}(n;N), a(n;N)]$, and of a departing customer leaving n in the queue $[\mathbf{d}(n;N), d(n;N)]$, are related by the following [from (4.1.7) and (4.1.12)]:

For $0 \le n < N$,

$$\mathbf{a}(n;N) = \frac{1}{1 - r(N;N)}\boldsymbol{\pi}(n;N), \tag{4.1.13a}$$

$$\mathbf{d}(n;N) = \frac{r(n;N)}{1 - r(N;N)}\mathbf{p}, \tag{4.1.13b}$$

$$a(n;N) = d(n;N) = \frac{r(n;N)}{1 - r(N;N)}, \tag{4.1.13c}$$

and finally,

$$a(N;N) = d(N;N) = 0. \tag{4.1.13d}$$

By virtue of the completeness of ME functions, as described in Section 3.2.1, the scalar equations are true for classes of service time distributions more general than ME. Thus (4.1.13c) and (4.1.13d) are valid for all M/G/1//N queues. Last, note that although $a(n;N)$ and $d(n;N)$ are equal, their vector counterparts are not. We show how these results carry over to the open queue in succeeding sections. ■

You may be wondering what terms (3) and (5) from Equations (4.1.11) contribute to the behavior of an M/ME/1 queue. After all, no customers are exchanged between S_1 and S_2 during these events. Their role is to give S_1 its nonexponential character, as seen by an outside observer.

4.2 Open M/ME/1 Queue

In Section 2.1.2 we showed how an M/M/1//N loop becomes an open M/M/1 queue when N becomes unboundedly large. In Section 3.5 we showed that a server with an unboundedly long queue generates a renewal process, and in particular, if the server is exponential, its departures are Poisson distributed. Recall from (3.1.4b) that $\Psi[\mathbf{V}]$ is the mean service time for S_1 and λ is the mean service rate for S_2 [see (1.1.4a) and surrounding discussion], so

$$\rho := \textbf{\textit{utilization factor}} = \lambda\Psi[\mathbf{V}] = \lambda\bar{x}.$$

Therefore, if the mean service time of our general server S_1 is less than the mean service time of S_2 [$\rho < 1$], the M/ME/1//N loop approaches an M/ME/1 open queue for very large N. In reality, the number of customers in a system is always finite, but if N is large enough, then the probability that all (or even most) of them will be at S_1 at any time is so small that such events can be neglected in any performance considerations. In that case, N can be replaced by infinity. The reader might ask, "What is meant by *so small*?" Recall the definition of the limit of a sequence of numbers (see any calculus book). Let $\{a_n \mid 0 \le n\}$ be such a sequence. Then if for every $\epsilon > 0$ there exists a unique number a such that for some N (possibly dependent on ϵ) the following is true.

$$|a - a_n| < \epsilon \qquad \forall\ n > N,$$

then

$$\lim_{n \to \infty} a_n := a$$

In our case, ϵ is "so small," that N might as well be ∞.

4.2.1 Steady-State M/ME/1 Queue

Before going on, we need some relationships among our matrix operators that we organize into the following two lemmas and a corollary. The first lemma is a variant of the ***Sherman-Morrison Formula*** [ShermanMorrison50], which itself is a special case of the *Woodbury formula*. These are of use to us in later chapters as well.

Lemma 4.2.1: Let $\mathbf{F}$ be any m-dimensional square matrix for which $\Psi[\mathbf{F}] \neq 1$. Then (recall that $\mathbf{Q} = \boldsymbol{\epsilon}'\mathbf{p}$, and thus $\mathbf{QFQ} = \Psi[\mathbf{F}]\,\mathbf{Q}$), $(\mathbf{I} - \mathbf{QF})$ is nonsingular and

$$(\mathbf{I} - \mathbf{QF})^{-1} = \mathbf{I} + \frac{1}{1 - \Psi[\mathbf{F}]}\mathbf{QF}. \tag{4.2.1a}$$

Similarly,

$$(\mathbf{I} - \mathbf{FQ})^{-1} = \mathbf{I} + \frac{1}{1 - \Psi[\mathbf{F}]}\mathbf{FQ}. \tag{4.2.1b}$$

This lemma is valid for any two vectors $\mathbf{x}$ and $\mathbf{y}$ for which $\mathbf{xy}' = 1$ and the scalar $\mathbf{xFy}' \neq 1$, but is used in this book only for $\mathbf{x} = \mathbf{p}$ and $\mathbf{y}' = \boldsymbol{\epsilon}'$. ■

The proof is evident by direct substitution.

> **Exercise 4.2.1:** Prove by direct multiplication that the expressions given in Equations (4.2.1) are the inverses of $(\mathbf{I} - \mathbf{FQ})$ and $(\mathbf{I} - \mathbf{QF})$.

The fact that $[\mathbf{I} - \mathbf{U}]$ is invertible is central to the development of this section and parts of Chapter 5. Therefore, we state and prove the following lemma.

Lemma 4.2.2: Let $\rho = \lambda\Psi[\mathbf{V}] \neq 1$; then

$$\mathbf{K} := [\mathbf{I} - \mathbf{U}]^{-1} \tag{4.2.2a}$$

exists, and the following relations are true:

$$\mathbf{K} = \lambda\left[\mathbf{I} + \frac{\lambda}{1-\rho}\mathbf{VQ}\right]\mathbf{V}\,\mathbf{A} = \lambda\mathbf{A}\,\mathbf{V}\left[\mathbf{I} + \frac{\lambda}{1-\rho}\mathbf{QV}\right] \tag{4.2.2b}$$

and

$$\mathbf{K} = \mathbf{I} + \lambda\mathbf{V} + \frac{\lambda^2}{1-\rho}\mathbf{VQV}. \tag{4.2.2c}$$

These relations are true even if $\rho > 1$, and even if ρ is complex. Only if $\rho = 1$ does $[\mathbf{I} - \mathbf{U}]$ fail to have an inverse. ■

Proof: From (4.1.4a) we have $\mathbf{A} = \mathbf{I} + (\mathbf{1}/\lambda)\mathbf{B} - \mathbf{Q}$ and $\mathbf{U} = \mathbf{A}^{-1}$. Observe that (4.2.2b) can be proven directly by multiplying the middle or right expression by $(\mathbf{I} - \mathbf{U})$ and noting that $\mathbf{A}(\mathbf{I} - \mathbf{U}) = (\mathbf{I} - \mathbf{U})\mathbf{A} = (1/\lambda)\mathbf{B} - \mathbf{Q}$. However, (4.2.2c) is messier, and it is informative to prove it by deduction so the reader can discover how such formulas are found in the first place.

$$\mathbf{I} - \mathbf{U} = \mathbf{U}(\mathbf{A} - \mathbf{I}) = \mathbf{U}\frac{1}{\lambda}(\mathbf{B} - \lambda\mathbf{Q}) = \frac{1}{\lambda}\mathbf{U}\mathbf{B}(\mathbf{I} - \lambda\mathbf{V}\mathbf{Q}).$$

By symmetry,

$$\mathbf{I} - \mathbf{U} = (\mathbf{A} - \mathbf{I})\mathbf{U} = \frac{1}{\lambda}(\mathbf{B} - \lambda\mathbf{Q})\mathbf{U} = \frac{1}{\lambda}(\mathbf{I} - \lambda\mathbf{Q}\mathbf{V})\mathbf{B}\mathbf{U}.$$

We next take the inverse of both sides to get

$$\mathbf{K} = (\mathbf{I} - \mathbf{U})^{-1} = \lambda(\mathbf{I} - \lambda\mathbf{V}\mathbf{Q})^{-1}\mathbf{V}\mathbf{A} = \lambda\mathbf{A}\mathbf{V}(\mathbf{I} - \lambda\mathbf{Q}\mathbf{V})^{-1}.$$

Using the last equation together with (4.2.1) for $\mathbf{F} = \lambda\mathbf{V}$, we get (4.2.2b). Finally, we get (4.2.2c) by substituting $\mathbf{A} = \mathbf{I} + (1/\lambda)\mathbf{B} - \mathbf{Q}$ into (4.2.2b).

As one further comment, note that $\mathbf{A}$, $\mathbf{V}$, and $\mathbf{Q}$ do not commute with each other, so the order in which they appear is important. **QED**

The equations for $\mathbf{K}$ are explicit in terms of known quantities, and therefore exist as long as $\rho \neq 1$, so $[\mathbf{I} - \mathbf{U}]$ does indeed have an inverse. This also proves that if $\rho = 1$, then $\mathbf{U}$ has an eigenvalue equal to 1.

Several expressions that prove useful in Chapter 5 are given in the following.

Corollary 4.2.2: Multiplying the right-most term in (4.2.2b) on the right with $\boldsymbol{\epsilon}'$ yields

$$\lambda\mathbf{A}\mathbf{V}\boldsymbol{\epsilon}' = (1 - \rho)\mathbf{K}\boldsymbol{\epsilon}', \tag{4.2.3a}$$

and multiplying the second last term on the left with $\mathbf{p}$ gives

$$\lambda\mathbf{p}\mathbf{V}\mathbf{A} = (1 - \rho)\mathbf{p}\mathbf{K}. \tag{4.2.3b}$$

Similarly, it follows directly from (4.2.2c) that

$$\mathbf{p}\mathbf{K} = \mathbf{p}\left[\mathbf{I} + \frac{\lambda}{1 - \rho}\mathbf{V}\right] \tag{4.2.3c}$$

and

$$\mathbf{K}\boldsymbol{\epsilon}' = \left[\mathbf{I} + \frac{\lambda}{1 - \rho}\mathbf{V}\right]\boldsymbol{\epsilon}'. \tag{4.2.3d}$$

The last expression we need is $\Psi[\mathbf{K}]$. Using either of the last two equations, we get

$$\Psi[\mathbf{K}] = 1 + \frac{\rho}{1-\rho} = \frac{1}{1-\rho}, \tag{4.2.3e}$$

a rather simple expression but a nonetheless important result. ■

We are now prepared to look at the M/ME/1 queue. The open queue is described by the following probabilities for $\rho < 1$. From Theorem 4.1.2:

$$r(n) := \lim_{N\to\infty} r(n;N) = \left[\lim_{N\to\infty} r(0;\, N)\right] \Psi[\mathbf{U}^n], \tag{4.2.4a}$$

and

$$\boldsymbol{\pi}(n) := \lim_{N\to\infty} \boldsymbol{\pi}(n;N) = \left[\lim_{N\to\infty} r(0;\, N)\right] \mathbf{p}\,\mathbf{U}^n. \tag{4.2.4b}$$

Both depend on (4.1.6g)

$$[r(0)]^{-1} = \lim_{N\to\infty} [r(n;\, N)]^{-1} = \lim_{N\to\infty} \Psi[\mathbf{K}(N)].$$

For the moment, let $\mathbf{X}$, if it exists, be defined by

$$\mathbf{X} := \lim_{n\to\infty} \mathbf{K}(N),$$

Using (4.1.6e), we can write

$$\mathbf{X} = \lim_{N\to\infty} \mathbf{K}(N+1) = \lim_{N\to\infty} [\mathbf{I} + \mathbf{U}\mathbf{K}(N)] = \mathbf{I} + \mathbf{U} \lim_{N\to\infty} \mathbf{K}(N)) = \mathbf{I} + \mathbf{U}\mathbf{X}.$$

Solving for $\mathbf{X}$, we get

$$\mathbf{X} = (\mathbf{I} - \mathbf{U})^{-1}.$$

But that's what we defined as $\mathbf{K}$ in (4.2.2a). Therefore, when the limit exists (i.e., when $\rho < 1$), we have:

$$\lim_{N\to\infty} \mathbf{K}(N) = \mathbf{K}. \tag{4.2.4c}$$

Equations (4.2.4) and Theorem 4.1.2 together lead to the following.

Theorem 4.2.3: The steady-state vector and scalar probabilities of finding n customers in an M/ME/1 queue are

$$\boldsymbol{\pi}(n) = (1-\rho)\mathbf{p}\mathbf{U}^n \tag{4.2.5a}$$

and

$$r(n) = (1-\rho)\Psi[\mathbf{U}^n]. \tag{4.2.5b}$$

$\rho = 1 - r(0)$ is the probability that S_1 is busy. To efficiently compute all the above, the recursive formula $\boldsymbol{\pi}(n) = \boldsymbol{\pi}(n-1)\mathbf{U}$ for $n > 0$ should be used, starting with $\boldsymbol{\pi}(0) = (1-\rho)\mathbf{p}$. Then use $r(n) = \boldsymbol{\pi}(n)\boldsymbol{\epsilon}'$. ■

It is easy to argue that $r(N;N)$ [from (4.1.7b)] goes to 0 as N goes to infinity whenever ρ is less than 1 (i.e., S_2 is always busy). We can then extend Theorem 4.1.4 to the open M/G/1 queue, expressed by the following:

Theorem 4.2.4: Let $\mathbf{a}(n)$ and $\mathbf{d}(n)$ be the open M/G/1 queue equivalents to $\mathbf{a}(n;N)$ and $\mathbf{d}(n;N)$ Then for $(\rho < 1)$,

$$\mathbf{a}(n) = \lim_{N\to\infty} \mathbf{a}(n;N) \quad \text{and} \quad \mathbf{d}(n) = \lim_{N\to\infty} \mathbf{d}(n;\ N).$$

Therefore,

$$a(n) = d(n) = r(n)$$

and the vectors,

$$\mathbf{a}(n) = \boldsymbol{\pi}(n).$$

However, $\mathbf{d}(n) = r(n)\mathbf{p} \neq \boldsymbol{\pi}(n)$. ■

This well-known result is discussed, for instance, in [COOPER81]. Cooper refers to the ***outside observer***, whereas we also use the term ***random observer***. The two concepts are not the same, but the so-called ***PASTA*** property (*Poisson Arrivals See Time Averages*) equates the two. A random observer looks at the system *randomly*. That is, the times between her viewings are exponentially distributed, so her observation times constitute a Poisson process. The outside observer views the system continuously, in effect taking time averages. The equality of their long-term averages was first proven by C. Palm [PALM43] (see also [KHINCHINE60]). Therefore we tend to use the terms interchangeably. [See, however, the discussion surrounding Equations (1.1.1).] Note that $a(n)$, $d(n)$, and $r(n)$ are not equal to each other for the open G/M/1 queue. This is discussed fully in Chapter 5.

To close this section, we mention that $\mathbf{K}$, as the limit of $\mathbf{K}(N)$, exists whenever all the eigenvalues of $\mathbf{U}$ are less than 1 in magnitude. We assume without proof that this occurs whenever $\rho < 1$. In any case, Equations (4.2.2) and (4.2.3) are valid as long as $\mathbf{U}$ has no unit eigenvalues, and thus when $\rho \neq 1$. In Chapter 5 we look at this problem more closely, and in Chapter 7 we show that for more complicated queues, $\mathbf{U}$ always has a unit eigenvalue (in fact, 1 may be a multiple eigenvalue).

4.2.2 System Times: Pollaczek-Khinchine Formulas

The prototypical question asked in relation to queueing theory is: "How long can a customer expect to wait for service from a busy server?" The M/G/1 queue provides an unusually simple answer. This result is amazingly simple, considering that all attempts to find similar answers for somewhat more complicated systems have failed in the 70 or more years since Pollaczek [POLLACZEK30] and Khinchine [KHINCHINE32] separately found that the mean queue length and mean system time for the steady-state open M/G/1 queue depend only on ρ and the first and second moments of S_1's pdf. Even the closed M/G/1//N loop does not share the simple result. These formulas are derived here.

4.2.2.1 Mean Queue Length

The mean queue length of a general server with Poisson arrivals can be calculated directly from (4.2.5):

$$\bar{q} := \sum_{n=1}^{\infty} n\, r(n) = (1-\rho)\Psi\left[\sum_{n=1}^{\infty} n\mathbf{U}^n\right]. \tag{4.2.6a}$$

From the properties of the geometric series, we know that

$$\sum_{n=1}^{\infty} n\mathbf{U}^n = (\mathbf{I}-\mathbf{U})^{-1}(\mathbf{I}-\mathbf{U})^{-1}\mathbf{U} = \mathbf{K}\,\mathbf{K}\,\mathbf{U}.$$

We also know that $\mathbf{KU} = \mathbf{UK} = \mathbf{K} - \mathbf{I}$, so (4.2.3c) and (4.2.3d) can be used to reduce the mean queue-length formula to

$$\bar{q} = (1-\rho)\mathbf{pK}(\mathbf{K}-\mathbf{I})\boldsymbol{\epsilon}' = (1-\rho)\Psi\left[\left(\mathbf{I} + \frac{\lambda}{1-\rho}\mathbf{V}\right)\left(\frac{\lambda}{1-\rho}\mathbf{V}\right)\right]$$

$$= \lambda\Psi\left[\mathbf{V} + \frac{\lambda}{1-\rho}\mathbf{V}^2\right]. \tag{4.2.6b}$$

But $\Psi[\lambda\mathbf{V}] = \rho$, and $\Psi\left[\mathbf{V}^2\right] = \mathbb{E}[X^2]/2$, [from (3.1.9)], so we get the Pollaczek-Khinchine (P-K) formula:

$$\bar{q} = \rho + \frac{\lambda^2}{1-\rho}\frac{\mathbb{E}[X^2]}{2}. \tag{4.2.6c}$$

Another form for the P-K formula, which is perhaps more enlightening, can be written by recalling the definition of variance $[\sigma^2 = \mathbb{E}[X^2] - \bar{x}^2]$ and the squared coefficient of variation $[C_v^2 = \sigma^2 / \bar{x}^2]$. Then

$$\bar{q} = \frac{\rho}{1-\rho} + \frac{\rho^2}{1-\rho}\frac{C_v^2 - 1}{2}. \tag{4.2.6d}$$

Let T_s be the random variable denoting the time a customer spends in the system. The mean time he spends in S_1 or its queue is given by ***Little's formula*** [Equation (2.1.7)], namely,

$$\mathbb{E}[T_s] = \frac{\bar{q}}{\lambda} = \frac{\bar{x}}{1-\rho} + \frac{\bar{x}\rho}{1-\rho}\frac{C_v^2 - 1}{2}. \tag{4.2.6e}$$

In this form, for a given ρ and $\bar{x}$, it is clear that if C_v^2 is greater than 1, the mean queue length and the mean time in the subsystem will be longer than that for an M/M/1 queue (for which $C_v^2 = 1$), whereas if C_v^2 is less than 1, $\bar{q}$ and $\mathbb{E}[T_s]$ will be shorter. See Figures 1.1.2 and 1.1.3 for well-behaved examples.

$\mathbb{E}[T_s]$ can be written in yet another form, one that can be interpreted directly. From (4.2.6c) we get

$$\mathbb{E}[T_s] = \bar{x} + \frac{\rho}{1-\rho}\left[\frac{\mathbb{E}(X^2)}{2\bar{x}}\right]. \tag{4.2.6f}$$

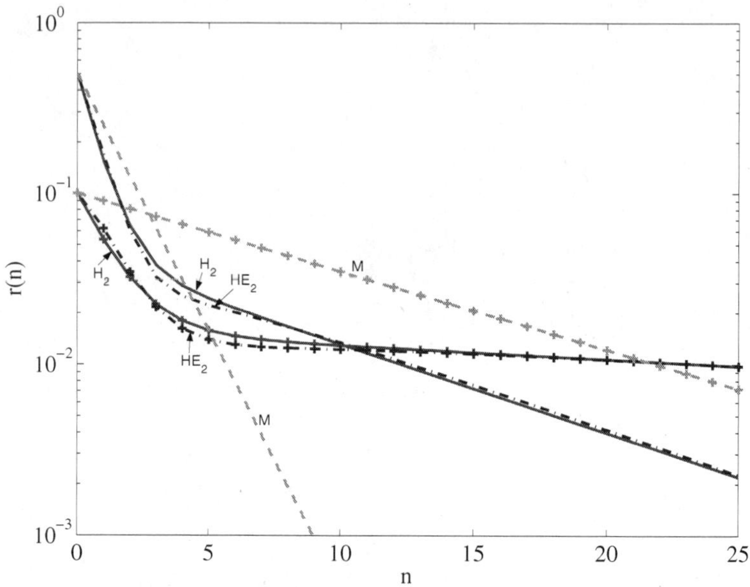

Figure 4.2.1: M/G/1 Queue-length probabilities (on a log scale) for two pairs of H_2, and two hyper-Erlangian functions with the same first three moments. In all cases, $\bar{x} = 1$, $C_v^2 = 10$, and $\mathbf{E}(X^3) = 330.0$. The pair that starts higher corresponds to $\rho = 0.5$, and the other pair has $\rho = 0.9$. The M/M/1 queue ($C_v^2 = 1$) is included for comparison.

This can be understood in the following way. Suppose a customer arrives at an empty queue needing a time x to be served. While he is being served, λx more customers arrive. It will take on average $(\lambda x)\bar{x}$ amount of time before the last of them begins service. But in that interval of time, another $\rho x \lambda$ (we have made use of $\rho = \lambda \bar{x}$) will have arrived, and they will have to wait an average of $\rho x \lambda \bar{x}$ time before the last one of them is processed. Continuing in this way and adding all the delays, we get $(1+\rho+\rho^2+\rho^3+\cdots)x = x/(1-\rho)$. We see that the ubiquitous term $1/(1-\rho)$ is due to the propagated delay due to an initial delay. In Theorem 3.5.4 we showed that the mean residual time $\bar{x}_r$ is given by the expression in square brackets above.

We also show in Theorem 4.3.1 below that the mean time remaining for the customer in service when a new customer arrives is the same $\bar{x}_r$. Thus (4.2.6f) tells us that an arriving customer will take on average $\bar{x}$ to be served, *plus* if the server is busy when he arrives $[\rho]$ he will have to wait, on average $\bar{x}_r/(1-\rho)$ before he begins service. We give one cautionary reminder that Equations (4.2.6) are true only for the steady-state M/G/1 open queue.

A point to be made concerning the P-K formula is the following. Although it is true that all M/G/1 queues have the same $\bar{q}$ and mean system time for a given λ, $\bar{x}$, and C_v^2, that does not imply that other properties are the same. For instance, different distributions yield different queue-length probabilities, as we show in the next example.

Example 4.2.1: In Sections 3.2.1.2 and 3.2.3.1 we presented the H_2 function and a 4-state hyper-Erlangian which can be made to have the same first three moments. We have calculated $r(n)$ from (4.2.5b) using the two functions with $\bar{x} = 1$, $C_v^2 = 10$, and $\mathbb{E}(X^3) = 330.0$, and for $\rho = 0.5$ and 0.9. The results of these calculations are shown in Figure 4.2.1. Later, when we discuss ***buffer overflow*** and ***customer loss*** we show that the difference can be important. ▲

> **Exercise 4.2.2:** Evaluate the mean system times $\mathbb{E}[T_s]$ for queueing systems with mean service time of 1, and with the following values of C_v^2, the squared coefficient of variation: 0, 0.25, 0.50, 1.0, 2.0, 5.0, and 10.0. Use enough values of ρ between 0 and 1 to draw curves for all of them that appear visually smooth. Make sure that they all have the same value at $\rho = 0$, namely, $\bar{x}$, which in this case equals 1.

4.2.2.2 Queue-Length Probabilities of M/PT/1 Queues

For a given ρ, the shortest queue length and system time occur for the deterministic distribution, where $C_v^2 = 0$, but there is no longest mean queue length, because one can always find a distribution whose coefficient of variation exceeds any number. In fact, there exist distributions that have infinite variance, examples of which were given in Section 3.3. In that section we introduced the family of Power-Tail (PT) distributions and their Truncated (TPT) relatives. We showed that if $\alpha \le 2$ then the PT distribution has infinite variance, and it would take an infinite number of samples to exhibit that. Therefore, systems that exhibit PT behavior can never reach their steady state. Yet, for $\alpha > 1$ the steady-state M/PT/1 solution exists. How can that be if $\bar{q} = \infty$? In Figure 4.2.2 we plot $r(n)$ and $n^\alpha\, r(n)$ versus n for several values of ρ. The graphs indicate that for all $\rho < 1$ $n^\alpha\, r(n)$ approaches a constant value for n large enough. (Well, it *does* show it for $\rho < 0.8$ but if the graph were extended to larger n then all the curves would level off.) In other words,

$$r(n) \Longrightarrow \frac{c(\rho)}{n^\alpha}. \tag{4.2.7}$$

It is well known that as long as $\alpha > 1$,

$$\sum_{n=1}^{\infty} \frac{c(\rho)}{n^\alpha} < \infty;$$

that is, the series converges. We ignore the possibility of $\alpha \le 1$ because that would imply an infinite mean service time, in which case $\rho = \lambda\bar{x} = \infty$, no solution.

Now consider the mean queue length. Equation (4.2.6a) converges if and only if

$$\sum_{n=1}^{\infty} n \frac{c(\rho)}{n^\alpha} = \sum_{n=1}^{\infty} \frac{c(\rho)}{n^{\alpha-1}} < \infty$$

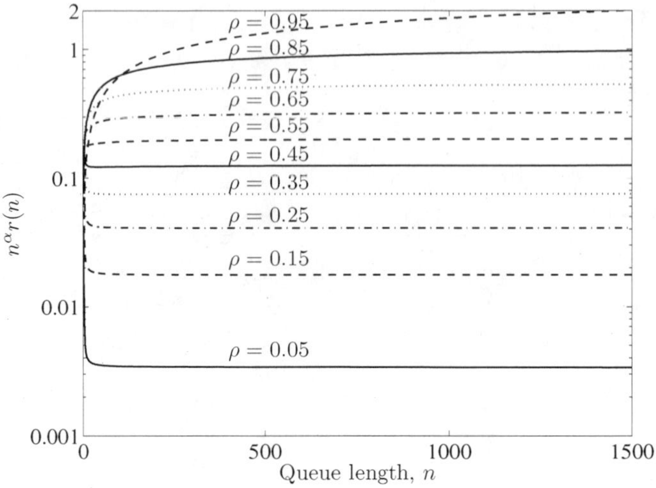

Figure 4.2.2: M/PT/1 Queue-length probabilities, $n^\alpha\, r(n)$ (on a log scale) versus n for various values of ρ. The PT function is that given by (3.3.18) with $\alpha = 1.4$ and $\theta = 0.5$. The calculation would require the use of infinite matrices, therefore the actual calculation was made with the truncated version for $T = 30$. For this range of $n \leq 1500$ there would be no visible difference using any other $T > 30$.

which is true only if $\alpha - 1 > 1$, or $\alpha > 2$. Conversely, if $\alpha \leq 2$ then we get an infinite variance, and thus an infinite queue length, in agreement with the P-K formula, (4.2.6b). for a discussion of the occurence of large queues, see [AsmussenKluppelberg97].

To be honest, the curves in Figure 4.2.2 were actually calculated based on a TPT30 distribution (i.e., a truncated power tail with $T = 30$). Any other $T > 30$ would yield almost exactly the same curves for $n < 1500$. If we would have extended the curves for larger n we would have seen $n^\alpha\, r(n)$ begin to drop to 0 above some $N(T)$. We have not examined the behavior of $N(T)$ as a function of T except to note that it monotonically increases to ∞ with increasing T. In any case, we see that $r(n)$ is independent of T for $n < N(T)$. This shows us that one cannot distinguish between TPTs and the full PT unless one observes long enough for very long queues to occur. This agrees with the discussion in Section 3.3 concerning the range of the distribution.

4.2.2.3 Throughput

We have developed the mathematical properties of $\mathbf{K}$ sufficiently to be able to find the limit of $\Lambda(N)$ in (4.1.8a) without any effort. We also point out in passing, that although $\mathbf{U}$ and $\mathbf{K}(N)$ do not commute, $\mathbf{U}$ and $\mathbf{K}$ do. When ρ is less than 1, we have [from (4.1.8a), (4.2.2a) and (4.2.3e)]

$$\lim_{n\to\infty} \Lambda(N) = \frac{\lambda}{\rho}\frac{\Psi\,[\mathbf{UK}]}{\Psi\,[\mathbf{K}]} = \frac{\lambda}{\rho}\frac{\Psi\,[\mathbf{K}-\mathbf{I}]}{\Psi\,[\mathbf{K}]} = \frac{\lambda}{\rho}(1-\rho)\left(\frac{1}{1-\rho} - 1\right) = \lambda.$$

So, as in the M/M/1//N queue [Equation (2.1.6c)], the ***throughput*** of the system is limited by the capacity of the slower server S_2. When ρ is greater than 1, the problem is more difficult. We deal with it in Chapter 5.

4.2.2.4 Z-Transform

Pollaczek and Khinchine separately derived an expression for the ***Z-transform***, also known as the ***generating function***, of the set of queue-length probabilities. We first derive the vector z-transform and then reproduce the P-K formula. First define the row vector (not to be confused with the exit vector $\mathbf{q}'$)

$$\mathbf{q}(z) := \sum_{n=o}^{\infty} \boldsymbol{\pi}(n) z^n = (1-\rho)\mathbf{p} \sum_{n=o}^{\infty} z^n \mathbf{U}^n = (1-\rho)\mathbf{p}(\mathbf{I} - z\mathbf{U})^{-1}. \quad (4.2.8a)$$

This expression can be manipulated into a form that makes use of the properties of $\mathbf{V}$, as given in (3.1.9) and (3.1.10). First note that

$$(\mathbf{I} - z\mathbf{U}) = \frac{1}{\lambda}\mathbf{UB}[\mathbf{I} + \lambda(1-z)\mathbf{V} - \lambda\mathbf{VQ}].$$

Next, let $s = \lambda(1-z)$, and define

$$\mathbf{D}(s) := [\mathbf{I} + s\mathbf{V}]^{-1}. \quad (4.2.8b)$$

This matrix shows up often, and from (3.1.10), is related to the Laplace transform by the following:

$$d(s) := \Psi[\mathbf{D}(s)] = B^*[\lambda(1-z)]. \quad (4.2.8c)$$

We manipulate the equation before (4.2.8b) to a form in which Lemma 4.2.1 can be applied, so it follows that

$$\mathbf{I} - z\mathbf{U} = \frac{1}{\lambda}\mathbf{UBD}^{-1}(\mathbf{I} - \lambda\mathbf{DVQ}).$$

Before going on, note that $\lambda\mathbf{pDVQ} = \Psi[\lambda\mathbf{DV}]\,\mathbf{p}$, and from (4.2.8b) that $\lambda\mathbf{DV} = (\mathbf{I} - \mathbf{D})/(1-z)$. We must now take the inverse of $(\mathbf{I} - z\mathbf{U})$ to get

$$(\mathbf{I} - z\mathbf{U})^{-1} = (\mathbf{I} - \lambda\mathbf{DVQ})^{-1}\lambda\mathbf{DVA}.$$

Then as long as $\Psi[\lambda\mathbf{DV}] \neq 1$, Lemma 4.2.1 applies, so (4.2.8a) yields

$$\mathbf{q}(z) = (1-\rho)\mathbf{p}\left(\mathbf{I} + \frac{1}{1 - \Psi[\lambda\mathbf{DV}]}\lambda\mathbf{DVQ}\right)\lambda\mathbf{DVA}$$

$$= (1-\rho)\left(1 + \frac{\Psi[\lambda\mathbf{DV}]}{1 - \Psi[\lambda\mathbf{DV}]}\right)\lambda\mathbf{pDVA}.$$

By virtue of the fact that $\Psi[\lambda\mathbf{DV}] = (1-d)/(1-z)$, we finally get (after simplifying the expression in the large parentheses)

$$\mathbf{q}(z) = \frac{1-\rho}{1-\Psi[\lambda\mathbf{DV}]}\lambda\mathbf{pDVA} = \frac{(1-\rho)(1-z)}{d-z}\lambda\mathbf{pDVA}. \tag{4.2.8d}$$

This vector z-transform contains the information concerning the internal states of S_1. The sum of its components corresponds to the P-K transform formula. Using Lemma 4.1.1, it easily follows that

$$Q(z) := \mathbf{q}(z)\boldsymbol{\epsilon}' = \frac{(1-\rho)(1-z)}{d(s)-z}d(s) = \frac{(1-\rho)(1-z)B^*(s)}{B^*(s)-z} \tag{4.2.8e}$$

[where again, $s = \lambda(1-z)$]. The rightmost term is the expression normally referred to as the P-K formula. It is not easy to use because it is indeterminate at $z = 1$, for then $s = 0$ and $B^*(0) = 1$. In fact, (4.2.8a) is surely the easiest form to use for evaluation. From this equation,

$$Q(z) = (1-\rho)\Psi\left[(\mathbf{I}-z\mathbf{U})^{-1}\right] \tag{4.2.8f}$$

(the matrix equivalent of the z-transform of the geometric distribution), and from (4.2.2a) and (4.2.3e) it is obvious that $Q(1) = 1$. This must necessarily be true, because by the definitions (4.2.8a) and (4.2.8e) $Q(1)$ is the sum of the queue-length probabilities, which must be 1. The usefulness of the z-transform comes from the ability to get the mean queue length and higher moments without evaluating an infinite sum. In our case the infinite sums are geometric in form and are evaluable, so the potential advantage is limited.* However, we do that next.

It is well known that the derivative of $Q(z)$ evaluated at $z = 1$ is $\bar{q}$, and the variance of the queue length is $\sigma_q^2 = Q''(1) - \bar{q}(\bar{q}-1)$. Now from (4.2.8f),

$$\bar{q} = \left(\frac{dQ(z)}{dz}\right)_{z=1} = (1-\rho)\Psi\left[(\mathbf{I}-\mathbf{U})^{-2}\mathbf{U}\right] = (1-\rho)\Psi[\mathbf{KKU}],$$

the same expression that led to the derivation of (4.2.6b). It is also straightforward to find the expression for Q'', which is

$$\left(\frac{d^2Q(z)}{dz^2}\right)_{z=1} = 2(1-\rho)\Psi\left[\mathbf{KK}^2\mathbf{U}^2\right] = 2(1-\rho)\Psi\left[\mathbf{K}(\mathbf{K}-\mathbf{I})^2\right]$$

$$= 2(1-\rho)\Psi\left[\mathbf{K}^3 - 2\mathbf{K}^2 + \mathbf{K}\right].$$

The last two terms in the rightmost Ψ brackets are simple enough to evaluate, and the first one can be evaluated by doing the following:

$$\Psi\left[\mathbf{K}^3\right] = \mathbf{pKKK}\boldsymbol{\epsilon}'$$

*We should point out, however, that $Q(z) = \sum_{n=o}^{\infty} r(n)z^n$ and $r(n) \geq 0$ for all n. Therefore it follows that $Q(z) \geq 0$ for $z \geq 0$. Then (4.2.8f) might be used in the future to find those properties $\mathbf{U}$ must have to guarantee this.

$$= \mathbf{p}\left[\mathbf{I} + \frac{\lambda}{1-\rho}\mathbf{V}\right]\left[\mathbf{I} + \lambda\mathbf{V} + \frac{\lambda^2}{1-\rho}\mathbf{VQV}\right]\left[\mathbf{I} + \frac{\lambda}{1-\rho}\mathbf{V}\right]\boldsymbol{\epsilon}'.$$

It is straightforward, if a bit tedious, to multiply out all terms and regroup them to get

$$Q''(1) = \frac{2}{1-\rho}\Psi\left[(\lambda\mathbf{V})^2\right] + \frac{2}{1-\rho}\Psi\left[(\lambda\mathbf{V})^3\right] + 2\left(\frac{\Psi\left[(\lambda\mathbf{V})^2\right]}{1-\rho}\right)^2.$$

Further manipulation yields

$$\sigma_q^2 = \rho(1-\rho) + \frac{3-2\rho}{1-\rho}\Psi\left[(\lambda\mathbf{V})^2\right] + \frac{2}{1-\rho}\Psi\left[(\lambda\mathbf{V})^3\right] + \left(\frac{\Psi\left[(\lambda\mathbf{V})^2\right]}{1-\rho}\right)^2. \tag{4.2.9a}$$

We put this into another form by making use of the fact that $\Psi\left[(\lambda\mathbf{V})^2\right] = \rho^2 + \rho^2(C_v^2 - 1)/2$. Then

$$\sigma_q^2 = \frac{\rho(1-2\rho^2+2\rho^3)}{(1-\rho)^2} + \frac{\rho^2(3-5\rho+4\rho^2)}{(1-\rho)^2}\left(\frac{C_v^2-1}{2}\right) + \frac{\rho^4}{(1-\rho)^2}\left(\frac{C_v^2-1}{2}\right)^2 + \frac{2}{1-\rho}\Psi\left[(\lambda\mathbf{V})^3\right]. \tag{4.2.9b}$$

The next two equations give expressions for two special cases. For exponential servers, $C_v^2 = 1$ and $\Psi\left[(\lambda\mathbf{V})^n\right] = \rho^n$, so

$$\sigma_q^2 = \frac{\rho}{(1-\rho)^2}.$$

For the deterministic distribution $C_v^2 = 0$, and $\Psi\left[(\lambda\mathbf{V})^n\right] = \rho^n/n!$, so

$$\sigma_q^2 = \frac{\rho(12-18\rho+10\rho^2-\rho^3)}{12(1-\rho)^2}.$$

We have seen that (4.2.8f) is easy enough to use, although a bit tedious, to get the moments of the queue length. Use of (4.2.8e) is considerably harder and even more tedious to use. In either case, even the second moment is not particularly informative for general analysis, so we leave it for now. However, in the following section we surprisingly find a better use of (4.2.8f).

4.2.3 System Time Distribution

The P-K transform formulas (4.2.8) turn out to have more significance than that implied in the preceding section. Following standard texts, we now show that $Q(z)$ is also the Laplace transform $B_s^*(s)$ of the system time pdf, $b_s(x)$, where $s = \lambda(1-z)$. Then we will go even further (thanks to Appie van de Liefvoort, who first recognized it [LIEFVOORT90]) and find the matrix generator $\langle\, \mathbf{p_s}\,,\, \mathbf{B_s} \,\rangle$ of the system time distribution itself.

Recall the definition of system time (or total, or response time) from the end of Section 2.1.3, and define the steady-state distribution.

Definition 4.2.1

X_s := r.v for the time a customer spends at S_1 from the moment he arrives until the moment he completes service.

$B_s(x) := \mathbb{P}\mathbf{r}(X_s \le x)$. That is, $B_s(x)$ is the PDF for system time, $b_s(x)$ is its derivative, and $R_s(x) = 1 - B_s(x)$ is the probability that the customer will still be in the subsystem at time x. □

From Theorem 4.2.4 we know that the steady-state probability of finding n customers at S_1 $[r(n)]$, is the same as the probability that a departing customer will leave n customers behind $[d(n)]$. Now, because the arrival process to S_1 is Poisson, the probability that n customers will arrive in the time interval x (the time spent there by our now-departing customer), is given by (3.5.16b). Therefore, the probability that he will leave n customers behind, irrespective of how long he was at S_1, is

$$d(n) = r(n) = \int_0^\infty \frac{(\lambda x)^n}{n!} e^{-x\lambda} b_s(x)\, dx.$$

Next, insert this into the expression for $Q(z)$ [Equations (4.2.8a) and (4.2.8e)], to get

$$Q(z) = \sum_{n=0}^\infty z^n r(n) = \sum_{n=0}^\infty \int_0^\infty \frac{(\lambda x z)^n}{n!} e^{-x\lambda} b_s(x) dx$$

$$= \int_0^\infty \sum_{n=0}^\infty \frac{(\lambda x z)^n}{n!} e^{-x\lambda} b_s(x) dx = \int_0^\infty e^{\lambda x z} e^{-x\lambda} b_s(x) dx.$$

Finally, we identify the Laplace transform in the following theorem.

Theorem 4.2.5: The Laplace transform for the steady-state system-time distribution in an M/G/1 queue is given by

$$B_s^*[\lambda(1-z)] = Q(z) = \int_0^\infty e^{-\lambda(1-z)x} b_s(x) dx, \tag{4.2.10a}$$

and from (4.2.8f), we have for M/ME/1 queues,

$$B_s^*(s) = (1-\rho)\Psi\left[(\mathbf{I} - z\mathbf{U})^{-1}\right], \tag{4.2.10b}$$

where $s = \lambda(1-z)$. In particular (for $z = 0$), $B_s^*(\lambda) = (1-\rho)$. ■

This is a most interesting result, but remember that this simple expression occurred for two special reasons. First, $d(n)$ and $r(n)$ are equal, and second, the Poisson arrival process and the Laplace transform are both generated by the exponential function. We cannot expect such simple results for the G/G/1 queue. In attempting an alternative derivation using the arrival probabilities (which also satisfy Theorem 4.2.4) we get a result that so far has not been shown equal to (4.2.10b). We postpone this derivation until the end of the next section, after we have discussed residual times.

Equation (4.2.10b) can be used to find a vector-matrix pair that generates the moments of $B_s(x)$, and thus, by (3.1.7c), (3.1.8b), (3.1.9) and (3.1.10), the same pair will be a faithful representation of $b_s(x)$ itself, as well as $B_s^*(s)$. First recall that the Laplace transform is also known as the moment generating function, in that its n-th derivative evaluated at $s = 0$ is $(-1)^n$ times the n-th moment. That is,

$$\mathbb{E}[T_s^n] = (-1)^n \left(\frac{d^{(n)} B_s^*(s)}{ds^n}\right)_{s=0} = \int_0^\infty x^n\, b_s(x)\, dx.$$

Next, given that $s = \lambda\,(1 - z)$, note that

$$\frac{d}{ds} = \frac{dz}{ds}\frac{d}{dz} = -\frac{1}{\lambda}\frac{d}{dz},$$

so (clearly, $z = 1$ when $s = 0$), using (4.2.10b), and recalling that $\mathbf{K} = (\mathbf{I} - \mathbf{U})^{-1}$ [see Equations (4.2.2)], we have

$$\left(\frac{dB_s^*(s)}{ds}\right)_{s=0} = -\frac{1}{\lambda}(1-\rho)(-1)\Psi\left[(\mathbf{I} - z\mathbf{U})^{-2}(-\mathbf{U})\right]_{z=1}$$

$$= -\frac{1}{\lambda}(1-\rho)\Psi\left[(\mathbf{I} - \mathbf{U})^{-2}\mathbf{U}\right] = -(1-\rho)\Psi\left[\mathbf{K}\frac{\mathbf{KU}}{\lambda}\right].$$

Clearly, the n-th differentiation with respect to s introduces two minus signs that cancel, an additional factor of n/λ, and another power of $-\mathbf{UK}$ inside the Ψ brackets. Thus in general we get

$$\left(\frac{d^{(n)} B_s^*(s)}{ds^n}\right)_{s=0} = (-1)^n(1-\rho)n!\,\Psi\left[\mathbf{K}\left(\frac{\mathbf{KU}}{\lambda}\right)^n\right]$$

$$= (-1)^n n!\,[(1-\rho)\mathbf{pK}]\left(\frac{\mathbf{KU}}{\lambda}\right)^n \boldsymbol{\epsilon}'.$$

Now define

$$\mathbf{p_s} := (1-\rho)\mathbf{pK} \tag{4.2.11a}$$

[which from (4.2.3b) can also be written as $\mathbf{p_s} := \lambda\mathbf{pVA}$] and

$$\mathbf{V_s} := \frac{1}{\lambda}\mathbf{KU}. \tag{4.2.11b}$$

Then the equations preceding (4.2.11a) lead to the familiar-looking expression

$$\mathbb{E}[T_s^n] = n!\Psi_s\left[\mathbf{V_s^n}\right] := n!\,\mathbf{p_s}\,\mathbf{V_s^n}\,\boldsymbol{\epsilon}'. \tag{4.2.12a}$$

The resemblance of this equation to (3.1.9) is not superficial. Recall that $\mathbf{p_s}\,\boldsymbol{\epsilon}' = 1$ from (4.2.3b), allowing us to say that $\langle\mathbf{p_s}\,,\,\mathbf{V_s}\rangle$ is a matrix representation of, or generates, the system time distribution. By virtue of Theorem 3.1.1 we have the following.

Theorem 4.2.6: Let $\mathbf{p_s}$ and $\mathbf{V_s}$ and $\Psi_s[\cdot]$ be defined by (4.2.11a), (4.2.11b), and (4.2.12a), respectively; then (where $\mathbf{B_s} = \mathbf{V_s}^{-1}$)

$$\mathbb{E}[T_s^n] = n!\Psi_s[\mathbf{V_s}^n],$$

$$b_s(x) = \Psi_s[\mathbf{B_s}\exp(-x\mathbf{B_s})], \tag{4.2.12b}$$

$$B_s^*(s) = \Psi_s\left[(\mathbf{I} + s\mathbf{V_s})^{-1}\right]. \tag{4.2.12c}$$

Thus the vector-matrix pair $\langle \mathbf{p_s}, \mathbf{B_s} \rangle$ generates a faithful representation of the distribution of system times in a steady-state M/ME/1 open queue. ■

It should be clear from these discussions that the mean system time $\mathbb{E}[X_s]$ is the same as $\mathbb{E}[T_s]$ of (4.2.6e).

We now find explicitly simple forms for $\mathbf{B_s}$ and $\mathbf{V_s}$. From (4.2.11b),

$$\mathbf{B_s} = \mathbf{V_s}^{-1} = \lambda\mathbf{A}(\mathbf{I} - \mathbf{U}) = \lambda(\mathbf{A} - \mathbf{I}) = \mathbf{B} - \lambda\mathbf{Q}. \tag{4.2.13a}$$

Also, from (4.2.2c), and noting once again that $\mathbf{KU} = \mathbf{K} - \mathbf{I}$,

$$\mathbf{V_s} = \frac{1}{\lambda}(\mathbf{K} - \mathbf{I}) = \mathbf{V} + \frac{\lambda}{1-\rho}\mathbf{VQV}. \tag{4.2.13b}$$

One can also solve for $\mathbf{K}$ in terms of $\mathbf{V_s}$ to get

$$\mathbf{K} = (\mathbf{I} + \lambda\mathbf{V_s}). \tag{4.2.13c}$$

This, together with (4.2.11a) and (4.2.12c), shows again that $B_s^*(\lambda) = 1 - \rho$.

Note that (4.2.3c) yields an expression for $\mathbf{p_s}$ that has a clear physical meaning. Using (3.5.12a), and $\rho = \lambda\Psi[\mathbf{V}]$, we get

$$\mathbf{p_s} = (1-\rho)\mathbf{p} + \lambda\mathbf{pV} = (1-\rho)\mathbf{p} + \rho\boldsymbol{\pi}_\mathbf{r}. \tag{4.2.13d}$$

$(1-\rho)$ is the probability that S_1 will be empty when a customer arrives, ρ is the probability that it will not be empty, and $[(\boldsymbol{\pi}_\mathbf{r})_i]$ from (3.5.10b) is the probability that phase i will be busy upon the customer's arrival, given that at least one customer is already there. Therefore $(\mathbf{p_s})_i$ is the probability that phase i will be busy immediately after an arrival, irrespective of S_1's condition before the arrival. It would be nice to find such a simple interpretation of $\mathbf{B_s}$.

Example 4.2.2: We have used $\langle \mathbf{p_s}, \mathbf{B_s} \rangle$ from Equations (4.2.11) to generate $b_s(x)$ for the open M/E_2/1 queue ($N = \infty$) by directly evaluating (4.2.12b) for many values of x, using the algorithm described in Section 3.1.4. We set $\bar{x} = 1$, and selected various values for ρ. The results are shown in Figure 4.2.3. When ρ is very small, then $b_s(x)$ is very peaked, just as is $E_2(x)$. In fact, the curve labeled $\rho = 0.1$ is extremely close to the Erlangian-2 distribution,

$$E_2(x) = 4xe^{-2x},$$

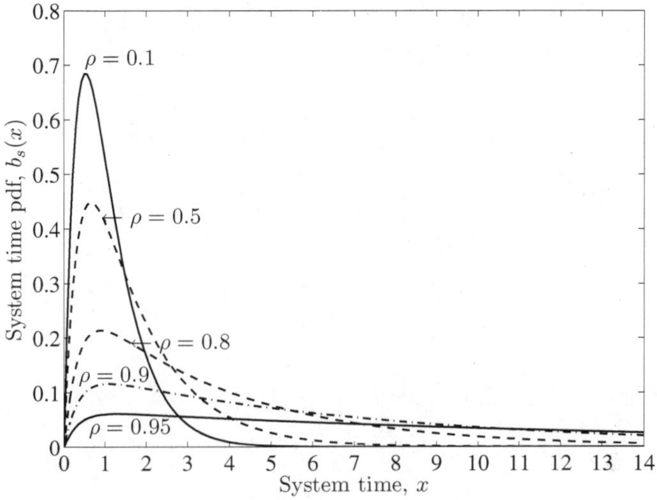

Figure 4.2.3: System time density function $b_s(x)$ for the M/E_2/1 queue, with $\rho = 0.1, 0.5, 0.8, 0.9$, and 0.95. For small ρ, $b_s(x)$ tends to look like the service-time density function, $4x\exp(-2x)$, whereas for ρ close to 1, it looks very much like the interarrival time density function $\lambda\exp(-\lambda x)$, except near $x = 0$.

which peaks at $x = 0.5$. When ρ is close to 1, $b_s(x)$ looks more like the interarrival distribution $\lambda\exp(-\lambda x)$. The curve labeled $\rho = 0.95$ does not seem to support this. Bear in mind, however, that in general, $b_s(0) = (1-\rho)b(0)$, which in this case is 0, while the exponential has a value of λ at the origin. Note that the curve rises rapidly from 0 and then gently decays close to the exponential curve. Another interesting feature of this figure is that all the curves peak at approximately the same place ($x = 0.5$). It seems that for small x, $b_s(x)$ retains the shape of $b(x)$ for all ρ. ▲

It should be interesting to study $b_s(x)$ further, using other pdfs. The reader must not be too quick to generalize from what is learned from the exponential and Erlangian-2 distributions.

Exercise 4.2.3: Using the definitions given by Equations (4.2.11) and $s = \lambda(1-z)$, manipulate (4.2.10b) directly to get (4.2.12c). Also, show that $b_s(0) = (1-\rho)b(0)$. Furthermore, prove by direct algebraic manipulation that $\mathbb{E}[X_s] = \mathbb{E}[T_s]$; that is, show that (4.2.12a) for $n = 1$ and (4.2.6e) yield the same result. [Hint: Use (4.2.13b) and (4.2.13d) in (4.2.12a).]

4.2.4 Buffer Overflow and Customer Loss

In Section 2.1.4 we discussed the overflow probabilities for the M/M/1 queue, and the customer loss probabilities for the M/M/1/N queue. Before we generalize to the M/G/1 and M/G/1/N queues, the reader should review that section. We note that in telecommunications applications, a customer is called a ***packet*** or ***cell***.

In this section we set up the formulas for determining the ***overflow probability*** $P_o(N)$ and the ***customer loss*** probability $P_f(N)$. As in Section 2.1.4, $P_o(N)$ is the probability that an M/G/1 queue will be at least as long as N when a customer arrives, causing him to be placed in a ***backup buffer***. $P_f(N)$ is the probability that an M/G/1/N queue will be full when a customer arrives, thereby causing that customer to be lost, or what is mathematically equivalent, have to return to the queue at S_2. First we find $P_o(N)$.

Buffer Overflow Probabilities

From Theorems 4.2.3 and 4.2.4, we know that $a(n) = r(n) = (1-\rho)\Psi[\mathbf{U}^n]$. Then, following Equations (2.1.8), we have

$$P_o(N) = \sum_{n=N}^{\infty} a(n) = (1-\rho)\sum_{n=N}^{\infty} \Psi[\mathbf{U}^n] = (1-\rho)\Psi\left[\sum_{n=N}^{\infty} \mathbf{U}^n\right]$$

$$= (1-\rho)\Psi\left[\mathbf{U}^N \sum_{n=0}^{\infty} \mathbf{U}^n\right] = (1-\rho)\Psi\left[\mathbf{U}^N(\mathbf{I}-\mathbf{U})^{-1}\right] = (1-\rho)\Psi\left[\mathbf{U}^N\,\mathbf{K}\right].$$

Although it is not clear which expression is more useful, we can use (4.2.3d) to get

$$P_o(N) = (1-\rho)\Psi\left[\mathbf{U}^N\,\mathbf{K}\right] = (1-\rho)\Psi\left[\mathbf{U}^N\right] + \lambda\Psi\left[\mathbf{U}^N\mathbf{V}\right]. \qquad (4.2.14a)$$

This compares with (2.1.8d).

Given that $\mathbf{U}$ is a matrix, it is not easy to see just how $P_o(N)$ varies with N. However, from the spectral decomposition theorem [see (1.3.8b)], we know that for N large enough

$$\mathbf{U}^N \longrightarrow s^N\,\mathbf{v}_\mathbf{s}'\,\mathbf{u}_\mathbf{s}, \qquad (4.2.14b)$$

where s is the largest eigenvalue of $\mathbf{U}$, with eigenvectors $\mathbf{v}_\mathbf{s}'$ and $\mathbf{u}_\mathbf{s}$. If the service time distribution is well behaved in the sense of Definition 3.3.1, then this equation will be accurate enough for reasonable size N. To get an idea of what size that might be, let s_1 be the second largest eigenvalue. Then we would expect that $|s_1/s|^N \ll 1$. When we insert (4.2.14b) into the expression for $P_o(N)$ we get

$$P_o(N) = (1-\rho)\Psi\left[\mathbf{U}^N\,\mathbf{K}\right] \longrightarrow (1-\rho)[(\mathbf{p}\,\mathbf{v}_\mathbf{s}')(\mathbf{u}_\mathbf{s}\,\mathbf{K}\,\boldsymbol{\epsilon}')]s^N, \qquad (4.2.14c)$$

where the expression in square brackets is independent of N.

Computational Note: At times it is necessary to evaluate expressions of the form $\mathbf{U}^N$. If N is very large this can be computationally expensive, particularly if $m = \text{Dim}(\mathbf{U})$ is also large. This has a complexity of order $O(N\,m^3)$. If all powers of $\mathbf{U}$ up through N are needed, then one must either perform the $O(N\,m^3)$ operations by recursively evaluating the expression $\mathbf{U}^{n+1} = \mathbf{U}\,\mathbf{U}^n$ for $1 \le n < N$, or do a spectral decomposition of $\mathbf{U}$. The latter procedure is very convenient if it can be done to satisfactory accuracy (not trivial), but it too can be computationally expensive, particularly if m is large. If instead, what is needed are expressions of the form $\mathbf{U}^n\,\boldsymbol{\epsilon}'$, then the recursive expression, $\mathbf{U}^{n+1}\boldsymbol{\epsilon}' = \mathbf{U}\,(\mathbf{U}^n\boldsymbol{\epsilon}')$, is only of order $O(N\,m^2)$.
In many cases (as in this section) $\mathbf{U}^N$ is needed for only one, or a few, very large values of N. In that case, the calculation can be performed in $O(\lg_2(N)\,m^3)$ steps using the following procedure. Compute the sequence $\mathbf{U}$, $\mathbf{U}^2$, $\mathbf{U}^4$, $\mathbf{U}^8$, ... , $\mathbf{U}^n$, where $n = 2^j$ is the largest integer such that $n \le N$ (each matrix is the square of the previous one). This takes only $j = \lceil \lg(N) \rceil - 1$ multiplications. One then takes the product of a subset of these matrices to yield $\mathbf{U}^N$. The matrices in the subset are those corresponding to 1's in the base-2 representation of N. An example should make this clear. Let $N = 1000 = (1111101000)_2$. Then

$$\mathbf{U}^{1000} = \mathbf{U}^{512}\,\mathbf{U}^{256}\,\mathbf{U}^{128}\,\mathbf{U}^{64}\,\mathbf{U}^{32}\,\mathbf{U}^{8},$$

a total of $9 + 5 = 14$ multiplications. One can sometimes find better combinations if one tries hard enough, but this should be satisfactory for our purposes.

As with the M/M/1 queue, $P_o(N)$ approaches a geometric function and the discussion at the end of Section 2.1.4 also applies here. That is, one can "throw buffer storage" at the overflow problem. The analysis is not quite so simple here because $s \ne \rho$, although it is always less than 1 if ρ is. But if the service time distribution has very high variance, s may be much closer to 1 than ρ is. We look at this in the following exercise.

Exercise 4.2.4: The primary buffer of a network router has enough space for 100 packets, and $\rho = 0.9$. Assume that the packets are arriving in a Poisson stream. What fraction of the arriving packets will find the buffer full and have to be placed in a backup buffer? Do the calculations for the following service-time distributions.

- Exponential;
- Erlangian-2;
- $H_2(x)$ of (3.2.8e), with $C_v^2 = 10$ and $p = 0.1$;
- $HE_2(x)$ of (3.2.16f), with the same first 3 moments as $H_2(x)$;
- $b_+(x)$ of Example 3.2.4.

How much primary buffer would have to be added to each to reduce the probability of overflow by a factor of 10? How much buffer would have to be added to each to get the same P_o as for the E_2 distribution? And last, in each case, how much would the router have to be sped up to give the same overflow probability as for E_2?

What we have said so far applies to well-behaved functions. What happens if the service time distribution is subexponential (see Definition 3.3.1), and in particular, power-tailed? Such distributions, if they can be represented exactly, must have infinite dimensional representations. Therefore $\mathbf{U}$ must have an infinite number of eigenvalues, all less than 1 in value. In this case, the value 1 is an ***accumulation point*** in the sense that there must be an infinite number of points arbitrarily close to it. As a trivial example, consider the set $S = \{s_n \,|\, s_n = 1 - 1/n\}$. For every $\epsilon > 0$, no matter how small, there are an infinite number of points in S such that $|1 - s_n| < \epsilon$. It is not necessary to understand this more deeply, except to see what it does to Equation (4.2.14b). There is no N large enough for this to be a reasonable approximation. Therefore, PT distributions never show the geometric behavior that allows buffer overflow to be controlled easily.

But what about TPTs? In this case $\mathbf{U}$ is finite-dimensional, and there exists a largest eigenvalue, but it is so close to 1, and to many other eigenvalues that (4.2.14b) may not apply for any N of physically reasonable size. Consequently we must try elsewhere for some idea as to how M/TPT/1 queues behave. We already did this in Section 4.2.2.2, where we saw from some numerical calculations [namely (4.2.7)] that $r(n) \Longrightarrow c(\rho)/n^\alpha$. Because $r(n) = a(n)$, we get

$$P_o(N) = \sum_{n=N}^{\infty} a(n) \Longrightarrow c(\rho) \sum_{n=N}^{\infty} \frac{1}{n^\alpha} = \mathrm{O}\left(\frac{1}{N^{\alpha-1}}\right)$$

which certainly is *not* geometric. Recall from Section 2.1.4 that if one doubles the size of the primary buffer of an M/M/1 queue, one in effect squares the probability of overflow. So, if $P_o(N)$ is small, then $P_o(2N)$ will be significantly smaller. But here,

$$\frac{P_o(N)}{P_o(2N)} \Longrightarrow \frac{(2N)^{\alpha-1}}{N^{\alpha-1}} = 2^{\alpha-1}.$$

So, if $\alpha = 1.4$ (a typical value found in telecommunications systems) then we get only a 32% reduction in overflow probability ($2^{.4} = 1.3195$). This is not a very effective way to improve service. Note that even if $\alpha > 2$ (the distribution has a finite variance), $P_o(N)$ is not reduced by nearly as much as for well-behaved distributions.

The above statements carry over to TPTs if the range of the distribution is large enough (see the discussion in Section 3.3.6.1). The reader should test this out in the following exercise.

Exercise 4.2.5: Redo all of Exercise 4.2.4 using the TPT distributions taken from Example 3.3.4. Let $\theta = 0.5$, $\alpha = 1.4$, and thus $\gamma = (1/\theta)^{1/\alpha}$. Perform the calculations for $T = 10$, 20, 30, and 40. You should be able to show that the overflow probabilities do not change appreciably with T when T is large enough, even though C_T^2 grows unboundedly with increasing T. Repeat the calculations for $\alpha = 2.4$. Here C_∞^2 is finite, but the buffer problem remains. In all cases calculate the range of the distributions $[x_r(T) = \gamma^T/\mu(T)]$.

Customer Loss Probabilities

Calculating the loss probabilities $P_f(N)$ requires finding the steady-state arrival probabilities for the M/G/1/N queue. Definition 2.1.4 for $r_f(n;\, N)$ and $a_f(n;\, N)$ is directly applicable here, and we can even extend them to the vector probabilities, $\boldsymbol{\pi}_{\mathbf{f}}(n;\, N)$ and $\mathbf{a}_{\mathbf{f}}(n;\, N)$.

Definition 4.2.2

$[\boldsymbol{\pi}_{\mathbf{f}}(n;\, N)]_i$:= *probability that a random observer of an* M/G/1/N *queue will see* n *customers at* S_1*, with the active customer being at phase* i. Clearly, $r_f(n;\, N) = \boldsymbol{\pi}_{\mathbf{f}}(n;\, N)\boldsymbol{\epsilon}'$.

$[\mathbf{a}_{\mathbf{f}}(n;\, N)]_i$:= *probability that a customer, arriving at an* M/G/1/N *queue will find* n *customers already at* S_1*, with the active customer being at phase* i. Clearly, $a_f(n;\, N) = \mathbf{a}_{\mathbf{f}}(n;\, N)\boldsymbol{\epsilon}'$.

If the arriving customer sees N customers already at S_1 (i.e., the buffer is full), then he is lost (or he returns to S_2). Therefore,

$$P_f(N) = a_f(N;\, N).$$

Recall that the subscript, 'f' stands for ***finite buffer***. □

Fortunately for us, for Poisson arrivals, an arriving customer sees the same thing as a random observer. In fact, by the same argument given at the beginning of Section 2.1.4, the M/G/1/N and M/G/1//N queues satisfy

$$\mathbf{a}_{\mathbf{f}}(n;\, N) = \boldsymbol{\pi}_{\mathbf{f}}(n;\, N) = \boldsymbol{\pi}(n;\, N). \tag{4.2.15}$$

Only $\mathbf{a}(n; N)$ is different by a normalization factor because $\mathbf{a}(N; N) = \mathbf{o}$ (an arriving customer cannot see N customers at the queue because he is one of them).

From Theorem 4.1.2, we have

$$P_f(N) = r(N; N) = \lambda r(0; N)\Psi\left[\mathbf{U}^{N-1}\mathbf{V}\right] = r(0; N)\Psi\left[\mathbf{U}^N(\lambda\mathbf{A}\,\mathbf{V})\right].$$

But $\lambda\mathbf{AV}\boldsymbol{\epsilon}' = (1-\rho)\mathbf{K}\boldsymbol{\epsilon}'$, from (4.2.3a), so

$$P_f(N) = (1-\rho)r(0; N)\Psi\left[\mathbf{U}^N\,\mathbf{K}\right]. \tag{4.2.16}$$

Interestingly enough, this only differs from $P_o(N)$ by the factor $r(0; N)$, which for well-behaved distributions is approximately $(1-\rho)$ when N is large. That is,

$$\frac{P_f(N)}{P_o(N)} = r(0; N) \longrightarrow (1-\rho).$$

Everything we said about the behavior of $P_o(N)$ for large N carries over to $P_f(N)$, reduced by the factor $r(0; N)$. Thus $P_f(N) < P_o(N)$ for all N and all $\rho < 1$. For $\rho \geq 1$ $P_o(N)$ is not defined (no steady state), but $P_f(N)$ still is. The following exercises show the differences.

Exercise 4.2.6: Redo all of Exercise 4.2.4, but for $P_f(N)$. Compare the two sets of results.

TPT service time distributions also cause problems for control of customer loss, as can be seen by doing the following.

Exercise 4.2.7: Redo all of Exercise 4.2.5, but for $P_f(N)$. Compare the two sets of results.

Often a system must be designed so that no more than a fraction p_ℓ of packets should be lost. Then the question becomes "How big must the buffer be?" In the section surrounding (2.1.10b) we showed that for any single-server queue ρ could be greater than 1 and still have a stable queue if $p_\ell > 0$, but only up to $\rho < \rho_m = 1/(1-p_\ell)$. In this case, ρ and p_ℓ are assumed given, and one evaluates (4.2.16) for multiple values of N until one finds that largest N for which $P_f(N) \leq p_\ell$. This issue is explored in the following exercise.

Exercise 4.2.8: Consider the question presented in the previous paragraph. Suppose some application can afford a 2% loss ($p_\ell = .02$). Find the buffer size needed to satisfy this constraint for the five service time distributions given in Exercise 4.2.4. Do this for enough values of $0 < \rho < \rho_m$ to draw a smooth curve. Note that all the curves blow up at $\rho = \rho_m$. Produce another graph where the Y-axis is $(\rho_m - \rho) * N$. Here, the curves should be finite at $\rho = \rho_m$.

Exercise 4.2.9: Redo Exercise 4.2.8, but now for the service time distributions given in Exercise 4.2.5. What is the behavior of $(\rho_m - \rho) * N$ as ρ approaches ρ_m? Is it still finite?

4.2.5 Distribution of Interdeparture Times

We have developed enough results to be able to look once again at departures from S_1. As in Section 2.1.6, we place our observer just outside the exit of S_1 and have her measure the time between departures. The problem is more complicated only because S_1 now represents some general server. It is useful, then, to review Section 2.1.5 before going on.

We ask the following question. Given that a customer, call him C_1, has just left S_1, how long will it be before the next one, call him C_2, leaves? We can assume that our observer has been sitting for a long time, so the system is in its steady state. Also, she has no idea how many customers are at S_1, but if the system is closed, she knows what N is.

Definition 4.2.3

$X_d(N)$:= *r.v. denoting the time between departures from* S_1 *of a steady-state* $M/ME/1//N$ *queue.*

$X_d := X_d(\infty)$.

$B_d(x;\, N) := \mathbf{Pr}(X_d(N) \leq x) =$ *PDF for the interdeparture times of a steady-state* $M/ME/1//N$ *loop.* The process begins immediately after customer C_{i-1} leaves S_1, and ends as soon as customer C_i leaves. Customer C_i may not yet have arrived at S_1 when C_{i-1} left. (In that case, C_{i-1} left behind an empty queue.) $b_d(x;\, N)$ is the derivative of $B_d(x;\, N)$, and $R_d(x; N) = 1 - B_d(x; N)$ is the probability that the second customer is still in the subsystem or has not yet arrived at time x. The subscript d reminds us that this is a ***d***eparture process. □

We are assuming that i is large enough so that the interdeparture times are identically distributed. However, we postpone considering the correlation of successive departures until Section 8.3.5. Only two things are possible. Either S_1 is busy and C_i must be served from the beginning, or S_1 is idle and our patient observer must wait for C_i to arrive before being completely served. The probability that the latter will happen is $d(0; N)$ [Equation (4.1.13c)], while the vector probability for the former to happen is $[1 - d(0;\, N)]\mathbf{p}$. Following this description, the pdf for the process can be found by taking the convolution of the pdf's of S_1 and S_2, but instead, we will give a matrix representation of the process that is more useful and more picturesque.

Look at Figure 4.2.4. Consider S_1 and S_2 together as one subsystem. S_2 is only an exponential server with service rate λ, therefore we can assume that service begins there at the moment of the previous departure with probability $d(0; N)$. The dimension of this composite subsystem is $m + 1$, corresponding

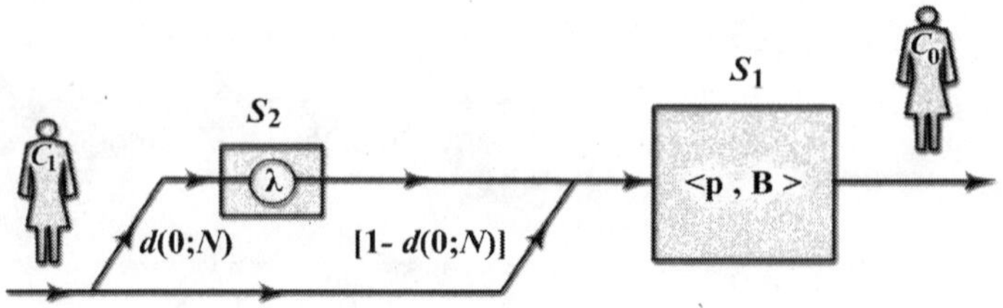

Figure 4.2.4: Pictorial representation of the departure process from S_1 in an M/G/1//N loop. Dependence on the number of customers is implicitly given through the steady-state probabilities at departure times. Given that customer C_{i-1} has just left, C_i must first enter [**p**], and travel through S_1 before leaving [**B**], or if S_1 is empty, C_i must finish being served by S_2 and then go to S_1 to be served. The probability that no one is at S_1 at the moment of a departure $d(0;N)$ is given by (4.1.13c).

to the possibility that C_i can either be at one of m phases in S_1 or at the one phase in S_2. This is a ***sum space representation*** [the two subspaces, of dimension 1 and m, are concatenated to produce one $(m+1)$-dimensional space]. In Chapter 7, we are forced to use a ***product space representation*** to describe the status of customers at two general subsystems. In this representation, the first component refers to the one phase in S_2 and the next m components (which we replace by an m-vector) refer to the m phases in S_1. The initial vector for the composite subsystem is given by

$$\mathbf{p_d}(N) := [d(0;N), \{1 - d(0;N)\}\mathbf{p}]. \tag{4.2.17a}$$

If the queue at S_1 is not empty the moment after the departure, then C_i enters according to $\mathbf{p}$.

The transition matrix $\mathbf{P_d}$ is easy enough to write down once we recognize that a customer goes from 0 to i with probability p_i, and goes from $i > 0$ to j with probability P_{ij}, where $\mathbf{p}$ and $\mathbf{P}$ are the same objects we used previously to represent S_1. Therefore,

$$\mathbf{P_d} = \begin{bmatrix} 0 & \mathbf{p} \\ \mathbf{o}' & \mathbf{P} \end{bmatrix} \quad \text{and} \quad \mathbf{M_d} = \begin{bmatrix} \lambda & \mathbf{o} \\ \mathbf{o}' & \mathbf{M} \end{bmatrix}.$$

These formulas are to be interpreted in the following way. 0 is a 1×1 matrix filling the element $(1,1)$. $\mathbf{p}$ is a $1 \times m$ matrix filling elements $(1,2)$ to $(1, m+1)$. $\mathbf{o}'$ is an $m \times 1$ matrix of 0's, filling elements $(2,1)$ to $(m+1,1)$. Finally, $\mathbf{P}$ is an $m \times m$ matrix filling the rest of $\mathbf{P_d}$. We follow the discussion and procedure described in Sections 3.1.2 and 3.1.3 to get the process-rate and process-time matrices $\mathbf{B_d}$ and $\mathbf{V_d}$. Let $\mathbf{I_d}$ be the identity matrix of dimension $m+1$; then

$$\mathbf{B_d} = \mathbf{M_d}(\mathbf{I_d} - \mathbf{P_d}) = \begin{bmatrix} \lambda & -\lambda\mathbf{p} \\ \mathbf{o}' & \mathbf{B} \end{bmatrix}. \tag{4.2.17b}$$

One can easily prove by direct matrix multiplication that its inverse is

$$\mathbf{V_d} = \mathbf{B_d}^{-1} = \begin{bmatrix} 1/\lambda & \mathbf{pV} \\ \mathbf{o}' & \mathbf{V} \end{bmatrix}. \tag{4.2.17c}$$

Now that we have a matrix representation of the departure time distribution, generated by $\langle \mathbf{p_d}, \mathbf{B_d} \rangle$ (or $\langle \mathbf{p_d}, \mathbf{V_d} \rangle$), we can find its moments, and even the pdf itself. First, let us find the mean interdeparture time when there are N customers in the loop. From Theorem 3.1.1, Equation (3.1.9),

$$\mathbb{E}[X_d(N)] := \int_0^\infty x\, b_d(x; N)\, dx = \mathbf{p_d}(N)\, [\mathbf{V_d}]\boldsymbol{\epsilon}'_{\boldsymbol{d}}$$

$$= [d(0; N),\ \{1 - d(0; N)\}\mathbf{p}] \begin{bmatrix} 1/\lambda & \mathbf{pV} \\ \mathbf{o}' & \mathbf{V} \end{bmatrix} \boldsymbol{\epsilon}'_{\boldsymbol{d}}$$

$$= \left[\frac{d(0; N)}{\lambda},\ d(0; N)\mathbf{pV} + \{1 - d(0; N)\}\mathbf{pV}\right] \boldsymbol{\epsilon}'_{\boldsymbol{d}} = \left[\frac{d(0; N)}{\lambda},\ \mathbf{pV}\right] \boldsymbol{\epsilon}'_{\boldsymbol{d}}.$$

Given that $\rho = \lambda\bar{x}$, the mean time reduces to the following simple expression (compare with (2.1.19b).

$$\mathbb{E}[X_d(N)] = \frac{1}{\lambda}[d(0; N) + \rho]. \tag{4.2.18a}$$

$d(0; N)$ can be calculated from (4.1.13c), at the same time that the other properties of the steady-state M/G/1//N queue are computed, which as usual, we leave as an exercise. An interesting aspect of this representation is that the departure time's dependence on N appears only in $\mathbf{p_d}(N)$.

Before finding the equation for the pdf, we find the mean interdeparture time for the open system. We already know from (4.2.5b) and Theorem 4.2.4 that $\lim_{N\to\infty} d(0; N) = 1 - \rho$ as long as $\rho < 1$, so

$$\mathbb{E}[X_d] := \lim_{N\to\infty} \mathbb{E}[X_d(N)] = \frac{1}{\lambda}(1 - \rho + \rho) = \frac{1}{\lambda} \quad \text{for } \rho < 1. \tag{4.2.18b}$$

Actually, (4.2.18a) is valid for all ρ. If ρ is greater than 1, then $d(0; N)$ goes to 0 as N grows larger, so in this case,

$$\mathbb{E}[X_d] := \lim_{N\to\infty} \mathbb{E}[X_d(N)] = \frac{1}{\lambda}(0 + \rho) = \bar{x} \quad \text{for } \rho > 1. \tag{4.2.18c}$$

Surprised? Of course not. After all, $\mathbb{E}[X_d]$ is the reciprocal of the mean departure rate, and as long as ρ is less than 1, what goes in must come out, so the arrival rate equals the departure rate (in the steady state, of course). We already saw this for the M/M/1 queue in (2.1.20a). If $\rho > 1$ then the departure rate is limited by the service rate of S_1. Note that the departure and arrival rates are equal to each other for all N, but they only equal λ for the open queue. In any closed network, even the busiest server will be idle some of the time, so the throughput will be less than maximum in proportion to the time it is not busy.

We can find the second moment in a similar fashion. First observe that

$$\mathbf{V_d}\,\boldsymbol{\epsilon}'_{\boldsymbol{d}} = \begin{bmatrix} \frac{1}{\lambda} + \bar{x} \\ \\ \mathbf{V}\boldsymbol{\epsilon}' \end{bmatrix} = \frac{1}{\lambda}\begin{bmatrix} 1+\rho \\ \\ \lambda\mathbf{V}\boldsymbol{\epsilon}' \end{bmatrix}.$$

Then, making use of the fact that $\mathbf{p_d}(N)\mathbf{V_d}^2\boldsymbol{\epsilon}'_{\boldsymbol{d}} = [\mathbf{p_d}(N)\mathbf{V_d}][\mathbf{V_d}\boldsymbol{\epsilon}'_{\boldsymbol{d}}]$, and using the expression preceding (4.2.18a), we get

$$\mathbf{p_d}(N)\mathbf{V_d}^2\boldsymbol{\epsilon}'_{\boldsymbol{d}} = \frac{1}{\lambda^2}[d(0;\,N),\,\lambda\mathbf{pV}]\begin{bmatrix} 1+\rho \\ \lambda\mathbf{V}\boldsymbol{\epsilon}' \end{bmatrix}$$

$$= \frac{1}{\lambda^2}\left(d(0;N)(1+\rho) + \lambda^2\Psi\left[\mathbf{V}^2\right]\right).$$

Next recall that $\mathbb{E}[X^2] = 2\Psi\left[\mathbf{V}^2\right]$. The equivalent formula must be true for the departure process, so

$$\mathbb{E}[X_d(N)^2] = \frac{1}{\lambda^2}\left(2d(0;N)(1+\rho) + \lambda^2\mathbb{E}[X^2]\right).$$

The variance is easy to get now.

$$\sigma_d^2(N) = \mathbb{E}[X_d(N)^2] - (\mathbb{E}[X_d(N)])^2$$

$$= \frac{1}{\lambda^2}\left(2d(0;N)(1+\rho) + \lambda^2[\mathbb{E}[X^2] - \bar{x}^2 + \bar{x}^2] - [d(0;N)+\rho]^2\right).$$

Further trivial manipulation yields the next expression, where $\boldsymbol{\sigma^2}$ is the variance for S_1.

$$\sigma_d^2(N) = \frac{1}{\lambda^2}\left(1 - [1 - d(0;N)]^2 + \lambda^2\sigma^2\right). \tag{4.2.19a}$$

The open system limit is straightforward, because $d(0;N)$ approaches $1-\rho$ as N goes to infinity. So

$$\sigma_d^2 := \lim_{N\to\infty}\sigma_d^2(N) = \frac{1}{\lambda^2}\left(1 - \rho^2 + \lambda^2\sigma^2\right). \tag{4.2.19b}$$

Recall that the squared coefficient of variation for any process is defined to be the ratio of variance and mean squared. Thus, given $\mathbb{E}[X_d] = 1/\lambda$ from (4.2.18b),

$$C_d^2 := 1 - \rho^2 + \rho^2 C_v^2 = 1 + \rho^2(C_v^2 - 1). \tag{4.2.19c}$$

In this form we can see that for all $\rho < 1$, C_d^2 is less (greater) than 1 whenever C_v^2 is less (greater) than 1. This expression can be manipulated into the following form,

$$C_d^2 = C_v^2 - (1-\rho^2)(C_v^2 - 1), \tag{4.2.19d}$$

which implies that if C_v^2 is greater (less) than 1, C_d^2 is less (greater) than C_v^2. Both sets of inequalities can be summarized by the single statement: "For all $\rho < 1$, C_d^2 lies between C_v^2 and 1." The squared coefficient of variation for the departure process is some sort of average of the squared coefficients of variation for the interarrival distribution ($C_v^2 = 1$ for exponential distributions) and the service time distribution C_v^2.

We are almost ready to find the density function itself. Recall from Theorem 3.1.1 that because $\langle \mathbf{p_d}(N), \mathbf{B_d} \rangle$ generates $b_d(x; N)$, they are related by (3.1.7d), or

$$b_d(x; N) = \mathbf{p_d}(N)[\mathbf{B_d} \exp(-x\mathbf{B_d})]\boldsymbol{\epsilon}'_{\mathbf{d}}. \tag{4.2.20}$$

We can make use of this formula by either finding a similarity transformation matrix that diagonalizes $\mathbf{B_d}$, or by replacing exp(·) with its Taylor expansion and substituting a general expression for ${\mathbf{B_d}}^n$ (assuming that we can find one). We do the latter here. First, from (4.2.17b) let us look at the square of $\mathbf{B_d}$:

$${\mathbf{B_d}}^2 = \begin{bmatrix} \lambda^2 & -\lambda^2 \mathbf{p} \left(\mathbf{I} + \frac{1}{\lambda}\mathbf{B}\right) \\ \mathbf{o}' & \mathbf{B}^2 \end{bmatrix}.$$

If the reader cannot guess at a general expression for the n-th power of $\mathbf{B_d}$, then calculating and examining ${\mathbf{B_d}}^3$ should give sufficient hint. We leave that step out and write the expression directly. Before we do that, we are beginning to see that the matrix expressions can become rather large and cumbersome, so for convenience, we define the matrix $\mathbf{X}$ for this section only.

$$\mathbf{X} := \left(\mathbf{I} - \frac{1}{\lambda}\mathbf{B}\right)^{-1}.$$

Then the n-th power of $\mathbf{B_d}$ is

$${\mathbf{B_d}}^n = \begin{bmatrix} \lambda^n & -\lambda^n \mathbf{p} \sum_{k=o}^{n-1} \left(\frac{1}{\lambda}\mathbf{B}\right)^k \\ \mathbf{o}' & \mathbf{B}^n \end{bmatrix}$$

$$= \begin{bmatrix} \lambda^n & -\lambda^n \mathbf{p}\mathbf{X} \left(\mathbf{I} - \left(\frac{1}{\lambda}\mathbf{B}\right)^n\right) \\ \mathbf{o}' & \mathbf{B}^n \end{bmatrix}. \tag{4.2.21a}$$

The proof is by induction and is left as an exercise.

Exercise 4.2.10: Prove by induction that (4.2.21a) is true for all $n > 0$. That is, multiply either of the two matrix expressions by $\mathbf{B_d}$ and show that the resulting expression is of the same form, with the index n increased by 1.

The process of summing all the terms of the form $(1/n!)(-x\mathbf{B_d})^n$ is not difficult, because it can be done element by element, or block by block. First, define the $(m+1)\times(m+1)$ matrix, $\mathbf{R_d}(x) := \exp(-x\mathbf{B_d})$ [recall the reliability matrix function of Equations (3.1.6)], then

$$[\mathbf{R_d}(x)]_{ij} = [\exp(-x\mathbf{B_d})]_{ij} = \sum_{n=o}^{\infty} \frac{(-x)^n}{n!} [(\mathbf{B_d})^n]_{ij} \,.$$

For instance,

$$[\mathbf{R_d}(x)]_{11} = \sum_{n=o}^{\infty} \frac{(-x)^n}{n!}\lambda^n = e^{-x\lambda}$$

and

$$[\mathbf{R_d}(x)]_{j1} = 0 \quad \text{for } 1 < j \leq m+1.$$

The elements $(1,2)$ to $(1,m+1)$ are best treated as a block; call it $\mathbf{g}$. Then

$$\mathbf{g} = -\sum_{n=o}^{\infty} \frac{(-x\lambda)^n}{n!}\mathbf{pX}\left(\mathbf{I} - \left(\frac{1}{\lambda}\mathbf{B}\right)^n\right)$$

$$= \mathbf{pX}\sum_{n=o}^{\infty}\left(\frac{(-x\mathbf{B})^n}{n!} - \frac{(-x\lambda)^n}{n!}\mathbf{I}\right) = \mathbf{pX}\left(\exp(-x\mathbf{B}) - e^{-x\lambda}\mathbf{I}\right).$$

The block of all elements for which both i and j are greater than 1 is $\exp(-x\mathbf{B})$. We put these all together in the following expression.

$$\mathbf{R_d}(x) = \begin{bmatrix} e^{-x\lambda} & \mathbf{pX}\left(\exp(-x\mathbf{B}) - e^{-x\lambda}\mathbf{I}\right) \\ \mathbf{o}' & \exp(-x\mathbf{B}) \end{bmatrix}. \tag{4.2.21b}$$

We next calculate $\mathbf{B_d}\exp(-x\mathbf{B_d})$ as the last step before evaluating (4.2.20). This is not particularly hard to do, and comes out to be

$$\mathbf{B_d}\mathbf{R_d}(x) = \begin{bmatrix} \lambda e^{-x\lambda} & \mathbf{pX}\left(\mathbf{B}\exp(-x\mathbf{B}) - \lambda e^{-x\lambda}\mathbf{I}\right) \\ \mathbf{o}' & \mathbf{B}\exp(-x\mathbf{B}) \end{bmatrix}.$$

We multiply on the right with $\boldsymbol{\epsilon}'_\mathbf{d}$ to get the following column vector:

$$\mathbf{B_d}\mathbf{R_d}(x)\boldsymbol{\epsilon}'_\mathbf{d} = \begin{bmatrix} \lambda e^{-x\lambda} + \Psi[\mathbf{XB}\exp(-x\mathbf{B})] - \Psi[\mathbf{X}]\,\lambda e^{-x\lambda} \\ \mathbf{B}\exp(-x\mathbf{B})\boldsymbol{\epsilon}' \end{bmatrix}.$$

Notice that up to now, N does not appear at all, so this expression is good for all N, even in the limit. We are now ready to evaluate (4.2.20) using (4.2.17a).

$$b_d(x;N) = \mathbf{p_d}(N)[\mathbf{B_d}\mathbf{R_d}(x)]\boldsymbol{\epsilon}'_\mathbf{d}$$

$$= d(0;\ N)\left(\lambda e^{-x\lambda} + \Psi[\mathbf{XB}\exp(-x\mathbf{B})] - \Psi[\mathbf{X}]\,\lambda e^{-x\lambda}\right)$$

$$+ [1 - d(0;N)]\Psi[\mathbf{B}\exp(-x\mathbf{B})]$$

$$= b(x) + d(0;N)\left(\Psi[\mathbf{I}-\mathbf{X}]\,\lambda e^{-x\lambda} + \Psi[(\mathbf{X}-\mathbf{I})\mathbf{B}\exp(-x\mathbf{B})]\right).$$

But from the definition of $\mathbf{X}$,

$$\mathbf{I} - \mathbf{X} = \mathbf{I} - \left(\mathbf{I} - \frac{1}{\lambda}\mathbf{B}\right)^{-1} = \left(\mathbf{I} - \frac{1}{\lambda}\mathbf{B}\right)^{-1}\left(\mathbf{I} - \frac{1}{\lambda}\mathbf{B} - \mathbf{I}\right)$$

$$= \left(\mathbf{I} - \frac{1}{\lambda}\mathbf{B}\right)^{-1}\left(-\frac{1}{\lambda}\mathbf{B}\right) = -\left(\lambda\mathbf{V}\left(\mathbf{I} - \frac{1}{\lambda}\mathbf{B}\right)\right)^{-1} = (\mathbf{I} - \lambda\mathbf{V})^{-1}.$$

Therefore, recalling that $d(0;N)$ is given by Theorem 4.1.4,

$$b_d(x;N) = b(x) + d(0;N)$$
$$\times \left(\Psi\left[(\mathbf{I}-\lambda\mathbf{V})^{-1}\right]\lambda e^{-x\lambda} - \Psi\left[(\mathbf{I}-\lambda\mathbf{V})^{-1}\mathbf{B}\exp(-x\mathbf{B})\right]\right). \qquad (4.2.22a)$$

In particular, for $x = 0$,

$$b_d(0;N) = [1 - d(0;N)]b(0). \qquad (4.2.22b)$$

This formula is as simple as it can get in terms of its dependence on the customer population, so there is no real gain in writing down the limit as N goes to infinity. We point out, though, that [as with the mean interdeparture time (4.2.18)] when ρ is less than 1, $d(0;\ N)$ is replaced by $1-\rho$, but that does not simplify (4.2.22) any, except when $x = 0$, for then $b_d(0) = \rho b(0)$. If ρ is greater than 1, then $d(0;N)$ goes to 0 for large N, so $b_d(x) = b(x)$, as expected. Also, note that because $b(x)$ and $b_d(x)$ are both density functions, the integral from 0 to infinity of each function is 1. Therefore, the integral of the term multiplying $d(0;N)$ must be 0. In other words, the two terms inside the large parentheses contribute opposing changes to $b(x)$ that exactly cancel out upon integration. This can be shown directly by first recognizing that

$$\int_0^\infty \mathbf{B}\exp(-x\mathbf{B})dx = \mathbf{I}.$$

There is one other limit that is interesting. Under very light loads (i.e., when ρ is very small), $\lambda\mathbf{V}$ is also very small. In this case, $(\mathbf{I}-\lambda\mathbf{V})$ drops out, $d(0;N)$ can be replaced by 1, and we end up with the reasonable result that $b_d(x;N) \to \lambda e^{-x\lambda}$. We see, then, that as ρ increases from 0 to 1, the interdeparture distribution gradually changes from the arrival distribution to the service distribution. "Exponential in $\to$ exponential out (EIEO)" is valid only under light loads.

Example 4.2.3: We have used $\langle\, \mathbf{p_d}\,,\ \mathbf{B_d}\,\rangle$ from (4.2.17) to generate $b_d(x)$ for the open M/E_2/1 queue ($N = \infty$) by directly evaluating (3.1.7d) for many values of x, using the algorithm described in Section 3.1.4. Just as with Figure 4.2.3, we set $\bar{x} = 1$ and selected various values for ρ. The results are shown in Figure 4.2.5. This figure looks similar to Figure 4.2.3; however, note that their dependence on ρ is completely inverted relative to each other, although they are extremely close for $\rho = 0.5$. When ρ is very close to 1, $b_d(x)$ is very peaked, just as is $E_2(x)$. In fact the curve labeled $\rho = 0.95$ is virtually indistinguishable from the same Erlangian-2 distribution, given above, which peaks at $x = 0.5$. When ρ is very small, $b_d(x)$ will look more like the interarrival distribution $\lambda\exp(-\lambda x)$. The curve labeled $\rho = 0.1$ does not seem to support this. Bear in mind, analogous to the system-time distribution, that in general, $b_d(0) = \rho b(0)$, which in this case is 0, whereas the exponential has a value of λ at the origin. Note that the curve rises rapidly from 0 and then gently decays close to the exponential curve. Another interesting feature that this figure shares with Figure 4.2.3 is that all the curves peak at approximately the same place ($x = .5$). Again, it seems that for small x, $b_d(x)$ retains the shape of $b(x)$ for all ρ. ▲

It would be interesting to find out if this "peaking" property is typical of interdeparture distributions for all M/G/1 queues.

We have one question to ask before moving on. Why should EIEO be true for an open system *even* if S_1 is exponential, as was proven in Chapter 2, Equation (2.1.20b) (it was *not* true for the closed system)? After all, our representation of the departure process has dimensions equal to the sum of the dimensions of S_1 and S_2, which in the case of the M/M/1 queue should be 2. Of course, we would expect (4.2.22) to duplicate (2.1.20b) for the open

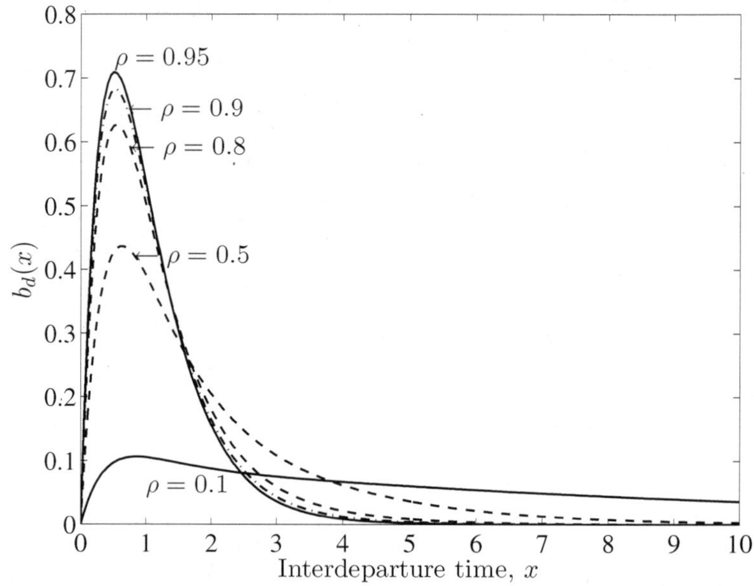

Figure 4.2.5: Interdeparture time density function, $b_d(x)$ for the M/E_2/1 queue, with $\rho = 0.1$, 0.5, 0.8, 0.9, and 0.95. For small ρ, except near $x = 0$, $b_d(x)$ tends to look like the interarrival distribution $\lambda \exp(-\lambda x)$, but for ρ close to 1, it looks very much like the service-time density function, $4x \exp(-2x)$.

system, which it does if S_1 is 1-dimensional. In that case, $\mathbf{B}$ goes to μ, $\lambda\mathbf{V}$ goes to ρ, and $b(x)$ becomes $\mu e^{-x\mu}$. Put this all together with the fact that $d(0; N)$ goes to $1-\rho$ and the negative term in the large brackets of (4.2.22b) exactly cancels $b(x)$, leaving $b_d(x) = \lambda e^{-x\lambda}$. But this argument does not give us much insight. Another view is to look at the matrix representation of $b_d(x)$. Note that the initial vector for the open system $[1-\rho, \rho]$ is a left eigenvector of $\mathbf{B_d}$, with eigenvalue λ. That is,

$$[1-\rho, \rho] \begin{bmatrix} \lambda & -\lambda \\ 0 & \mu \end{bmatrix} = \lambda[1-\rho, \rho].$$

We discussed minimal representations in Section 3.4.1, where we showed by example that the dimension of the invariant subspaces of $\mathbf{p}$ and $\boldsymbol{\epsilon}'$ determine the dimension of the minimal representation. In this case, given that the equation above is true, from Theorem 3.1.1, we have for the M/M/1 queue,

$$b_d(x) = \mathbf{p_d B_d} \exp(-x\mathbf{B_d})\boldsymbol{\epsilon}'_{\boldsymbol{d}} = \lambda \mathbf{p_d I_d} \exp(-x\lambda \mathbf{I_d})\boldsymbol{\epsilon}'_{\boldsymbol{d}} = \lambda e^{-x\lambda} \mathbf{p_d} \boldsymbol{\epsilon}'_{\boldsymbol{d}} = \lambda e^{-x\lambda}.$$

Whenever either $\boldsymbol{\epsilon}'$ or the entrance vector is an eigenvector of the generating matrix, $\mathbf{B}$ or $\mathbf{V}$, the resulting pdf is exponential [Neuts81]. In Section 8.3.5.4 we prove that EIEO is, in fact, only true as the M/M/1 queue reaches its steady state.

4.3 M/G/1 Queue Dependence On n

In Chapter 3 we discussed the idea of residual times, where what can be predicted about the future is contained in what is known about the system now, and is summarized by the residual vector [Equations (3.5.10) to (3.5.13)]. In particular, if nothing is known about the internal state of S_1 (except that it is busy), the mean time until a customer leaves is given by (3.5.12b), with pdf given by (3.5.13). We can extend this to the M/ME/1//N loop and the M/ME/1 queue in the following way.

4.3.1 Residual Time as Seen by a Random Observer

Suppose that a random observer comes to view S_1 without knowing anything about its past history except that n customers are there at present. The probability that she will find n customers there is $r(n;N)$, but we can actually give an expression for the internal state of S_1 at the moment she arrives.

Definition 4.3.1

$\boldsymbol{\pi}_{\mathbf{r}}(n;N)$:= *residual probability vector of the state* S_1 *is in when a random observer first arrives, given that there are n customers in a steady-state M/ME/1//N queue.* $\boldsymbol{\pi}_{\mathbf{r}}(n;N)\,\boldsymbol{\epsilon}' = 1$. $[\boldsymbol{\pi}_{\mathbf{r}}(n;N)]_i$ is the probability that the customer in service in S_1 will be at phase i when the observer comes. There is no internal state if $n=0$, but for convenience we let $\boldsymbol{\pi}_{\mathbf{r}}(0;N) = \mathbf{p}$. □

From (4.1.6a) and (4.1.6b), we have

$$\boldsymbol{\pi}_{\mathbf{r}}(n;N) = \frac{\boldsymbol{\pi}(n;N)}{r(n;N)} = \frac{\mathbf{p}\mathbf{U}^n}{\Psi\left[\mathbf{U}^n\right]} \quad \text{for } 0 \le n < N \tag{4.3.1a}$$

and

$$\boldsymbol{\pi}_{\mathbf{r}}(N;N) = \frac{\mathbf{p}\mathbf{U}^{N-1}\mathbf{V}}{\Psi\left[\mathbf{U}^{N-1}\mathbf{V}\right]}. \tag{4.3.1b}$$

These vectors serve as the initial vectors for the process of the active customer completing service. Thus

$$\langle\, \boldsymbol{\pi}_{\mathbf{r}}(n;N)\,,\ \mathbf{B} \,\rangle$$

is the generator of the distribution function of the r.v. $X_r(n;\, N)$, the time remaining for the one in service, given that the random observer has found n customers at S_1. For instance, the density function for this process is given by the expression

$$b_r(x; n; N) := \boldsymbol{\pi}_{\mathbf{r}}(n; N)\mathbf{B}\exp(-x\mathbf{B})\boldsymbol{\epsilon}' = \frac{\Psi\left[\mathbf{U}^n\mathbf{B}\exp(-x\mathbf{B})\right]}{\Psi\left[\mathbf{U}^n\right]} \tag{4.3.2a}$$

for $0 < n < N$, and

$$b_r(x; N; N) := \frac{\Psi\left[\mathbf{U}^{N-1}\mathbf{V}\mathbf{B}\exp(-x\mathbf{B})\right]}{\Psi\left[\mathbf{U}^{N-1}\mathbf{V}\right]} = \frac{\Psi\left[\mathbf{U}^{N-1}\exp(-x\mathbf{B})\right]}{\Psi\left[\mathbf{U}^{N-1}\mathbf{V}\right]}. \tag{4.3.2b}$$

These formulas are not as hard to compute as they look. First, the vectors $\mathbf{pU}^n$ can be calculated recursively, and in any case are needed to compute the steady-state probabilities. Second, $\exp(-x\mathbf{B})\boldsymbol{\epsilon}'$ can be calculated recursively by the algorithm given in Section 3.1.4.

The mean time remaining for the one in service is

$$\mathbb{E}[X_r(n;\, N)] = \frac{\Psi\left[\mathbf{U}^n\mathbf{V}\right]}{\Psi\left[\mathbf{U}^n\right]} \quad \text{for } \; 0 < n < N \tag{4.3.3a}$$

$$\mathbb{E}[X_r(N;\, N)] = \frac{\Psi\left[\mathbf{U}^{N-1}\mathbf{V}^2\right]}{\Psi\left[\mathbf{U}^{N-1}\mathbf{V}\right]}. \tag{4.3.3b}$$

In particular, $\mathbb{E}[X_r(0;\, N)] = \Psi\left[\mathbf{V}\right] = \bar{x}$.

The mean residual time [from (3.5.12b)] is of interest because it can differ enormously from the mean service time. It is not hard to find examples where the queue-length dependent residual times differ as much from $\mathbb{E}[X_r]$ and each other as $\mathbb{E}[X_r]$ differs from $\bar{x}$.

Example 4.3.1: As can be seen in Figure 4.3.1, for even the simplest nonexponential distribution (the Erlangian-2), $\mathbb{E}[X_r(n; N)]$ can vary greatly. The value at $n = 0$ corresponds to the mean service time, which we have set equal to 1. The average value of the queue-length times, weighted over the $r(n; N)$s, we show below, turns out to be equal to the mean residual time, $\mathbb{E}[X_r]$. Therefore, the weighted average is independent of ρ and N. The big drop in all curves between 19 and 20 is real. Note that all of these numbers would be equal to each other and to $\bar{x}$ if this were an M/M/1 queue. ▲

The procedure we have applied to $b_r(x; n; N)$ and $\mathbb{E}[X_r(n; N)]$ can also be applied to the Laplace transform. Thus,

$$B_r^*(s;\, n;\, N) := \boldsymbol{\pi}_{\mathbf{r}}(n; N)[\mathbf{I} + s\mathbf{V}]^{-1}\boldsymbol{\epsilon}'. \tag{4.3.3c}$$

This function actually has an interesting physical meaning. Recall that $B^*(\lambda)$ is the probability that a customer who has just started service will finish before the next customer comes, [see discussion after Theorem 3.1.1, and (2.1.1b)], $B_r^*(\lambda; n; N)$ must be the probability that the customer in service at S_1 when a random observer starts looking (and sees n customers there), will finish

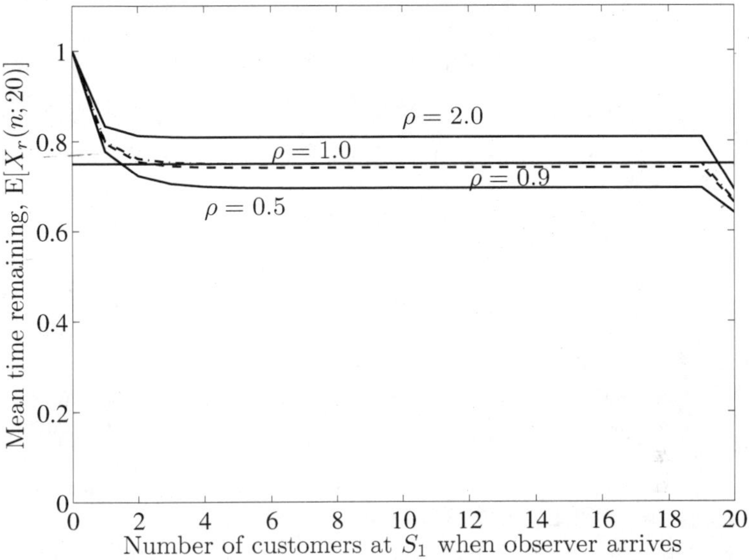

Figure 4.3.1: Mean time remaining for the customer in service, as seen by a random observer, as a function of the number of customers at S_1 when she starts observing. The service distribution is an E_2 function, with a mean service time of $\bar{x} = 1.0$. Thus we have an M/E_2/1/ /20 loop. The curves for four different values of ρ are presented. In all cases, the expected time until completion for a customer who just began service is 1.0. If the random observer takes no notice of the length of the queue, the mean time until completion is $\bar{x}_r = 0.75$. If she does note the length of the queue, the mean time to completion is given by $\mathbb{E}[X_r(n;\, N)]$.

service before the next customer arrives. Let us state this more precisely. Let X_2 be the time until the next customer arrives. Then

$$C_r(n;\, N) := \mathbb{P}\mathbf{r}[X_r(n; N) \leq X_2] = B_r^*(\lambda;\, n;\, N). \tag{4.3.3d}$$

Exercise 4.3.1: Let S_1 be an Erlangian-2 server with mean service time equal to 1. Calculate $b_r(0; n; N)$ $(0 < n \leq N)$, for the four systems with $\rho = 0.5$, 0.9, 1.0, and 2.0. Plot all your answers on the same graph $[b_r(0; n; N)$ versus $n]$. Also draw as a horizontal line

$$b_r(0) = \frac{\mathbf{pVB}\boldsymbol{\epsilon}'}{\Psi\,[\mathbf{V}]} = \frac{1}{\bar{x}},$$

which in this case is equal to 1. Note that $b(0) = 0$.

Exercise 4.3.2: Let S_1 be the H_2 server of Exercise 4.1.2. Do the same as in Example 4.3.1. In this case, the mean residual time is $1090/361 = 3.019391$ (over three times greater than the mean service time of S_1).

4.3.2 Weighted Averages of Matrix Operators

As can be seen from (4.3.1a), (4.3.2a), and (4.3.3a), or should be obvious from the last two exercises, the queue-length-dependent behavior does not depend on the total number of customers in the system, as long as they are not all at S_1. We next show that the "average" residual time, given that S_1 was busy when observation began, is the mean residual time, again independent of N. In fact, the average density function is the same as the mean residual distribution given in (3.5.13). Quite often, a matrix operator can be associated with some random variable. For instance, the service time X, and $\mathbf{V}$. We do this by examining the "average" of any matrix operator. First define for any square matrix $\mathbf{F}$,

$$\bar{F}_r(n;N) := \boldsymbol{\pi}_\mathbf{r}(n;N)\mathbf{F}\boldsymbol{\epsilon}' = \frac{\Psi\left[\mathbf{U}^n\mathbf{F}\right]}{\Psi\left[\mathbf{U}^n\right]} \quad \text{for } 0 \le n < N$$

and

$$\bar{F}_r(N;N) := \boldsymbol{\pi}_\mathbf{r}(N;N)\mathbf{F}\boldsymbol{\epsilon}' = \frac{\Psi\left[\mathbf{U}^{N-1}\mathbf{V}\mathbf{F}\right]}{\Psi\left[\mathbf{U}^{N-1}\mathbf{V}\right]}.$$

Then, for instance, from (4.3.3), $\mathbb{E}[X_r(n;\, N)] = \bar{V}_r(n;N)$. Next recall that $\mathbf{K} = [\mathbf{I} - \mathbf{U}]^{-1}$. Then by inserting (4.2.2b) into (4.1.6f), and observing that $\mathbf{U}^{N-1} = \mathbf{U}^N\,\mathbf{A}$, we have

$$\mathbf{K}(N) = \lambda\mathbf{AV} + \frac{\lambda^2}{1-\rho}\mathbf{AVQV} - \frac{\lambda^2}{1-\rho}\mathbf{U}^N\mathbf{AVQV}. \tag{4.3.4a}$$

Then from Lemma 4.1.1, it easily follows that

$$\mathbf{p}[\mathbf{K}(N) - \mathbf{I}] = \frac{\lambda}{1-\rho}\left(1 - \Psi\left[\mathbf{U}^{N-1}\lambda\mathbf{V}\right]\right)\mathbf{pV}. \tag{4.3.4b}$$

(In case you were not able to answer it, the equation in Exercise 4.1.3 follows directly from this.) Note that the expression in the round parentheses is a scalar, and that $\mathbf{pV}$ is proportional to $\boldsymbol{\pi}_\mathbf{r}$ as defined by (3.5.10b), so (4.3.4b) can be rewritten as

$$\mathbf{p}[K(N) - \mathbf{I}] = \Psi\left[\mathbf{K}(N) - \mathbf{I}\right]\boldsymbol{\pi}_\mathbf{r}. \tag{4.3.4c}$$

We can now state the following theorem.

Theorem 4.3.1: Let $\mathbf{F}$ be any matrix operator for properties of a steady-state M/ME/1//N queue [e.g., $\mathbf{V}$ or $\exp(-x\mathbf{B})$]. The weighted average of $\mathbf{F}$ as seen by a random observer, given that S_1 is busy, is independent of N and is equal to $\boldsymbol{\pi}_{\mathbf{r}}\mathbf{F}\boldsymbol{\epsilon}'$, where $\boldsymbol{\pi}_{\mathbf{r}}$ is given by (3.5.10b). That is, the "expected value of" $\mathbf{F}$ (call it $\bar{F}_r$), is

$$\bar{F}_r := \frac{\sum_{n=1}^{N} \bar{F}_r(n;N)\, r(n;N)}{1 - r(0;N)} = \frac{\mathbf{pVF}\boldsymbol{\epsilon}'}{\mathbf{pV}\boldsymbol{\epsilon}'} = \frac{\Psi\,[\mathbf{VF}]}{\Psi\,[\mathbf{V}]} = \boldsymbol{\pi}_{\mathbf{r}}\mathbf{F}\boldsymbol{\epsilon}'. \quad (4.3.5a)$$

The result is independent of N, thus it is also true for open systems (i.e., when $N \to \infty$). ■

Proof: First note that $1 - r(0;N) = \Psi\,[\mathbf{K}(N) - \mathbf{I}]\,/\,\Psi\,[\mathbf{K}(N)]$, and for $n < N$ that

$$r(n;N)\bar{F}_r(n;N) = \frac{\Psi\,[\mathbf{U}^n\mathbf{F}]}{\Psi\,[\mathbf{K}(N)]},$$

with a similar expression for $n = N$. Then

$$\sum_{n=1}^{N} \bar{F}_r(n;N) r(n;N) = \frac{\Psi\,[(\mathbf{K}(N) - \mathbf{I})\mathbf{F}]}{\Psi\,[\mathbf{K}(N) - \mathbf{I}]}.$$

The theorem follows directly from (4.3.4c). **QED**

We next state as a corollary that the "average" residual time and density are the same as the mean residual time and density discussed in Chapter 3.

Corollary 4.3.1: The mean time (appropriately averaged over the steady-state queue-length probabilities) a randomly arriving observer of an M/G/1 queue (either open or closed) will have to wait for the customer who is presently in service at S_1 to complete service is given by $\bar{V}_r$ and is equal to $\bar{x}_r$, the mean residual time of S_1. That is, if we let $\mathbf{F} = \mathbf{V}$ in (4.3.5a), we get:

$$\bar{x}_r = \frac{\Psi[\mathbf{VV}]}{\Psi[\mathbf{V}]} = \frac{\mathbb{E}(X^2)}{2\bar{x}}.$$

Furthermore, the time remaining is distributed according to (3.5.13). Finally, the mean residual vector [Equation (3.5.10b)] is the same for all N and satisfies

$$\boldsymbol{\pi}_{\mathbf{r}} = \frac{\sum_{n=1}^{N} r(n;N)\boldsymbol{\pi}_{\mathbf{r}}(n;N)}{1 - r(0;N)} = \frac{1}{\Psi[\mathbf{V}]}\mathbf{pV}. \quad (4.3.5b)$$

■

Proof: Let $\mathbf{F} = \mathbf{V}$ in (4.3.5a) to get the mean time, and let $\mathbf{F} = \mathbf{B}\exp(-x\mathbf{B})$ for the distribution; then compare with (3.5.10b) and (3.5.13). **QED**

This applies to the Laplace transform as well. If our observer knows nothing about S_1 except that someone is in service, then the probability, C_r, that service will complete before another customer arrives (see (3.5.3d)) is given by

$$C_r = \boldsymbol{\pi}_{\mathbf{r}}[\mathbf{I} + \lambda\mathbf{V}]^{-1}\boldsymbol{\epsilon}' = \frac{1}{\bar{x}}\Psi\left[\mathbf{V}(\mathbf{I} + \lambda\mathbf{V})^{-1}\right].$$

But $\lambda\mathbf{V}(\mathbf{I} + \lambda\mathbf{V})^{-1} = \mathbf{I} - (\mathbf{I} + \lambda\mathbf{V})^{-1}$, so

$$C_r = \frac{1-\delta}{\rho}, \tag{4.3.5c}$$

where $\delta = B^*(\lambda) = \Psi\left[(\mathbf{I} + \lambda\mathbf{V})^{-1}\right]$. As already discussed, δ is also the probability that S_1 will finish before S_2, given that they started at the same time.

We have seen that even if a random observer does not know when a customer started service, she can get some inkling of the internal state of S_1 by observing the number of customers in its queue. Let us suppose that the random observer decides to become a customer and wishes to pass through S_1 without pre-empting the customer presently in service. Then she must wait a mean time of $\mathbb{E}[X_r(n;N)]$. If, in addition she must wait at the end of the queue, she will have to wait an additional time of $(n-1)\bar{x}$. She also knows that the customer in service will finish before the next customer arrives with probability, $B_r^*(\lambda;n;N)$. If this readily available information (i.e., n, the queue length at time of first observation) is ignored, she is left with the "residual results" of renewal theory, $C_r(0)$ and the P-K formula. We mention that parts of these results, in particular, $\boldsymbol{\pi}_r\mathbf{B}\exp(-\mathbf{B}x)\boldsymbol{\epsilon}' = b_r(x)$ [from Corollary 4.3.1 and (3.5.13)] were derived using renewal theory by S. M. Ross [Ross96]. The results here are more general.

4.3.3 Waiting Time as Seen by an Arriving Customer

In the preceding section we viewed the M/G/1//N queue as an observer who did not affect the behavior of the system. It is perhaps more interesting to view the system from the customer's vantage point. The two viewpoints are different in principle, because a customer both observes those in front and affects those behind. (See, e.g., [MelamedWhitt90] and [Wolff82] for other thoughts on the subject.)

The items we need to examine this question were set up in Section 4.1.3. We already know $a(n;N)$ and $\mathbf{a}(n;N)$ (Theorem 4.1.4), the scalar and vector probabilities that, upon arriving at S_1, a customer will find n other customers already there. Because $\mathbf{a}(n;N)\boldsymbol{\epsilon}' = a(n;N)$, the i-th component of the unit vector, $[\mathbf{a}(n;N)/a(n;N)]$, is the conditional probability that an arriving customer will find S_1 in state i, given that n customers are there already. But this normalized vector is identical to (4.3.1a), so aside from the fact that an arriving customer cannot find N customers ahead of him at S_1, we have proven the following.

Theorem 4.3.2: In an M/G/1 queue (both open or closed) and $n < N$ given, a newly arrived customer and a random observer will find S_1 in the same state. Thus (4.3.1a), (4.3.2a), and (4.3.3a) are valid for the arriving customer as well as for the random observer. ∎

Note that this theorem is not necessarilly true for queues that are not of M/G/1-type.

Be reminded that although a customer has the same probability of finding n customers in S_1 when he arrives as when he leaves, the internal state will be different. The internal state seen by the arriving customer is proportional to $\boldsymbol{\pi}(n; N)$, whereas that for the departing customer is always $\mathbf{p}$ (the next customer in the queue enters S_1).

Now that we know that our random observer sees the same thing as the customers in the system, it pays to elaborate some on the equations of the preceding section. On the one hand, the outsider cannot make any use of the system's facilities without changing the steady-state solution. On the other hand, the customers cannot refuse to make use of the facilities without destroying the steady state. Therefore, even though both may have "inside information" as to expected waiting times, they cannot act upon it without changing the system's subsequent behavior. In any case it is good to know what one is in for.

When a customer arrives at S_1 with n customers already there, he must wait for the one in service to complete, and for $n-1$ additional customers to start and finish. The distribution of time that he must wait is identical to that for the n-th renewal epoch Y_n of a generalized renewal process, as discussed in Section 3.5. All n customers have pdfs generated by the same matrix, $\mathbf{B}$, but the first one has a starting vector given by (4.3.1a) as opposed to $\mathbf{p}$ for the other customers. Thus the mean waiting time for the new customer conditioned on the number already in the queue (call it $\mathbb{E}[X_w(n)]$) is [see (4.3.3a)]

$$\mathbb{E}[X_w(n)] = \mathbb{E}[X_r(n)] + (n-1)\bar{x}, \qquad 0 < n < N. \tag{4.3.6a}$$

The total time he will spend in the system averages to

$$\mathbb{E}[X_s(n)] = \mathbb{E}[X_w(n)] + \bar{x} = \mathbb{E}[X_r(n)] + n\bar{x}. \tag{4.3.6b}$$

Continuing in this way, we see that the variance of his waiting time can be written as

$$\sigma_w^2(n) = \frac{\Psi\left[\mathbf{U}^n(2\mathbf{V}^2 - \mathbf{V}\mathbf{Q}\mathbf{U}^n\mathbf{V})\right]}{\Psi\left[\mathbf{U}^n\right]} + (n-1)\sigma^2 \tag{4.3.6c}$$

where $\sigma^2 = \Psi\left[(2\mathbf{V}^2 - \mathbf{V}\mathbf{Q}\mathbf{V})\right]$ is the variance of the service time distribution. To get the variance of his total system time (again, conditioned on n), simply add one more σ^2 to (4.3.6c). These equations are easy enough to compute, especially if one is calculating the steady-state queue-length probabilities anyway. The higher moments are also accessible, but more difficult.

Exercise 4.3.3: Continuing Exercise 4.2.3, calculate $\mathbb{E}[X_w(n)]$, $\sigma_w^2(n)$, and the squared coefficient of variation, $C_w^2(n) := \sigma_w^2(n)/(\mathbb{E}[X_w(n)])^2$. Plot your answers for $C_w^2(n)$ versus n $(0 < n < N)$. Also plot the equivalent points for the M/M/1//N queue for comparison $[C_w^2(n) = 1/n]$.

Exercise 4.3.4: Do the same as in Exercise 4.3.3, except let S_1 be the hyperexponential server of Exercise 4.1.2.

4.3.4 System Time of an Arriving Customer

We saw in Section 4.2.3 that a departing customer leaves behind the same number of customers as a random observer finds, thus we were able to derive the system time distribution. We should also be able to derive the same expression from the arriving customer's point of view. At present we cannot quite make it, but we do come up with some interesting results.

First we derive the mean system time $\mathbf{E}[X_s]$, which we already know from the P-K formula to be the same as $\mathbf{E}[T_s]$ in (4.2.6e). If a customer arrives with no one at S_1 [which he does with probability $(1-\rho)$], he can expect to spend an average of $\bar{x} = \Psi[\mathbf{V}])$ units of time before leaving. However, if there are n customers there already $[r(n)]$, he must first wait for the one in service to finish ($\mathbf{E}[X_r(n)]$), and then n more customers (including himself) must finish $[n\bar{x}]$. That is,

$$\mathbf{E}[T_s] = (1-\rho)\bar{x} + \sum_{n=1}^{\infty} r(n)\mathbf{E}[X_r(n)] + \bar{x}\sum_{n=1}^{\infty} n\, r(n).$$

But from Corollary 4.3.1, for the open system ($N = \infty$), the middle term must be equal to the probability that S_1 is already busy $[\rho]$, times the mean residual time (i.e., $\rho\mathbf{E}[X_r]$), and the last sum is $\bar{q}$ [Equation (4.2.6b)]. So

$$\mathbf{E}[T_s] = (1-\rho)\bar{x} + \rho\mathbf{E}[X_r] + \bar{x}\bar{q} = (1-\rho)\bar{x} + \rho\mathbf{E}[X_r] + \rho\mathbf{E}[T_s],$$

where we have used the fact that $\bar{q} = \lambda\mathbf{E}[T_s]$ and $\rho = \lambda\,\bar{x}$. Next, solving for $\mathbf{E}[T_s]$, we get

$$\mathbf{E}[T_s] = \bar{x} + \frac{\rho}{1-\rho}\mathbf{E}[X_r].$$

Because $\mathbf{E}[X_r] = \mathbf{E}[X^2]/[2\bar{x}] = \bar{x}(C_v^2+1)/2$, this leads to the same answer as (4.2.6e).

It is not easy to get the distribution of the system time this way because, as we saw in Chapter 3, it is not easy to work with the convolutions of functions. We can, however, get an expression for the Laplace transform (LT) of $b_s(x)$. Recall that the LT of a convolution of two pdfs is equal to the product of their LTs, and that the LT of the sum of two functions is equal to the sum of their LTs. First, let $B_r^*(s;n)$ be the LT of $b_r(x;n)$, then by an argument analogous to the one used in this section to get $\mathbf{E}[T_s]$,

$$B_s^*(s) = (1-\rho)B^*(s) + \sum_{n=1}^{\infty} r(n)\boldsymbol{\pi}_{\mathbf{r}}(n)(\mathbf{I}+s\mathbf{V})^{-1}\boldsymbol{\epsilon}'[B^*(s)]^n.$$

This can be simplified using (4.2.5a) and (4.3.1a) to

$$B_s^*(s) = (1-\rho)B^*(s) + (1-\rho)\Psi\left[\sum_{n=1}^{\infty}[B^*(s)]^n\mathbf{U}^n(\mathbf{I}+s\mathbf{V})^{-1}\right].$$

For any $\mathbf{F}$ for which $(\mathbf{I}-\mathbf{F})^{-1}$ exists,

$$\sum_{n=1}^{\infty}\mathbf{F}^n = \mathbf{F}\sum_{n=o}^{\infty}\mathbf{F}^n = \mathbf{F}(\mathbf{I}-\mathbf{F})^{-1},$$

so this can be summed as

$$\begin{aligned}B_s^*(s) &= (1-\rho)B^*(s) + (1-\rho)\Psi\left[B^*(s)\,\mathbf{U}[\mathbf{I}-B^*(s)\,\mathbf{U}\,]^{-1}(\mathbf{I}+s\mathbf{V})^{-1}\right]\\ &= (1-\rho)B^*(s)\left(1+\Psi\left[\mathbf{U}(\mathbf{I}-B^*(s)\mathbf{U})^{-1}(\mathbf{I}+s\mathbf{V})^{-1}\right]\right).\end{aligned}$$

Now the mean system time for a customer is equal to the convolution of his waiting time, with the time for him to receive service, so the LT of his waiting (or queueing) time is

$$B_w^*(s) = (1-\rho)\left(1+\Psi\left[\mathbf{U}(\mathbf{I}-B^*(s)\mathbf{U})^{-1}[\mathbf{I}+s\mathbf{V}]^{-1}\right]\right).$$

On the other hand, for any $\mathbf{F}$, $\sum_{n=1}^{\infty}\mathbf{F}^n = \sum_{n=o}^{\infty}\mathbf{F}^n - \mathbf{I}$, so

$$B_s^*(s) = (1-\rho)\Psi\left[[\mathbf{I}-B^*(s)\mathbf{U}]^{-1}(\mathbf{I}+s\mathbf{V})^{-1}\right].$$

This equation looks fairly simple, but it is not nearly as easy to use as (4.2.10b) or (4.2.12c), because s appears in the expression in an implicit way through $B^*(s)$. As mentioned earlier, we cannot at present show the two expressions to be equal by purely algebraic means.

Exercise 4.3.5: Use this expression to show that $B_s^*(0) = 1$, and that its derivative evaluated at $s = 0$ does indeed yield $\mathbb{E}[T_s]$.

4.4 Relation To Standard Solution

From this book's point of view, Theorems 4.1.2 and 4.2.2 [Equations (4.1.7) and (4.2.5)] are quite sufficient for studying the steady-state M/ME/1 queue. However, it is always informative to connect to the formulas used by other methods. We do that here, after establishing some matrix relations. Some of these relations are important, some are interesting, and some are just true. But queues have never been analyzed in the way presented here, so it is not clear just which formulas will prove to be useful ultimately. Therefore, we are including as many as we run across as we go.

4.4.1 Exponential Moments, $\alpha_k(s)$, and Their Meaning

Let us look at Equations (4.2.8b) and (4.2.8c). Recalling that $\mathbf{D}(s) = (\mathbf{I} + s\mathbf{V})^{-1}$, and $d(s) = \Psi[\mathbf{D}(s)]$, it follows that

$$\frac{d}{ds}\mathbf{D}(s) = -\mathbf{V}(\mathbf{I} + s\mathbf{V})^{-2} = -\mathbf{V}\mathbf{D}(s)^2$$

and

$$\frac{d}{ds}d(s) = -\Psi\left[\mathbf{V}\mathbf{D}(s)^2\right].$$

In general,

$$\left(\frac{d}{ds}\right)^k d(s) = (-1)^k k!\Psi\left[\mathbf{V}^k\mathbf{D}(s)^{k+1}\right].$$

On the other hand, $d(s) = B^*(s) = \int_0^\infty e^{-sx}b(x)dx$, and

$$\left(\frac{d}{ds}\right)^k d(s) = \left(\frac{d}{ds}\right)^k \int_0^\infty e^{-sx}b(x)dx = (-1)^k \int_0^\infty x^k e^{-sx}b(x)dx.$$

Therefore,

$$k!\Psi\left[\mathbf{V}^k\mathbf{D}(s)^{k+1}\right] = \int_0^\infty x^k e^{-sx}b(x)dx.$$

Define the ***exponential moments*** as given in [KLEINROCK75],

$$\alpha_k(s) := \int_0^\infty \frac{(sx)^k}{k!}e^{-sx}b(x)dx. \tag{4.4.1a}$$

When no confusion is likely to arise, the dependence of $\mathbf{D}$ on the parameter s, is suppressed [i.e., $\mathbf{D}(s)$ and $\mathbf{D}$ are the same thing]. Then

$$\alpha_k(s) = \Psi\left[(s\mathbf{V}\mathbf{D})^k\mathbf{D}\right]. \tag{4.4.1b}$$

These functions have physical meanings. The term, $(sx)^k\exp(-sx)/k!$, in (4.4.1a) is the Poisson probability with arrival rate s that k customers will arrive in time interval x. $[b(x)\,dx]$ can be thoght of as the probability that a service time will take a time within dx of x. Therefore, $\alpha_k(s)$ is the probability that k customers will arrive after a customer begins being served and before he is finished. It follows, then, that $\sum_{k=0}^\infty \alpha_k = 1$. This can be shown directly from (4.4.1a), because

$$\sum_{k=0}^\infty \alpha_k(s) = \int_0^\infty \sum_{k=0}^\infty \left[\frac{(sx)^k}{k!}\right] e^{-sx}b(x)dx = \int_0^\infty e^{sx}e^{-sx}b(x) = 1.$$

We have used the fact that the sum in square brackets is the Taylor expansion for e^{sx}. We can also easily get the mean number of arrivals.

$$\sum_{k=0}^\infty k\,\alpha_k(s) = \int_0^\infty \sum_{k=1}^\infty k\left[\frac{(sx)^k}{k!}\right] e^{-sx}b(x)dx$$

$$= \int_{\text{o}}^{\infty} sx \sum_{k=\text{o}}^{\infty} \left[\frac{(sx)^k}{k!} \right] e^{-sx} b(x)dx = s \int_{\text{o}}^{\infty} x\, b(x)dx = s\bar{x},$$

where we have used $k/k! = 1/(k-1)!$.

Exercise 4.4.1: Show by direct computation, using (4.4.1b) that

$$\sum_{k=\text{o}}^{\infty} \alpha_k(s) = 1 \quad \text{and} \quad \sum_{k=\text{o}}^{\infty} k\alpha_k(s) = s\Psi[\mathbf{V}].$$

This is identical to the results when using the integral definition of α_k, recognizing that $\Psi[\mathbf{V}] = \mathbb{E}[X] = \bar{x}$.

Next define:

$$d_k(s) := \Psi\left[\mathbf{D}(s)^k\right]. \tag{4.4.1c}$$

From (4.2.8c), it follows that $d(s) = d_1(s) = \alpha_{\text{o}}(s)$, and that $d_{\text{o}}(s) = 1$. A little manipulation lets us see that

$$s\mathbf{VD}(s) = \mathbf{I} - \mathbf{D}(s),$$

so (using the binomial expansion) we get a relationship between the α's and the d's,

$$\alpha_k(s) = \Psi\left[(\mathbf{I}-\mathbf{D})^k\mathbf{D}\right] = \Psi\left[\sum_{j=\text{o}}^{k} \binom{k}{j} (-1)^j \mathbf{D}^{j+1}\right]$$

$$= \sum_{j=\text{o}}^{k} \binom{k}{j} (-1)^j d_{j+1}(s). \tag{4.4.2a}$$

4.4.2 Connection to Laguerre Polynomials

The d_k's can be written in terms of the α_k's, leading to perhaps a more interesting result. From $\mathbf{D} = \mathbf{I} - s\mathbf{VD}$, we can write for $d_k(s)$,

$$d_{k+1}(s) = \Psi\left[(\mathbf{I} - s\mathbf{VD})^k\mathbf{D}\right] = \sum_{j=\text{o}}^{k} \binom{k}{j} \Psi\left[(-s\mathbf{VD})^j\mathbf{D}\right]$$

$$= \sum_{j=\text{o}}^{k} \binom{k}{j} (-1)^j \alpha_j(s). \tag{4.4.2b}$$

Next substitute the original definition for α_j from (4.4.1a) to get

$$d_{k+1}(s) = \int_{\text{o}}^{\infty} \left[\sum_{j=\text{o}}^{k} \binom{k}{j} \frac{(-sx)^j}{j!} \right] e^{-sx} b(x)dx. \tag{4.4.2c}$$

It is somewhat surprising to find that the expression in brackets is the ***Laguerre polynomial*** of order j, $[L_j(sx)]$, which satisfies the following orthogonality condition (see a book such as [AbramowitzStegun64] for full information)

$$\int_0^\infty L_j(x)L_k(x)e^{-2x}\,dx = \delta_{jk}. \tag{4.4.3}$$

The Laguerre polynomials form a complete set, in that any *appropriately well-behaved* function of x can be expanded by them in much the same way that periodic functions can be expanded in a Fourier series of sines and cosines. That is, we can say the following. Equation (4.4.2c) can be rewritten as

$$d_{k+1}(s) = \int_0^\infty L_k(sx)e^{-sx}b(x)dx, \tag{4.4.4a}$$

which by the completeness property of orthogonal polynomials, lets us formally write

$$b(x) = s\sum_{k=0}^{\infty} d_{k+1}(s)L_k(sx)e^{-sx}. \tag{4.4.4b}$$

This leads to the sum rule,

$$\int_0^\infty b^2(x)dx = s\sum_{k=0}^{\infty}[d_k(s)]^2. \tag{4.4.4c}$$

These equations are true for any $s > 0$, which allows us to make the statement that every theorem proved by the method of Laguerre functions is automatically true here, too. (See, e.g., [AbateChoudhuryWhitt96] and [Keilson-Nunn79] for examples of the use of Laguerres in queueing theory.)

The Laguerre polynomials are often used to approximate functions, but in a context where a least squares fit is meaningful. Such fits do not guarantee that a finite (truncated) sum of L_k's, as in (4.4.4a) will be positive for all x, whereas any approximation to $b(x)$ must be greater than 0 for all x to be physically meaningful, so if one is to try this approximation method, great care must be taken.

Exercise 4.4.2: Prove that (4.4.4b) is identically true in the formal sense. That is, replace d_k by (4.4.1c), substitute for $L_k(sx)$, and manipulate to get (3.1.7d). Similarly, use (4.4.3) and (4.4.4b) to prove (4.4.4c).

There is one last set of functions of s to be defined. We use $s\mathbf{VD}(s) = \mathbf{I} - \mathbf{D}(s)$, to write

$$\gamma_n(s) := \Psi\left[(s\mathbf{VD})^n\right] = \Psi\left[(\mathbf{I}-\mathbf{D})^n\right]. \tag{4.4.5a}$$

Just as with (4.4.2a), we use the binomial theorem to get a relation between the d's and the γ's,

$$\gamma_k(s) = \Psi\left[\sum_{j=0}^{k}\binom{k}{j}(-1)^j\mathbf{D}^j\right] = \sum_{j=0}^{k}\binom{k}{j}(-1)^j d_j(s). \qquad (4.4.5b)$$

The equivalent to (4.4.2b) is

$$d_k(s) = \Psi\left[\sum_{j=0}^{k}\binom{k}{j}(-s\mathbf{VD})^j\right] = \sum_{j=0}^{k}\binom{k}{j}(-1)^j\gamma_j(s). \qquad (4.4.5c)$$

The relation between the $\alpha' s$ and the $\gamma' s$ is found by replacing the last $\mathbf{D}$ in (4.4.1b) with $\mathbf{I} - s\mathbf{V}D$ to get

$$\alpha_k(s) = \gamma_k(s) - \gamma_{k+1}(s). \qquad (4.4.6a)$$

It is not hard to prove by induction that

$$\gamma_k(s) = 1 - \sum_{j=0}^{k-1}\alpha_j(s) = \sum_{j=k}^{\infty}\alpha_j(s). \qquad (4.4.6b)$$

This tells us that $\gamma_k(s)$ is the probability that "at least k customers will arrive during one service time." It is left for Exercise 4.4.3 to prove that

$$\gamma_{k+1}(s) = s\int_0^\infty \frac{(sx)^k}{k!}e^{-sx}R(x)\,dx, \qquad (4.4.6c)$$

where $R(x) = \int_x^\infty b(t)\,dt$.

Exercise 4.4.3: Prove (4.4.6c) by first substituting (4.4.1a) into (4.4.6b), identifying the sum as the ***incomplete gamma function***, $\Gamma(k, x)$, which can then be replaced by its integral representation,

$$\Gamma(k, x) := \int_x^\infty e^{-t}t^{k-1}\,dt.$$

Finally, change the order of integration and end up with (4.4.6c). By the way, $\Gamma(k, x)$, from its definition, must be proportional to the reliability function for the Erlangian-k distribution. That is,

$$\Gamma(k, x) = k!\int_x^\infty E_k(t)\,dt = k!\,R_k(x).$$

Exercise 4.4.4.: Use their matrix definitions [Equations (4.4.1b), (4.4.1c), and (4.4.5a)] to prove the following sum rules for α, d, and γ.

$$\sum_{k=o}^{\infty} \alpha_k(s) = 1, \tag{4.4.7a}$$

$$\sum_{k=o}^{\infty} d_k(s) = 1 + \frac{1}{s} b(0), \tag{4.4.7b}$$

and

$$\sum_{k=o}^{\infty} \gamma_k(s) = 1 + s\bar{x}. \tag{4.4.7c}$$

These equations can also be proven using their integral definitions, (4.4.1a), (4.4.4a), and (4.4.6c) if one is careful about $k = 0$.

Exercise 4.4.5: Using any of the formulas just established, find explicit expressions for $d_k(s)$, $\alpha_k(s)$, and $\gamma_k(s)$ for: (1) an exponential server with service rate β; (2) a server with hyperexponential-2 distribution; and (3) an Erlangian-2 server. Verify explicitly that in all three cases the sum rules of Equations (4.4.7) are valid.

4.4.3 Connection to Standard Solution

The standard solution of the steady-state M/G/1 queue is actually an algorithm involving the α_n's. To reproduce those results, we must rearrange (4.1.7) and (4.2.5a), which means that we must do something with $\Psi[\mathbf{U}^n]$. First recall that $\mathbf{V} = \mathbf{B}^{-1}$, and from (4.1.4) and (4.2.8b) that $\mathbf{A} = \mathbf{I} + \mathbf{B}/\lambda - \mathbf{Q}$, $\mathbf{U} = \mathbf{A}^{-1}$, and $\mathbf{D}(\lambda) = (\mathbf{I} + \lambda\mathbf{V})^{-1}$. Then

$$\mathbf{A} = \frac{1}{\lambda}\mathbf{B}[\mathbf{I} + \lambda\mathbf{V} - \lambda\mathbf{V}\mathbf{Q}] = \frac{1}{\lambda}\mathbf{B}[\mathbf{I} + \lambda\mathbf{V}][\mathbf{I} - \lambda\mathbf{D}\mathbf{V}\mathbf{Q}].$$

With the aid of Lemma 4.2.1, we can write

$$\mathbf{U} = [\mathbf{I} - \lambda\mathbf{D}\mathbf{V}\mathbf{Q}]^{-1}\lambda\mathbf{D}\mathbf{V} = \left(\mathbf{I} + \frac{1}{1-\gamma_1(\lambda)}\lambda\mathbf{D}\mathbf{V}\mathbf{Q}\right)\lambda\mathbf{D}\mathbf{V}.$$

Let

$$\mathbf{C} := \lambda\mathbf{D}\mathbf{V} = \mathbf{I} - \mathbf{D}, \tag{4.4.8a}$$

which means [from (4.4.5a)] that $\gamma_n(\lambda) = \Psi[\mathbf{C}^n]$. Then

$$\mathbf{U} = \mathbf{C} + \frac{1}{1-\gamma_1}\mathbf{C}\mathbf{Q}\mathbf{C} \tag{4.4.8b}$$

and ($\mathbf{pCQ} = \mathbf{pC}\boldsymbol{\epsilon}'\mathbf{p} = \Psi[\mathbf{C}]\,\mathbf{p} = \gamma_1\mathbf{p}$)

$$\mathbf{pU} = \mathbf{pC} + \frac{\gamma_1}{1-\gamma_1}\mathbf{pC} = \frac{1}{1-\gamma_1}\mathbf{pC}. \tag{4.4.8c}$$

It simply follows that $\Psi[\mathbf{U}] = \gamma_1/(1-\gamma_1)$. Next, look at

$$\begin{aligned}\mathbf{pU}^2 = \mathbf{pUU} &= \frac{1}{1-\gamma_1}\mathbf{pC}\left[\mathbf{C} + \frac{1}{1-\gamma_1}\mathbf{CQC}\right]\\ &= \frac{1}{1-\gamma_1}\mathbf{pC}^2 + \frac{\gamma_2}{(1-\gamma_1)^2}\mathbf{pC},\end{aligned}$$

which yields $\Psi\left[\mathbf{U}^2\right] = \gamma_2/(1-\gamma_1)^2$. From this it can be seen that successive applications of (4.4.7a) to $\mathbf{pU}^n$ will lead to a series expansion in terms of $\mathbf{pC}^k$. Therefore, let

$$\mathbf{pU}^n = \sum_{k=1}^{n} a_k^{(n)}\mathbf{pC}^k, \tag{4.4.9a}$$

which leads to

$$\Psi[\mathbf{U}^n] = \sum_{k=1}^{n} a_k^{(n)}\gamma_k. \tag{4.4.9b}$$

On the one hand,

$$\mathbf{pU}^{n+1} = \sum_{k=1}^{n+1} a_k^{(n+1)}\mathbf{pC}^k,$$

and on the other hand,

$$\begin{aligned}\mathbf{pU}^{n+1} = \mathbf{pU}^n\mathbf{U} &= \sum_{k=1}^{n} a_k^{(n)}\mathbf{pC}^k\left[\mathbf{C} + \frac{1}{1-\gamma_1}\mathbf{CQC}\right]\\ &= \sum_{k=1}^{n} a_k^{(n)}\mathbf{pC}^{k+1} + \sum_{k=1}^{n} a_k^{(n)}\gamma_{k+1}\mathbf{pC}.\end{aligned}$$

For these two expressions to be identically equal, we must have

$$a_{k+1}^{(n+1)} = a_k^{(n)} \quad \text{for } 1 \le k \le n \tag{4.4.9c}$$

and

$$a_1^{(n+1)} = \frac{1}{1-\gamma_1}\sum_{k=1}^{n} a_k^{(n)}\gamma_{k+1}. \tag{4.4.9d}$$

The penultimate equation implies that $a_k^{(n)} = a_j^{(m)}$ as long as $n-k = m-j$. In particular,

$$a_k^{(n)} = a_1^{(n-k+1)}. \tag{4.4.9e}$$

We come up with an interesting relation by putting (4.4.9c) into (4.4.9d),

$$a_1^{(n+1)} = \frac{1}{1-\gamma_1}\sum_{k=1}^{n} a_{k+1}^{(n+1)}\gamma_{k+1} = \frac{1}{1-\gamma_1}\left(\sum_{k=2}^{n+1} a_k^{(n+1)}\gamma_k + a_1^{(n+1)}\gamma_1 - a_1^{(n+1)}\gamma_1\right)$$

$$= \frac{1}{1-\gamma_1}\left(\sum_{k=1}^{n+1} a_k^{(n+1)}\gamma_k - a_1^{(n+1)}\gamma_1\right).$$

Next bring the extra term on the right-hand side to the left-hand side of the equation, clear fractions, and cancel like terms to get, for $n > 1$,

$$a_1^{(n+1)} = \sum_{k=1}^{n+1} a_k^{(n+1)}\gamma_k = \Psi\left[\mathbf{U}^{n+1}\right]. \tag{4.4.10a}$$

The relationship with $\Psi\left[\mathbf{U}^{n+1}\right]$ comes from comparing with (4.4.9b). For convenience, let $u_1 := 1/(1-\gamma_1)$, and for $n > 1$,

$$u_n := \Psi\left[\mathbf{U}^n\right],$$

then with the aid of (4.4.9b) and (4.4.9e), (4.4.10a) can be rewritten as

$$u_n = \sum_{k=1}^{n} \gamma_k u_{n-k+1} \quad \text{for } n > 1, \tag{4.4.10b}$$

and, as previously noted, $\Psi[\mathbf{U}] = \gamma_1/(1-\gamma_1) = \gamma_1 u_1$. The standard solution as given in standard texts such as [ALLEN90] is expressed in terms of the $\alpha_n(\lambda)$'s. Therefore, manipulate the above (n is replaced by $n+1$), and get

$$u_{n+1} = \sum_{k=1}^{n+1} \gamma_k u_{n-k+2} = \gamma_1 u_{n+1} + \sum_{k=2}^{n+1} \gamma_k u_{n-k+2}$$

$$= \gamma_1 u_{n+1} + \sum_{k=1}^{n} \gamma_{k+1} u_{n-k+1}.$$

Next bring the loose term over to the left, recall that $\alpha_o = 1-\gamma_1$, and substitute (4.4.6a) to get

$$\alpha_o u_{n+1} = \sum_{k=1}^{n} u_{n-k+1}(\gamma_k - \alpha_k) = u_n - \sum_{k=1}^{n} u_{n-k+1}\alpha_k.$$

This is next rearranged to give

$$u_n = \alpha_o u_{n+1} + \sum_{k=1}^{n} u_{n-k+1}\alpha_k = \sum_{k=o}^{n} u_{n-k+1}\alpha_k.$$

We are almost there now. Note that for an open system, $r(n) = r(0)u_n$, for $n > 1$, and $r(1) = r(0)\gamma_1 u_1$. So, upon multiplying by $r(0)$, we get

$$r(n) = r(0)\alpha_n u_1 + \sum_{k=o}^{n-1} r(n-k+1)\alpha_k = r(0)\alpha_n u_1 + \sum_{k=o}^{n} r(n-k+1)\alpha_k - r(1)\alpha_n.$$

But $r(0)\alpha_n u_1 - r(1)\alpha_n = r(0)\alpha_n[1/\alpha_o - \gamma_1/\alpha_o] = r(0)\alpha_n$. Therefore,

$$r(n) = r(0)\alpha_n + \sum_{k=o}^{n} r(n-k+1)\alpha_k = r(0)\alpha_n + \sum_{k=1}^{n+1} r(k)\alpha_{n-k+1}. \tag{4.4.10c}$$

This, together with the fact that $r(0) = 1 - \rho$, is the recursive formula given in most books. Its physical interpretation is as follows, using the meaning of (4.4.1a). The steady-state probability that n customers will be found at S_1 is equal to the probability that when no customers are present, n customers arrive before any of them finish $[r(0)\alpha_n]$, plus the probability that there are $0 < k \leq n+1$ customers present $[r(k)]$ and $n - k + 1$ arrive before any finish $[\alpha_{n-k+1}]$.

The closed system is somewhat more difficult. We have shown that for all $0 \leq n < N$, $r(n; N)$ is proportional to $r(n)$, therefore we need only evaluate $\Psi\left[\mathbf{U}^{N-1}\mathbf{V}\right]$ by a separate means, and renormalize. That is, given that Equations (4.1.7) are true, $r(N;N) = \lambda r(0;N)\Psi\left[\mathbf{U}^{N-1}\mathbf{V}\right]$, and $r(n;N) = r(0;N)u_n$ for $n < N$. So

$$\frac{1}{r(0;N)} = \Psi\left[\mathbf{U}^{N-1}\mathbf{V}\right] + 1 + \sum_{n=1}^{N-1} u_n.$$

Finally, note that $\lambda\mathbf{AV} = \mathbf{I} + \lambda\mathbf{V} - \lambda\mathbf{QV}$, so

$$b_n := \Psi\left[\mathbf{U}^{n-1}\lambda\mathbf{V}\right] = \Psi\left[\mathbf{U}^n\lambda\mathbf{AV}\right] = \Psi\left[\mathbf{U}^n(\mathbf{I} + \lambda\mathbf{V} - \lambda\mathbf{QV})\right]$$
$$= u_n + b_{n+1} - \rho u_n,$$

which yields the simple recursive relation, starting with $b_1 = \rho$,

$$b_{n+1} = (1-\rho)u_n - b_n. \tag{4.4.11}$$

This last formula is not usually included in standard texts but is valid for all M/G/1/ /N queues.

As a final thought on this subject, note that the b_N's not only give the steady-state probabilities that all N customers are at S_1, $[r(N;N)]$, they also yield the residual waiting times for $n < N$ in the queue. That is, from (4.3.3a),

$$\mathbb{E}[X_r(n < N;\, N)] = \frac{b_{n+1}}{\lambda u_n}. \tag{4.4.12}$$

Equation (4.3.3b) must still be calculated by a different algorithm.

4.4.4 M/M/X//N Approximations to M/ME/1//N Loops

It is not our purpose here to search for approximations to the equations we have worked so hard to derive. Rather, we wish to explore the extent of robustness of ***Jackson networks*** (see, e.g., [BASKETETAL75], [LIPSKY-CHURCH77], [LAZOWSKAETAL84], [KANT92], and the entire issue of *Computing Surveys*, 3 [DENNING78]). The loop with two load-dependent servers, which we described in Section 2.1.5 and assigned the symbol M/M/X/ /N, can be viewed as a Jackson network with two service centers. In fact, Equations (2.1.11) were deliberately written in a form that reflects the product-form solution one sees in more general networks. One of the great attributes of Jackson networks is their ability to describe the steady-state behavior of a whole network, based on the properties of the individual service centers (the set of load-dependent service rates). Most important, the properties ascribed to each service center do not depend on the properties of other servers or the system as a whole. Of course, we are accomplishing the same thing in this book, but we have found it necessary to give each subsystem properties that must be expressed by a nontrivial matrix rather than a simple set of scalars. We point out that the M/M/X/ /N loop, unlike our M/ME/1/ /N formulation, simply does not have the structure to distinguish residual processes, or other transient properties, from those of the steady state. Therefore, we only compare the steady-state behaviors here.

Suppose that we observe a system which is exactly described by an M/G/1/ /N loop over a very long period of time. How would one measure the ***load dependence*** of a server? A natural and self-consistent definition, or defining measurement procedure, would be as follows (thanks to Victor Wallace for the underlying idea). Let t be the total time that the system has been under observation, and as we did in Section 1.1.1, let $N_i(t)$ be the number of customers who have left S_i in that time. If t is indeed very large, we would expect the ratio of $N_1(t)$ to $N_2(t)$ to be very close to 1, close enough so that we can assume that they are equal to each other, and drop the subscript. Then the system throughput is measured as

$$\Lambda(N) \approx \frac{N(t)}{t}. \tag{4.4.13a}$$

Next, we define the following measurable quantities.

Definition 4.4.1

$N_i(n;t)$:= *number of departures from* S_i *in the time interval,* t*, which occurred while there were* n *customers there (counting the one who left).* Every time a customer leaves S_i, the observer, noting how many customers were there just before the departure, increments that counter by 1. □

Then we can say that

$$\sum_{n=1}^{N} N_i(n;t) = N(t). \tag{4.4.13b}$$

Definition 4.4.2

$T_i(n;t)$:= *total time that there were* n *customers at* S_i. Every time a customer enters or leaves a subsystem, the observer notes how many customers were there just before that event and adds the amount of time since the previous arrival or departure to the appropriate counter. Of course, an arrival to one subsystem occurs at the same time as the departure from the other subsystem, so two counters are modified simultaneously. □

We then have

$$\sum_{n=o}^{N} T_i(n;t) = t \quad \text{for } i = 1,\ 2. \tag{4.4.13c}$$

The best we can say about load-dependent service rates is to describe them as "the rate at which customers leave a subsystem for a given queue length." So we use the following, consistent with the definitions we gave in Section 2.1.5 (for arbitrary load dependence).

$$\mu(n) \approx \frac{N_1(n;t)}{T_1(n;t)} \tag{4.4.14a}$$

and

$$\lambda(k) \approx \frac{N_2(k;t)}{T_2(k;t)}. \tag{4.4.14b}$$

These parameters are similar to those considered by J. P. Buzen's ***operational analysis*** (e.g., [BuzenDenning]). We assume that t is so large that the steady-state probabilities we have previously derived for various events are very close to the measured relative frequencies of those events. From our rules and definitions, $T_1(n;t)$ must be approximately equal to the probability that there are n customers at S_1, multiplied by the total time that the system was observed. That is,

$$T_1(n;t) \approx r(n;N)\,t. \tag{4.4.15a}$$

Also, after some thought, the reader should be able to accept the following formula:

$$N_1(n;t) \approx d(n-1;N)\,N(t). \tag{4.4.15b}$$

The r's and d's were defined in Definitions 4.1.1 and 4.1.5, respectively. Remember that $d(n;N)$ is the probability that a customer will leave n other customers behind, but N_1 and N_2 are defined as including the departing customer, hence the $n-1$ in (4.4.15b). The equivalent formulas for S_2 are (k is the number at S_2)

$$T_2(k;t) \approx r(N-k;N)\,t \tag{4.4.16a}$$

and

$$N_2(k;\,t) \approx d_2(k-1;\,N)\,N(t).$$

The symbol $d_2(k-1;N)$ is borrowed from Section 5.1.2 and is the probability that a customer when departing S_2 will leave behind $k-1$ customers. Clearly, that same customer will arrive at S_1, finding $N-k$ customers already there. (Let's see: there are $k-1$ at S_2, $N-k$ at S_1, and 1 traveling, giving a total of $k-1+N-k+1=N$, right.) Therefore, $d_2(k-1;N) = a(N-k,N)$, and we can write

$$N_2(k;\,t) \approx a(N-k;\,N)\,N(t). \tag{4.4.16b}$$

We are now ready to put things together. Using Equations (4.4.13a) and (4.4.15) in (4.4.14a) yields

$$\mu(n) = \frac{d(n-1;\,N)\,N(t)}{r(n;\,N)\,t} = \frac{d(n-1;\,N)}{r(n:\,N)}\,\Lambda(N).$$

But from (4.1.13c) and (4.1.8b), and noting that $1/\bar{x}_2 = \lambda$, we have

$$\mu(n) = \frac{r(n-1;\,N)}{r(n;\,N)}\,\frac{\Lambda(N)}{1-r(N;\,N)} = \lambda\frac{r(n-1;\,N)}{r(n;\,N)}. \tag{4.4.17a}$$

Similarly, we can work on S_2.

$$\lambda(k) = \frac{a(N-k;\,N)\,N(t)}{r(N-k;\,N)\,t} = \lambda. \tag{4.4.17b}$$

We have again made use of (4.1.13c). Thus we see that S_2 is indeed a load-independent server, just as we theorized, but S_1 is more complicated, as we would have expected.

Before we look at (4.4.17a) more closely, let us see what these service rates give us for probabilities when we use them in Equations (2.1.11). For the moment, let us call these probabilities $r_a(n; N)$ (a is for ***a***pproximation). Then

$$\lambda(N-n)\, r_a(n; N) = \mu(n+1)\, r_a(n+1;\, N).$$

Put in Equations (4.4.17), to get

$$\lambda\, r_a(n;\, N) = \lambda \frac{r(n;\, N)}{r(n+1;\, N)} r_a(n+1; N)$$

or

$$\frac{r(n; N)}{r_a(n; N)} = \frac{r(n+1; N)}{r_a(n+1; N)} \quad \text{for } 0 \le n < N. \tag{4.4.18}$$

The r_a's are proportional to the r's, term by term, and both sets sum to 1. Therefore they must be equal, term by term. Thus we have proven that for any M/G/1//N loop, we can find appropriate μ's that yield identical steady-state probabilities for an M/M/X//N loop. Is this truly miraculous? **NO**. All we did was find N numbers, $[\mu(n)]$, which would let us generate $N+1$ other numbers $[r(n; N)]$, constrained to sum to 1. In other words, the product-form solution has so many unspecified parameters that it can fit anything. The real test of the model comes when we see if the same parameters can be used to model a system that has been changed slightly.

Let us look again at (4.4.17a). From (4.1.7a) and (4.1.7b) we can write the following.

$$\mu(n) = \lambda \frac{\Psi\left[\mathbf{U}^{n-1}\right]}{\Psi\left[\mathbf{U}^{n}\right]} \quad \text{for } 1 \le n < N, \tag{4.4.19a}$$

but

$$\mu(N) = \frac{\Psi\left[\mathbf{U}^{N-1}\right]}{\Psi\left[\mathbf{U}^{N-1}\mathbf{V}\right]}. \tag{4.4.19b}$$

These equations tell us that if we tested a system with, say, four customers, and then asked how the system would behave if we added one more customer, we could use some of the same parameters, but we would have to change $\mu(4)$, as well as find a value for $\mu(5)$. In other words, from an M/M/C//N point of view, the properties ascribed to S_1 depend on the system's population to a certain extent.

We can ask what happens if we change the behavior of another server somewhat. In our M/ME/1//N loop the only thing we can do to S_2 is change λ. Suppose that we again tested a system with four customers, and then asked how the system would behave if λ were changed somewhat. Everything seems to be constant, but the matrix $\mathbf{U}$ depends on λ in a nontrivial way.

Example 4.4.1: Let us look at $\mu(1)$ from (4.4.19a), for an M/E_2/1//N queue. In that case (see Exercise 3.1.1)

$$\langle\, \mathbf{p}\,,\, \mathbf{B}\,\rangle = \langle\, [1\ 0],\ \mu \begin{bmatrix} 1 & -1 \\ 0 & 1 \end{bmatrix} \rangle,$$

so (recall that $\mathbf{Q} = \boldsymbol{\epsilon}'\,\mathbf{p}$)

$$\mathbf{A} = \mathbf{I} + \frac{1}{\lambda}\mathbf{B} - \boldsymbol{\epsilon}'\,\mathbf{p} = \begin{bmatrix} 1 & 0 \\ 0 & 1 \end{bmatrix} + \frac{\mu}{\lambda} \begin{bmatrix} 1 & -1 \\ 0 & 1 \end{bmatrix} - \begin{bmatrix} 1 & 0 \\ 1 & 0 \end{bmatrix}.$$

We know that $\bar{x}_1 = 2/\mu$; therefore, $\rho = \lambda \bar{x}_1 = 2\lambda/\mu$. Thus we can write

$$\mathbf{A} = \begin{bmatrix} \frac{2}{\rho} & -\frac{2}{\rho} \\ -1 & 1 + \frac{2}{\rho} \end{bmatrix}$$

and

$$\mathbf{U} = \mathbf{A}^{-1} = \frac{\rho}{2} \begin{bmatrix} 1 + \frac{\rho}{2} & 1 \\ \frac{\rho}{2} & 1 \end{bmatrix}.$$

Of course, $\Psi\,[\mathbf{U}] = \mathbf{p}\,\mathbf{U}\,\boldsymbol{\epsilon}'$, so (4.4.19a) for $n = 1$ becomes

$$\bar{x}_1\, \mu(1) = \frac{4}{4 + \rho}.$$

We see even in this simplest of all nontrivial queues, that a load-dependent exponential approximation to a (load-independent) nonexponential server depends heavily on parameters of other parts of the system, as represented here by ρ. For instance, when $\rho = 0$, we get $\mu(1) = 1/\bar{x}_1$, which is what one would expect. But for $\rho = 1$, $\mu(1) = 0.8/\bar{x}_1$. For yet larger values of ρ (remember that for closed systems, ρ can take on any nonnegative value), $\mu(1)$ will be even smaller. Similar comments can be made for $\mu(k)$, $k > 1$. ▲

Our conclusion is that Jackson networks, due to their parametric richness, are robust enough to fit the measurements of any given network of service centers. This can be most useful, because one is often overcome with a flood of data in measuring the performance of complex systems, and the product-form solution provides a framework on which the data can be *hung*, to test self-consistency and provide meaning. They also warn us not to try too hard to get more out of a system near saturation. However, one must be very cautious in using the same data in extrapolating to other systems if the systems do not satisfy the assumptions that went into the derivation of the product-form solution. In short, Jackson network model *explains* everything, but its predictions are no better than the assumptions that go into it.

4.5 Transient Behavior of M/ME/1 Queues

It is in the discussion of non-steady-state properties of queues that LAQT shows its unique value, for we see that all events correspond to some linear matrix operation on a state vector. The approach is quite general, but for now we limit ourselves to those topics covered in Section 2.3. Before reading further, the reader should go back to that section, as well as Section 3.1, and review the material contained therein, carefully.

4.5.1 First-Passage Processes for Queue Growth

To evaluate the time it takes for a queue to grow to a given length, we must first find out how long it takes the queue to go from n to $n+1$ for the first time. The procedure we must use is in the same spirit as Section 2.3.1, but more complex. Not only can the external state of the system (i.e., the number of customers at S_1) change by one unit at a time, up or down, as in Chapter 2, but it can also remain constant, as in Chapter 3. Furthermore, we must keep track of the internal state of the system as the queue grows. Because n can never exceed the total number in the system, N plays no role in this process (unless S_2 is a load-dependent server, a subject we could cover with equal ease). Therefore, this section is equally valid for open and closed systems. Unfortunately, we have to be satisfied with recursive formulas for the parameters of interest rather than the nice explicit expressions we were able to get for the M/M/1 queue. We are not making the claim that explicit expressions do not exist, but merely that we have not found them as yet. Very little work has been done with these formulas up to now, so there is every reason to hope that an adventurous, algebraically oriented researcher will find one in the future.

4.5.1.1 Conditional Probabilities for Queue Growth

Before even looking at times for ***first passage***, we must first find out the probability that the system will be in state j when it reaches queue length $n+1$ for the first time after starting in $\{i;\, n\}$. On first thought this seems to be a trivial question. It certainly is trivial for decreasing lengths, because a decrease can only occur immediately after a departure, subsequent to which, another customer enters S_1, putting the system in ***internal state*** $\mathbf{p}$. By this we mean the following. "The probability that the system is in state $\{i;\, n\}$ is p_i." We use the two expressions synonymously.

What we just said about decreasing lengths would seem to be true for increasing lengths as well. For then, an increase can only occur immediately after an arrival to S_1, and that does not change the internal state at all. Ah, but many things may have happened before that final arrival sent the system from n to $n+1$. Suppose that initially the system has n customers at S_1 and the active customer is at phase i. That is, the system is in state $\{i;\, n\}$. Define the conditional probability matrix.

Definition 4.5.1

$\mathbf{H_u}(n)$:= *probability matrix of first passage from n to $n+1$* That is, $[\mathbf{H_u}(n)]_{ij}$ is the probability that S_1 will be in state j when its queue goes from n to $n+1$ for the first time, given that it started in state $\{i;\, n\}$. As in Section 2.3, the subscript **u** stands for *up*. Recall that a subscript is **boldfaced**, if and only if the object to which it is attached is a vector or matrix. □

We assert that the queue must grow to $n+1$ some day, so the sum across each row must be 1:

$$\mathbf{H_u}(n)\,\boldsymbol{\epsilon}' = \boldsymbol{\epsilon}' \quad \text{for all } \; n \;\geq\; 0. \tag{4.5.1}$$

Thus $\mathbf{H_u}(n)$ is isometric. We prove this algebraically after we have found a recursive formula for the $\mathbf{H_u}$'s. For the remainder of this section we usually drop the subscript when there is no ambiguity. The following discussion is similar to the material in Section 4.1.2 related to Figure 4.1.2.

Given that our system is initially in state $\{i;\, n\}$, the first event can occur in only two ways: either a completion occurs in S_1, with probability $[(\mathbf{M}+\lambda\mathbf{I})^{-1}\mathbf{M}]_{ii}$, or there is a completion at S_2, with probability $[(\mathbf{M}+\lambda\mathbf{I})^{-1}\lambda]_{ii}$. Next look at Figure 4.5.1. If the event occurred in S_2, a customer will arrive at S_1, increasing the number there by one without changing the internal state. This corresponds to the solid arrow going diagonally upward and to the right (labeled I, $a \to d$). If the event occurred in S_1, one of two things could happen. Either the active customer goes from i to some other phase, say k (with probability P_{ik}), thereby leaving the system in the same external state $[n]$, or he could leave S_1 (with probability q_i) and be replaced by a new customer who would then go to phase k (with probability p_k), putting the system in state $\{k;\, n-1\}$. If the former is the case, it is like starting over again, and given that the system now starts in state $\{k;\, n\}$, it will find itself in external state $n+1$ for the first time with probability $[\mathbf{H}(n)]_{kj}$ of being in internal state j. This sequence of events corresponds to the solid vertical arrow, followed by the wavy arrow pointed diagonally upward to the right (labeled II, $a \to c \to f$).

Recall from Chapter 2 that a wavy arrow represents the infinity of possible ways to get from the tail to the head, and a solid arrow corresponds to a direct, single process. The last case puts the system in state $\{k;\, n-1\}$, from which it must eventually get back to $\{l;\, n\}$ for some l, and then finally to $\{j;\, n+1\}$. This is represented in Figure 4.5.1 by the path labeled III ($a \to b \to e \to g$), which is the solid arrow pointing diagonally to the left, followed by two successive wavy arrows diagonally upward to the right.

The three sequences of events are mutually exclusive, and exhaustive, but remember to sum over all possible intermediate states k and l. They clearly are mutually exclusive. We show that they are exhaustive by proving that the sum of the three sets of initial probability matrices is isometric, which is the same as showing that customer surely went somewhere. Look at the following. The (ij)-th component of each of the three terms is the probability of taking path I, II, or III, respectively, ending in internal state j, after starting in state

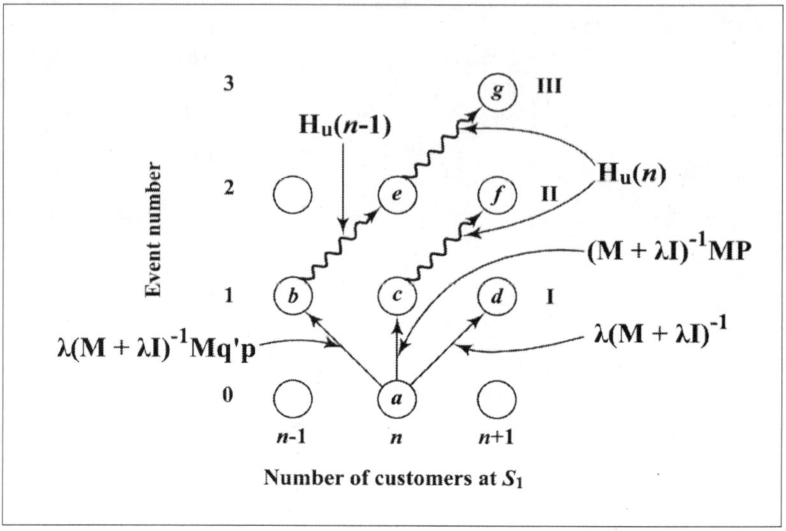

Figure 4.5.1: Time-dependent state transition diagram for both the open and closed M/ME/1 queues, showing what a system must do to go from n to $n+1$ for the first time. Path I is $(a \rightarrow d)$, path II is $(a \rightarrow c \rightarrow f)$, and path III is $(a \rightarrow b \rightarrow e \rightarrow g)$.

i.

$$\begin{aligned}\mathbf{X} &:= (\lambda\mathbf{I}+\mathbf{M})^{-1}\lambda + (\lambda\mathbf{I}+\mathbf{M})^{-1}\mathbf{MP} + (\lambda\mathbf{I}+\mathbf{M})^{-1}\mathbf{Mq}'\mathbf{p} \\ &= (\lambda\mathbf{I}+\mathbf{M})^{-1}[\lambda\mathbf{I} + \mathbf{MP} + \mathbf{Mq}'\mathbf{p}].\end{aligned}$$

We wish to show that $\mathbf{X}\boldsymbol{\epsilon}' = \boldsymbol{\epsilon}'$. Recall that $\mathbf{p}\boldsymbol{\epsilon}' = 1$, and that $\mathbf{q}' = (\mathbf{I}-\mathbf{P})\boldsymbol{\epsilon}'$, so $\mathbf{P}\boldsymbol{\epsilon}' + \mathbf{q}'\,\mathbf{p}\boldsymbol{\epsilon}' = \boldsymbol{\epsilon}'$. Therefore,

$$\begin{aligned}\mathbf{X}\boldsymbol{\epsilon}' &= (\lambda\mathbf{I}+\mathbf{M})^{-1}[\lambda;\, \boldsymbol{\epsilon}' + \mathbf{M}(\mathbf{P}+\mathbf{q}'\,\mathbf{p})\boldsymbol{\epsilon}'] = (\lambda\mathbf{I}+\mathbf{M})^{-1}[\lambda\boldsymbol{\epsilon}' + \mathbf{M}\boldsymbol{\epsilon}'] \\ &= (\lambda\mathbf{I}+\mathbf{M})^{-1}[\lambda\mathbf{I}+\mathbf{M}]\boldsymbol{\epsilon}' = \boldsymbol{\epsilon}'.\end{aligned}$$

Thus we have indeed proven that $\mathbf{X}$ is isometric, which in turn means that we have included all possible events.

We now write the matrix equation for $\mathbf{H}(n)$.

$$\mathbf{H}(n) = (\lambda\mathbf{I}+\mathbf{M})^{-1}\left[\lambda\mathbf{I} + \mathbf{MPH}(n) + \mathbf{Mq}'\mathbf{pH}(n-1)\mathbf{H}(n)\right].$$

The three terms on the right correspond to processes (I), (II), and (III), respectively. Remember that matrix multiplication is the same as summing over all intermediate states, k and l. Next we multiply both sides from the left by $(\lambda\mathbf{I}+\mathbf{M})$, collect all terms proportional to $\mathbf{H}(n)$, and get for $n > 0$:

$$[\mathbf{M} + \lambda\mathbf{I} - \mathbf{MP} - \mathbf{Mq}'\mathbf{pH}(n-1)]\mathbf{H}(n) = \lambda\mathbf{I}. \qquad (4.5.2a)$$

Note from (3.1.3) and (4.1.3a) that $\mathbf{B} = \mathbf{M} - \mathbf{MP}$, $\mathbf{Mq}' = \mathbf{B}\boldsymbol{\epsilon}'$, and from Lemma 3.5.1 that $\mathbf{Q} = \boldsymbol{\epsilon}'\,\mathbf{p}$. We then make these substitutions, divide both sides of the equation by λ, and then solve for $\mathbf{H}(n)$, to get the desired recursive formulas for $n > 1$,

$$\mathbf{H_u}(n) = \lambda[\lambda\mathbf{I} + \mathbf{B} - \mathbf{BQH_u}(n-1)]^{-1}. \tag{4.5.2b}$$

From the definition of $\mathbf{A}$ in (4.1.4a) and Lemma 4.1.1, this can also be written as

$$\mathbf{H_u}(n) = [\mathbf{A} + \mathbf{Q} - \mathbf{AQH_u}(n-1)]^{-1}. \tag{4.5.2c}$$

It is not known whether the form for $\mathbf{H_u}(n)$ that contains $\mathbf{A}$ will ultimately be more convenient than that which contains $\mathbf{B}$, so we use whichever seems more useful.

The formula, when only one customer is at S_1, is slightly different. If the customer should leave, S_1 remains idle until another customer arrives and enters, $[\mathbf{p}]$. After that, the system eventually gets to $n = 2$. The equation for this is

$$\mathbf{H}(1) = \lambda(\lambda\mathbf{I} + \mathbf{M})^{-1} + (\lambda\mathbf{I} + \mathbf{M})^{-1}\mathbf{MPH}(1) + (\lambda\mathbf{I} + \mathbf{M})^{-1}\mathbf{Mq'pH}(1).$$

[Compare this with (4.5.2a) before going on.] We easily solve for $\mathbf{H_u}(1)$, getting

$$\mathbf{H_u}(1) = \lambda[\lambda\mathbf{I} + \mathbf{B} - \mathbf{BQ}]^{-1} = [\mathbf{A} + \mathbf{Q} - \mathbf{AQ}]^{-1}. \tag{4.5.2d}$$

As with all recursive relations, we must start with a nonrecursive equation, which we easily get by noting that

$$\mathbf{H_u}(0) = \mathbf{p}.$$

But we can make believe that state $\{\cdot;\, 0\}$ has internal states [we already did this in (4.1.1)]; then we can use

$$\mathbf{H_u}(0) = \mathbf{Q}, \tag{4.5.2e}$$

and thus, because $\mathbf{Q}^2 = \mathbf{Q}$, (4.5.2d) becomes a special case of (4.5.2c).

We next show that $\mathbf{H_u}(1)\boldsymbol{\epsilon}' = \boldsymbol{\epsilon}'$, and by induction, using (4.5.2c), prove that (4.5.1) is true for all n. First note that for any matrix $\mathbf{D}$, if $\mathbf{D}\boldsymbol{\epsilon}' = \boldsymbol{\epsilon}'$, then its inverse satisfies $\mathbf{D}^{-1}\boldsymbol{\epsilon}' = \boldsymbol{\epsilon}'$. We say, then, that if $\mathbf{D}$ is isometric, so is $\mathbf{D}^{-1}$. Therefore, if $[\mathbf{A} + \mathbf{Q} - \mathbf{AQ}]\boldsymbol{\epsilon}' = \boldsymbol{\epsilon}'$, its inverse, $\mathbf{H}(1)$, satisfies $\mathbf{H}(1)\boldsymbol{\epsilon}' = \boldsymbol{\epsilon}'$. But the *if* condition is obviously true, because $\mathbf{Q}\,\boldsymbol{\epsilon}' = (\boldsymbol{\epsilon}'\,\mathbf{p})\,\boldsymbol{\epsilon}' = \boldsymbol{\epsilon}'\,(\mathbf{p}\,\boldsymbol{\epsilon}') = \boldsymbol{\epsilon}'$. Next assume that $\mathbf{H}(k)\,\boldsymbol{\epsilon}' = \boldsymbol{\epsilon}'$ for all $k = 1, 2, \ldots, n-1$, and rewrite (4.5.2c) as

$$\mathbf{H}(n)\,[\mathbf{A} + \mathbf{Q} - \mathbf{AQH}(n-1)] = \mathbf{I}.$$

Then multiply both sides on the right with $\boldsymbol{\epsilon}'$. The left-hand side of the resulting equation gives

$$\mathbf{H}(n)[\mathbf{A}\,\boldsymbol{\epsilon}' + \boldsymbol{\epsilon}' - \mathbf{AQH}(n-1)\boldsymbol{\epsilon}'] = \mathbf{H}(n)[\mathbf{A}\,\boldsymbol{\epsilon}' + \boldsymbol{\epsilon}' - \mathbf{AQ}\,\boldsymbol{\epsilon}']$$
$$= \mathbf{H}(n)[\mathbf{A}\,\boldsymbol{\epsilon}' + \boldsymbol{\epsilon}' - \mathbf{A}\,\boldsymbol{\epsilon}'] = \mathbf{H}(n)\boldsymbol{\epsilon}',$$

and the right-hand side yields $\mathbf{I}\,\boldsymbol{\epsilon}' = \boldsymbol{\epsilon}'$. Therefore, we have proven our assertion that $\mathbf{H}(n)$ is isometric for all n. In effect, we have proven the following (perhaps obvious) theorem.

Theorem 4.5.1: For any M/G/1//N queue, and for any ρ, if at any time there are $n < N$ customers in the queue of S_1, then given enough time, the queue will eventually have $n+1$ customers in it [i.e., $\mathbf{H_u}(n)\,\boldsymbol{\epsilon}' = \boldsymbol{\epsilon}'$]. ■

This might be called the "pessimist's theorem," because it implies that no matter how bad things are now (long queue), if our random observer waits long enough, she will certainly see it get worse some day (longer queue). There are at least two weaknesses to this argument, however. First of all, the theorem assumes that conditions will remain the same for time immemorial, the ***homogeneous*** assumption. Second, the pessimist is assuming that the random observer will live long enough to see things get worse. This is an important reason for studying non-steady-state behavior. For if "some day" is longer than say, the age of the universe, who cares? In Chapter 2 we calculated what this time would be for an exponential queue [Equations (2.3.2)], and saw that this could be long indeed if $\rho < 1$. See a related discussion in Section 3.3.6 on the St. Petersburg Paradox and PT distributions.

We now show how to calculate mean ***first-passage times*** for general queues in the next section, after saying some final remarks about the first-passage matrices. Equation (4.5.2d) seems simple enough, so we might be encouraged to substitute it into (4.5.2b) or (4.5.2c) to get an explicit formula for $\mathbf{H_u}(2)$, but the resulting expression does not simplify greatly. For higher n it is even messier. It is better to think of these formulas as a recursive definition of the ($\mathbf{H_u}$)s, and to use (4.5.2b) or (4.5.2c) to numerically compute them recursively when explicit examples are needed. Note that in general, the ($\mathbf{H_u}$)s are all different, although they do approach a limit for large n.

From these matrices one can also find the probability matrices of first passage from n to $n+l$, for any n and l.

Definition 4.5.2

$\mathbf{H_u}(n \to n+l)$:= *probability matrix of* ***first passage*** *from n to $n+l$*, $l \geq 1$. That is, $[\mathbf{H_u}(n \to n+l)]_{ij}$ is the probability that S_1 will be in state j when its queue goes from n to $n+l$ for the first time, given that it started in state i with n customers. In particular, $\mathbf{H_u}(n \to n+1) = \mathbf{H_u}(n)$. □

The ***first-passage matrix*** of going from n to $n+2$ is simply

$$\mathbf{H_u}(n \to n+2) = \mathbf{H_u}(n)\mathbf{H_u}(n+1),$$

and in general,

$$\begin{aligned}\mathbf{H_u}(n \to n+l+1) &= \mathbf{H_u}(n \to n+l)\mathbf{H_u}(n+l)\\ &= \mathbf{H_u}(n)\mathbf{H_u}(n+1)\cdots\mathbf{H_u}(n+l).\end{aligned} \tag{4.5.3}$$

Would the author be presumptuous in declaring it obvious that $\mathbf{H_u}(n \to n+l)$ is isometric?

A particularly interesting matrix (it is actually a vector) is the probability of first passage from $0 \to n$. It is given by

$$\mathbf{p_u}(n) := \mathbf{p}\mathbf{H_u}(1)\mathbf{H_u}(2)\cdots\mathbf{H_u}(n-1). \tag{4.5.4}$$

Here too, it is clear that $\mathbf{p_u}(n)\boldsymbol{\epsilon}' = 1$ for all n, so Theorem 4.5.1 extends to the statement: "given enough time, every possible queue length will be experienced at least once." But what is "enough time?" We discuss this vector further when we actually define it in Definition 4.5.4.

The first-passage matrices may not appear to be very interesting in their own right, but they are needed for calculating first-passage times, as shown in the next section.

4.5.1.2 Mean First-Passage Time for Queue Growth

This section is a direct generalization of the material in Section 2.3.1. By arguments similar to those required to derive (4.5.2), one can derive the mean time for the queue to grow from n to $n+1$ for the first time. First define the vector $\boldsymbol{\tau}'_{\mathbf{u}}(n)$.

Definition 4.5.3

$\boldsymbol{\tau}'_{\mathbf{u}}(n) :=$ ***mean first-passage time vector from n to n+1***. The i-th component is the mean time it takes for the queue at S_1 to have $n+1$ customers for the first time, having started in state $\{i;\, n\}$. □

Look once more at Figure 4.5.1. Suppose that there are n customers in the queue at S_1, and the active customer is at phase i. From that figure, one of three things will happen next. The mean time until the next event is given by $1/(\lambda + \mu_i) = [(\lambda\mathbf{I} + \mathbf{M})^{-1}\boldsymbol{\epsilon}']_i$. If the event that occurs is an arrival from S_2, [path I], the process is over. If, however, the event is internal to S_1, [path II], the system will go to state $\{j,\, n\}$ with probability given by $[(\lambda\mathbf{I} + \mathbf{M})^{-1}\mathbf{MP}]_{ij}$, and then will take another $[\boldsymbol{\tau}'_{\mathbf{u}}(n)]_j$ to accomplish the task. Worse yet, if the event results in a departure from S_1, as shown in path III, the system, finding itself in some state $\{j;\, n-1\}$ with probability $[(\lambda\mathbf{I} + \mathbf{M})^{-1}\mathbf{Mq}'\mathbf{p}]_{ij}$, must first get back to length n in time $[\boldsymbol{\tau}'_{\mathbf{u}}(n-1)]_j$ and then on to $n+1$. But this long excursion of going down and back up puts the system into state k with probability $[(\lambda\mathbf{I} + \mathbf{M})^{-1}\mathbf{Mq}'\mathbf{p}\mathbf{H_u}(n-1)]_{ik}$. (At last we see the need for a first-passage matrix.) The three processes together lead to the following vector equation.

$$\boldsymbol{\tau}'_{\mathbf{u}}(n) = (\lambda\mathbf{I} + \mathbf{M})^{-1}\boldsymbol{\epsilon}' + (\lambda\mathbf{I} + \mathbf{M})^{-1}\mathbf{MP}\boldsymbol{\tau}'_{\mathbf{u}}(n)$$
$$+(\lambda\mathbf{I} + \mathbf{M})^{-1}\mathbf{Mq}'\mathbf{p}[\boldsymbol{\tau}'_{\mathbf{u}}(n-1) + \mathbf{H_u}(n-1)\boldsymbol{\tau}'_{\mathbf{u}}(n)].$$

Next, premultiply both sides of the equation by $(\lambda\mathbf{I} + \mathbf{M})$, bring all terms proportional to $\boldsymbol{\tau}'_{\mathbf{u}}(n)$ to the left-hand side, and get

$$[\lambda\mathbf{I} + \mathbf{M} - \mathbf{MP} - \mathbf{Mq}'\mathbf{p}\mathbf{H_u}(n-1)]\boldsymbol{\tau}'_{\mathbf{u}}(n) = \boldsymbol{\epsilon}' + \mathbf{Mq}'\mathbf{p}\boldsymbol{\tau}'_{\mathbf{u}}(n-1).$$

This formula has several familiar components. Recall that $\mathbf{M} - \mathbf{MP} = \mathbf{B}$, $\mathbf{Mq}'\mathbf{p} = \mathbf{BQ}$, and thus from (4.5.2b) the term in brackets is λ times the inverse of $\mathbf{H_u}(n)$. This, then, gives us the important recursive equation for the $\boldsymbol{\tau}'_{\mathbf{u}}(n)$'s.

$$\boldsymbol{\tau}'_{\mathbf{u}}(n) = \frac{1}{\lambda}\boldsymbol{\epsilon}' + \frac{1}{\lambda}\mathbf{H_u}(n)\mathbf{BQ}\boldsymbol{\tau}'_{\mathbf{u}}(n-1), \quad \text{with } \boldsymbol{\tau}'_{\mathbf{u}}(0) := \frac{1}{\lambda}\boldsymbol{\epsilon}'. \tag{4.5.5}$$

To get these formulas we had to divide by λ, premultiply both sides by $\mathbf{H_u}(n)$, and make use of the isometric property of $\mathbf{H_u}(n)$.

Before going on, let us use the following theorem to summarize what we have done so far.

Theorem 4.5.2: For any M/ME/1//N queue, and for any ρ, the first-passage matrices $\mathbf{H_u}(n)$, and mean first-passage time vectors $\boldsymbol{\tau}'_{\mathbf{u}}(n)$, are recursively given by (4.5.2) and (4.5.5), and can be calculated efficiently in the following way:

$$\mathbf{H_u}(0) = \mathbf{Q}, \qquad \boldsymbol{\tau}'_{\mathbf{u}}(0) = \frac{1}{\lambda}\boldsymbol{\epsilon}'.$$

For $n = 1, 2, \ldots,$

$$\mathbf{H_u}(n) = \lambda[\lambda\mathbf{I} + \mathbf{B} - \mathbf{BQH_u}(n-1)]^{-1}$$

and

$$\boldsymbol{\tau}'_{\mathbf{u}}(n) = \frac{1}{\lambda}\boldsymbol{\epsilon}' + \frac{1}{\lambda}\mathbf{H_u}(n)\mathbf{BQ}\boldsymbol{\tau}'_{\mathbf{u}}(n-1).$$

These objects are the same for all N as long as $n < N$, and thus the theorem is true for the open system ($N \to \infty$) as well. The first-passage matrices are isometric, (i.e., $\mathbf{H_u}(n)\boldsymbol{\epsilon}' = \boldsymbol{\epsilon}'$). ■

Example 4.5.1: We have computed $\boldsymbol{\tau}'_{\mathbf{u}}(n)$ of the M/E_2/1 queue for various values of ρ and have plotted the results in Figure 4.5.2. Note that $\boldsymbol{\tau}'_{\mathbf{u}}(n)$ has two components, so there are two curves for each ρ. The most obvious feature is that for a given value of n, smaller ρ leads to longer times for the queue at S_1 to grow by 1. Next, for a given ρ, the mean time it takes to grow by 1 increases with n, and if $\rho < 1$, the increase is exponential. This is caused by the fact that for large n, the queue can drop much farther before it finally goes up (remember, the first-passage times include possible excursions down to 0). For $\rho > 1$, the curve approaches a constant, because the queue is not likely to drop very far before going up. The curve for $\rho = 1$ appears to be linear, just as it is in the M/M/1 case.

The third feature we see is the separation of the two components of $\boldsymbol{\tau}'_{\mathbf{u}}(n)$. The mean first-passage time to grow by 1 is a weighted average of the two components, depending on the state the system was in when the process began. If the process begins at the moment a customer enters S_1, then $\mathbf{p} = [1,\ 0]$, and the growth time follows the curve labeled $[\boldsymbol{\tau}'_{\mathbf{u}}(n)]_1$. Note that the curves for the two components actually diverge as n gets bigger. If a customer starts at phase 2, he has a higher probability of leaving before another customer

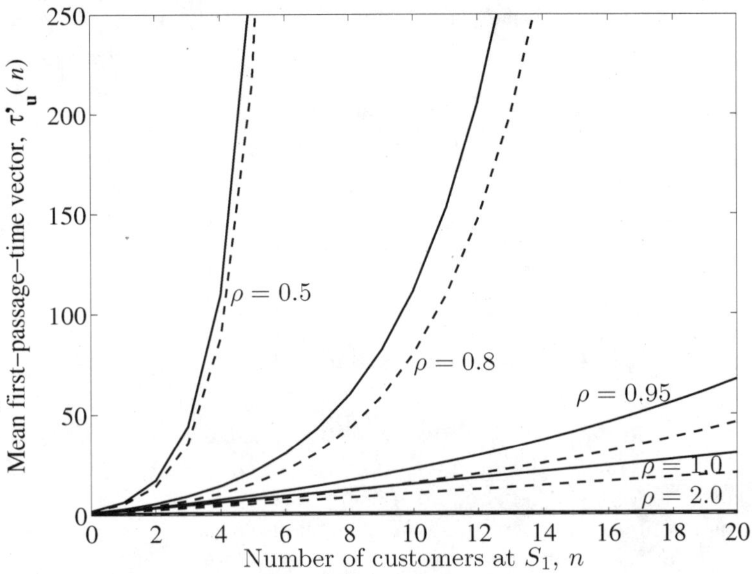

Figure 4.5.2: The two components of mean first-passage time vector $\boldsymbol{\tau}'_{\mathbf{u}}(n)$, as a function of the number of customers at S_1, for the M/E_2/1 queue. There are five sets of curves, corresponding to $\rho = 0.5$, 0.8, 0.95, 1.0, and 2.0. If the process starts when a customer first enters, he goes to phase 1, and when finished there, goes to phase 2, after which he leaves. If a new customer arrives before the active customer leaves, the process ends (the queue has grown by 1). Otherwise, the process continues, with possibly many events occurring. For all ρ and n, $[\boldsymbol{\tau}']_1$ (dashed lines) lies below $[\boldsymbol{\tau}']_2$ (solid lines). The curves corresponding to $\rho = 2$ are not negligible. For $n \geq 20$, their values are constant at 0.809 and 1.118, respectively.

arrives, thereby leaving the queue with only $n - 1$ customers. Therefore, it will take longer to recover if n is larger. ▲

It would be most interesting to study first-passage times for other distributions, because very little is known about this type of behavior.

The first-passage time vectors do not by themselves give us the times we are looking for. We must first decide what state we are in when the process begins. In Chapter 2 this was no problem, in as much as we only had to know the number in the queue. Now unfortunately, we must make some statement as to the initial internal state of S_1. Once we do this (whether the system is open or closed, irrespective of whether ρ is less than, equal to, or greater than 1), we can then calculate such things as

1. The mean first-passage time of going from n to $n + 1$, given that the customer in service has just begun;

2. The mean first-passage time to $n+1$, as seen by a random observer who sees n customers there initially;

3. The mean first-passage time to $n + 1$, given that there are n customers in the queue, and the last customer just arrived;

4. The mean first-passage time from n to $n+1$, given that the queue was originally empty;

5. The mean time for a queue to grow to n for the first time, given that a customer has just arrived at an empty queue.

(Note that items 1 to 4 yield identical results for the M/M/1 queue.) For instance, the internal state of S_1 immediately after a customer departs and a new customer enters is the entrance vector $\mathbf{p}$. Therefore, the first item of the list above can be calculated as follows.

Corollary 4.5.2a: The mean time for an M/ME/1 queue to grow to $n+1$ for the first time, given that n customers are there at the beginning, and the customer in service at S_1 has just begun, is given by

$$\mathbf{p}\boldsymbol{\tau}'_{\mathbf{u}}(n).$$

This is the same as the ***mean first-passage time to*** $n+1$, given that a customer has just left behind n customers. It is also the same as the "mean time for S_1 to return to queue length $n+1$ for the first time, given that it just dropped to n." There are, no doubt, other equivalent statements. The state the system will be in when this occurs is given by

$$\mathbf{p}\mathbf{H}_{\mathbf{u}}(n).$$

Thus the expression

$$\mathbf{p}\boldsymbol{\tau}'_{\mathbf{u}}(n) + \mathbf{p}\mathbf{H}_{\mathbf{u}}(n)\boldsymbol{\tau}'_{\mathbf{u}}(n+1)$$

is the mean first-passage time to $n+2$, given that service has just begun with $n \leq N-2$ customers. ■

Another interesting passage time is given by item 2 above. The condition as stated there is insufficient to derive an expression. After all, what was the history of the queue before the random observer arrived? We could assume that the system has been in operation for a long time, long enough to be near its steady state. This was discussed in Section 4.3.1 in analyzing residual times. We follow that section here. Thus the random observer will find the system in the composite state described by the vector [see (4.3.1a)]

$$\frac{1}{r(n;N)}\boldsymbol{\pi}(n;N) = \boldsymbol{\pi}_{\mathbf{r}}(n) = \frac{1}{\Psi\left[\mathbf{U}^n\right]}\mathbf{p}\mathbf{U}^n.$$

The residual vector appears again. Note that this vector does not depend on N, except that n must be less than N. If $n=N$, the queue can never rise above N anyway. We can state the time for this process by the following.

Corollary 4.5.2b: The mean time for a steady-state M/ME/1 queue to grow to $n+1$ for the first time, as seen by a random observer who finds n customers there already, is given by

$$\boldsymbol{\pi}_{\mathbf{r}}(n)\,\boldsymbol{\tau}'_{\mathbf{u}}(n) \quad \text{for } 0 \leq n < N$$

(yes, it is true for $n = 0$). After the system finally gets to $n+1$, it will be in state

$$\boldsymbol{\pi}_{\mathbf{r}}(n)\,\mathbf{H}_{\mathbf{u}}(n).$$

The expression

$$\boldsymbol{\pi}_{\mathbf{r}}(n)\boldsymbol{\tau}'_{\mathbf{u}}(n) + \boldsymbol{\pi}_{\mathbf{r}}(n)\mathbf{H}_{\mathbf{u}}(n)\,\boldsymbol{\tau}'_{\mathbf{u}}(n+1)$$

is the mean first-passage time from n to $n+2$, as seen by a random observer. ■

In Section 4.3.2 we showed that an arriving customer will see much the same thing as a random observer if he remembers not to count himself as a member of the queue. Thus a newly arriving customer will find S_1 in state $\boldsymbol{\pi}_{\mathbf{r}}(n)$, given that there are already n customers there. In other words, he becomes the $(n+1)$st customer. Thus he will *not* see the same mean passage times as did the random observer, because he is part of the action. In fact, he may not even be around long enough to see the queue grow longer than it was when he first arrived. For instance, suppose that a customer arrives at an empty queue. Then he himself enters S_1 and puts it in state $\boldsymbol{\pi}_{\mathbf{r}}(0) = \mathbf{p}$. If he finishes service before the next customer arrives, he will not be around to see the queue grow to 2, even though it will eventually happen [in mean time $\mathbf{p}\boldsymbol{\tau}'_{\mathbf{u}}(1)$]. We state this result as yet another corollary. The reader should compare this with the previous one to be sure that the differences are clear.

Corollary 4.5.2c: The mean time for a steady-state M/ME/1 queue to grow to $n+1$ for the first time, given that the n-th customer has just arrived, is given by

$$\boldsymbol{\pi}_{\mathbf{r}}(n-1)\boldsymbol{\tau}'_{\mathbf{u}}(n) \quad \text{for } 0 < n < N$$

(no, it is not true for $n = 0$). After the queue length finally reaches $n+1$, it will be in state

$$\boldsymbol{\pi}_{\mathbf{r}}(n-1)\mathbf{H}_{\mathbf{u}}(n).$$

The expression

$$\boldsymbol{\pi}_{\mathbf{r}}(n-1)\,\boldsymbol{\tau}'_{\mathbf{u}}(n) + \boldsymbol{\pi}_{\mathbf{r}}(n-1)\,\mathbf{H}_{\mathbf{u}}(n)\,\boldsymbol{\tau}'_{\mathbf{u}}(n+1)$$

is the mean first-passage time for the queue to grow from n to $n+2$, given that a customer has just arrived. ■

The most important variation on the theme of this section is the first-passage time starting with an empty subsystem, or starting with the arrival of a customer to an empty subsystem. We assume the former, but the two differ only by the mean time until a customer arrives, which is $1/\lambda$. This is the process that corresponds to the queue growth discussed in Section 2.3.1 for the M/M/1 queue. To do this, we need two new types of objects.

Definition 4.5.4

$\mathbf{p_u}(n)$:= *probability vector for first passage from* 0 *to* n. Component $[\mathbf{p_u}(n)]_i$ is the probability that a customer will be in state i when the queue at S_1 reaches length n for the first time, given that the queue was initially empty. □

This vector was actually introduced in (4.5.4), but we were not ready to use it then.

Definition 4.5.5

$t_u(n)$:= *mean first-passage time for the queue at* S_1 *to grow from* n *to* $n+1$, *given that the queue was originally empty, and a customer has just arrived.* The process begins at the moment the queue reaches length n. □

This more or less corresponds to Definition 2.3.1 for $\boldsymbol{\tau}_\mathbf{u}(n)$, but an M/M/1 queue has no internal states (or rather, only one internal state), so it did not make any difference when service began.

We can describe this process through the eyes of the random observer. At some time in the past she observed that the queue at S_1 was empty (no one was being served). She then watched the queue, and when it finally reached the length n, she turned on her timer. At that moment, the system was in state $\mathbf{p_u}(n)$. This is the initial vector for what follows. When the queue finally reaches length $n+1$, she turns off the timer. The mean time that her timer shows is $t_u(n)$.

Let us suppose that there is no one at S_1 initially, then in mean time, $t_u(0) = 1/\lambda$, the first customer will arrive, putting the system into internal state $\mathbf{p_u}(1) = \mathbf{p}$. Eventually, the queue will grow to 2 for the first time, in mean time, $t_u(1) = \mathbf{p}\boldsymbol{\tau}'_\mathbf{u}(1)$, at which time the system will be in internal state $\mathbf{p_u}(2) = \mathbf{p}\mathbf{H_u}(1)$. At some time in the future the queue will get to 3 for the first time, taking on average $t_u(2) = \mathbf{p_u}(2)\boldsymbol{\tau}'_\mathbf{u}(2)$ units of time. At that moment the system will find itself in internal state $\mathbf{p_u}(3) = \mathbf{p}\mathbf{H_u}(1)\mathbf{H_u}(2) = \mathbf{p_u}(2)\mathbf{H_u}(2)$. The sequence continues until the number of customers at S_1 reaches N. The total time it takes to go from 0 to n is the sum of the t'_us.

Example 4.5.5: In Figure 4.5.3, we plotted the components of $\mathbf{p_u}(n)$ as a function of n for the M/E_2/1 queue. It is not easy to understand what is going on here, because the process is so complicated. The residual vector (Definition 4.3.1) $\boldsymbol{\pi}_\mathbf{r}(n)$ is quite different from this. In the residual process, a random observer (and for the M/G/1 queue, an arriving customer) will find a steady-state system in vector state $\boldsymbol{\pi}_\mathbf{r}(n)$ as given by (4.3.1), assuming that there were n customers there already. The vector $\mathbf{p_u}(n)$ refers only to the customer whose arrival brings the queue to length n for the first time, given that the queue started at 0. Thus this special customer found $n-1$ customers there already when he arrived. ▲

Definition 4.5.6

$t(0 \to n)$:= ***mean first-passage time from 0 to n***. This is the

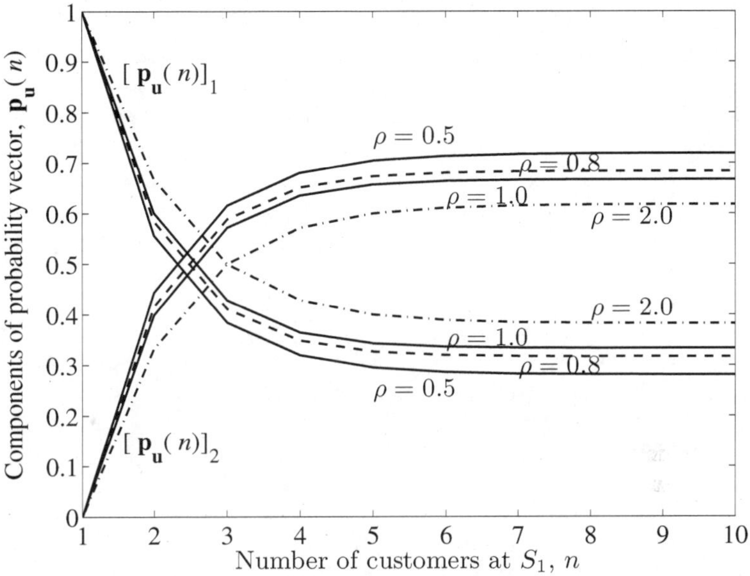

Figure 4.5.3: Components of $\mathbf{p_u}(n)$, the probability vector of first passage from 0 to n, versus n, for the M/E_2/1 queue. If a customer arrives at an empty queue, he will certainly go to phase 1. Thus all curves start with $[1,\ 0]$. The two sets of curves are mirror images of each other about the line $\mathbf{p_u}(n) = 1/2$, because for any n, the sum of the two components is 1. For all ρ, the vectors reach their asymptotic values before $n = 10$. Compare with the mean residual vector $\boldsymbol{\pi_r} = [0.5,\ 0.5]$.

mean time it will take the queue at S_1 to grow to length n, given that S_1 was initially empty. This is the same as Definition 2.3.2. □

This process is summarized by the final corollary of this section.

Corollary 4.5.2d: The mean time for an M/ME/1 queue (open or closed) to grow from n to $n+1$ for the first time, given that S_1 was initially empty, starting with $t_u(0) = 1/\lambda$, is

$$t_u(n) := \mathbf{p_u}(n)\boldsymbol{\tau}'_\mathbf{u}(n), \qquad n = 1,\ 2, \ldots. \tag{4.5.6a}$$

Starting with $\mathbf{p_u}(1) := \mathbf{p}$, the internal state of the system at the moment of first passage to n, $\mathbf{p_u}(n)$ is given recursively by

$$\mathbf{p_u}(n) = \mathbf{p_u}(n-1)\mathbf{H_u}(n-1), \qquad n = 1,\ 2, \cdots \tag{4.5.6b}$$

The mean first-passage time from 0 to n is the same as (2.3.3a), namely

$$t(0 \to n) = \sum_{l=o}^{n-1} t_u(l). \tag{4.5.7}$$

Compare this with (2.3.3a). These formulas are independent of N and are true as long as $n \le N$. ■

Example 4.5.3: The overall behavior of $t(0 \to n)$ for the M/E_2/1 queue is similar to that for the M/M/1 queue, given in Figure 2.3.2. In Figure 4.5.4 we have plotted the two types on the same graph so they can be compared. Although similar, they have distinct differences. As n gets larger, the two curves separate from each other, and the closer ρ gets to 1, the greater the separation, with the E_2 curve lying below the M/M/1 curve. When ρ is much greater than 1, the growth is dominated by the difference of the arrival and service rates, but there *is* a difference, depending on the pdf of S_1. For the M/H_2/1 queue, the differences are more pronounced, and the corresponding curves end up above those for the M/M/1 queue. ▲

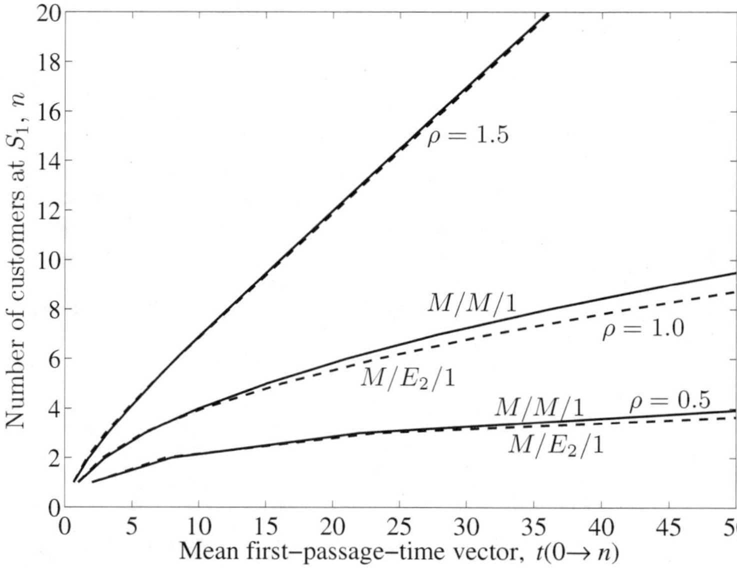

Figure 4.5.4: Comparison of the mean first-passage times from 0 to n, $t(0 \to n)$, between the M/M/1 queue and the M/E_2/1 queue, for ρ =0.5, 1.0, and 1.5. In all cases, the curve corresponding to E_2 ends up lower, but the two do cross.

Is this property dependent on C_v^2? The reader should explore the behavior of this process for other distributions, considering that so little is known about this subject.

Note that the first-passage processes we have been discussing allow the queue at S_1 to empty any number of times before finally reaching its goal. In the third subsection of Section 4.5.3 we study the first excursion to n during a ***busy period***. In that case we find the *probability* that the queue will reach length n before it empties, because it is not certain to do so. We have to develop some other expressions first.

4.5.2 Formal Procedure for Finding System Parameters

After reading the preceding section, the reader must have become familiar with how to set up the expressions needed to calculate various system parameters. We now outline a formal procedure for doing this. First, based on the given conditions, or initial assumptions, one finds the ***initial vector*** $\mathbf{p_i}$, that describes the internal state of the system initially (e.g., the $\mathbf{p_u}$'s). Then, depending on the process of interest, ***propagation matrices***, $\mathbf{S_p}$, are found (e.g., the first-passage matrices). Finally, the ***final vector***, $\mathbf{v'_f}$, that contains the kind of information desired (e.g., $\boldsymbol{\tau}'$ for mean times and $\boldsymbol{\epsilon}'$ for probabilities), is found. The desired scalar property (call it g) is then given by

$$g = \mathbf{p_i S_p v'_f}. \tag{4.5.8a}$$

The initial and final vectors are commonly made of propagation matrices post- or premultiplying other initial or final vectors, whereas propagation matrices are usually products of other propagation matrices. In this way one can build up an unlimited sequence of conditions and results without difficulty. Also, the boundary between $\mathbf{i}$ and $\mathbf{p}$, or $\mathbf{p}$ and $\mathbf{f}$, is not necessarily unique, nor is it important to try to find a definition that makes them unique.

The reader should peruse through the material already covered, to see if this scheme holds true everywhere. In doing so you will notice that almost always, an initial vector can be written as the entrance vector of S_1, $[\mathbf{p}]$, postmultiplied by a propagation matrix (call it $\mathbf{S_i}$). Also, almost always, the final vector can be written as some other propagation matrix (call it $\mathbf{S_f}$), premultiplying $\boldsymbol{\epsilon}'$. This leads to

$$g = \mathbf{p S_i S_p S_f} \boldsymbol{\epsilon}' = \Psi\left[\mathbf{S_i S_p S_f}\right]. \tag{4.5.8b}$$

We now see why the $\Psi[\,\cdot\,]$ operator appears in so many places and why it is such a useful object.

4.5.3 Properties of the k-Busy Period

Everything that goes up must come down; well, almost everything. Whenever S_1 is emptied of customers ($n = 0$), we say that "a busy period has ended." If observation began with some initial conditions (call them collectively $\{\cdots\}$), then we have a "$\{\cdots\}$-busy period." As described in Section 2.3.2, if a customer has just arrived at an empty subsystem, we simply have the beginning of a ***busy period***. Clearly, studying busy periods requires studying queue-length reduction.

We proceed in analogy with Section 4.5.1. However, not all objects will work out in the same way. The $\mathbf{H_d}$ matrices are much simpler than the $\mathbf{H'_u}$s. However, the $\boldsymbol{\tau}'_\mathbf{d}$ vectors depend explicitly on N, as well as n; thus length reduction processes are somewhat more complicated to express. The reason for this, as we presently show, is that in its attempt to go up, the queue can never drop below 0, and thus is bounded by its own length. In trying to shrink, the queue can falter and grow to any length before finally coming down. A ceiling of N is imposed by the system's finite population, and the higher the ceiling, the longer it takes to get down to 0. Actually, first-passage processes to go from n to $n-1$ depend on $N-n$, so unless S_2 is load dependent, the problem is not that bad.

We have one last point before going on. In dealing with a growing queue, we had to start at 0. Similarly, in studying the decreasing queue, the recursive equations must start at N. But where does one start in an open system?

4.5.3.1 Conditional Probabilities for Queue Decrease

The first-passage matrices from n to $n-1$ can be written down with some thought and no algebra. A decrease in queue length can only occur after a departure. Immediately after that a new customer (provided that n was greater than 1 originally) enters S_1, putting the system in internal state $\mathbf{p}$. Given that this is independent of the state the system was in initially, our desired matrix must be $\mathbf{Q}$. However, we go through a full algebraic derivation, because we have do it anyway when we derive the corresponding first-passage times. Define the following matrix for an M/ME/1/ /N loop.

Definition 4.5.7

$\mathbf{H_d}(n;N) :=$ *probability matrix of first passage from n to $n-1$*. Component $[\mathbf{H_d}(n;N)]_{ij}$ is the probability of finding the system in state $\{j;\ n-1;\ N\}$, given that the queue at S_1 has reached length $n-1$ for the first time, after starting in state $\{i;\ n;\ N\}$. □

Next look at Figure 4.5.5. This diagram is similar to Figure 4.5.1, but here the wavy lines go from higher to lower n. It also includes the possibilities when all customers are already at S_1 $[n=N]$. Clearly, if all customers are at S_1, the next event must be there, and either the customer in service stays in S_1, $[\mathbf{P}]$, and then eventually leaves $[\mathbf{H_d}(N;N)]$, or leaves directly, and is replaced by the next customer $[\mathbf{q'p}]$. Thus

$$\mathbf{H_d}(N;N) = \mathbf{P}\mathbf{H_d}(N;N) + \mathbf{q'p}.$$

Now solve for $\mathbf{H_d}(N;N)$ to get, using (3.1.1b):

$$\mathbf{H_d}(N;N) = (\mathbf{I}-\mathbf{P})^{-1}\mathbf{q'p} = \boldsymbol{\epsilon}' p = \mathbf{Q}, \tag{4.5.9a}$$

as expected. For any other $n > 0$ (we drop the $\mathbf{d}$ for now), Figure 4.5.5 implies that

$$\mathbf{H}(n;N) = (\lambda\mathbf{I}+\mathbf{M})^{-1}\mathbf{Mq'p} + (\lambda\mathbf{I}+\mathbf{M})^{-1}\mathbf{MPH}(n;N)$$
$$+\lambda(\lambda\mathbf{I}+\mathbf{M})^{-1}\mathbf{H}(n+1;N)\mathbf{H}(n;N).$$

Once more, left-multiply both sides by $(\lambda\mathbf{I}+\mathbf{M})$, yet again recognize that $\mathbf{Mq'p} = \mathbf{BQ}$, and that $\mathbf{M}-\mathbf{MP} = \mathbf{B}$, to get

$$[\lambda\mathbf{I}+\mathbf{B}-\lambda\mathbf{H}(n+1;N)]\mathbf{H}(n;N) = \mathbf{BQ}. \tag{4.5.9b}$$

Let us look at this equation for $n = N-1$, and make use of (4.5.9a).

$$[\lambda\mathbf{I}+\mathbf{B}-\lambda\mathbf{Q}]\mathbf{H}(N-1;N) = \mathbf{BQ},$$

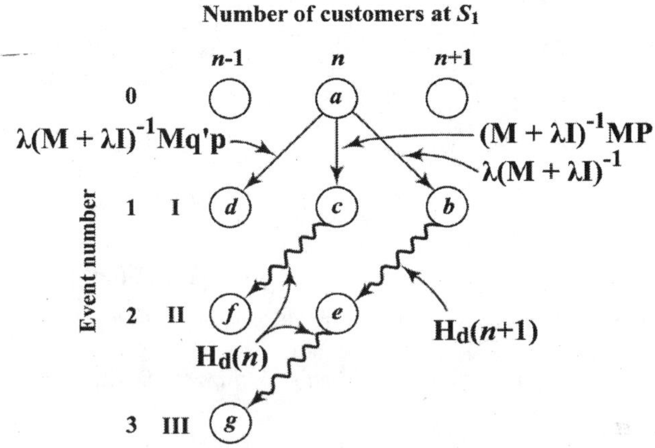

Figure 4.5.5: Time-dependent state transition diagram for both the open and closed M/ME/1 queues, showing what a system must do to go from n to $n-1$ for the first time, as long as $n < N$. Path I is $(a \to d)$, path II is $(a \to c \to f)$, and path III is $(a \to b \to e \to g)$.

but the expression in brackets is, from (4.1.4a), none other than $\lambda\mathbf{A}$ from the s.s. queue, so $\lambda\mathbf{A}\mathbf{H_d}(N-1;N) = \mathbf{BQ}$, or

$$\mathbf{H_d}(N-1;N) = \frac{1}{\lambda}\mathbf{UBQ}.$$

But from Lemma 4.1.1 the right-hand side is $\mathbf{Q}$, so we have

$$\mathbf{H_d}(N-1;N) = \mathbf{Q}. \tag{4.5.10a}$$

Let us look again at (4.5.9b). If $\mathbf{H_d}(n+1;N) = \mathbf{Q}$, then by the same arguments which gave us (4.5.10a), it follows that $\mathbf{H_d}(n;N)$ also equals $\mathbf{Q}$, so by induction, we have proven what we expected for all $N \geq 2$,

$$\mathbf{H_d}(n;N) = \mathbf{Q} \quad \text{for } 1 < n \leq N. \tag{4.5.10b}$$

Because $\mathbf{Q}$ is isometric, so, obviously, are the $\mathbf{H_d}$'s.

4.5.3.2 Mean First-Passage Times for Queue to Drop

We start this section with the prerequisite definition.

Definition 4.5.8

$\boldsymbol{\tau}'_{\mathbf{d}}(n;N)$:= *mean first-passage time vector from n to n-1.* $[\boldsymbol{\tau}'_{\mathbf{d}}(n;N)]_i$ is the mean time for the queue at S_1 to reach $n-1$ for the first time, given that the system started in state $\{i;\ n;\ N\}$. Note that these vectors depend on N as well as n. □

Let us again start with $n = N$. Then we have exactly what we had in Section 3.1.1. As with (3.1.2a),

$$\boldsymbol{\tau}'_{\mathbf{d}}(N;N) = \mathbf{M}^{-1}\boldsymbol{\epsilon}' + \mathbf{P}\,\boldsymbol{\tau}'_{\mathbf{d}}(N;N).$$

We solve for $\boldsymbol{\tau}'_{\mathbf{d}}(N;N)$ to get the same as (3.1.2b),

$$\boldsymbol{\tau}'_{\mathbf{d}}(N;N) = \mathbf{V}\,\boldsymbol{\epsilon}'. \tag{4.5.11a}$$

Now on to the general case. Following our familiar course, we can write

$$\begin{aligned}\boldsymbol{\tau}'_{\mathbf{d}}(n;N) &= (\lambda\mathbf{I}+\mathbf{M})^{-1}\boldsymbol{\epsilon}' + (\lambda\mathbf{I}+\mathbf{M})^{-1}\mathbf{MP}\,\boldsymbol{\tau}'_{\mathbf{d}}(n;N)\\ &\quad + \lambda(\lambda\mathbf{I}+\mathbf{M})^{-1}[\boldsymbol{\tau}'_{\mathbf{d}}(n+1;N) + \mathbf{Q}\,\boldsymbol{\tau}'_{\mathbf{d}}(n;N)].\end{aligned}$$

Regrouping, and so on, gives the following equality.

$$[\lambda\mathbf{I}+\mathbf{M}-\mathbf{MP}-\lambda\mathbf{Q}]\boldsymbol{\tau}'_{\mathbf{d}}(n;N) = \boldsymbol{\epsilon}' + \lambda\boldsymbol{\tau}'_{\mathbf{d}}(n+1;N).$$

This leads to the recursive formula

$$\boldsymbol{\tau}'_{\mathbf{d}}(n;N) = \frac{1}{\lambda}\mathbf{U}\,\boldsymbol{\epsilon}' + \mathbf{U}\,\boldsymbol{\tau}'_{\mathbf{d}}(n+1;N), \tag{4.5.11b}$$

where the reader is reminded that $\mathbf{U} = \mathbf{A}^{-1}$ is given by (4.1.4). We are fortunate that all the first-passage matrices are equal to each other, for now we can actually find an explicit formula for the $\boldsymbol{\tau}'_{\mathbf{d}}$'s. First let $n = N-1$ in (4.5.11b), and use (4.5.11a) to get

$$\boldsymbol{\tau}'_{\mathbf{d}}(N-1;\,N) = \frac{1}{\lambda}\mathbf{U}[\mathbf{I}+\lambda\mathbf{V}]\boldsymbol{\epsilon}'.$$

Similarly, for $n = N-2$,

$$\boldsymbol{\tau}'_{\mathbf{d}}(N-2;N) = \frac{1}{\lambda}\mathbf{U}[\mathbf{I}+\mathbf{U}+\lambda\mathbf{UV}]\boldsymbol{\epsilon}'.$$

In general, one can write, and check by direct substitution into (4.5.11b), that

$$\boldsymbol{\tau}'_{\mathbf{d}}(N-l;N) = \frac{1}{\lambda}\mathbf{U}[\mathbf{I}+\mathbf{U}+\mathbf{U}^2+\cdots+\mathbf{U}^{l-1}+\lambda\mathbf{U}^{l-1}\mathbf{V}]\boldsymbol{\epsilon}'.$$

Compare the expression in brackets with (4.1.6d) and (4.1.6e) to get

$$\boldsymbol{\tau}'_{\mathbf{d}}(N-l;N) = \frac{1}{\lambda}\mathbf{UK}(l)\boldsymbol{\epsilon}' = \frac{1}{\lambda}[\mathbf{K}(l+1)-\mathbf{I}]\boldsymbol{\epsilon}', \tag{4.5.12}$$

where $l = N-n$. Yes, we are already familiar with $\mathbf{K}(N)$, the normalization matrix of the steady-state M/ME/1//N queue.

We could go through the gamut of initial vectors, as we did in the second part of Section 4.5.1, but for now let us only consider $\mathbf{p_i} = \mathbf{p}$ (i.e., the customer in service at S_1 has just begun). Note that this is the *down* vector analogue to $\mathbf{p_u}(n)$ in (4.5.4), because all the $\mathbf{H_d}$'s are equal to $\mathbf{Q}$.

Definition 4.5.9

$t_d(n;N)$:= *mean first-passage time from n to n-1.* This is the mean time it will take for the queue at S_1 to drop to $n-1$ for the first time, given that it started with queue length n and the active customer had just begun service. The "given" part can also be worded as "given that a customer has just departed, leaving n customers behind." Implicit in this is the assumption that the queue can never exceed N. □

From its definition, it follows that

$$t_d(n;N) := \mathbf{p}\boldsymbol{\tau}'_{\mathbf{d}}(n;N) = \frac{1}{\lambda}\left[\Psi\left[\mathbf{K}(N-n+1)\right]-1\right]$$

$$= \frac{1}{\lambda}\left[\frac{1}{r(0;N-n+1)}-1\right] = \frac{1-r(0;N-n+1)}{\lambda\, r(0;N-n+1)}. \tag{4.5.13}$$

This is a rather interesting result. It says, in words, that the mean time to go from n to $n-1$ for the first time in an M/G/1//N queue $[t_d(n,N)]$, can be expressed in terms of properties of the steady-state M/G/1//$(N-n+1)$ queue with the same ρ. It is equal to $1/\lambda$ times the ratio of the steady-state probability that S_1 would be busy to the probability that it would be idle. Furthermore, as long as N is finite, it is true for all ρ.

Of particular interest is the case where $n=1$, for that corresponds to the mean time of a busy period of an M/G/1//N loop. This was discussed in the first part of Section 2.3.2 in the context of the M/M/1//N loop, but now we have a more general theorem for M/G/1 queues. First,

$$\boldsymbol{\tau}'_{\mathbf{d}}(1;N) = \frac{1}{\lambda}[\mathbf{K}(N)-\mathbf{I}]\boldsymbol{\epsilon}', \tag{4.5.14a}$$

then we get an expression that is valid for any G/G/1† queue:

$$t_d(1;N) = \frac{1}{\lambda}\frac{1-r(0;N)}{r(0;N)} = \frac{1}{\lambda}\frac{\textit{s.s. prob. that } S_1 \textit{ is busy}}{\textit{s.s. prob. that } S_1 \textit{ is idle}}. \tag{4.5.14b}$$

The rightmost expression does not explicitly depend upon N. It shows that the ratio of probabilities is the expected number of customers who will be served in a busy period. We proved this formula in (2.3.7d), but in a different way.

The k-busy period for the M/G/1//N loop requires some extra explanation beyond that given in Definition 2.3.4, because we must define the starting state.

Definition 4.5.10

$t(k\to 0;N)$ = *mean time for the k-busy period of an* M/G/1//N *loop.* This is the mean time for the queue at S_1 to drain (drop to 0) given that there were k customers there initially, and the one in service had just begun. □

†The expression, 'GI/G/1' is also commonly used, where 'GI' stands for *General Independent.* Unless otherwise stated, we assume that the arrivals are independent (they constitute a renewal process), so we usually use 'G' in this book.

This mean time is given by (2.3.8a), namely,

$$t(k \to 0; N) = \sum_{n=1}^{k} t_d(n; N). \tag{4.5.15}$$

There are other variations of the busy period, but they only differ in the first term of the sum. For instance, a random observer could come upon a system that has been in operation for an indefinite period, noting that there are k customers at S_1 when she starts her clock. Then the mean time until the queue drops to $k-1$ for the first time is $\boldsymbol{\pi}_{\mathbf{r}}(k; N)\boldsymbol{\tau}'_{\mathbf{d}}(k; N)$, and the mean time to drop to 0 is

$$\boldsymbol{\pi}_{\mathbf{r}}(k; N)\boldsymbol{\tau}'_{\mathbf{d}}(k; N) + t(k-1 \to 0; N).$$

This is a very common process. It corresponds to the request one often gets that "I'd like to see you as soon as you are free." Remember, in this case, the server must not only finish that work which is on hand, but also everything that comes before it finishes.

We close out this section with an examination of the open M/G/1 queue. To do this we must let N become unboundedly large. Now, this requires taking the limit for $N \to \infty$,

$$\mathbf{K} = \lim_{N\to\infty} \mathbf{K}(N).$$

This limit only exists for $\rho < 1$, but when it does exist, it is given in various forms by (4.2.2), and $\Psi[\mathbf{K}] = 1/(1-\rho)$, from (4.2.3e). Therefore, from (4.2.3c) and (4.5.12),

$$\boldsymbol{\tau}'_{\mathbf{d}}(n) := \lim_{N\to\infty} \boldsymbol{\tau}'_{\mathbf{d}}(n; N) = \frac{1}{\lambda}[\mathbf{K} - \mathbf{I}]\boldsymbol{\epsilon}' = \frac{1}{1-\rho}\mathbf{V}\boldsymbol{\epsilon}'. \tag{4.5.16a}$$

So the mean first-passage vector from n to $n-1$ for an open queue is independent of n. Also,

$$t_d(n) := \lim_{N\to\infty} t_d(n; N) = \frac{\bar{x}}{1-\rho}. \tag{4.5.16b}$$

This well-known result tells us that the mean time for a busy period is the same for all M/G/1 queues with the same mean service time, and is equal to the mean system time for the equivalent M/M/1 queue. We would expect this term to be independent of n, because all finite queue lengths are equidistant from their infinite roof. But why does it not depend on the particular pdf of S_1? We saw in Section 2.3.2 that the length of the busy period depends upon the idle time, and thus the interarrival distribution, and the mean service time, but not the service time distribution.

4.5.3.3 Probability That Queue Will Reach Length n

We closely parallel the discussion in the second part of Section 2.3.2, with the added complication that we must keep track of internal states. The consequent matrice $\mathbf{W}_{\mathbf{u}}(n)$, is similar t $\mathbf{H}_{\mathbf{u}}(n)$. In fact, they satisfy the same recursive equations, but they have different initial matrices, and $\mathbf{W}_{\mathbf{u}}(n)$ turns out not to be isometric. Define the following for $k < n < N$:

Definition 4.5.11

$\mathbf{W_u}(n;k)$:= *probability matrix that the queue will go from* n *to* $n+1$ *without dropping to* k. $\mathbf{W_u}(n;k)$ assumes the following initial conditions. Given an M/ME/1//N loop, there are $n < N$ customers at S_1, and the active customer is at phase i. The process ends when either the queue grows to $n+1$, or shrinks to $k < n$. If it is the former, then $[\mathbf{W_u}(n;k)]_{ij}$ is the probability that the system will be in state $\{j;\, n+1;\, N\}$. □

In other words, $[\mathbf{W_u}(n;\, k)]_{ij}$ is the probability that the system will go from $\{i;\, n;\, N\}$ to $\{j;\, n+1;\, N\}$ for some (any) j without going to $\{\cdot\,,\, k;\, N\}$. Component i of vector $\mathbf{W_u}(n;k)\boldsymbol{\epsilon}'$ is the probability of going from $\{i;\, n;\, N\}$ to any internal state of $n+1$ customers, without dropping to k. But this process is not certain to happen, so it cannot have probability 1, thus $\mathbf{W_u}(n;k)$ is not isometric.

This process, and in fact all first-passage processes, fall into the class of ***taboo processes*** (or ***tabu processes***). For such processes, the entire state space of the system is partitioned into three (disjoint) subsets. The process begins with the system in a single state in one of the subsets, and ends when the system finds itself in any one of the states of the other two subsets. In our case, subset 1 consists of all internal states corresponding to queue lengths of $k+1$, $k+2$, ..., $n-1$, and n, whereas subset 2 is all the states with queue length $< k$. Subset 3 consists of all the states with queue length $> n$. It is "tabu' to enter subset 3, and the process is a success if it ends in subset 2. The initial state is $\{i;\, n;\, N\}$, which is an element of subset 1. This concept is much broader than we need. In fact, it obscures the underlying view in LAQT, that all internal states belonging to one queue length should always be treated as a whole.

There is a natural scalar that goes with matrix $\mathbf{W_u}(n;k)$, which we now define.

Definition 4.5.12

$W_u(n;k)$:= *probability that the queue at* S_1 *will rise from* n *to* $n+1$ *without first dropping to* k*, given that the active customer has just begun service*. We call this "the scalar probability associated with $\mathbf{W_u}(n;k)$." From its definition it is clear that

$$W_u(n;k) := \mathbf{p}\mathbf{W_u}(n;k)\boldsymbol{\epsilon}' = \Psi\left[\mathbf{W_u}(n;k)\right]. \tag{4.5.17}$$

Each of the $\mathbf{W}$ matrices we presently introduce has an analogous W scalar counterpart. □

Fortunately, Figure 4.5.1 is applicable to deriving the relationships among the $\mathbf{W_u}(n;k)$s. First look at $\mathbf{W_u}(k+1;k)$. [$\mathbf{W_u}(k;k)$ must be $\mathbf{0}$, because the system is already at its lower bound.] There are two successful paths available in this case. Either an arrival occurs, putting the system in state $\{i;\, n+1\}$ immediately, or there is an internal transition, after which the queue eventually rises to $n+1$ without ever having a departure. Thus

$$\mathbf{W_u}(k+1;k) = \lambda(\lambda\mathbf{I}+\mathbf{M})^{-1} + (\lambda\mathbf{I}+\mathbf{M})^{-1}\mathbf{M}\mathbf{P}\mathbf{W_u}(k+1;k).$$

Multiply by $(\lambda\mathbf{I}+\mathbf{M})$, collect terms, and get

$$\mathbf{W_u}(k+1;k) = \left(\mathbf{I} + \frac{1}{\lambda}\mathbf{B}\right)^{-1} = \lambda(\lambda\mathbf{I}+\mathbf{B})^{-1}. \tag{4.5.18a}$$

We are now ready to treat the general case. Here all three types of events can occur, because the queue at S_1 can drop by 1 and still go back up. We write, for $n > k+1$ (while momentarily dropping the subscript $\mathbf{u}$),

$$\mathbf{W}(n;k) = \lambda(\lambda\mathbf{I}+\mathbf{M})^{-1} + (\lambda\mathbf{I}+\mathbf{M})^{-1}\mathbf{MPW}(n;k) \\ + (\lambda\mathbf{I}+\mathbf{M})^{-1}\mathbf{Mq'pW}(n-1;k)\mathbf{W}(n;k).$$

The usual manipulations lead to the following recursive formulas. For fixed k, and $n > k+1$,

$$\mathbf{W_u}(n;k) = \lambda\left[\lambda\mathbf{I}+\mathbf{B}-\mathbf{BQW_u}(n-1;k)\right]^{-1}. \tag{4.5.18b}$$

So, for instance,

$$\mathbf{W_u}(k+2;k) = \lambda\left[\lambda\mathbf{I}+\mathbf{B}-\mathbf{BQ}(\lambda\mathbf{I}+\mathbf{B})^{-1}\right]^{-1}.$$

A comparison of (4.5.18b) with (4.5.2b) shows that $\mathbf{W_u}(n;k)$ and $\mathbf{H_u}(n)$ satisfy the same recursive formula, yet they are not equal. In particular, $\mathbf{W_u}(n;k)$ is not isometric, even though $\mathbf{H_u}(n)$ is. This apparent dilemma is easily resolved when we recognize that the two sets of matrices have different first matrices in their recursive construction, Equations (4.5.2e) and (4.5.18a). Recall that we proved by induction that $\mathbf{H_u}(n)$ is isometric. First we showed that $\mathbf{H_u}(0)\boldsymbol{\epsilon}' = \boldsymbol{\epsilon}'$, and second, showed that if it was true for $\mathbf{H_u}(n)$, then it must be true for $\mathbf{H_u}(n+1)$. We could show the second part of the proof for $\mathbf{W_u}(n;k)$, but we cannot satisfy the first condition. For $\mathbf{W_u}(k+1;k)$ to be isometric, we must have $\mathbf{B}\boldsymbol{\epsilon}' = \mathbf{o}'$, which in turn implies that $b(x)$, the pdf for S_1, is identically 0 everywhere, an impossibility.

Now we are prepared to find the object described in the title of this section. Let us define the following multistep matrix.

Definition 4.5.13

$\mathbf{W_u}(n \to n+l;k) :=$ *probability matrix that the number of customers at S_1 will grow from n to $n+l$ without dropping to k.* The process starts with the system in state $\{i;\, n\}$, and stops when the system is either in some state with $n+l$ customers, or in some state with $k < n$ customers. $[\mathbf{W_u}(n \to n+l;k)]_{ij}$ is the probability that the system will be in state $\{j;\, n+l\}$ when the process ends. $W_u(n \to n+l;k) := \Psi\left[\mathbf{W_u}(n \to n+l;k)\right]$ is the associated scalar probability. □

$[\mathbf{W_u}(n \to n+l;k)\boldsymbol{\epsilon}']_i$ is the probability that the process will end with $n+l$ customers at S_1, given that it started in internal state i, and $[\mathbf{I} - \mathbf{W_u}(n \to n+l;k)]\boldsymbol{\epsilon}'_i$ is the probability that the process will end with only k customers in the queue.

By their very definitions, we know that

$$\mathbf{W_u}(n \to n+1; k) = \mathbf{W_u}(n; k). \tag{4.5.19a}$$

In analogy with the discussion surrounding (2.3.10a), we see that in order to go up two steps without dropping to k, we must first go up one step without dropping to k, and then go to the second step. Therefore,

$$\mathbf{W_u}(n \to n+2; k) = \mathbf{W_u}(n; k)\mathbf{W_u}(n+1, k) = \mathbf{W_u}(n \to n+1; k)\mathbf{W_u}(n+1; k),$$

or in general,

$$\mathbf{W_u}(n \to n+l+1; k) = \mathbf{W_u}(n \to n+l; k)\mathbf{W_u}(n+l; k). \tag{4.5.19b}$$

This recursive expression is all that is needed to calculate everything, but it can also be written in the alternative form

$$\mathbf{W_u}(n \to n+l+1; k) = \mathbf{W_u}(n; k)\mathbf{W_u}(n+1; k)\cdots\mathbf{W_u}(n+l; k). \tag{4.5.19c}$$

Keep in mind that these matrices do not commute with each other, so the order of multiplication is important.

It is time to summarize the results of this section in a theorem.

Theorem 4.5.3: For any k and n such that $0 \le k < n < N$, the matrices $\mathbf{W_u}(n; k)$ and $\mathbf{W_u}(n \to n+l; k)$ are recursively given by the following procedure. From (4.5.18a)

$$\mathbf{W_u}(k+1;\, k) = \lambda(\lambda\mathbf{I} + \mathbf{B})^{-1}.$$

Next, from (4.5.18b), for $l = 1, 2, \ldots, N-k-1$,

$$\mathbf{W_u}(k+l+1;\, k) = \lambda[\lambda\mathbf{I} + \mathbf{B} - \mathbf{BQW_u}(k+l;\, k)]^{-1}.$$

For any $n > k$, [Equation (4.5.19a)], set

$$\mathbf{W_u}(n \to n+1; k) = \mathbf{W_u}(n; k),$$

and for $l = 1, 2, \ldots, N-n-1$,

$$\mathbf{W_u}(n \to n+l+1; k) = \mathbf{W_u}(n \to n+l; k)\mathbf{W_u}(n+l; k)$$

[from (4.5.19b)]. Given any initial vector $\mathbf{p_I}$, the conditional scalar probabilities of queue growth as defined in this section are given by

$$\mathbf{p_I}\mathbf{W_u}(n; k)\boldsymbol{\epsilon}' \quad \mathit{aand} \quad \mathbf{p_I}\mathbf{W_u}(n \to n+l;\, k)\boldsymbol{\epsilon}'.$$

All of these equations are valid for any ρ, and for both open and closed M/ME/1 systems (as long as $n + l \le N$). ■

There are numerous variations that one can pursue, but by far the most important and most interesting is the "probability that the queue at S_1 will grow to at least n during a ($k = 1$) busy period." Here we want to see the queue reach n without going to 0. Because the busy period is so special, we will provide special treatment.

Definition 4.5.14

$\mathbf{W_u}(n)$:= *probability matrix that the queue at S_1 will rise from n to n+1 customers during a busy period.* This is the same as the probability that the queue will get to some state with $n+1$ customers before it empties, given that the system started with n customers, that is, $\mathbf{W_u}(n) = \mathbf{W_u}(n;\, 0)$. □

Definition 4.5.15

$\mathbf{W_u}(1 \to n)$:= *probability matrix that the queue length at S_1 will reach at least n during a busy period.* The component definitions are the same as those given in Definitions 4.5.11 and 4.5.13, with $k = 0$. $W_u(1 \to n) = \Psi\left[\mathbf{W_u}(1 \to n)\right]$ is the associated scalar probability. □

That is, these matrices satisfy the following equations,

$$\mathbf{W_u}(n) := \mathbf{W_u}(n; 0), \tag{4.5.20a}$$

$$\mathbf{W_u}(1 \to n) := \mathbf{W_u}(1 \to n; 0), \tag{4.5.20b}$$

and $W_u(1 \to n)$ is the same as that defined in the second part of Section 2.3.2. That is, it is the (scalar) probability that the queue at S_1 will grow at least to n during a busy period. Then, by definition, $W_u(1;1) = 1$. Recall that a busy period begins with the arrival of a customer at an empty server, thus the system is initially put into internal state $\mathbf{p}$, with queue length $n = 1$. Then we can state the busy period corollary to Theorem 4.5.3.

Corollary 4.5.3: For any n such that $1 < n < N$, the probability that the queue at S_1 will reach at least n during a busy period can be calculated in the following way. Let

$$\mathbf{W_u}(1) = \lambda(\lambda\mathbf{I} + \mathbf{B})^{-1};\;\; \mathbf{W_u}(1 \to 2) = \mathbf{W_u}(1);$$

$$W_u(1 \to 2) = \Psi\left[\mathbf{W_u}(1 \to 2)\right].$$

Then for $n = 2, 3, \ldots, N-1$,

$$\mathbf{W_u}(n) = \lambda\left[\lambda\mathbf{I} + \mathbf{B} - \mathbf{BQW_u}(n-1)\right]^{-1}, \tag{4.5.21a}$$

$$\mathbf{W_u}(1 \to n+1) = \mathbf{W_u}(1 \to n)\mathbf{W_u}(n), \tag{4.5.21b}$$

with associated scalar probabilities

$$W_u(1 \to n+1) = \Psi\left[\mathbf{W_u}(1 \to n+1)\right]. \tag{4.5.21c}$$

The results are independent of N as long as it is recognized that the queue can never exceed N. Thus the open system satisfies the same formulas; just let $N \to \infty$. ■

Example 4.5.4: We have calculated $W_u(1 \rightarrow n)$ for the M/E_2/1 queue and have plotted the results as a function of n, for various values of ρ, in Figure 4.5.6. We see that if $\rho \leq 1$, the probability goes to 0 as n increases, but for $\rho > 1$, $W_u(1 \rightarrow n)$ asymptotically approaches a value greater than 0. This value is the probability that the busy period will never end. We have also bothered to compare with the M/M/1 queue, as given by Equations (2.3.11) in Figure 4.5.7. Note that for $\rho < 1$ the two queues have similar behavior, but they do cross. For larger n, the M/M/1 queue has a slightly higher probability of growing longer. We would expect this, because the mean queue length for the steady-state M/M/1 queue is longer than that for the M/E_2/1 queue. One should not draw any conclusions about this without first studying other distributions.

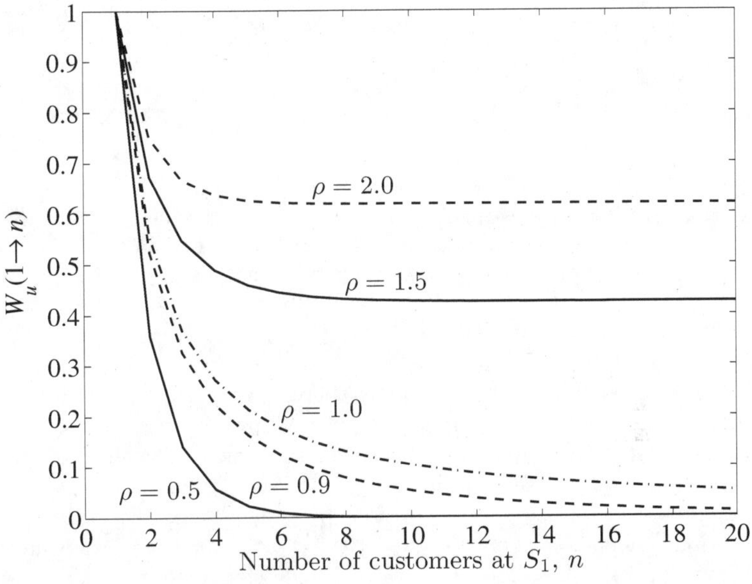

Figure 4.5.6: Probability $W_u(1 \rightarrow n)$ that the number of customers at an M/E_2/1 queue will rise to at least n during a busy period versus n, for ρ =0.5, 0.9, 1.0, 1.5, and 2.0. Obviously, the probability that it will reach at least length one, is 1, for all ρ. For $\rho > 1$ there is a finite probability that the queue will grow forever (if you can find an infinite number of customers). The larger ρ is, the larger that probability.

An unexpected result shows up when ρ is greater than 1. In that case, the open M/ME/1 system can never reach a steady state. We know from (2.3.11c) that the probability that the busy period will never end is $1 - 1/\rho$ for the M/M/1 queue, which for $\rho = 1.5$ is 0.3333, the asymptotic value of that curve. However, for the M/E_2/1 queue the asymptotic value is approximately 0.42, or over 30% higher! This seems to be counterintuitive (if one can have intuition about these things), but after some thought we give the following explanation.

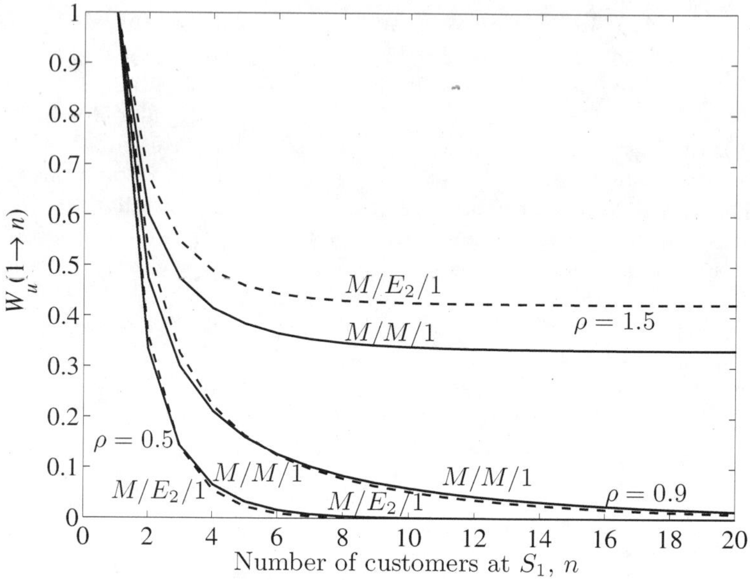

Figure 4.5.7: Comparison of the probability $W_u(1 \to n)$ between the M/M/1 and M/E_2/1 queues versus n, for ρ =0.5, 0.9, and 1.5. The curves for the E_2 queue are the same as those in Figure 4.5.6. For $\rho < 1$ the two curves are close for all n, but for $\rho = 1.5$, the two differ by over 30%. See the text and Figure 4.5.8 for more information.

First note that in the D/D/1 queue there is never any waiting when ρ is less than 1, but there is no chance whatever that the busy period will end when ρ is greater than 1. In these examples, when ρ is greater than 1, the probability that the queue will drain becomes vanishingly small as the queue length increases, hence the rapid approach to the asymptotic value for both distributions (once the queue reaches 10, for $\rho = 1.5$, there is no hope that it will ever drain). Therefore, it is only for short queues that there is some reasonable probability of dropping to 0. For this to happen, the customers who are in the queue must put a smaller demand on the server than is average. Now, the probability that a given customer will make a demand that is far below the mean is much less for Erlangian distributed service times than it is for exponential service times. Therefore, it is less likely to drain.

Consider the other extreme. We can construct distributions in which the vast majority of customers ask for a negligible amount of service time, but once in a while a customer with an enormous demand arrives. In such a case, the probability that the queue will contain only customers with small demands is close to 1, and therefore the queue will probably drain. ▲

In the next example we study the busy period behavior for various distributions, but only for $\rho = 1.5$.

Example 4.5.5: In Figure 4.5.8 we show $W_u(1 \to n)$ for various Erlangians up to $E_{30}(x)$, as well as a hyperexponential-2 distribution with $C_v^2 = 5.039$.

All distributions have a mean of 1. These results are consistent with our arguments in this and the preceding paragraph. The $H_2(x)$ function is of the type in which 90% of the customers have small demands. This is connected to C_v^2, but is not completely dependent on it. So we can only hazard a general statement which says that the probability that the busy period will end tends to increase with C_v^2. Indeed, the Erlangians have $C_v^2 = 1/n$; thus all the curves we present in this figure satisfy the rule. ▲

The above examples lead us to the following observation. The P-K formula in (4.2.6d) tells us that for $\rho < 1$ the bigger C_v^2 is, the more likely it is for the queue to grow very large (big jobs kill). The example tells us that for $\rho > 1$, the bigger C_v^2 is, the more likely it will be for the busy period to end (small jobs save). Remember, large C_v^2 implies the occurrence of jobs that are much bigger than the mean. But to compensate for this, there must also be more jobs that are much smaller than the mean. We warn the reader that this is only a speculation, and the subject requires further study.

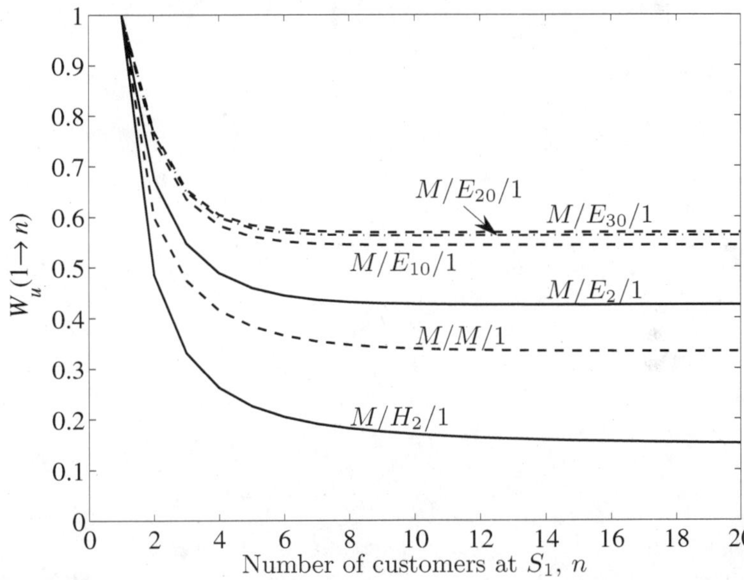

Figure 4.5.8: Probability that the population at S_1 in an M/ME/1 queue will rise to at least n during a busy period, for the exponential, four different Erlangians, and a hyperexponential-2 distribution. Erlangians have a squared coefficient of variation, $C_v^2 = 1/n$, and the hyperexponential function has a $C_v^2 = 5.039$. All have a mean service time of 1, and $\rho = 1.5$. These curves satisfy the rule that the probability for the busy period to end, $[1 - W_u(1 \to \infty)]$, increases with C_v^2.

Very little research has been done on these equations, thus we know of no explicit formulas for the various **W** matrices except for the M/M/1 queue. Surely with some effort, such expressions will be forthcoming. In the meantime, we continue deriving yet more equations, which might leave the reader feeling somewhat overwhelmed. If that is the case, review Section 2.3 yet again, and return here knowing that at the end of the next section the most important equations are summarized in an easy-to-follow algorithm in Theorem 4.5.4.

4.5.3.4 Maximum Queue Length of a Busy Period

In the preceding section we examined the probability that an M/G/1 queue would reach at least n. This did not preclude the possibility that the queue would go even higher. Now we are interested in the probability that the queue will reach exactly n, and no more. In Equation (2.3.16b) we surmised that this probability should be equal to the probability of reaching at least n, minus the probability of reaching at least $n+1$. However, we go through a more tedious process, because that will prove itself useful in studying the busy period of S_2 (i.e., the ME/M/1 queue). Again, in analogy to the third part of Section 2.3.2, we must combine what we just found, with the probability that the queue will decrease to 0 without exceeding n. The reader has presumably become so good at this that we can race through quickly. First define the following matrix, for $1 \leq n \leq k \leq N$.

Definition 4.5.16
$\mathbf{W_d}(n; k)$:= *probability matrix of dropping from* n *to* $n-1$, *without exceeding* $k \geq n$. Note the slight difference in definition between this *down* operator and its counterpart *up* operator described in Definition 4.5.11. In the *up* case, the queue was not allowed to drop as low as k, whereas here, the queue must not exceed k. $W_d(n; k) := \Psi[\mathbf{W_d}(n; k)]$ is the associated scalar probability. Strictly speaking, we should include $\mathbf{W_d}$'s dependence on N, as we did in Definition 2.3.8. But as long as $k < N$, $\mathbf{W_d}(n; k)$ does not depend upon N. □

As with the M/M/1//N queue and the first part of Section 4.5.3, for $\mathbf{H_d}(N; N)$, $\mathbf{W_d}(N; N) = \mathbf{Q}$. In fact,

$$\mathbf{W_d}(n; N) = \mathbf{H_d}(n; N) = \mathbf{Q} \quad \text{for all } n \leq N, \tag{4.5.22a}$$

because the queue can never exceed length N in any case. The same cannot be said when $k < N$, for here (using Figure 4.5.5 and recalling that $\mathbf{Mq'p} = \mathbf{BQ}$)

$$\mathbf{W_d}(k; k) = (\lambda\mathbf{I} + \mathbf{M})^{-1}\mathbf{BQ} + (\lambda\mathbf{I} + \mathbf{M})^{-1}\mathbf{MPW_d}(k; k)$$

or,

$$\mathbf{W_d}(k; k) = (\lambda\mathbf{I} + \mathbf{B})^{-1}\mathbf{BQ} = (\mathbf{I} + \lambda\mathbf{V})^{-1}\mathbf{Q} \quad \text{for } k < N. \tag{4.5.22b}$$

Finally, using the same arguments as those required to derive (2.3.12b), we have for $0 < n \leq k < N$,

$$\begin{aligned}\mathbf{W_d}(n-1; k) &= [\lambda\mathbf{I} + \mathbf{B} - \lambda\mathbf{W_d}(n; k)]^{-1}\mathbf{BQ} \\ &= [\mathbf{I} + \lambda\mathbf{V} - \lambda\mathbf{VW_d}(n; k)]^{-1}\mathbf{Q}.\end{aligned} \tag{4.5.22c}$$

Note that all these matrices have $\mathbf{Q}$ as a multiplying factor. This means that $\mathbf{W_d}(n;k)$ is not invertible (unless S_1 is of dimension 1) and in fact is of rank 1. $\mathbf{Q}$ has such unique properties that it is useful to have it appear explicitly whenever possible. We can do this by introducing an auxiliary matrix function which, when right-multiplied by $\mathbf{Q}$, will yield $\mathbf{W_d}(n;k)$. Also observe from (4.5.22b) that $\mathbf{W_d}(k;k)$ is the same for all $k < N$. Therefore [from (4.5.22c)],

$$\mathbf{W_d}(k-1;\, k) = [\lambda \mathbf{I} + \mathbf{B} - \lambda \mathbf{W_d}(k;\, k)]^{-1}\mathbf{BQ}$$

is also independent of k. Then, by induction, we can show that for all $k_1,\, k_2 \geq l$,

$$\mathbf{W_d}(k_1 - l; k_1) = \mathbf{W_d}(k_2 - l; k_2).$$

This means we can define for $k < N$,

$$\mathbf{Z}(0) := (\mathbf{I} + \lambda \mathbf{V})^{-1}, \tag{4.5.23a}$$

and recursively define for $l = 1, 2, \ldots,$

$$\mathbf{Z}(l) := [\lambda \mathbf{I} + \mathbf{B} - \lambda \mathbf{Z}(l-1)\mathbf{Q}]^{-1}\mathbf{B} = [\mathbf{I} + \lambda \mathbf{V} - \lambda \mathbf{V}\mathbf{Z}(l-1)\mathbf{Q}]^{-1}. \tag{4.5.23b}$$

It can be proven by direct substitution into (4.5.22b) and (4.5.22c) that

$$\mathbf{W_d}(n;\, k) = \mathbf{Z}(k-n)\mathbf{Q}, \quad \text{for } 1 \leq n \leq k < N, \tag{4.5.23c}$$

and for $k = N$, we use (4.5.22a). We make use of these equations below.

The obvious definition of the matrix that carries the queue from n to $n-l$ is given by the following.

Definition 4.5.17

$\mathbf{W_d}(n \to n-l; k)$:= *probability matrix of dropping from n to n - l, without exceeding k, where* $N \geq k \geq n$.

The associated scalar, the *down* equivalent of Definition 4.5.13, is given by $W_d(n \to n-l; k) := \Psi\,[\mathbf{W_d}(n \to n-l; k)]$. Also,

$\mathbf{W_k}(k \to 0)$ =*Probability matrix that the queue will go all the way from k to* 0 *without exceeding* $k < N$. □

From their definitions, we can say that $\mathbf{W_d}(k \to k-1; k) = \mathbf{W_d}(k; k)$, and for $k < N$,

$$\mathbf{W_d}(k \to 0) \;=\; \mathbf{W_d}(k;k)\mathbf{W_d}(k-1;k)\cdots\mathbf{W_d}(1;k), \tag{4.5.24a}$$

and for $k = N$,

$$\mathbf{W_d}(N \to 0) = \mathbf{Q}. \tag{4.5.24b}$$

We must make one clarifying remark before going on. Recall that we used the artificial convention that when no one was at S_1, we would make believe that the system was in internal state $\mathbf{p}$. If we instead use the realistic convention that an empty queue has only one state, we have the following column vectors.

$$\mathbf{w}'_{\mathbf{d}}(1;k) = [\mathbf{I} + \lambda\mathbf{V} - \lambda\mathbf{V}\mathbf{W_d}(2;\, k)]^{-1}\boldsymbol{\epsilon}' \quad \text{for } 1 < k < N. \tag{4.5.25a}$$

We also have

$$\mathbf{w}'_{\mathbf{d}}(1;N) = \mathbf{w}'_{\mathbf{d}}(N \to 0) = \boldsymbol{\epsilon}'. \tag{4.5.25b}$$

Note that these equations are for $n = 1$ only, because that is the only time the empty queue is reached.

To go from the artificial to the real convention, one merely right-multiplies with $\boldsymbol{\epsilon}'$ ($\mathbf{Q}\,\boldsymbol{\epsilon}' = \boldsymbol{\epsilon}'$). For instance,

$$\mathbf{w}'_{\mathbf{d}}(1;k) = \mathbf{W}_{\mathbf{d}}(1;k)\boldsymbol{\epsilon}',$$

and conversely,

$$\mathbf{W}_{\mathbf{d}}(1;k) = \mathbf{w}'_{\mathbf{d}}(1;k)\mathbf{p}.$$

The distinction between the vector and matrix objects becomes meaningful when the arrival process is not Poisson, for then, even when the queue is empty, the arrival process is in some state. We show this in Chapter 5.

Equation (4.5.24a) simplifies considerably when Equations (4.5.23) are substituted into it, for now we have (using the real convention)

$$\mathbf{w}'_{\mathbf{d}}(k \to 0) = \mathbf{Z}(0)\mathbf{Q}\,\mathbf{Z}(1)\cdots\mathbf{Q}\,\mathbf{Z}(k-1)\boldsymbol{\epsilon}' \quad \text{for } k < N.$$

But recall from Lemma 3.5.1 that $\mathbf{Q^2} = \mathbf{Q}$, and for any square matrix, $\mathbf{D}, \mathbf{QDQ} = \Psi\left[\mathbf{D}\right]\mathbf{Q}$. Also note that $\Psi\left[\mathbf{DQ}\right] = \Psi\left[\mathbf{QD}\right] = \Psi\left[\mathbf{D}\right]$, so

$$W_d(n;k) = Z(k-n) := \Psi\left[\mathbf{W}_{\mathbf{d}}(n;k)\right] = \Psi\left[\mathbf{Z}(k-n)\right]. \tag{4.5.26a}$$

All this leads to, for $k < N$,

$$\mathbf{w}'_{\mathbf{d}}(k \to 0) = \left[Z(1)\,Z(2)\,\cdots\,Z(k-1)\right](\mathbf{I} + \lambda\mathbf{V})^{-1}\boldsymbol{\epsilon}', \tag{4.5.26b}$$

which is a vector.

The object in brackets is a product of scalars, and thus is itself a scalar, so the vectors $[\mathbf{w}'_{\mathbf{d}}(k \to 0)$ for $1 \le k < N]$ are all proportional to the same vector $\mathbf{v}' := (\mathbf{I} + \lambda\mathbf{V})^{-1}\boldsymbol{\epsilon}'$. This vector is interesting in its own right, because from (3.1.10), it is the generator of the Laplace transform of S_1 [i.e., $\mathbf{pv}' = \mathbf{B}^*(\lambda)$]. But what is more relevant to our discussion, is that $\mathbf{pv}'$ is the probability that S_1 will complete service before S_2, given that they started at the same time! In fact, for any initial condition described by $\mathbf{p_i}$, $\mathbf{p_i v}'$ is the probability that S_1 will finish before S_2. Sometimes one wonders if the Laplace transform is a mathematical trick to divert us from getting a physical insight as to what is going on. D. G. Kendall [KENDALL64] apparently shared this view in stating the desire of "... raising the Laplacian curtain which has hitherto obscured much of the queue-theoretic scene."

We see that (4.5.24) to (4.5.26) actually depend on N in an obvious but nontrivial way. We do not make the notation any more complicated than it is at present, because these matrices are of secondary importance to the last defined function of this chapter. It was actually defined in Section 2.3.2 for the M/M/1 queue. The same definition for the M/ME/1//N queue suffices here as well. The object of interest is a scalar, because we both start and end with no one at S_1. Define the following scalar.

Definition 4.5.18

$W_m(k;N)$:=probability that the queue at S_1 will reach a maximum of k during a busy period of an M/ME/1//N loop. For this process to occur, the queue must grow from 0 to k without ever returning to 0, $[\mathbf{pW_u}(1 \to k)]$, and then it must reduce to 0 without ever exceeding k, $[\mathbf{w}'_\mathbf{d}(k \to 0)]$. □

Therefore, we have

$$W_m(k;N) = \mathbf{pW_u}(1 \to k)\mathbf{w}'_\mathbf{d}(k \to 0), \tag{4.5.27a}$$

which upon using (4.5.26) yields

$$W_m(k;N) := \left(\prod_{l=1}^{k-1} Z(l)\right) \Psi\left[\mathbf{W_u}(1 \to k)(\mathbf{I} + \lambda\mathbf{V})^{-1}\right], \tag{4.5.27b}$$

and by putting (4.5.24b) into (4.5.27a) for $k = N$,

$$W_m(N;N) := \Psi\left[\mathbf{W_u}(1 \to N)\right] = W_u(1 \to N). \tag{4.5.27c}$$

With some practice, one can figure out what process is going on just by looking at the terms in the equation. For instance, in (4.5.27b), the term inside the Ψ brackets is the probability that the queue will get to k, $[\mathbf{W_u}(1 \to k)]$, and then drop back to $k-1$, $[(\mathbf{I} + \lambda\mathbf{V})^{-1}]$. ‡ Then the queue works its way back to 0 without ever exceeding k $[Z(1), Z(2), \ldots, Z(k-1)]$.

We are indeed fortunate to find $Z(\cdot)$s that are so simple. For more complicated systems (either load-dependent, M/ME/C, or ME/ME/1), we do not find such simple equations for these processes, although the general formalism is the same. We are still left with the question of how Equation (2.3.16b) connects ***up*** and ***down operators***. Recall that

$$W_m(k;N) = W_u(1 \to k) - W_u(1 \to k+1),$$

thus, from (4.5.21b), (4.5.27a), and (4.5.26b), we can write

$$\begin{aligned} W_m(k;N) &= \mathbf{pW_u}(1 \to k)\mathbf{w}'_\mathbf{d}(k \to 0) \\ &= \mathbf{pW_u}(1 \to k)[\mathbf{I} - \mathbf{W_u}(k)]\boldsymbol{\epsilon}'. \end{aligned} \tag{4.5.28a}$$

A sufficient condition for this to be true is for the following equation to be true.

$$\begin{aligned} [\mathbf{I} - \mathbf{W_u}(k)]\boldsymbol{\epsilon}' &= \mathbf{w}'_\mathbf{d}(k \to 0) \\ &= [Z(1)\, Z(2) \cdots Z(k-1)]\,(\mathbf{I} + \lambda\mathbf{V})^{-1}\boldsymbol{\epsilon}'. \end{aligned} \tag{4.5.28b}$$

It would be nice if we could prove this equality algebraically, for it might give us some further insights into *up* and *down* processes.

We now show how this all fits together in the following summary algorithm/theorem.

‡Remember, this is the operator which finds the probability that S_1 will finish before S_2.

Theorem 4.5.4: For any M/ME/1//N loop, and for any ρ, the busy-period queue-length probabilities of Definitions 4.5.15 and 4.5.18 can be calculated using Equations (4.5.21), (4.5.23), and (4.5.27) [or (4.5.28a)], in the following way.

BEGIN PROCEDURE

* Set

. $\mathbf{Z}(0) = (\mathbf{I} + \lambda\mathbf{V})^{-1}$,

. $\mathbf{W_u}(0) = \mathbf{0}$,

. $\mathbf{w_u}(1 \to 1) = \mathbf{p}$

. $z(1) = 1$,

. $W_m(1) = \Psi\left[(\mathbf{I} + \lambda\mathbf{V})^{-1}\right]$,

. $W_u(1 \to 1) = 1$.

. FOR $n = 1$ TO $NMAX$, DO

. $\mathbf{Z}(n) := [\mathbf{I} + \lambda\mathbf{V} - \lambda\mathbf{V}\mathbf{Z}(n-1)\mathbf{Q}]^{-1}$,

. $\mathbf{W_u}(n) = \lambda[\lambda\mathbf{I} + \mathbf{B} - \mathbf{B}\mathbf{Q}\mathbf{W_u}(n-1)]^{-1}$,

. $\mathbf{w_u}(1 \to n+1) = \mathbf{w_u}(1 \to n)\mathbf{W_u}(n)$,.

. $Z(n) = \Psi[\mathbf{Z}(n)]$

. $z(n+1) = z(n)Z(n)$

. $W_u(1 \to n+1) = \mathbf{w_u}(1 \to n+1)\boldsymbol{\epsilon}'$

. $W_m(n+1) = z(n+1)\mathbf{w_u}(1 \to n+1)(\mathbf{I} + \lambda\mathbf{V})^{-1}\boldsymbol{\epsilon}'$.

. END FOR

END PROCEDURE

For any M/ME/1//N loop, with $N \geq 2$, the probability that the queue at S_1 will contain at least n customers at one time during a busy period is given by the sequence

$$1,\ W_u(1 \to 2),\ W_u(1 \to 3),\ \ldots,\ W_u(1 \to N-1),\ W_u(1 \to N).$$

The probability that the largest queue length during a busy period will be n is given by the sequence

$$W_m(1),\ W_m(2),\ \ldots,\ W_m(N-1),\ W_u(1 \to N).$$

(Note: The last term in the sequence is correct.) ∎

In both sequences, the dependence on N is determined by how one ends the sequence. For the open queue, the sequences never end, but when $\rho \leq 1$ they tend to 0. If $\rho > 1$, then $W_u(1 \to N)$ will not approach 0, but instead will approach

$$\lim_{N\to\infty} W_u(1 \to N) = \text{probability that a busy period will never end.}$$

Example 4.5.6: We have calculated the W_m's, once again for the M/E_2/1/20 queue, and compared them with the corresponding values for the M/M/1/20 queue for three different values of ρ. The results are presented in Figure 4.5.9. For any given ρ, when n is small, the curve for the exponential distribution is higher than that for the E_2. But because the sum over all integer points must be 1, the two curves cross somewhere, and for large n, the curve for E_2 is higher. We give the same warning here as we did for the other curves. Although the two distributions yield similar results, one should look for other distributions that could give radically different results. ▲

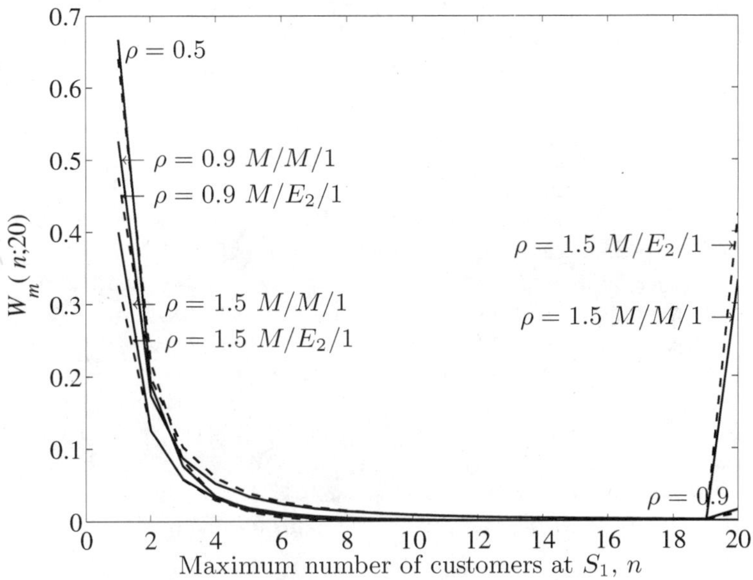

Figure 4.5.9: Probability $W_m(n; 20)$ as a function of n, for both the M/M/1 and M/E_2/1 queues. Three sets of curves are shown, for $\rho = 0.5$, 0.9, and 1.5. The curves for the M/M/1 queue are the same as those in Figure 2.3.4 as long as $n < 20$. The value at $n = 20$ corresponds to the probability that the queue will exceed 19 during a busy period for any loop where $N \geq 20$, so for $\rho > 1$ it is quite significant. Even for $\rho = 0.9$, this probability is not negligible. The sum over all integer points must be 1.

As a final comment, note that $N = 1$ is a trivial case, for then the queue will always grow to 1, and never grow further before the busy period ends. For $N = 2$, we have

$$W_m(1) = \Psi\left[(\mathbf{I} + \lambda\mathbf{V})^{-1}\right]$$

and

$$W_m(2) = \lambda\Psi\left[(\lambda\mathbf{I} + \mathbf{B})^{-1}\right].$$

The first equation, as we have noted before, is the probability that S_1 will finish before S_2, and of course, the second term is the probability that S_2 will finish before S_1. Their sum must be 1, which is easily shown by the following:

$$\begin{aligned}(\mathbf{I} + \lambda\mathbf{V})^{-1} + \lambda(\lambda\mathbf{I} + \mathbf{B})^{-1} &= (\mathbf{I} + \lambda\mathbf{V})^{-1} + \lambda\mathbf{V}(\mathbf{I} + \lambda\mathbf{V})^{-1} \\ &= [\mathbf{I} + \lambda\mathbf{V}](\mathbf{I} + \lambda\mathbf{V})^{-1} = \mathbf{I},\end{aligned}$$

followed by $\Psi[\mathbf{I}] = 1$.

4.5.4 Mean Time to Failure with Backup and Repair

Our emphasis so far has been on viewing customers as individuals who go around in circles demanding service, one at a time, from two different subsystems. An increasingly important application, with a completely different emphasis than we usually see in queueing theory texts, occurs in reliability theory, where one asks such questions as: "how long it will take before a subsystem has fewer functional components than is acceptable?" We are ready to set up the procedure by which such questions can be analyzed, using the material already discussed in this chapter. We are even prepared to solve many of the simpler problems, although the question of how one deals with multiple components functioning simultaneously must wait until Chapter 6. It is most important to note that the procedures we discuss now generalize directly once we have set up the structure for parallel processing.

Consider the following. Suppose that we have several identical appearing devices (terminals, computers, automobiles, VLSI chips, etc.). Once one of them is turned on, it continues to run until it fails (breaks down, or something). Assume that the lifetime of one of these devices is described by the function $R_1(t)$. As you already know, this is the reliability function for S_1, which is where the name came from. That is, $R_1(t)$ is the probability that the device will still be functioning t units of time after it was first turned on, and $b_1(t) = -R_1'(t)$ is the pdf of the failure time. If only one device is available, the ***Mean Time To Failure*** (MTTF) is the expected life of the device, namely,

$$T_1 := \int_0^\infty t\, b_1(t)\, dt = \int_0^\infty R(t)\, dt.$$

(It is easy to show, and is well known, that the two integrals are always equal.)

Let there now be several devices available, and as soon as the first one fails, a second one is started up. The second one is referred to as a ***cold backup*** (cold, because it does not start up until the first one fails). If the first one is discarded, the pdf of the time until both have failed is the convolution of $b_1(t)$ with itself, with an MTTF of $2T_1$. Suppose, instead, that the broken one is immediately sent to the repair shop (with only one repairman), where the time it takes to fix it is distributed according to the pdf $b_2(x)$. As soon as it is repaired, it is returned to the pool of available devices, as good as new [its reliability function $R_1(t)$ is the same as it was the first time through]. The question to be answered is: "how long will it take to reach the unfortunate state where all the devices are in the repair shop?" Thus we have described the title of this section.

Let us call the process above, scheme (1). There are numerous variations that one can play on this scheme, some of which are: (2) failure occurs when only one (or in general, k) device(s) is (are) still functioning; (3) a backup must always be running, whether it is being used or not, even while the primary device is still functioning (hot backup, or parallel redundancy); and (4) the system has been running for some unknown time before questions are asked (residual times). Schemes (2) and (4) can be treated with material that we already have prepared in this chapter, but scheme (3) must wait until Chapter

6 and the M/G/C//N queue.

By now it should be clear to the reader that if we let S_1 represent $b_1(t)$, and $b_2(x)$ is exponentially distributed with mean $1/\lambda$, then we are looking at an M/ME/1//N loop, where N is the total number of devices (i.e., $N-1$ backups). Following scheme (1), suppose that initially all devices are functional, and one of them is started. Then the initial vector is $\mathbf{p}$ itself. The MTTF in this circumstance is the same as the mean time for the N-busy period, $t(N \to 0; N)$, as given in Definition 4.5.10. The ***utilization parameter*** ρ is less meaningful in this context. It is still λT_1, which is now the ratio of the mean lifetime to the mean repair time of a single device. We are not particularly interested in systems where ρ is close to 1, nor do open systems have much relevance (an infinite number of backups? Well, maybe in inventory problems where new parts are being manufactured continuously). Instead, we might expect ρ to be much greater than 1, because it usually takes much less time to repair a device than it did for it to break in the first place (retail commercial products such as children's toys excepted).

Let us first examine our equations for $N = 1$. Here repair time is of no significance (once you start falling, if you do not have a spare parachute, it is no use telling you that your failed parachute "can be mended in no time at all, after you land"), so as we said before, $MTTF(1) = T_1$.

The case where $N = 2$ is most enlightening. As before, the mean time for the first one to fail is T_1, but now the race is on to see if the first device can be repaired before the second one fails. According to (4.5.15),

$$MTTF(2) = t_d(1;2) + t_d(2;2).$$

But from (4.5.11a),

$$t_d(2;2) = \mathbf{p}\boldsymbol{\tau}'_{\mathbf{d}}(2;2) = \mathbf{pV}\boldsymbol{\epsilon}' = T_1$$

(of course), and from (4.5.12),

$$t_d(1;2) = \mathbf{p}\boldsymbol{\tau}'_{\mathbf{d}}(1;2) = \frac{1}{\lambda}\Psi\left[\mathbf{U}(\mathbf{I}+\lambda\mathbf{V})\right].$$

We played with expressions similar to this in Section 4.4.3. Look at (4.4.8b), where $\mathbf{C} = \lambda\mathbf{VD} = \mathbf{I} - \mathbf{D}$, $\mathbf{D} = (\mathbf{I}+\lambda\mathbf{V})^{-1}$, $\gamma_1 = \Psi[\mathbf{C}] = 1 - \Psi[\mathbf{D}]$, and

$$\mathbf{pU}(\mathbf{I}+\lambda\mathbf{V}) = \frac{1}{1-\gamma_1}\mathbf{pCD}^{-1} = \lambda\Psi[\mathbf{D}]\,\mathbf{pV}.$$

Therefore, $t_d(1;2) = T_1/\Psi[\mathbf{D}]$, so

$$MTTF(2) = T_1\left(1 + \frac{1}{\Psi[\mathbf{D}]}\right). \tag{4.5.29a}$$

As expected, the MTTF is proportional to the mean uptime of one device, but it also depends on the term $1/\Psi[\mathbf{D}]$, which can be interpreted as the expected number of times the broken device will be repaired before the good one fails, given that both processes began simultaneously. First, we show that $\Psi[\mathbf{D}]$ is truly the probability that repair will occur before backup failure.

Given that two processes (call them S_1 and S_2) begin simultaneously,

$$X := \mathbb{P}\mathbf{r}(S_1 \text{ will finish before } S_2) = \int_0^\infty b_1(t) R_2(t)\, dt.$$

But in our case, S_2 is exponentially distributed, so $R_2(t) = \exp(-\lambda t)$, and from (3.1.10),

$$X = \int_0^\infty e^{-\lambda t} b_1(t) dt = B^*(\lambda) = \Psi\left[(\mathbf{I} + \lambda \mathbf{V})^{-1}\right] = \Psi[\mathbf{D}].$$

Thus we have shown that the Laplace transform and the definition of X are the same. Which interpretation is more basic to our understanding of this process? Well, (4.5.29a) is also the expression for the MTTF of a **G**/G/1//2 queue, but in that case, altough the expression for X will still hold, there will be no Laplace transform to interpret, because in that more general case R_2 is not exponential.

Let us look at (4.5.29a) one more time before going on to $N > 2$. Note that if there is no repair ($\lambda = 0$), then $X = 1$, and $MTTF(2) = 2T_1$, as already predicted. On the other hand, if repair is instantaneous (and breakdown can never occur instantaneously), then $X = 0$ and $MTTF(2) = \infty$, also as expected. A third possibility, implied by the parenthetical statement, is the probability that breakdown *can* occur instantaneously. This would happen, for instance, if the backup part was already faulty. We have almost completely ignored this possibility in our discussions, but it is easily handled. It corresponds to $R_1(0) = 1 - \alpha < 1$, and to a service time matrix, $\mathbf{V}$, which has a 0 eigenvalue. Such distributions are referred to as ***defective distributions*** [FELLER71] and can be handled by a pdf of the form

$$b_1(x) = \alpha\delta(x - 0_+) + (1 - \alpha) f_1(x),$$

where α is the probability that a part is faulty to begin with, and f_1 is the pdf for parts that are not faulty. δ is the ***Dirac delta function***, which is described in detail in (3.2.5), and in (5.1.12a) and following. If we put this into the equation for X, and note that at least $R_2(0) = 1$, we get

$$X = \alpha + (1 - \alpha) \int_0^\infty f_1(x) R_2(x) dx. \tag{4.5.29b}$$

From this we see that even if repair is almost instantaneous (assume that instantaneous breakdown occurs before instantaneous repair), X must be greater than α, and

$$MTTF(2) \le T_1 \left(1 + \frac{1}{\alpha}\right) < \infty.$$

This implies that the behavior of $b_1(x)$ for very small x (even if there is no instantaneous breakdown) could be critical for estimating the mean time to failure of a system.

We were able to find a convenient expression for $MTTF(2)$, but for $N > 2$ it becomes more tedious. Because (4.5.12) is fairly simple, we now seek a general expression that is not recursive. From (4.5.12) and (4.5.13) we know that $t_d(N-l;N) = \Psi[\mathbf{UK}(l)]/\lambda$. Therefore from (4.5.15),

$$MTTF(N) = t(N \to 0; N) = \frac{1}{\lambda}\sum_{k=1}^{N} t_d(k;N) = \frac{1}{\lambda}\sum_{k=1}^{N} \Psi[\mathbf{UK}(N-k)].$$

Now let $l = N - k$; then

$$MTTF(N) = \frac{1}{\lambda}\sum_{l=o}^{N-1} \Psi[\mathbf{UK}(l)]. \tag{4.5.30a}$$

We actually have worked with something like this already, in Section 4.3.1. There, in (4.3.4b) we showed that (we have replaced N with $l+1$)

$$\mathbf{p}[\mathbf{K}(l+1) - \mathbf{I}] = \frac{1}{1-\rho}\left(1 - \Psi\left[\mathbf{U}^l\lambda\mathbf{V}\right]\right)\lambda\mathbf{pV}.$$

But $\mathbf{K}(l+1) - \mathbf{I} = \mathbf{UK}(l)$, so if we postmultiply with $\boldsymbol{\epsilon}'$, we get

$$\Psi[\mathbf{UK}(l)] = \frac{\rho}{1-\rho}\left(1 - \lambda\Psi\left[\mathbf{U}^l\mathbf{V}\right]\right).$$

When this is placed in (4.5.30a), and we use the fact that [see (4.1.6f)]

$$\sum_{l=o}^{N-1} \mathbf{U}^l = \mathbf{K}(\mathbf{I} - \mathbf{U}^N),$$

with $\mathbf{K} = (\mathbf{I} - \mathbf{U})^{-1}$ [from (4.2.2a)], we get

$$\begin{aligned} MTTF(N) &= \frac{1}{\lambda}\frac{\rho}{1-\rho}\left(N - \lambda\Psi\left[\sum_{l=o}^{N-1}\mathbf{U}^l\mathbf{V}\right]\right) \\ &= \frac{NT_1}{1-\rho} - \frac{\rho}{1-\rho}\Psi\left[\mathbf{K}(\mathbf{I} - \mathbf{U}^N)\mathbf{V}\right]. \end{aligned}$$

Now, from its definition, we know that $\mathbf{KU} = \mathbf{K} - \mathbf{I}$, and by postmultiplying (4.2.3b) with $\mathbf{U}$, we know that $\mathbf{pKU} = [\lambda/(1-\rho)]\mathbf{pV}$, so with some awkward manipulation, we get the following expression.

$$MTTF(N) = \frac{N-\rho}{1-\rho}T_1 - \frac{\lambda}{1-\rho}\Psi\left[\mathbf{V}^2\right] + \frac{\rho}{1-\rho}\Psi\left[\mathbf{KU}^N\mathbf{V}\right]. \tag{4.5.30b}$$

This expression is deceptive in that it seems to be telling us that the MTTF depends on $\Psi\left[\mathbf{V}^2\right]$, when it really does not, at least not for small N. When N is small, the last term can be manipulated so that it cancels the middle term, as well as the dependence on $1/(1-\rho)$, as can clearly be seen from the expressions we already derived for $MTTF(1)$ and $MTTF(2)$. However, it does tell us this much for $\rho < 1$. For then, $\mathbf{U}^N$ gets to be negligibly small for large N, and thus $MTTF(N)$ grows as $NT_1/(1-\rho)$. Anyway, either (4.5.30a) or (4.5.30b) can be used to calculate $MTTF(N)$ in general.

From what we have seen in this section, there are unlimited variations one can pursue based on what has been done. We have already suggested a few. We elaborate further here. For instance, suppose that a system has N devices, and one has just failed, leaving behind k good ones. What is the $MTTF$ then? The answer is $t(k \to 0; N)$, from (4.5.15). But what if you, as the new manager have just arrived, and do not know when the last breakdown occurred; what is the $MTTF$ then? You are the random observer, and the system was in state $\boldsymbol{\pi}_\mathbf{r}(k)$ (see Corollary 4.5.2b) when you arrived. Thus the MTTF is the mean time to drop from k to $k-1$, and thence to 0:

$$MTTF = \boldsymbol{\pi}_\mathbf{r}(k)\, \boldsymbol{\tau}'_\mathbf{d}(k;\ N) + t(k-1 \to 0;\ N).$$

Suppose, instead, that you must change your plans once you are down to your last device; what is the MTTF then? Just subtract $t_d(1; N)$ from the above.

Now take a different viewpoint. What is the probability that the system will fail (down to your last device) before it ever gets back to full strength? Maybe you should quit now. This probability is given in Definition 4.5.17 and is

$$\boldsymbol{\pi}_\mathbf{r}(k)\, \mathbf{W}_\mathbf{d}(k \to 1; N-1)\, \boldsymbol{\epsilon}'.$$

(Note the $N-1$.) By definition, $\mathbf{W}_\mathbf{d}$ deals with *not exceeding*, while we are seeking the probability of *not reaching*. So we did find an additional use for the $\mathbf{W}_\mathbf{d}$ matrices.

The open system also has some application in this context. Suppose that instead of repairing devices, you go out and buy new ones when old ones break. There is an unlimited supply of these devices on the market, but it takes time to do this. If you work for a public university, the longest part of this task is getting the purchase order approved. Because of the uncertain delay, you try to have k devices on hand. The mean time until you run out of devices is given by the k-busy period, which for the M/G/1 system is [from (4.5.16b)]

$$\lim_{N\to\infty} t(k \to 0; N) = \frac{kT_1}{1-\rho}.$$

and so on and on and on.

We have seen an inkling of the power of LAQT in being able to separate the initial conditions from the transition period from the final result. Now what remains is for us to extend the procedure to include other, and more general systems, which we do in the following chapters.

Chapter 5

G/M/1 QUEUE

Thou com'st in such a questionable shape.
Hamlet, Act I, Scene IV

If we knew what we were doing, it wouldn't be called research, would it?
Albert Einstein

In Chapter 4 we talked about a closed loop made up of two subsystems, S_1 and S_2, where each subsystem was equivalent to a matrix representation of some general distribution $b_i(x)$. The notation for such a loop is $G_2/G_1/1//N$, where the N stands for the number of customers in the loop. However, we only treated the case where $G_2 = M$ [i.e., $b_2(x)$ is an exponential function]. In that case we found that an arriving customer would find n customers already in S_1 with the same probability as he would leave n behind. Furthermore, we showed that except for the fact that $d(N;N) = a(N;N) = 0$, these probabilities are proportional to the random observer's probability of finding n customers there. We also argued that the "finite waiting room," M/G/1/N queue (i.e., where S_1 could hold no more than N customers, thereby forcing all extra arrivals to disappear), yielded the same results as M/G/1//N, by virtue of the memoryless property of S_2. The behavior of the open M/G/1 system came easily (provided that the utilization parameter ρ was less than 1) by letting N become unboundedly large. In that case, given that S_2 was the slower server, the probability that it would ever be idle went to zero. Then it became a "constant" source of customers to S_1, with independent, exponentially distributed interarrival times, that is, a Poisson process. Finally, we showed that the three queue length probabilities, $a(n)$, $d(n)$, and $r(n)$, are all equal.

In this chapter we turn things upside down by letting ρ be greater than 1. Now, S_1 is the slower server, and in the limit as N goes to infinity, becomes a non-Poisson source of customers to S_2, with interarrival times distributed according to $b_1(x)$. We find that the limit, which yields the G/M/1 open queue (at S_2), does not come so easily, that the finite waiting room G/M/1/N does not give the same results as the closed G/M/1//N loop, nor do the arriving or departing customers see the same thing as our random observer. The formulas are sufficiently simple that we can hope to gain physical insight into the behavior of steady-state queues generally.

L. Lipsky, *Queueing Theory*, DOI 10.1007/978-0-387-49706-8_5,

This subject has been covered in many monographs. For instance, Kleinrock [KLEINROCK75] gives a classic solution of the G/M/1 queue that is in the same form as our scalar solution. Cohen [COHEN82] covers many aspects of the subject, and Ross [ROSS92] provides an alternate approach using renewal theory. The formulas given here extend the results in [CARROLLLIPVDL82] and [NEUTS82].

5.1 Steady-State Open ME/M/1 Queue

We make considerable use of the equations of Chapter 4. Therefore are forced to retain the definition of ρ as $\lambda\bar{x}$, which could also be written as $\bar{x}_1/\bar{x}_2$, because $1/\lambda = \bar{x}_2$. Clearly, as we show presently, the utilization of S_2 in an open G/M/1 queue is given by $\bar{x}_2/\bar{x}_1$, which is $1/\rho$. One must remember to replace ρ by $1/\rho$ when comparing formulas given in this chapter to those given in the general literature. To emphasize this difference, we here use the symbol ϱ (\varrho in LaTeX) as the ***utilization parameter***. That is,

$$\varrho := \frac{1}{\rho} = \frac{\bar{x}_2}{\bar{x}_1}.$$

We have to make some other notational changes; the first, referring to $\{\cdot;\ \cdot;\ \cdot\}$, we give now.

Definition 5.1.1

$\{i;\ k;\ N\}$ describes the state of the system, where N is the total number of customers in the system, k is the number of customers at S_2 (therefore there are $N-k$ customers at S_1), and i is the phase in S_1 that is busy. We might say that $i \in \Xi$ is an ***internal state*** of the system, and that $\{k;\ N\}$ is an ***external state*** of the system. □

The only change in notation from Section 4.1.1 is that now k stands for the number of customers at S_2, rather than S_1. This the notation used throughout this chapter.

Rather than introduce a collection of new notations, we modify previous symbols. For instance, the $\mathbf{d}(n; N)$ of Chapter 4 (the vector probability that a customer will leave n customers behind when departing S_1) is now written as $\mathbf{d}_1(n; N)$, and we make three new definitions.

Definition 5.1.2

$\mathbf{d_2}(k; N)$:= *steady-state vector probability that a customer will leave k customers behind when departing S_2.* Given that a customer has just left S_2 in an ME/M/1//N loop with nothing else known (another viewpoint of the steady state), $[\mathbf{d_2}(k; N)]_i$ is the probability that k customers are still at S_2, and the active customer at S_1 is at phase i. $d_2(k; N) := \mathbf{d_2}(k; N)\boldsymbol{\epsilon'}$ is the steady-state scalar probability that a customer will leave k customers behind when departing S_2. □

We also say that this is the probability that the system will be in state $\{i;\ k;\ N\}$ immediately after a departure from S_2.

Definition 5.1.3

$\mathbf{a_2}(k; N)$:=*steady-state vector probability that a customer, upon arriving at* S_2*, will find k customers already there.* $[\mathbf{a_2}(k; N)]_i$ is the probability that there are now $k+1$ customers at S_2, and the active customer in S_1 is at phase i. $a_2(k; N) := \mathbf{a_2}(k; N)\boldsymbol{\epsilon}'$ is the associated scalar probability. □

We also say that this is the probability that the system will be in state $\{i;\ k+1;\ N\}$ immediately after an arrival to S_2.

Definition 5.1.4

$\boldsymbol{\pi_2}(k; N)$:=*steady-state vector probability that there are k customers at* S_2 *in an* ME/M/1/ /N *loop*. A random observer will find a long-running system in state $\{i;\ k;\ N\}$ with probability $[\boldsymbol{\pi_2}(k; N)]_i$. $r_2(k;\ N) := \boldsymbol{\pi_2}(k;\ N)\boldsymbol{\epsilon}'$ is the associated scalar probability. □

As long as we have a closed system (i.e., N is finite), an arrival to one queue corresponds exactly to a departure from the other queue, so for $n + k = N$, we have the following theorem:

Theorem 5.1.1 The steady-state vector probabilities for the $G/M/1//N$ queue follow directly from Equations (4.1.6) and Theorem 4.1.4, and are given by:

$$\mathbf{a_2}(k; N) = \mathbf{d_1}(n-1; N) = c(N)\Psi[\mathbf{U}^{N-k-1}]\mathbf{p}, \tag{5.1.1a}$$

$$\mathbf{d_2}(k;\ N) = \mathbf{a_1}(n-1; N) = c(N)\mathbf{p}\,\mathbf{U}^{N-k-1}, \tag{5.1.1b}$$

$$\mathbf{d_2}(N;\ N) = \mathbf{a_2}(N; N) = \mathbf{o}, \tag{5.1.1c}$$

where $0 \le k < N$, and

$$1/c(N) = [1 - r_1(N; N)] = \Psi[\mathbf{I} + \mathbf{U} + \mathbf{U}^2 + \cdots + \mathbf{U}^{N-1}]$$
$$= \Psi\left[(\mathbf{I} - \mathbf{U}^N)\mathbf{K}\right].$$

Also,

$$\boldsymbol{\pi_2}(k; N) := \boldsymbol{\pi_1}(N-k; N), \tag{5.1.1d}$$

The sum of the first argument of the left-hand side of (5.1.1a) and (5.1.1b), $[k]$, and the first argument on the right-hand side of those equations, $[n-1]$, is $N-1$. The "1" missing is our customer-observer. The scalar probabilities $r_2(k; N)$, $d_2(k; N)$, and $a_2(k; N)$ are, as usual, found from their vector counterparts by dotting with $\boldsymbol{\epsilon}'$. ■

There may be some confusion when dealing with vector probabilities. As before, $[\boldsymbol{\pi_1}(n; N)]_i$ is the steady-state probability of there being n customers at S_1 with phase i (in S_1) busy. But the corresponding probability that there are k customers at S_2, and phase i in S_1 is busy, given by the ith component of the equation still refers to the internal status of S_1. After all, S_2 is represented by only one state, so it has no internal status. This becomes a bit sticky when $\varrho < 1$ (or when $\rho > 1$) and we go to the open system ($N \to \infty$), for then we would like to think that S_1 has somehow disappeared, and the arriving customers are of their own volition select their interarrival times from some nonexponential distribution. Conceptually, it is more useful to view S_1 as being *upstream* from S_2, with an inexhaustible supply of customers trying to get through its gates, one at a time, of course. In any case the events at S_1 have no inflence on what happens at S_2.

It would seem that this notational change is unnecessary, and indeed it is, but only as long as we are dealing with a closed system. In Chapter 4, with $\rho < 1$, we let N go to infinity, holding n constant. In this chapter, with $1/\rho = \varrho < 1$, we want to let N go to infinity, holding k constant. This subtle difference is best handled by our change of notation. Note that under these conditions, with n fixed, $\mathbf{d_1}(n;N)$, $\mathbf{a_1}(n;N)$, $r_1(n;N)$, and $\boldsymbol{\pi_1}(n;N)$ all go to 0 as N increases to infinity, just as $\mathbf{d_1}(N-n;N)$, and so on did when ρ was less than 1.

5.1.1 Steady-State Probabilities of the G/M/1 Queue

We can see from (4.2.2a) and (4.2.2b) that $\mathbf{K}$ exists whether ρ is greater than or less than 1 (it only lacks definition when $\rho = 1$, in which case neither the M/G/1 nor the G/M/1 queue has a steady-state solution). The problem is that when $\rho > 1$, the limit of $\mathbf{K}(N)$ [Equation (4.2.4c)] does not exist! We must be more careful in taking the limit. Let $\{s_i\}$ be the set of eigenvalues of $\mathbf{A}$, where $\{\mathbf{u_i}\}$, and $\{\mathbf{v_i'}\}$ are the sets of left and right eigenvectors of $\mathbf{A}$, respectively. Define s to be the eigenvalue of smallest magnitude, with corresponding eigenvectors $\mathbf{u}$ and $\mathbf{v}'$. That is,

$$|s| = \min_{i=1}^{m} |s_i|.$$

For simplicity, assume that the eigenvalues are distinct (although what follows only needs the fact (known from other sources) that s is unique, positive, and less than 1). Then from the spectral decomposition theorem [Equation (1.3.8a)],

$$\mathbf{A} = \sum_{i=1}^{m} s_i \mathbf{v_i'} \mathbf{u_i},$$

so (recall that $\mathbf{U}$ is the inverse of $\mathbf{A}$)

$$\mathbf{U}^N = \sum_{i=1}^{m} \left(\frac{1}{s_i}\right)^N \mathbf{v_i'} \mathbf{u_i}. \tag{5.1.2a}$$

Then it follows that

$$s^N \mathbf{U}^N = \mathbf{v}'\,\mathbf{u} + \sum_{i^*=1}^{m} \left(\frac{s}{s_i}\right)^N \mathbf{v_i'}\,\mathbf{u_i}, \tag{5.1.2b}$$

where i^* stands for all terms excluding the term that corresponds to s. The limit is now straightforward, because $|s\,/\,s_i|$ is less than 1 for all i,

$$\lim_{N\to\infty} s^N \mathbf{U}^N = \mathbf{v}'\mathbf{u}. \tag{5.1.2c}$$

We are almost ready to move ahead, but first look at [from (4.1.6d)]

$$s^N \mathbf{K}(N) = s^N[\mathbf{I} + \mathbf{U} + \mathbf{U}^2 + \cdots + \mathbf{U}^{N-1} + \lambda \mathbf{U}^{N-1}\mathbf{V}].$$

Note that for all N greater than 0,

$$[\mathbf{I} + \mathbf{U} + \mathbf{U}^2 + \cdots + \mathbf{U}^{N-1}](\mathbf{I} - \mathbf{U}) = \mathbf{I} - \mathbf{U}^N,$$

and because $\mathbf{K} = (\mathbf{I} - \mathbf{U})^{-1}$ exists, we have

$$s^N \mathbf{K}(N) = s^N[(\mathbf{I} - \mathbf{U}^N)\mathbf{K} + \mathbf{U}^N(\lambda \mathbf{A}\mathbf{V})].$$

At last we are ready to let N go to infinity. Note that (we are assuming that) $0 < s < 1$, thus the term $s^N\mathbf{K}$ goes to 0, leaving us with

$$\mathbf{F} := \lim_{N\to\infty} s^N \mathbf{K}(N) = \mathbf{v}'\mathbf{u}[-\mathbf{K} + \lambda \mathbf{A}\mathbf{V}]$$

$$= -\frac{\lambda^2}{1-\rho}\mathbf{v}'\mathbf{u}\mathbf{A}\mathbf{V}\mathbf{Q}\mathbf{V} = -\frac{\lambda^2}{1-\rho}\mathbf{v}'\mathbf{u}\mathbf{A}\mathbf{V}\boldsymbol{\epsilon}'\mathbf{p}\mathbf{V}, \tag{5.1.3a}$$

where we have made use of (4.2.2c). Equation (4.2.3a) finally comes in handy, for it allows us to replace $\lambda\mathbf{A}\mathbf{V}\boldsymbol{\epsilon}'$ with $(1-\rho)\mathbf{K}\boldsymbol{\epsilon}'$ to get

$$\mathbf{F} = -\lambda \mathbf{v}'\mathbf{u}\mathbf{K}\boldsymbol{\epsilon}'\mathbf{p}\mathbf{V}.$$

Ah, but $\mathbf{K}$ is a function of $\mathbf{U}$, so it has $\mathbf{u}$ as a left eigenvector, and

$$\mathbf{u}\mathbf{K} = [\mathbf{I} - \mathbf{U}]^{-1}\mathbf{u} = \left(1 - \frac{1}{s}\right)^{-1}\mathbf{u} = -\frac{s}{1-s}\mathbf{u}.$$

That leaves us with the simple expression (it really is simple)

$$\mathbf{F} = \left(\frac{\lambda s}{1-s}(\mathbf{u}\boldsymbol{\epsilon}')\right)\mathbf{v}'\mathbf{p}\mathbf{V}, \tag{5.1.3b}$$

where the expression in large parentheses is a scalar. The last preliminary step is to find $\Psi[\mathbf{F}]$, which is (remember that $1/\rho = \varrho < 1$)

$$\Psi[\mathbf{F}] = \left(\frac{\lambda s}{1-s}(\mathbf{u}\boldsymbol{\epsilon}')\right)\mathbf{p}\mathbf{v}'\mathbf{p}\mathbf{V}\boldsymbol{\epsilon}' = \frac{s(\mathbf{u}\boldsymbol{\epsilon}')(\mathbf{p}\mathbf{v}')}{(1-s)\varrho}. \tag{5.1.3c}$$

From Theorem 4.1.2 and (5.1.1d), for $k > 0$,

$$\boldsymbol{\pi}_2(k; N) = \frac{1}{\Psi[\mathbf{K}(N)]}\mathbf{p}\mathbf{U}^{N-k} = \frac{1}{\Psi[\mathbf{K}(N)]}\mathbf{p}\mathbf{U}^N\mathbf{A}^k.$$

Now multiply and divide by s^N and take the limit on N, while holding k fixed,

$$\boldsymbol{\pi}_2(k) := \lim_{N\to\infty}\left(\frac{s^N\mathbf{p}\mathbf{U}^N\mathbf{A}^k}{s^N\Psi[\mathbf{K}(N)]}\right) = \frac{1}{\Psi[\mathbf{F}]}\mathbf{p}\mathbf{v}'\mathbf{u}\mathbf{A}^k.$$

Remember now that $\mathbf{uA} = s\,\mathbf{u}$, and use (5.1.3c)

$$\boldsymbol{\pi}_2(k) = (1-s)\varrho\, s^{k-1}\frac{\mathbf{u}}{\mathbf{u}\boldsymbol{\epsilon}'}, \qquad k > 0. \tag{5.1.4a}$$

How interesting; all the vector probabilities for $k > 0$ are proportional to the same isometric vector.

This vector appears often, therefore it is given the special symbol

$$\hat{\mathbf{u}} := \frac{\mathbf{u}}{\mathbf{u}\boldsymbol{\epsilon}'}, \tag{5.1.4b}$$

where $\hat{\mathbf{u}}\boldsymbol{\epsilon}' = 1$. We next look at $k = 0$. Now we have

$$\boldsymbol{\pi}_2(0) = \frac{\lambda(1-s)}{\rho s}\hat{\mathbf{u}}\mathbf{AV} = \frac{1}{\bar{x}_1}(1-s)\hat{\mathbf{u}}\mathbf{V}. \tag{5.1.4c}$$

We must think about this for a moment before going on. Here we have a simple exponential server (S_2), with no customers present, yet it has some memory of when the last customer came. That is, the vector, $\boldsymbol{\pi}_2(0)$, has nontrivial components and is proportional to $\hat{\mathbf{u}}\mathbf{V}$, not $\hat{\mathbf{u}}$. (There is an analogy to this in quantum electrodynamics, where empty space, the "vacuum," has nontrivial properties, as well as in the pre-Einsteinian view of the *ether*.) Now we can appreciate the view that has S_1 upstream, busily generating customers for S_2, even though $k = 0$. We must never lose sight of the fact that it is the system as a whole that is in one state or another, not the subsystems by themselves. This is particularly true in the steady state, where the two subsystems have been exchanging customers for a long time. In our treatment of transient behavior, we see (perhaps) that the two subsystems gradually become interdependent as they exchange more and more customers.

The scalar probabilities $r_2(k)$ can now be found from Equations (5.1.4), because $r_2(k) = \boldsymbol{\pi}_2(k)\boldsymbol{\epsilon}'$. The formulas are summarized in the following.

Theorem 5.1.2 The steady-state probabilities of (a random observer) finding k customers in an open ME/M/1 queue as given by (5.1.4a) to (5.1.4c) can be written in the form ($\varrho = 1/\rho$):

$$\boldsymbol{\pi}_2(0) = (1-\varrho)\frac{\hat{\mathbf{u}}\mathbf{V}}{\hat{\mathbf{u}}\mathbf{V}\boldsymbol{\epsilon}'} \tag{5.1.5a}$$

and

$$\boldsymbol{\pi}_2(k) = (1-s)\varrho\, s^{k-1}\hat{\mathbf{u}} \quad \text{for } k > 0. \tag{5.1.5b}$$

The associated scalar probabilities are given by the following equations:

$$r_2(0) = 1-\varrho \tag{5.1.5c}$$

and

$$r_2(k) = (1-s)\varrho\, s^{k-1} \quad \text{for } k > 0. \tag{5.1.5d}$$

The parameter s (with its associated left eigenvector $\hat{\mathbf{u}}$) is the smallest positive eigenvalue satisfying $\hat{\mathbf{u}}\mathbf{A} = s\hat{\mathbf{u}}$, and $\hat{\mathbf{u}}\boldsymbol{\epsilon}' = 1$. Because of

(5.1.5d) it is known as the ***geometric parameter*** for the G/M/1 queue. The mean queue length $\bar{q}_2$ and mean system time $\mathbf{E}[T_2]$ are given below in Equations (5.1.7). ■

Proof: Note from (4.2.3a) that $\lambda \mathbf{AV}\boldsymbol{\epsilon}' = (1-\rho)\mathbf{K}\boldsymbol{\epsilon}'$, so on premultiplying by $\hat{\mathbf{u}}$ and rearranging,

$$\hat{\mathbf{u}}\mathbf{V}\boldsymbol{\epsilon}' = \frac{1-\varrho}{(1-s)\varrho\lambda}. \tag{5.1.5e}$$

The rest follows directly. **QED**

So the probabilities are geometrically distributed, just as in the M/M/1 queue, but with s instead of ϱ. Also, $r_2(0)$ does not satisfy the general expression but is what it should be, namely 1 minus the utilization $[\varrho]$ of S_2.

This well-known result is simple in form but is deceptively complicated in that the dependence of s on ϱ is not easy to get in general. Only when $b_1(x)$ is exponentially distributed does $s = \varrho$. It is known from other sources that s satisfies the following implicit relation. We state it as a corollary to Theorem 5.1.2 and prove it by purely algebraic means.

Corollary 5.1.2 The eigenvalue s is the smallest positive root of the following implicit equation,

$$\Psi\left[(\mathbf{I} + (1-s)\lambda\mathbf{V})^{-1}\right] = B^*[\lambda(1-s)] = s, \tag{5.1.6a}$$

where $B^*(\cdot)$ is the Laplace transform of $b_1(x)$, the pdf of S_1 (the interarrival time distribution). The associated eigenvector satisfies the equation

$$\hat{\mathbf{u}} = \lambda\mathbf{p}\mathbf{V}\left(\mathbf{I} + \lambda(1-s)\mathbf{V}\right)^{-1}. \tag{5.1.6b}$$

■

Proof: First we prove (5.1.6b). From its definition,

$$\hat{\mathbf{u}}\mathbf{A} = s\hat{\mathbf{u}} = \hat{\mathbf{u}}\left(\mathbf{I} + \frac{1}{\lambda}\mathbf{B} - \mathbf{Q}\right) = \hat{\mathbf{u}} + \frac{1}{\lambda}\hat{\mathbf{u}}\mathbf{B} - \mathbf{p}.$$

We have used the fact that $\hat{\mathbf{u}}\mathbf{Q} = \hat{\mathbf{u}}\boldsymbol{\epsilon}'\mathbf{p} = \mathbf{p}$. Next separate all terms that contain $\hat{\mathbf{u}}$ from those that do not.

$$\hat{\mathbf{u}}\left((1-s)\mathbf{I} + \frac{1}{\lambda}\mathbf{B}\right) = \mathbf{p}.$$

Now multiply both sides of the equation by $\lambda\mathbf{V}$:

$$\hat{\mathbf{u}}\left[\mathbf{I} + \lambda(1-s)\mathbf{V}\right] = \lambda\mathbf{p}\mathbf{V}. \tag{5.1.6c}$$

Multiplying both sides by the inverse of the matrix expression in large brackets yields (5.1.6b). Because $\hat{\mathbf{u}}\boldsymbol{\epsilon}' = 1$, Equation (5.1.6a) follows after some manipulation, by multiplying (5.1.6b) on the right with the vector $\boldsymbol{\epsilon}'$, noting that

$$\lambda \mathbf{V}\left[\mathbf{I}+\lambda(1-s)\mathbf{V}\right]^{-1} = \frac{1}{1-s}\left(\mathbf{I}-\left[\mathbf{I}+\lambda(1-s)\mathbf{V}\right]^{-1}\right).$$

Then, recalling (3.1.10), the matrix definition of the Laplace transform, the proof is completed. **QED**

It remains to verify that the probabilities sum to 1.

Exercise 5.1.1: Show that $\sum_{k=o}^{\infty} r_2(k) = 1$.

To find s, one must either solve an eigenvalue problem, or find the smallest positive root of (5.1.6a). In either case, numerical techniques are usually required. Once s is known, (5.1.6b) gives us $\hat{\mathbf{u}}$. As with many other objects we encounter in this book, $\hat{\mathbf{u}}$ has more information in it than that for which it was derived. In particular, it contains information regarding the arrival of the next customer. We discuss this further in the next section, after deriving the departure probabilities.

Exercise 5.1.2: The vector probabilities must also satisfy a sum rule. If a random observer watches S_1 without taking any notice of the number of customers at S_2, she sees customers perpetually coming and going, or equivalently (if she doesn't distinguish one customer from another), a single customer leaving and immediately returning to S_2, as described in Figure 3.5.3 with $\alpha = 1$. The steady-state vector for this process is given by Theorem 3.5.3a to be $\boldsymbol{\pi}_{\mathbf{r}}$. Therefore, prove by algebraic manipulation that

$$\sum_{k=o}^{\infty} \boldsymbol{\pi}_2(k) = \boldsymbol{\pi}_{\mathbf{r}} = \frac{\mathbf{p}\mathbf{V}}{\mathbf{p}\,\mathbf{V}\,\boldsymbol{\epsilon}'}.$$

Use Theorem 5.1.2 and (5.1.5e).

We next find the mean queue length and system time. Because the $r_2(k)$s are of geometric form, it is just as easy to get the z-transform of $\{r_2(k) \mid k \geq 0\}$ as it is to get $\bar{q}_2$ directly. By definition,

$$Q_2(z) = \sum_{k=0}^{\infty} z^k\, r_2(k) = 1 - \varrho + \frac{(1-s)\varrho}{s}\sum_{k=1}^{\infty}(zs)^k = 1 - \varrho + \frac{(1-s)\varrho\, z}{1-zs}.$$

We rewrite this in the form

$$Q_2(z) = 1 + \frac{(z-1)\varrho}{1-zs}. \qquad (5.1.7a)$$

Obviously, $Q_2(1) = 1$, and the derivative evaluated at $z = 1$ yields the mean queue length,

$$\bar{q}_2 = \left[\frac{d\,Q_2(z)}{dz}\right]_{z=1} = \frac{\varrho}{1-s}. \tag{5.1.7b}$$

As in Chapter 4 [Equation (4.2.6e)], we use ***Little's formula*** to get the mean system time (in this case, the arrival rate to S_2 is $1/\bar{x}_1$, and $\bar{x}_2$ is $1/\lambda$),

$$\mathbf{E}[T_2] = \bar{x}_1\bar{q}_2 = \frac{\bar{x}_2}{1-s} = \frac{1/\lambda}{1-s}. \tag{5.1.7c}$$

Again, this formula looks very similar to (2.1.7b) for the M/M/1 queue, except that s appears instead of ϱ. $\mathbf{E}[T_2]$ becomes unbounded when s approaches 1. The graph of (5.1.7c) for the D/M/1 queue was given in Figure 1.1.2, together with various M/G/1 queues.

It should be comforting to know that s/ϱ goes to 1 as ϱ approaches 1 from below. We explore the relation between ϱ and s further in Section 5.1.3.

Exercise 5.1.3: Verify that (5.1.7a) and (5.1.7b) are indeed true.

5.1.2 Arrival and Departure Probabilities

The hard work has already been done in preparing to take the limit as N goes to infinity of the arrival and departure probabilities. From Theorem 5.1.1 we have the following string of equalities.

$$\mathbf{a_2}(k;N) = \mathbf{d_1}(N-k-1;N) = \frac{r_1(N-k-1;N)}{1-r_1(N;N)}\mathbf{p} = \frac{r_2(k+1;N)}{1-r_2(0;N)}\mathbf{p}.$$

We already found the limits of both numerator and denominator for the last expression, and they are each finite [Equations (5.1.5c) and (5.1.5d)], so

$$\mathbf{a_2}(k) := \lim_{N\to\infty}\mathbf{a_2}(k;N) = \frac{1}{1-(1-\varrho)}[\varrho(1-s)]s^k\mathbf{p} = (1-s)s^k\mathbf{p}. \tag{5.1.8a}$$

The scalar probabilities obviously satisfy

$$a_2(k) = (1-s)s^k. \tag{5.1.8b}$$

We point out that (5.1.8a) and (5.1.8b) are valid for all k, even $k = 0$, which is not the case for $r_2(k)$ and $\boldsymbol{\pi_2}(k)$. Also, note that (not merely at $k = 0$) $a_2(k)$ does not equal $r_2(k)$, and $\mathbf{a_2}(k)$ is not even parallel to $\boldsymbol{\pi_2}(k)$! Well, it is not all that bad. After all $a_2(k)$ $(k \neq 0)$ is proportional to $r_2(k)$ [i.e., $a_2(k) = sr_2(k)/\varrho$, for all k greater than 0].

The $\mathbf{d_2}(k)$s can be found in a manner identical to that for $\mathbf{a_2}(k)$. From (5.1.1b) and (4.1.13a),

$$\mathbf{d_2}(k;N) = \frac{1}{1-r_2(0;N)}\boldsymbol{\pi_2}(k+1;N).$$

The limit follows directly. The different formulas are collected in the following theorem.

Theorem 5.1.3 The steady-state probabilities of queue lengths as seen by customers arriving to, and departing from an open ME/M/1 queue are given for all $k \geq 0$ by [repeating Equation (5.1.8a)]

$$\mathbf{a_2}(k) = (1-s)s^k \mathbf{p}, \tag{5.1.9a}$$

$$\mathbf{d_2}(k) = (1-s)s^k \hat{\mathbf{u}}, \tag{5.1.9b}$$

and

$$d_2(k) = a_2(k) = (1-s)s^k. \tag{5.1.9c}$$

Equation (5.1.9a) is so simple that we can immediately write down the probability that an arriving customer will find k or more customers already in the queue. That is,

$$P_{o2} := \mathbf{Pr}(K \geq k) = \sum_{\ell=k}^{\infty} a_2(\ell) = s^k. \tag{5.1.9d}$$

As in previous chapters, this is also referred to as the *overflow probability.*

Thus we have shown for this simple system that except for the M/M/1 queue, $\mathbf{a_2}(k)$, $\mathbf{d_2}(k)$, and $\boldsymbol{\pi_2}(k)$ are distinctly different. They are similar, but nonetheless different. ■

The form of (5.1.9c) is so familiar by now that one can truly say "it is obvious that" the sum of the $a_2(k)$s is 1, and the mean queue length seen by both a departing and an arriving customer is $s/(1-s)$. Although the difference seems minor, it is important to recognize that this quantity is not equal to the mean queue length as seen by our random observer, $\bar{q}_2$ [Equation (5.1.7b)]. As with the $a_2(k)$ and $r_2(k)$, they differ by the factor s/ϱ. It is (5.1.7b) that one uses in Little's formula to get the mean system time, as we did in (5.1.7c). We now use $a_2(k)$ to find $\mathbf{E}[T_2]$ from its definition. Given that S_2 is an exponential server, there is no distinction between its mean time and its residual time, so the care we had to take in Section 4.3.1 is not necessary here. If there are k customers at S_2 (including none) when a customer arrives, he will have to wait an average of $(k+1)\bar{x}_2$ units of time before leaving. The mean time averaged over all queue lengths is

$$\mathbf{E}[T_2] = \sum_{k=0}^{\infty} a_2(k)(k+1)\bar{x}_2 = (1-s)\bar{x}_2 \sum_{k=0}^{\infty}(k+1)s^k$$

$$= \frac{(1-s)\bar{x}_2}{s} \sum_{k=1}^{\infty} ks^k = \frac{\bar{x}_2}{1-s},$$

the same as (5.1.7c). Our purpose here was to prepare the reader to derive the system time distribution.

Exercise 5.1.4: In Exercises 2.1.7 through 2.1.9 we examined how and when one might improve service for an M/M/1 queue when the arrival rate gets too big. Here we look at one more simple possibility. Recall that for System (B) when a customer arrives at the dispatching point he is randomly sent to one or the other of the two queues (two M/M/1 queues, each with one half the arrival rate), but in System (C) the customers queue up at the dispatcher, and are later sent to the first available server (an M/M/2 queue). Consider the following dispatching procedure. When a customer arrives at the dispatching point he is immediately sent to the queue least recently visited. That is, customer 1 goes to server 1, customer 2 goes to server 2, customer 3 goes to server 1, and so on. What each queue sees is the arrival of customers separated by *two* exponential intervals. In other words, the arrival process is an Erlangian-2 renewal process. Call this double $E_2/M/1$ queue System (E). Redo Exercises 2.1.7 and 2.1.9 using System (E) and compare with Systems (A) through (D). You should find that T_E falls between T_B and T_C.

The time for a customer to go through an exponential server $k+1$ times, or equivalently, of $k+1$ customers going through one at a time, is distributed according to the Erlangian-(k+1) distribution $[E_{k+1}(x;\lambda)]$ whose pdf is given in (3.2.1a), and is $\lambda(\lambda x)^k e^{-\lambda x}/(k!)$. The weighted average over all k is, then,

$$b_{2s}(x) := \sum_{k=0}^{\infty} a_2(k) E_{k+1}(x;\lambda) = (1-s)\lambda \sum_{k=0}^{\infty} s^k \frac{(\lambda x)^k}{k!} e^{-\lambda x}$$

$$= (1-s)\lambda \left(\sum_{k=0}^{\infty} \frac{(\lambda s x)^k}{k!} \right) e^{-\lambda x},$$

or finally,

$$b_{2s}(x) = (1-s)\lambda e^{-(1-s)\lambda\, x}. \tag{5.1.10}$$

So the system time is exponentially distributed, with mean time equal to $1/[(1-s)\lambda]$ (but we already knew $\mathbb{E}[T_2]$).

5.1.3 Properties of Geometric Parameter s

Theorem 5.1.2 showed us that the behavior of the G/M/1 queue is dominated by the geometric parameter s. Even $\hat{\mathbf{u}}$ can be evaluated from (5.1.6b) if we know s. The value of s can be found from any one of the three equations: (1) (5.1.6a); (2) (3.1.10); or (3) $\hat{\mathbf{u}}\mathbf{A} = s\hat{\mathbf{u}}$, by a root-finding or other numerical technique. That is, for a given arrival process, with interarrival times generated by $\langle \mathbf{p}, \mathbf{B} \rangle$, and given λ, s is uniquely determined by any of these equations. The properties of s are best understood by thinking of it as a function of λ, or ρ, or better, ϱ. How one should calculate numerical values for s is a matter of taste and numerical analysis and is by and large outside the interests of this book, but we mention some points so that the reader may avoid possible pitfalls.

For convenience of description, in the rest of this section we make the following symbol changes. Recall that $\rho = \lambda T$, where

$$T := \bar{x}_1 = \Psi[\mathbf{V}].$$

We have already defined ϱ, which can now be written as

$$\varrho := \frac{1}{\rho} = \frac{1}{\lambda T}.$$

Therefore, we replace λ whenever it is to our convenience with $1/T\varrho$.

When S_1 Is Exponential

Let us start slowly and see what the three formulas tell us when S_1 is an exponential server. In that case, $\mathbf{B}$ becomes $\mu = 1/T$, $\mathbf{V}$ becomes T, $\mathbf{Q}$ becomes 1, and $\mathbf{A} = 1 + (1/\lambda)\mu - 1 = \varrho$. Thus the eigenvalue equation $\hat{\mathbf{u}}\mathbf{A} = s\hat{\mathbf{u}}$ reduces to $\varrho = s$. This obvious result tells us that the G/M/1 queue reduces to the M/M/1 queue when G is Poisson (that *is* obvious). Equation (5.1.6a) is not quite so simple. From that equation, $s = B^*[(1-s)\lambda] = B^*[(1-s)/(\varrho T)]$, so

$$s = \int_0^\infty \exp[-x(1-s)/\varrho T]\frac{e^{-x/T}}{T}dx = \frac{1/T}{1/T + (1-s)/(\varrho T)} = \frac{\varrho}{\varrho + (1-s)}.$$

After we clear fractions, we get $s\varrho + s(1-s) = \varrho$, or

$$(1-s)\varrho = (1-s)s.$$

Notice that although we get the root we are looking for, $s = \varrho$, we also get the meaningless, extraneous root $s = 1$, for all ϱ. This extraneous root always appears for any distribution, reflecting the fact that the integral of $b(x)$ is 1. It can get in the way when ϱ is close to 1, and can be a real drag when one is looking for heavy traffic performance, as we show presently. The third equation has the same difficulty, but we can get around that. First, (3.1.10) gives us the following when S_1 is exponential.

$$s = \Psi\left[(\mathbf{I} + (1-s)\lambda\mathbf{V})^{-1}\right] = \frac{1}{1 + (1-s)T/(\varrho T)},$$

which, indeed, leads to the same awkward equation we had before. Now let us play a little trick for any ME distribution, by noting that $s = \Psi[s\mathbf{I}]$ in (3.1.10), then (keep λ for the moment)

$$0 = \Psi\left[[\mathbf{I} + (1-s)\lambda\mathbf{V}]^{-1} - s\mathbf{I}\right] = \Psi\left[[\mathbf{I} + (1-s)\lambda\mathbf{V}]^{-1}[\mathbf{I} - s\mathbf{I} - (1-s)s\lambda\mathbf{V}]\right],$$

or

$$(1-s)\Psi\left[[\mathbf{I} + (1-s)\lambda\mathbf{V}]^{-1}[\mathbf{I} - \lambda s\mathbf{V}]\right] = 0.$$

Therefore, we can throw away the term $(1-s)$ before we begin. Finally, replace λ, clear fractions, and after some other trickery, get the following alternative equation,

$$\Psi\left[\mathbf{V}[\varrho T\mathbf{I} + (1-s)\mathbf{V}]^{-1}\right] = 1. \tag{5.1.11}$$

This form is about as good as we can get for the purposes we have in mind. In particular, we can see that when $\varrho = 0$, we must have $s = 0$, and if $s = 1$, ϱ must be 1 also. This is true for every G/M/1 queue, *except* for those for which the interarrival time distributons are ***defective***, or equivalently, have an ***initial impulse***, which we now discuss.

Defective Distributions

Distributions with an initial impulse are those for which $R(0) < 1$, or equivalently, $B(0) > 0$. When a customer finally gets to be served, he decides with probability $p = B(0)$ that he does not need any service. Such distributions are not uncommon. For instance, in reliability theory, this is the probability that a device will be faulty even though it is brand new, an important problem to worry about. Any distribution that has this property has a pdf of the form

$$b(x) = p\delta(x) + (1-p)b_a(x), \tag{5.1.12a}$$

where $b_a(x)$ is the pdf of those devices that function properly initially [i.e., $\int b_a(x)\,dx = 1$], and $\delta(x)$ is the ***Dirac delta function***, which has these properties:

$$\int_{-a}^{b} \delta(x)\,dx = 1 \qquad \text{for every} \quad a,\ b > 0,$$

or

$$f(0) = \int_{-\infty}^{\infty} f(x)\delta(x)\,dx$$

for all $f(x)$ which are continuous at $x = 0$, or

$$f(t) = \int_{-\infty}^{\infty} f(x)\delta(x-t)\,dx.$$

It can also be viewed as the derivative of the ***unit step function***, which satisfies

$$\Delta(t) = \int_{-\infty}^{t} \delta(x)\,dx$$

$$\Delta(t) = \begin{cases} 0 & \text{if} \quad t < 0 \\ \frac{1}{2} & \text{if} \quad t = 0 \\ 1 & \text{if} \quad t > 0 \end{cases}.$$

Pictorially think of $\delta(x)$ as a spike of infinite height with unit area and 0 width, or the limit of a family of very high but very narrow functions. One such example was given in Example 3.2.1 as the limit of the set of Erlangian-k distributions with the same mean. There are other ways to look at it.

Anyway, we can also write

$$B(x) = p + (1-p)B_a(x) \tag{5.1.12b}$$

and

$$R(x) = (1-p)R_a(x). \tag{5.1.12c}$$

This distribution has the following Laplace transform.

$$B^*(s) = \int_{0_-}^{\infty} e^{-sx}[p\delta(x) + (1-p)b_a(x)]\,dx = p + (1-p)B_a^*(s).$$

The LAQT treatment is as follows. Let $b_a(x)$ be generated by $\langle \mathbf{p_a}, \mathbf{V_a} \rangle$; then

$$\mathbf{V} = \begin{bmatrix} 0 & \mathbf{o} \\ \mathbf{o}' & \mathbf{V_a} \end{bmatrix} \quad \text{and} \quad \mathbf{p} = [p, (1-p)\mathbf{p_a}], \tag{5.1.13}$$

where $\mathbf{p_a}\,\boldsymbol{\epsilon}' = 1$. Be careful; $\mathbf{V}$ does not have an inverse, but luckily, (5.1.11), which we worked so hard to get, does not have $\mathbf{B}$ in it. The mean time T, for the process represented by $\langle \mathbf{p}, \mathbf{V} \rangle$, is related to the mean time T_a for the process $\langle \mathbf{p_a}, \mathbf{V_a} \rangle$ by the following.

$$T = \Psi[\mathbf{V}] = \mathbf{pV}\boldsymbol{\epsilon}' = (1-p)\mathbf{p_a V_a}\boldsymbol{\epsilon}' = (1-p)\Psi_a[\mathbf{V_a}] = (1-p)T_a.$$

If some customers take no time at all, the rest must take more time than the overall average, so $T_a > T$ if $p > 0$.

When (5.1.13) is substituted into (5.1.11), the following expression results.

$$(1-p)\Psi_a\left[\mathbf{V_a}[\varrho T\,\mathbf{I} + (1-s)\mathbf{V_a}]^{-1}\right] = 1. \tag{5.1.14a}$$

For $s = 1$, this equation yields

$$\frac{(1-p)}{\varrho T}\Psi_a[\mathbf{V_a}] = \frac{(1-p)T_a}{\varrho T} = \frac{T}{\varrho T} = 1;$$

that is, $\varrho = 1$, as before. But if $\varrho = 0$, then (5.1.14a) yields

$$(1-p)\Psi_a\left[\mathbf{V_a}[(1-s)\mathbf{V_a}]^{-1}\right] = \frac{1-p}{1-s} = 1,$$

or $s = p$. What this means is the following. Even though arrivals are infrequent (after all, ϱ is 0), when a customer *does* arrive, there is a finite probability [p] that he will be followed immediately by a second customer, and this second customer will have to wait for the first one to finish. It is even possible for a third (p^2) or fourth (p^3) or more customers to arrive together. This implies that even if the arrival rate is negligible, the waiting time T_{2w} (the time a customer must wait from the moment he arrives at S_2 until he begins to be served) will be greater than 0. From (5.1.7c), and (2.1.7c), the mean waiting time for a G/M/1 queue is given by

$$\mathbb{E}[T_{2w}] = \mathbb{E}[T_2] - \bar{x}_2 = \frac{s}{1-s}\bar{x}_2,$$

where the reader should remember that we are now looking at S_2, whereas in Chapter 2 we were looking at S_1. In the limit as the arrival rate goes to 0, we see that

$$\lim_{\varrho\to 0}\mathbb{E}[T_{2w}] = \frac{p}{1-p}\bar{x}_2 > 0 \quad \text{as long as } p < 1. \tag{5.1.14b}$$

Notice that this is equivalent to a ***bulk arrival process*** (or ***batch arrival process***) which is geometrically distributed; that is, given that an arrival has occurred, $(1-p)p^{j-1}$ is the probability that $j \geq 1$ customers have arrived together (in bulk).

As a final comment, if $b_a(x)$ is exponential, $b(x)$ is often referred to as a ***generalized exponential***, or ***degenerate hyperexponential*** distribution, and has been used as a test function for studying the performance of various systems (see e.g., [GUPTAETAL07]). It is convenient to use because it only depends on two parameters and can have arbitrarily large variance. But its singular behavior at $x = 0$ can lead to spurious results. For further discussion see "Distributions Coming from Singular **B** or **V**" following Figure 3.2.4.

Behavior of s As a Function of ϱ

In Chapter 4 we saw that the mean system time and mean queue length for an M/G/1 queue depend on the factor $1/(1-\rho)$. This was simple enough to visualize, but from (5.1.7c) for G/M/1 queues, the mean system time depends on the factor $1/(1-s)$. To visualize this we must first find how s varies with ϱ, which we now propose to do.

What we have discovered so far can best be summarized by Figure 5.1.1, where s is plotted as a function of ϱ. We are examining several distributions here, therefore we use the notation $s(\varrho; X)$, to indicate the dependence of s on ϱ for the distribution symbolized by X. For the M/M/1 queue $[X = M]$, $s(\varrho; M) = \varrho$, corresponding to the straight line from $(0,0)$ to $(1,1)$. If there is an initial impulse $[X = M_p]$, then $s(0) = p$. The M_p/M/1 queue with initial impulse p corresponds to the straight line from $(0,p)$ to $(1,1)$, or $s(\varrho; M_p) = p + (1-p)\varrho$.

For general interarrival time distributions $[X = G]$, $s(\varrho; G)$ also increases monotonically until it reaches $(1,1)$. We know that the larger s is, the longer will be the system time, from (5.1.7c). We also know that the system time can be reduced by regulating arrivals, and the most regular arrival pattern is the one where the time between arrivals is constant. In other words, the *deterministic distribution* $[X = D]$, given by

$$b_D(x) = \delta(x-T) \quad \text{or} \quad B_D(x) = \Delta(x-T),$$

should yield the smallest s for a given ϱ. Said yet another way, the D/M/1 queue has the shortest mean system time among all G/M/1 queues with the same ϱ. Unfortunately, there is no finite-dimensional representation of $B_D(x)$; therefore we have to resort to (3.1.10) to find the dependence of s on ϱ. From that equation (remembering that $\lambda T = 1/\varrho$),

$$s = \int_0^\infty e^{-\lambda(1-s)x}\delta(x-T)\,dx = e^{-(1-s)/\varrho}. \tag{5.1.14c}$$

Notice that $s = 1$ is a solution to this equation for all ϱ, but as we stated previously, this root has no physical significance except when $\varrho = 1$ also. It turns out that one can draw the graph of the relation between s and ϱ by solving for ϱ (one cannot solve explicitly for s). The function $\varrho = (s-1)/\log(s)$ yields the graph labeled D on Figure 5.1.1. This curve is the greatest lower bound for all possible distributions, for every ϱ between 0 and 1. That is, let $s(\varrho; G)$ be the geometric parameter corresponding to some general PDF, $B_G(x)$. Then

$$s(\varrho;\, G) \geq s(\varrho; D) \quad \text{for all } \; 0 \leq \varrho \leq 1.$$

Example 5.1.1: For comparison, we have plotted the geometric parameter for the uniform distribution $[X = U]$, the Erlangian-k, for $k = 2, 4, 8$ $[E_k]$, the Erlangian-2 with initial impulse $p = 0.1$ $[E_{2p}]$, and a hyperexponential-2 distribution with squared coefficient of variation [recall that $C_v^2 = \sigma^2/(\bar{x})^2$] equal to 10 $[H_2]$. Again, the uniform distribution required the use of (3.1.10), but the others, being proper ME distributions, were best suited for (5.1.14a).

Note that, indeed, all the curves satisfy the bound theorem just stated, and in fact, $s(\varrho; E_k)$ approaches $s(\varrho; D)$ from above for all ϱ, as $k \to \infty$:

$$\lim_{k\to\infty} [s(\varrho; E_k) - s(\varrho; D)] = 0_+, \quad \text{for all } \; 0 \leq \varrho \leq 1.$$

This equation indicates how the deterministic distribution is approximated arbitrarily closely by a family of finite-dimensional ME distributions. We can say that

$$\delta(x - T) = \lim_{m\to\infty} E_m(x; m/T),$$

where $E_m(x; \alpha)$ is defined in (3.2.1a). Therefore, in some sense, the deterministic distribution is an ME distribution because it is a member of the closure set. Further discussion in this vein requires more advanced mathematics than we ask for understanding this book, so we leave it to the experts. ▲

Behavior of s Near $\varrho = 0$ and $\varrho = 1$

It is commonly accepted that if the coefficient of variation for a given distribution is greater than 1, its geometric parameter will be greater than that for the M/M/1 queue [i.e., $s(\varrho; G) > \varrho$], and if $C_G^2 < 1$, we would expect $s(\varrho; G) < \varrho$. Although this is true for ϱ sufficiently close to 1, it need not be true for all ϱ. The function $s(\varrho; H)$, with $C_H^2 = 10$, clearly satisfies this rule. So does $s(\varrho; U)$, with $C_U^2 = 1/3$. However, $s(\varrho; E_{2p})$, for which $C_{2p}^2 = 2/3$, clearly does not, as seen by the crossing of the two curves corresponding to E_{2p} and M.

We cannot in general show how s varies explicitly with ϱ, except by direct numerical computation. However, we can see their relation more clearly near $\varrho = 0$ and 1, by expanding s in a Taylor series about each of those points. To do this, we need to know the derivatives of s with respect to ϱ there. We do not have an explicit relation between the two variables, so we must perform the differentiation implicitly. Consider the function, taken from (5.1.14a),

$$g(s;\, \varrho) := (1 - p)\Psi_a \left[\mathbf{V_a}[\varrho T\,\mathbf{I} + (1 - s)\mathbf{V_a}]^{-1}\right] - 1. \tag{5.1.15a}$$

For a given ϱ, the geometric parameter for the G/M/1 queue satisfies the equation: $g(s; \varrho) = 0$. In particular, we know that

$$g(p; 0) = 0 \quad \text{and} \quad g(1; 1) = 0. \tag{5.1.15b}$$

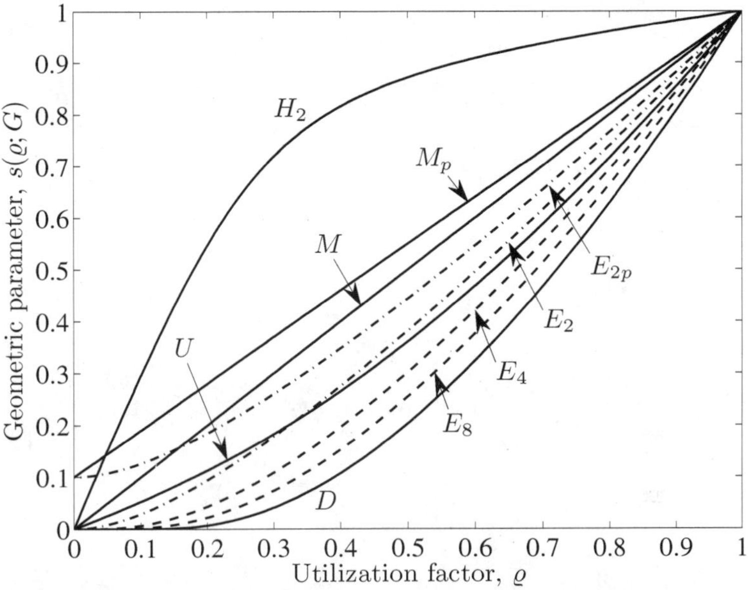

Figure 5.1.1: Dependence of s, the geometric parameter of the steady-state G/M/1 queue, on the utilization $\varrho = 1/\lambda T = \bar{x}_2/\bar{x}_1$ for various interarrival time distributions. The distributions and their labels are (M), exponential; (M_p), exponential with initial impulse, $p = 0.1$; (E_k), Erlangian-k, for $k = 2, 4, 8$; (E_{2p}), Erlangian-2 with initial impulse; (D), Deterministic; (U), uniform; and (H_2), hyperexponential-2, with $C_v^2 = 10$. All possible geometric parameters must be monotonically nondecreasing functions of ϱ, bounded from below by $s(\varrho; D)$, and bounded from above by $s = 1$. For all distributions $s(1; G) = 1$.

Next we can write

$$\frac{dg}{d\varrho} = \frac{\partial g}{\partial s}\frac{ds}{d\varrho} + \frac{\partial g}{\partial \varrho} = 0.$$

Therefore, we have

$$\frac{ds}{d\varrho} = -\frac{\partial g}{\partial \varrho} \Big/ \frac{\partial g}{\partial s}. \tag{5.1.16}$$

The higher derivatives can be computed by differentiating this expression over and over again. We spare the reader this tedium, and only quote the results. However, we go part of the way, so as to prove that all the derivatives of s evaluated at $\varrho = 1$ depend only on the moments of the distribution function. We also prove that all the derivatives of s evaluated at $\varrho = 0$ depend only on the value of $B(x)$ [or $R(x)$] and its derivatives at $x = 0_+$.

First, from Equations (5.1.12), we see that the kth derivatives of $R(x)$ and $b(x)$ are related to the derivatives of $R_a(x)$ and $b_a(x)$ by the following. For $k \geq 1$:

$$B^{(k)}(x) := \frac{d^k B(x)}{dx^k} = (1-p)B_a^{(k)}(x) = -(1-p)R_a^{(k)}(x), \tag{5.1.17a}$$

and for $x > 0$

$$b^{(k)}(x) = (1-p)b_a^{(k)}(x). \tag{5.1.17b}$$

Next note from its definition that $\Psi[\mathbf{V}^n] = (1-p)\Psi_a[\mathbf{V_a}^n]$, so, using (3.1.8b) and (3.1.9), we can write for $k, n \geq 0$

$$b^{(k)}(0_+) = -R^{(k+1)}(0_+) = (1-p)b_a^{(k)}(0) = (-1)^k\,(1-p)\Psi_a[\mathbf{B_a}^{k+1}], \tag{5.1.17c}$$

and (pick any pair)

$$\mathbb{E}[X^n] = n!\Psi[\mathbf{V}^n] = n!(1-p)\Psi_a[\mathbf{V_a}^n] = (1-p)\mathbb{E}[X_a^n]. \tag{5.1.17d}$$

Now we show the utility of (5.1.15a) (and LAQT) for finding the derivatives of functions. As we do so often, we define an auxiliary function that seems to be more general than we need, and then come up with simpler expressions than we otherwise would. Let

$$G(k,\, l;\, \varrho) := (1-p)\Psi_a\left[\mathbf{V_a}^k[\varrho T\,\mathbf{I} + (1-s)\mathbf{V_a}]^{-l}\right], \tag{5.1.18a}$$

for $k,\ l \geq 1$. We have suppressed the dependence on s, because it, in turn, also depends on ϱ. Then from (5.1.15a),

$$g(s;\, \varrho) = G(1, 1;\, \varrho) - 1. \tag{5.1.19}$$

Now we are ready to take partial derivatives.

$$\begin{aligned} G_s(k,\, l;\, \varrho) :&= \frac{\partial}{\partial s} G(k,\, l;\, \varrho) \\ &= l(1-p)\Psi_a\left[\mathbf{V_a}^{k+1}[\,\varrho T\,\mathbf{I} + (1-s)\mathbf{V_a}]^{-(l+1)}\right]. \end{aligned}$$

Thus

$$G_s(k, l;\, \varrho) = lG(k+1,\, l+1;\, \varrho). \tag{5.1.20a}$$

Similarly, we can show that

$$G_\varrho(k, l;\, \varrho) := \frac{\partial}{\partial \varrho} G(k, l;\, \varrho) = -lTG(k,\, l+1;\, \varrho). \tag{5.1.20b}$$

We can use these equations to differentiate over and over again. For instance, applying (5.1.20b) twice, we get

$$G_{\varrho\varrho}(k, l;\, \varrho) = l(l+1)T^2 G(k,\, l+2;\, \varrho),$$

and applying (5.1.20a) and (5.1.20b) once each, we get

$$G_{\varrho\, s}(k, l;\, \varrho) = G_{s\,\varrho}(k, l;\, \varrho) = -l^2\, TG(k+1, l+2;\, \varrho).$$

Notice that if we start with $l \geq k$, then no matter how many partial derivatives we take of both kinds, we will always end up with an expression where the second argument of G is greater than, or equal to, the first argument. As long our object is to differentiate $g(s;\varrho)$ (where $k=l=1$), this will always be the case.

Actually, we are only interested in the G's when $\varrho = 0$ ($s = p$) and $\varrho = 1$ ($s = 1$). Thus (use $\mathbf{V_a} = \mathbf{B_a}^{-1}$)

$$G(k,\, l;\, 0) = (1-p)\Psi_a \left[\mathbf{V_a}^k[(1-p)\mathbf{V_a}]^{-l}\right]$$

$$= (1-p)^{-(l-1)}\Psi_a \left[\mathbf{B_a}^{l-k}\right] \tag{5.1.21a}$$

(we have assumed that $l \geq k$) and

$$G(k,l;\, 1) = (1-p)T^{-l}\Psi_a \left[\mathbf{V_a}^k\right] = T^{-l}\Psi\left[\mathbf{V}^k\right]. \tag{5.1.21b}$$

Notice that all the G functions, evaluated at $\varrho = 0$, depend only on the scalars, $\Psi_a\left[\mathbf{B_a}^j\right]$ (for $j \geq 0$), which from (5.1.17c) tells us that they depend on $R(x)$ and its derivatives at $x = 0$ only. Also notice from (5.1.21b) that the value of G at $\varrho = 1$ does not explicitly depend on the initial impulse, as represented by p and a, and in fact, depends only on the moments of the interarrival time distribution. Although (5.1.21a) and (5.1.21b) only explicitly apply to ME distributions, (5.1.17c) and (5.1.17d) allow us to extend the equations to any distribution for which the appropriate objects exist:

$$G(k,\, l;\, 1) = \frac{\mathbb{E}[X^k]}{k!\, T^l}. \tag{5.1.21c}$$

and

$$G(k,l;0) = \frac{(-1)^{l-k}}{(1-p)^l} R^{(l-k)}(0_+). \tag{5.1.21d}$$

Such relations could have been derived without the aid of the ME formulas, but the mathematical difficulties would have been enormous. For instance, *l'Hospital*'s rule must be applied $k+1$ times just to get the kth derivative. The reader should try it and see.

Okay, let us see what all this has done for us. Return to (5.1.16), and use (5.1.19) and (5.1.20), to get

$$s'(\varrho;\, G) := \frac{ds}{d\varrho} = -\frac{G_\varrho(1,1;\varrho)}{G_s(1,1;\varrho)} = \frac{TG(1,2;\varrho)}{G(2,2;\varrho)}. \tag{5.1.22a}$$

For $\varrho = 1$, using (5.1.21b), we have (remember, $\Psi[\mathbf{V}] = \mathbb{E}[X] = T$)

$$s'(1;\, G) = T\frac{\Psi[\mathbf{V}]}{T^2} \times \frac{T^2}{\Psi[\mathbf{V}^2]} = \frac{T^2}{\Psi[\mathbf{V}^2]}. \tag{5.1.22b}$$

But $\Psi\left[\mathbf{V}^2\right] = \mathbb{E}[X^2]/2$, $\mathbb{E}[X^2] = T^2 + \sigma^2$, and $C_v^2 = \sigma^2/T^2$, so

$$s'(1;\, G) = \frac{2}{1 + C_v^2}. \tag{5.1.22c}$$

Given that $s'(1; M) = 1$, (5.1.22c) tells us that any interarrival time distribution that has a coefficient of variation less than (greater than) 1 will have a slope greater (less) than 1, and thus its geometric parameter must be below (above) that for the M/M/1 queue as they both approach $(1, 1)$. The largest slope attainable occurs for the deterministic distribution for which $C_v^2 = 0$ and $s'(1; D) = 2$; thus all other curves must lie above it (at least for ϱ near 1). In a similar fashion we can show that (pick one)

$$s'(0;\, G) = T\Psi_a\left[\mathbf{B_a}\right] = Tb_a(0) = \frac{Tb(0_+)}{1-p} = (1-p)T_a b_a(0). \qquad (5.1.22d)$$

Although the above equations appear to depend on two factors (T and $b(0)$) they actually are related and produce only one independent parameter. In studying the behavior of G/M/1 queues one commonly varies the arrival rate of customers, or equivalently, the interarrival time, without varying the interarrival time distribution. In Definition 3.2.1 we discussed what it means to have two distributions with the ***same shape***. We apply it to the expression $T\Psi_a\left[\mathbf{B_a}\right]$. First define the matrix,

$$\mathbf{B_{ao}} := T_a\mathbf{B_a},$$

with inverse $\mathbf{V_{ao}} = (1/T_{\mathrm{a}})\mathbf{V_a}$. Then, for instance, $\Psi_a[\mathbf{V_{ao}}] = 1$, and $\langle\mathbf{p_a},\, \mathbf{B_a}\rangle \sim \langle\mathbf{p_a},\, \mathbf{B_{oa}}\rangle$, from which is follows that $\langle\mathbf{p},\, \mathbf{B}\rangle \sim \langle\mathbf{p},\, \mathbf{B_o}\rangle$. In other words, the PDFs generated by these representations ($F(x)$ and $F_{\mathrm{o}}(x)$) look alike, as would be expected for some renewal process where the arrival rate is changed. Then (5.1.22d) yields

$$s'(0;\, G) = T\frac{1}{T_a}\Psi[\mathbf{B_{ao}}] = (1-p)\Psi[\mathbf{B_{ao}}] = (1-p)b_{ao}(0) = b_{\mathrm{o}}(0_+). \quad (5.1.22e)$$

We see from this that $s'(0;\, G)$ does not depend on T.

We now see how s behaves by expanding it in a Taylor series around 0 and 1. But keep in mind that these expansions are valid only if all the derivatives of $b(x)$ exist around $x = 0_+$. A Taylor series expansion near $\varrho = 0$ gives us

$$s(\varrho;\, G) \approx p + s'(0;\, G)\varrho + \frac{1}{2}s''(0;\, G)\varrho^2 + \cdots \qquad (5.1.23a)$$

and for ϱ near 1,

$$s(\varrho;\, G) \approx 1 - s'(1;\, G)(1-\varrho) + \frac{1}{2}s''(1;\, G)(1-\varrho)^2 + \cdots. \qquad (5.1.23b)$$

Equation (5.1.23a) tells us that if $p > 0$, then $s(\varrho; G) > s(\varrho; M)$ near $\varrho = 0$, and if $p = 0$, (5.1.22d) tells us that $s(\varrho; G)$ is greater (less) than $s(\varrho; M)$ if $Tb(0) > 1$ [$Tb(0) < 1$]. It follows from (5.1.14c) that

$$s(\varrho; D) \approx e^{1/\varrho} \quad \text{for small } \varrho, \qquad (5.1.23c)$$

therefore, all its derivatives are 0 at $\varrho = 0_+$. This does not actually violate Taylor's theorem, because $s(0_-; D)$ does not exist, so (5.1.23a) does not hold, but it does tell us that $s(\varrho; D)$ is very flat near 0, and thus bounds all other s functions from below (at least for ϱ near 0). The behavior of s near $\varrho = 1$ follows directly from (5.1.22c) and (5.1.23b). Easy manipulation yields

$$\frac{1-s}{1-\varrho} = \frac{2}{1+C_v^2} + \mathrm{O}[1-\varrho]. \tag{5.1.23d}$$

This tells us that as ϱ approaches 1, larger C_v^2 means larger s.

Note that the conditions required for s to be smaller than ϱ near 0, and the requirements that s be larger than ϱ near 1, are completely unrelated; thus it is possible to construct distribution functions whose geometric parameters cross the line $s = \varrho$, at least once, even with $p = 0$. In fact, we discussed one such function in Section 3.2.3.1, a hyper-Erlangian with 4 states. This family of functions satisfies $b(0) = 0$, but can have any mean and any squared coefficient of variation $C_v^2 \geq 1/2$. See Example 5.5.2 for further discussion. The behavior of $s(\varrho)$ for various values of C_v^2 is explored in the following exercise.

Exercise 5.1.5: Calculate the geometric parameter s as a function of ϱ, using $T = 1$ and $C_v^2 = 1, 2, 5, 10$ for the two distributions given in Chapter 3, Equations (3.2.7) and (3.2.14) (the hyperexponential and the hyper-Erlangian). This can be done by numerically solving (5.1.6a) for enough values of ϱ to produce a smooth curve. Draw the two sets of four curves on the same graph, together with the line $s = \varrho$. (The hyperexponential with $C_v^2 = 1$ should give this.) Note that for the hyper-Erlangian, when $C_v^2 > 1$, $s(\varrho)$ crosses $s = \varrho$, but for $C_v^2 = 1$ it asymptotically approaches the line from below as $\varrho \Rightarrow 1$ (i.e., it has the same slope at $\varrho = 1$). This must be true because of (5.1.22c).

We have done everything we can to state and prove the following theorem, which summarizes this section.

Theorem 5.1.4 For any steady-state G/M/1 queue, with utilization factor, $\varrho = 1/\rho = 1/\lambda T$, and geometric parameter $s(\varrho;\, G)$, given by Theorem 5.1.2, the following statements are true.

(a) $s(\varrho;\, G)$ depends only on $B(x)$ [or $R(x)$] and its derivatives near $\varrho = 0$.

(b) $s(\varrho;\, G)$ depends only on the moments of $b(x)$ near $\varrho = 1$.

(c) $s(\varrho; G)$ is bounded from below by $s(\varrho; D)$ for $0 \leq \varrho \leq 1$.

We have not actually proven (c) for all ϱ. ∎

This theorem has an important implication for dealing with approximations to density functions when applied to heavy traffic queues and reliability theory. Heavy traffic queues occur when ρ, or in this chapter, ϱ, is close to 1, and the common belief that approximation functions should fit the first few moments is vindicated here. However, as we have already pointed out in Section 4.5.4 and do again in Section 6.5.3, MTTF is more interested in small ϱ, for one expects the time to repair a device to be much less than the time it takes for it to break. Therefore, the behavior of the pdf near $x = 0$ plays a more important role than the moments! Furthermore, in real-life situations, decisions are usually made before problems become serious (well, they should be), so the intermediate region should be the most important. Conclusion? Both moments and derivatives are important.

For the record, we give explicit formulas for the second derivatives without forcing the reader to go through the tedious derivations (just looking at the formulas is bad enough):

$$s''(1 : G) = \frac{2T^2}{(\Psi[\mathbf{V}^2])^3}\left((\Psi[\mathbf{V}^2])^2 - T\Psi[\mathbf{V}^3]\right)$$

$$= \frac{4T^2}{\mathbb{E}[X^2]} - \frac{8}{3}\left(\frac{T}{\mathbb{E}[X^2]}\right)^3 \mathbb{E}[X^3] \tag{5.1.24a}$$

(depends only on the moments), and

$$s''(0; G) = \frac{T^2}{1-p}\left[\Psi_a[\mathbf{B_a}]^2 - \Psi_a[\mathbf{B_a}^2]\right] = \frac{T^2}{1-p}\left[[b_a(0)]^2 + (1-p)b'_a(0)\right]$$

$$= \frac{T^2}{(1-p)^3}\left[[b(0_+)]^2 + (1-p)b'(0_+)\right] \tag{5.1.24b}$$

[depends only on $R(0)$ and its derivatives].

Finally, we note that one can automate the numerical calculation of all the derivatives of $s(\varrho; G)$ at 0 and 1, with the aid of (5.1.22a), (5.1.20), and (5.1.21), but you probably have already been exposed to more information about the geometric parameter than you care to know.

We postpone examining system time behavior until Example 5.5.2 and Figures 5.5.2 and 5.5.3, where we discuss the mean time for a busy period. It is truly extraordinary that the mean system time and the mean time for a busy period are equal for any G/M/1 queue, so what is said for one is true for the other. This is in contrast with M/G/1 queues where the mean time for a busy period is independent of the service time distribution, and is equal to $\bar{x}/(1-\rho)$, the same as the system time for the M/M/1 queue.

5.1.4 Systems Where Interarrival Times Are Power-Tailed

In Section 3.3 we introduced PT distributions, showing that they have infinite moments, and can cause havoc with statistical measurements. In Section 4.2.2.2 we showed what must be reconsidered if the service-time distribution is PT in the M/G/1 queue. Here we see what must be done to analyze the PT/M/1 queue. The subject is discussed in detail in [Grein-Job-Lip99]. The figures are taken from that paper.

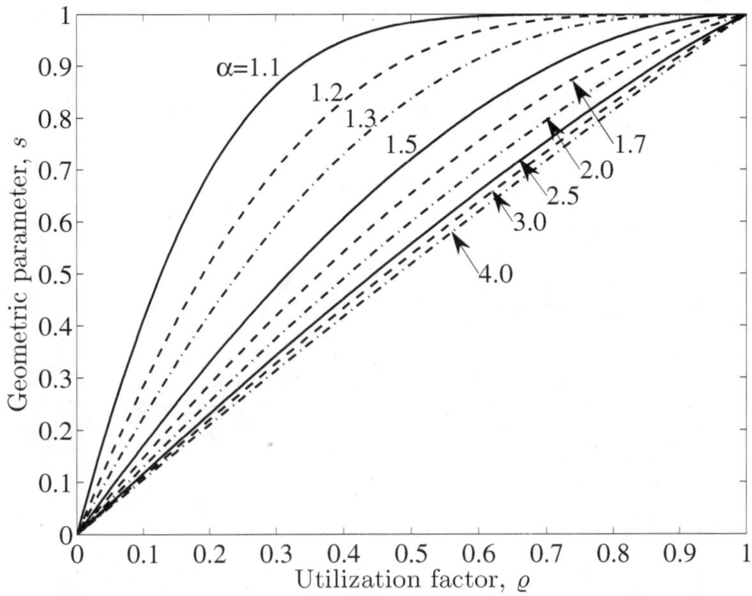

Figure 5.1.2: s as a function of ϱ for PT interarrival times with $\alpha \in [1.1, 1.2, 1.3, 1.5, 1.7, 2.0, 2.5, 3.0, 4.0]$ The PT function used is given in Section 3.3.6.2, where $\theta = 0.5$, and the number of terms T is large enough to be effectively ∞. For $\alpha > 2$ the slope at $\varrho = 1$ is positive, and for $\alpha = 4$ s is almost a straight line, similar to the M/M/1 queue. But for $\alpha < 2$, the slope of s is 0, and the smaller α, the longer s stays close to 1 for smaller and smaller values of ϱ. At $\varrho = 0$, s is well-behaved for all values of α (as long as $\alpha > 1$).

In the previous section we showed that the behavior of the geometric parameter s near $\varrho = 0$ depends on the derivatives of $R(x)$. PT distributions are certainly well behaved for small x, so there should be no problems for small ϱ. But near $\varrho = 1$, s depends on the moments of the distribution, and for PT distributions all moments $\mathbb{E}[X^\ell]$ are infinite for $\ell \geq \alpha$. In particular, if $1 < \alpha \leq 2$ (we must assume that $\alpha > 1$, otherwise the mean interarrival time would be infinite and we could not even define ϱ), then $C_v^2 = \infty$ and Equation (5.1.22c) tells us that the slope of s at $\varrho = 1$ is 0. In fact, according to Theorem 5.1.4, all the derivatives of s are 0. Therefore, a different analysis is necessary, at least near $\varrho = 1$.

In general it is not possible to find the Laplace transforms of PT distributions, but the ME representation of a truncated PT discussed in Section 3.3.6.2 makes it possible to numerically solve for s in (5.1.6a) as long as ϱ is not too close to 1. The results of a series of computations are presented in Figure 5.1.2 for various values of α, and $\theta = 0.5$. The value of T, the number of terms in the function, was chosen to be large enough so as not to affect the answer. The most significant feature is the behavior near $\varrho = 1$. As would be expected, as long as $\alpha > 2$ the slope of s there is positive. But for $\alpha < 2$ the slope is 0, also as expected for a function with infinite C_v^2. As α decreases, s

stays close to 1 for smaller values of ϱ.

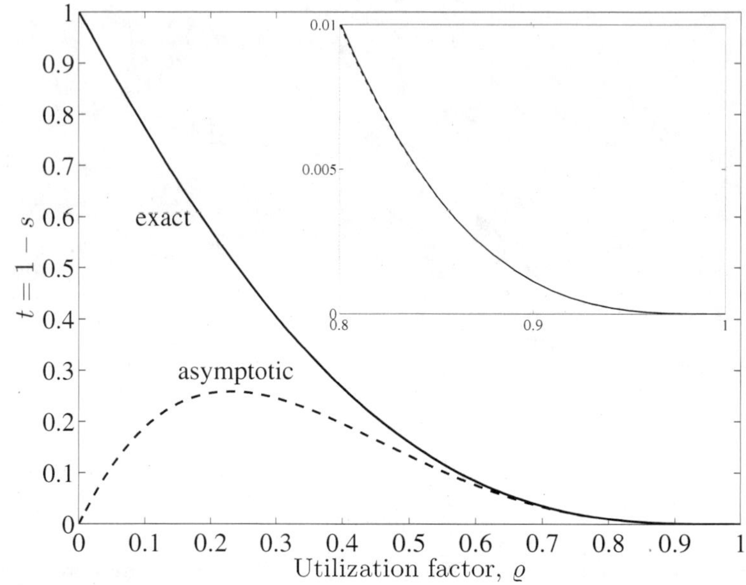

Figure 5.1.3: $\varrho - t$–Diagram, both for the exact and the asymptotic equations for a PT/M/1 queue, where $t := 1 - s$, $\alpha = 1.3$ and $\theta = 0.5$. From the inset, it is clear that the asymptotic Equation (5.1.26a) is an excellent approximation for ϱ as small as 0.8.

The fact that "s is very close to 1" is in itself not very informative. The question is "How close?" After all, it is $t := 1 - s$ that yields the information needed. From Equations (5.1.7b) and (5.1.7c), it is seen that $\bar{q}_2$ and $\mathbf{E}[T_2]$ depend inversely on t; that is, the smaller t is, the larger they are. Furthermore, the overflow probabilities, as given in (5.1.9d), are very dependent upon t. Note that

$$\lim_{t \to \infty} (1 + t)^{1/t} = e,$$

so we can write

$$P_{o2} = s^k = (1 - t)^k = [(1 - t)^{1/t}]^{kt} \approx e^{-kt}. \tag{5.1.25}$$

That is, unless $kt >> 1$ we can expect the queue to exceed length k often. If t is very small, then very large buffers are needed. The analysis of the behavior of t near $\varrho = 1$ is too involved to present here, but is given in detail in [Grein-Job-Lip99]. Let

$$\beta := \frac{1}{1 - \alpha}$$

Then they show that, near $\varrho = 1$,

$$t(\varrho) \Rightarrow C\,\varrho\,(1 - \varrho)^{\beta}, \quad \text{for} \quad 1 < \alpha < 2, \tag{5.1.26a}$$

where C is a constant that depends on α. From (5.1.17c), the mean system time approaches

$$\mathbb{E}[T_2] \Rightarrow \frac{1}{C(1-\varrho)^{\beta}}, \quad \text{for} \quad 1 < \alpha < 2. \tag{5.1.26b}$$

For $\alpha \leq 1$ the mean interarrival time is infinite, so the steady-state solution has no meaning (what is ϱ?). For $\alpha \geq 2$ the exponent, $1/(\alpha - 1)$, is replaced by 1, and the system behaves in a way similar to those with well-behaved arrival processes. But in the in-between range, (5.1.26b) tells us that $\mathbb{E}[T_2]$ blows up more rapidly than for non-PT renewal processes.

We have calculated $t(\varrho)$ for $\alpha = 1.3$ and presented it in Figure 5.1.3, together with the approximation above. Clearly, the approximation is good for ϱ as small as 0.6. In fact, the inset shows that the two curves are indistinguishable for the range $0.8 < \varrho \leq 1$. For larger α, the approximation breaks down closer to 1.

5.1.5 Buffer Overflow Probabilities for the G/M/1 Queue

The ***buffer overflow probability*** was already given by (5.1.9d). As described previously, there are times when it is imperative that no customers be lost, but a primary buffer may be expensive, and a backup buffer can be supplied. But putting customers into the backup buffer has its own costs. It may take time, effort and/or inconvenience to bring a customer from the backup to the primary. A simple example of this would be if a customer finds the buffer full, returns to his source, and continuously tries to enter the queue until he is successful. (Try getting an answer from a busy telephone answering service.) In this case, the source acts as the backup buffer. Another example would be the Ethernet, and even the Web under TCP control acts more or less in this mode, because no packets are lost, and all packets are sent as soon as they can be accepted. Other discussions were given in Sections 2.1.4 and 4.2.4. The following example explores another issue, showing that in this case (as in many others) the overflow probabilities depend on more than the mean and variance of a distribution.

Example 5.1.2: Suppose that a server is to be designed so that no more than 1.0% of arriving customers must use the backup buffer. Then for a given ϱ we must find that ℓ which satisfies

$$P_{o2} = .01 = s^{\ell}, \quad \text{that is} \quad \ell = \ln(.01)/\ln(s).$$

For a given ϱ, one can solve for s either by finding the smallest eigenvalue of $\mathbf{A}$, or by solving for s in (5.1.6a). We have done this for five different interarrival time distributions (not counting the exponential), and have displayed the results in Figures 5.1.4 and 5.1.5. One of the distributions is a TPT as given in Equations (3.3.21) with truncation $M = 32$, and $\alpha = 1.4$, and $\theta = 0.5$. This gives a squared coefficient of variation of $C_v^2 = 5033.44\ldots$. The other distributions are the hyperexponentials described in Section 3.2.1.2, with the same mean and variance as the TPT, and $p = 1/10^k$. The curves agree near

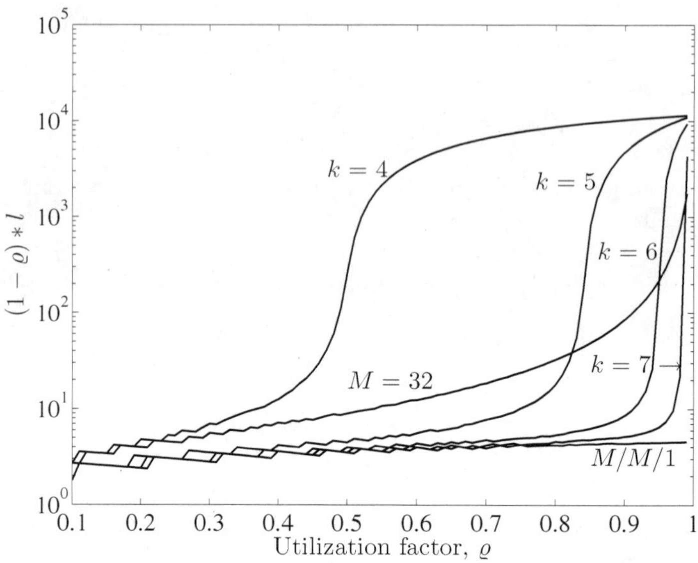

Figure 5.1.4: G/M/1 primary buffer size ℓ needed for overflow to be less than 1%, as a function of ϱ, for five interarrival time distributions with the same $C_v^2 \approx 5033$. Because the buffer size can become very large as ϱ approaches 1, the function actually plotted is $\log[(1-\varrho)\ell]$. All curves are finite at $\varrho = 1$, as shown in Figure 5.1.5. [See text and Equations (5.1.22).] The curve labeled $M = 32$, refers to a 32-term TPT interarrival time distribution. Four of the curves are for H_2 interarrival time distributions with $p = 10^{-k}$. The M/M/1 queue is included for comparison.

$\varrho = 0$ and $\varrho = 1$ but have nothing in common in between. This shows clearly that for at least some properties there is more to a distribution than merely mean and variance.

All the curves are equal at $\varrho = 1$ because of (5.1.22c) and (5.1.23b). From the above equation and (5.1.23b), we have

$$(1-\varrho)k = (1-\varrho)\ln(.01)/\ln(s) \approx \frac{(1-\varrho)\ln(.01)}{\ln[1-(1-\varrho)s'(1)]}.$$

And from (5.1.22c) and the fact that $\ln(1-x) \approx -x$, we have

$$\lim_{\varrho\to 1}(1-\varrho)k = \frac{\ln(.01)}{s'(1)} = \frac{\ln(.01)(1+C_v^2)}{2}.$$

In Figure 5.1.5, this is $\lim(1-\varrho)\,k = 11,572.236$.

As a final observation, the curves look jagged because k is an integer. Also, the slopes are slightly negative between jumps because of the factor $1-\varrho$. This material was taken from work by Fiorini and Hatem [FioriniLipHatem97], [Hatem97]. ▲

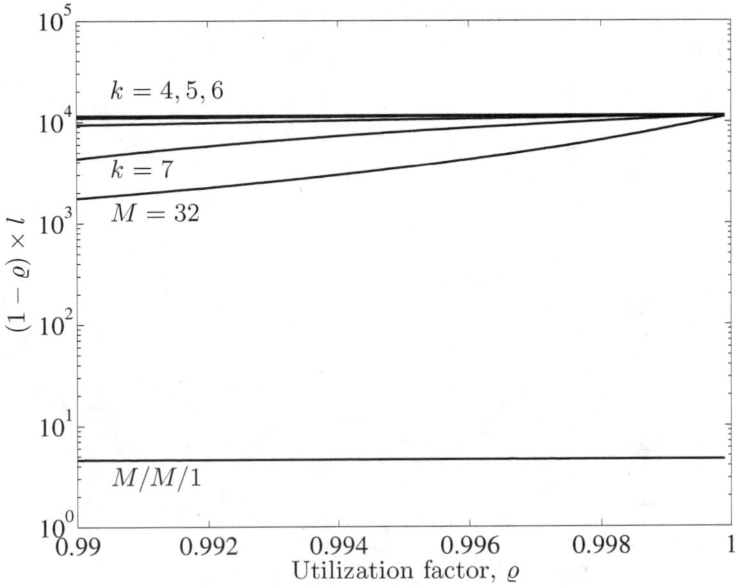

Figure 5.1.5: G/M/1 primary buffer size ℓ needed as ϱ approaches 1. The conditions are the same as those in Figure 5.1.4, i.e., ℓ is multiplied by $1-\varrho$ to yield finite values for their product. All the curves (excluding the one for the M/M/1 queue) are equal at $\varrho=1$ because they have the same C_v^2.

5.2 ME Representation of Departures

We now turn our attention to the behavior of customers leaving a service center. We already looked at this to some extent in Sections 2.1.6 and 4.2.5, in looking at the M/M/1 and M/G/1 queues. We do the same here for the G/M/1 queue, but first we look at arrivals to S_2 conditioned by departures from S_2. From the closed-loop point of view, arrivals to S_2 are the same as departures from S_1. There was no point in examining the equivalent question for the M/G/1 queue, because arrivals to the "G" queue (S_1) were governed according to the Poisson process, and thus no conditions could change that.

5.2.1 Arrival Time Distribution Conditioned by a Departure

We saw in Theorem 5.1.3 that all the steady-state vector departure probabilities $[\mathbf{d_2}(n)]$ are proportional to the same vector $\hat{\mathbf{u}}$. Thus at the moment a customer leaves S_2, S_1 will be found in that same state. We conclude, then, that the time until the next arrival to S_2 is generated by the vector-matrix pair $\langle\, \hat{\mathbf{u}}\, ,\, \mathbf{B}\,\rangle$. We must say a few words to distinguish this process from the interarrival process to S_2. The interarrival process refers to the distribution of times between arrivals to S_2, or the time until the next arrival, given that a customer has just arrived. It is the same as the time between departures from S_1, which is generated by $\langle\, \mathbf{p}, \mathbf{B}\,\rangle$. In this section we are interested in the time to the next arrival, given that a customer has just departed S_2 thus the change from $\mathbf{p}$ to $\hat{\mathbf{u}}$ as the initial, or startup, vector. For lack of a better symbol, we denote all properties of this process with the subscript ω. Thus X_ω is the r.v. denoting the time until the next arrival, given that a customer has just departed S_2, and $b_\omega(x)$ is its density function.

Consistent with Theorems 3.1.1 and 4.2.5 we describe this latest process by the following theorem.

Theorem 5.2.1 The arrival times for an open ME/M/1 queue, given that a customer has just left, is generated by the vector-matrix pair $\langle\, \hat{\mathbf{u}}\,,\, \mathbf{B}\rangle$ (or $\langle\, \hat{\mathbf{u}}\,,\, \mathbf{V}\rangle$), where $\hat{\mathbf{u}}$ is given by Corollary 5.1.2, and $\mathbf{B}$ is the service rate matrix for S_1. It then follows that (where $\Psi_\omega\,[\,\mathbf{X}\,] := \hat{\mathbf{u}}\mathbf{X}\,\boldsymbol{\epsilon}'$ for any $\mathbf{X}$)

$$\mathbb{E}[X_\omega^n] = n!\Psi_\omega\,[\mathbf{V}^n]\,, \tag{5.2.1a}$$

$$b_\omega(x) = \Psi_\omega\,[\mathbf{B}\exp(-x\mathbf{B})]\,, \tag{5.2.1b}$$

and

$$B_\omega^*(s) = \Psi_\omega\,\left[(\mathbf{I}+s\mathbf{V})^{-1}\right]. \tag{5.2.1c}$$

■

The proof follows from the definition of $\hat{\mathbf{u}}$ and Theorem 3.1.1.

Let us now examine this distribution further by calculating its mean and variance, and then see what we can do with its pdf. We can find $\mathbb{E}[X_\omega]$ by multiplying (5.1.6c) on the right with $\boldsymbol{\epsilon}'$. This process yields

$$1+(1-s)\lambda\hat{\mathbf{u}}\mathbf{V}\,\boldsymbol{\epsilon}' = \lambda\mathbf{p}\mathbf{V}\boldsymbol{\epsilon}' = 1+(1-s)\lambda\mathbb{E}[X_\omega] = \lambda\mathbb{E}[X_1] = 1/\varrho.$$

Upon solving for $\mathbb{E}[X_\omega]$ we get

$$\mathbb{E}[X_\omega] = \frac{1-\varrho}{(1-s)\varrho\,\lambda} = \frac{1-\varrho}{1-s}\,\mathbb{E}[X_1]. \tag{5.2.2a}$$

In general, $\mathbb{E}[X_\omega]$ is not equal to $\mathbb{E}[X_1]$. Of course, for the M/M/1 queue $s=\varrho$, so in that case, the two are equal. They are also equal in the limit as $\varrho\to 0$ (i.e., in the no-load limit), if there is no initial impulse. For then s also becomes 0. The heavy load limit is not so easy to find, because now both s and ϱ go to 1, and we are left with the indeterminate, 0/0. We can take the limit by going back to (5.1.6b). Now, remember that ϱ goes to 1, λ and $1/\mathbb{E}[X_1]$ become equal. Also, recall the definition of the mean residual vector $\boldsymbol{\pi}_\mathbf{r}$ from (3.5.10b). What we get is

$$\lim_{\varrho\to 1}\hat{\mathbf{u}} = \mathbf{p}(\mathbf{I}+0\mathbf{V})^{-1}\frac{1}{\mathbb{E}[X_1]}\mathbf{V} = \frac{1}{\Psi\,[\mathbf{V}]}\mathbf{p}\mathbf{V} = \boldsymbol{\pi}_\mathbf{r}. \tag{5.2.2b}$$

This is what a random observer sees upon visiting S_1 without noting its previous behavior. We would expect this, because a customer departing S_2 sort of randomly arrives at S_1. We also know that for the M/G/1 queue, a random observer and an arriving customer see the same thing at S_1. Why then, is this not true for the G/M/1 queue as well? First we show that the random observer still sees the arrival process to S_2 as being initiated by $\boldsymbol{\pi}_\mathbf{r}$ if she takes no note of how many customers are in the queue. What she sees is the vector average over all queue lengths. That is,

$$\boldsymbol{\pi}_{\mathbf{2r}} := \sum_{k=0}^{\infty} \boldsymbol{\pi}_\mathbf{2}(k) = \boldsymbol{\pi}_\mathbf{r}. \tag{5.2.2c}$$

Exercise 5.2.1: Prove that Equation (5.2.2c) is correct.

Next, recall that as long as $\mathbb{E}[X_1] > \mathbb{E}[X_2]$, as was the case in Chapter 4, S_2 is never idle, so its departing customers constitute a Poisson process, which is the equivalent of making random observations. But when $\mathbb{E}[X_2] > \mathbb{E}[X_1]$, as is the case in this chapter, then S_2 is idle some of the time, and its departing customers see only the sum from $k = 1$ to infinity of the above, or more correctly from (5.1.9b),

$$\sum_{k=0}^{\infty} \mathbf{d_2}(k) = \hat{\mathbf{u}}.$$

Alternatively we can argue given that S_1 has an unbounded number of customers and $\mathbf{a_{1r}}(n) = \boldsymbol{\pi}_\mathbf{1r}(n)$ (see Definition 4.3.1), (5.1.2c) implies that

$$\lim_{n\to\infty} \mathbf{a_{1r}}(n) = \lim_{n\to\infty} \frac{\mathbf{p}\mathbf{U}^n}{\Psi\left[\mathbf{U}^n\right]} = \hat{\mathbf{u}}.$$

Returning to the calculation of $\mathbb{E}[X_\omega]$ near $\varrho = 1$, we see from (5.2.2b) that

$$\lim_{\varrho\to 1} \mathbb{E}[X_\omega] = \lim_{s\to 1} \hat{\mathbf{u}}\mathbf{V}\boldsymbol{\epsilon}' = \boldsymbol{\pi}_\mathbf{r}\, \mathbf{V}\boldsymbol{\epsilon}' = \frac{\mathbb{E}[X_1^2]}{2\mathbb{E}[X_1]}.$$

Thus only when s and ϱ approach 1, does the mean time until the next arrival after a departure from S_2 equal the mean residual time of S_1. Only then do the random observer and the departing customer see the same thing.

We now find an expression for the variance and squared coefficient of variation for the process. First we need $\Psi_\omega\left[\mathbf{V}^2\right]$. We get this in the same way we found $\mathbb{E}[X_\omega]$. Multiply (5.1.6c) from the right by $\mathbf{V}\,\boldsymbol{\epsilon}'$, and then solve for the desired term.

$$\lambda^2\Psi_\omega\left[\mathbf{V}^2\right] = \frac{1}{1-s}\left(\lambda^2\Psi\left[\mathbf{V}^2\right] - \lambda\mathbb{E}[X_\omega]\right). \tag{5.2.3a}$$

We know that $\mathbb{E}[X_\omega^2] = 2\Psi_\omega\left[\mathbf{V}^2\right]$ and $\sigma_\omega^2 = \mathbb{E}[X_\omega^2] - (\mathbb{E}[X_\omega])^2$. Therefore,

$$\lambda^2\sigma_\omega^2 = \frac{1}{1-s}\left(\lambda^2\mathbb{E}[X^2] - 2\lambda\mathbb{E}[X_\omega]\right) - \lambda^2(\mathbb{E}[X_\omega])^2$$

$$= \frac{1}{1-s}\left(\lambda^2\sigma_1^2 + \rho^2 - 2\lambda\mathbb{E}[X_\omega] - (1-s)\lambda^2(\mathbb{E}[X_\omega])^2\right).$$

Next, from (5.2.2a) $\lambda\mathbb{E}[X_\omega] = (1-\varrho)/[(1-s)\varrho]$, and after some algebra, we have

$$\lambda^2\sigma_\omega^2 = \frac{\lambda^2\sigma_1^2}{1-s} + \frac{1-s\rho^2}{(1-s)^2}. \tag{5.2.3b}$$

Recall that C_i^2, the squared coefficient of variation, is the dimensionless ratio of variance to mean squared of any distribution $b_i(x)$. Therefore,

$$C_\omega^2 = \frac{\lambda^2\sigma_\omega^2}{\lambda^2(\mathbb{E}[X_\omega])^2} = \left(\frac{\lambda^2\sigma_1^2}{1-s} + \frac{\varrho^2-s}{(1-s)^2}\right)\left(\frac{1-s}{1-\varrho}\right)^2.$$

After performing a little cleanup, the following expression emerges:

$$C_\omega^2 = \frac{(1-s)C_1^2 + \varrho^2 - s}{(1-\varrho)^2}. \tag{5.2.3c}$$

From this we can tell that if S_1 is exponential, then $C_1^2 = 1$, $s = \varrho$, and $C_\omega^2 = 1$. But you knew that already. We also know from previous discussion that for low load $(s \to 0), C_\omega^2 \to C_1^2$. Under heavy load, the more detailed relation between s and ϱ which we did in Section 5.1.3 is needed before we can get a reasonable expression. Alternatively, by (5.2.2b) we can find what $b_\omega(x;\, s=1)$ itself is, and calculate C_ω^2 from it. That is what we do at the end of this section.

Our last task in this subsection is to find an expression for $b_\omega(x;s)$ itself. There are two approaches we take, neither of which yields analytically useful results, although both can be used computationally. First multiply (5.1.6b) on the right with $\mathbf{B}\exp(-x\mathbf{B})\boldsymbol{\epsilon}'$; then we get an explicit equation:

$$b_\omega(x;s) = \Psi_\omega\left[\mathbf{B}\exp(-x\mathbf{B})\right] = \lambda\Psi\left[[\mathbf{I} + \lambda(1-s)\mathbf{V}]^{-1}\exp(-x\mathbf{B})\right]. \tag{5.2.4a}$$

Our other approach is to use (5.1.6c). Again we multiply on the right with $\mathbf{B}\exp(-x\mathbf{B})$ to get the following,

$$b_\omega(x;\, s) + (1-s)\lambda R_\omega(x;s) = \lambda R_1(x), \tag{5.2.4b}$$

where we have made use of the definition of the reliability function given in (3.1.7b). This can be viewed as a differential equation in R_ω, because b_ω is its negative derivative, namely,

$$\frac{d}{dx}R_\omega(x;\, s) = (1-s)\lambda R_\omega(x;\, s) - \lambda R_1(x). \tag{5.2.4c}$$

The inhomogeneous term $R_1(x)$ is a known function of x, and $R_\omega(0;s) = 1$. For those who know something about solving differential equations, this formula has an interesting, if disconcerting property. Note that the coefficient of the homogeneous term is positive, namely, $(1-s)\lambda$. Thus the homogeneous solution $[R_H(x;s)]$ is a positive exponential, which increases unboundedly for large x. But $R_\omega(x;s)$ must go to zero for large x; therefore, the inhomogeneous solution $[R_I(x;s)]$ must have the value 1 at $x=0$, which then makes the homogeneous term drop out. Elaborating further, the general solution of (5.2.4c) must be of the form

$$R_\omega(x;\, s) = AR_H(x;\, s) + R_I(x;\, s),$$

where R_H is the general solution of (5.2.4c) with R_1 removed, A is an arbitrary constant, and R_I is any solution of the entire equation. The constant A is fixed by making $R_\omega(0;\, s) = 1$. Such a solution does not exist for arbitrary s, but only for that unique s less than 1 which satisfies (5.1.6a).

Exercise 5.2.2: Solve the differential equation (5.2.4c) for the case that S_1 is exponential and $R_\omega(0;\, s) = 1$, for any s [i.e., let $R_1(x) = e^{-x\mu}$]. Show that only if $s = \mu/\lambda$ does there exist a solution for which R_ω goes to 0 as x goes to infinity.

▲

The following expression can best summarize what we have discovered in this subsection. As s increases,

$$b_1(x) = b_\omega(x;\, 0) \;\rightarrow\; b_\omega(x;\, s) \;\rightarrow\; b_\omega(x;\, 1) = \frac{R_1(x)}{\mathbb{E}[X_\omega]}.$$

That is, as ϱ (and thus s) increases from 0 to 1, the distribution of arrival times for customers to an open G/M/1 queue that has just experienced a departure changes gradually from the interarrival process to the residual time distribution.

Example 5.2.1: It is no problem to calculate the pdf for the ω process. From Theorem 5.2.1 we know its generator; therefore, we have calculated $b_\omega(x)$ for the Erlangian-2 distribution, and show the results in Figure 5.2.1 for various values of $\varrho < 1$. We have held the interarrival times constant at $T_1 = \bar{x}_1 = 1$ and have varied λ, which equals $1/\varrho$. The smaller ϱ (and therefore s) is, the smaller b_ω at $x = 0$. This agrees with the relation we described above, because $b_1(0) = 0$ for all Erlangians. The curve labeled, $\lambda = 4$, is already close to $b_1(x) = 4x\exp(-2x)$. When ϱ is close to 1, $b_\omega(x)$ is close to $R_1(x) = (1 + 2x)\exp(-2x)$. There is one obvious unusual feature. All the curves seem to cross each other at the same point. We have expanded the box surrounding the crossing, and show it in the inset. The curves do indeed cross, and *exactly* at $x = 0.5$, with $b_\omega(0.5;\, s) = 2/e$. This happens to be exactly where $b_1(x)$ and $R_1(x)$ cross. That is, for all ϱ, $b_1(0.5) = R_1(0.5) = 2/e$. Any explanations? ▲

We can also calculate $C_\omega^2(s = 1)$ because we already know all the moments of $R_1(x)/\bar{x}_1$ from (3.3.12c) and (3.3.13). First we use (5.1.22d) and (5.1.24a) in (5.1.23a) to get a Taylor expansion of $1 - s$. Then, substituting this into (5.2.3c) we get

$$\left(C_\omega^2\right)_{s=1} = \frac{1}{3}\frac{\mathbb{E}[X_1^3]}{(\mathbb{E}[X_1])^3}\left(\frac{2}{1 + C_1^2}\right)^2 - 1.$$

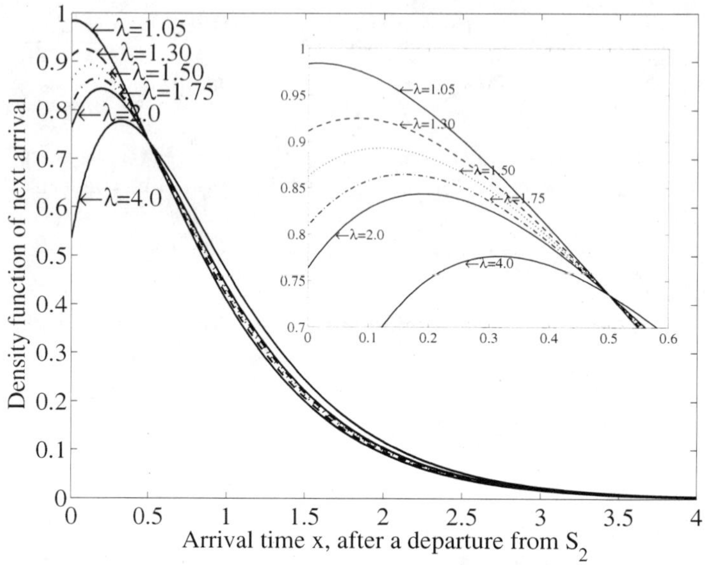

Figure 5.2.1: Distribution of arrival times, conditioned by departures from an E_2/M/1 queue, for various values of λ, the mean service rate of the lone exponential server in S_2. The mean interarrival time for all cases is held fixed at $T_1 = 1$. Thus $\lambda = 1/\varrho$. Note the multiple crossing, which is shown in detail in the inset graph. To within the numerical accuracy of our calculations, all the curves cross at $x = 0.5$.

Note the appearance of the third moment of S_1 in the expression. If S_1 is an exponential server, then $C_1^2 = 1$, and $\mathbb{E}[X_1^3]/(\mathbb{E}[X_1])^3 = 6$, so $C_\omega^2 = 1$ as well, (of course).

5.2.2 Distribution of Interdeparture Times

We spent considerable space in the preceding section discussing a process that does not seem to be of enormous interest to queueing practitioners. However, several of the formulas derived there are useful here, as we explore the behavior of customers departing the G/M/1 queue. We have already discussed this process twice before, in Sections 2.1.6 and 4.2.5, in conjunction with the M/M/1 and M/G/1 queues. The method presented here is similar to that already used in those sections; however, the results are considerably different and thus warrant a fresh analysis.

Let us follow the argument we used in Section 4.2.5 in examining Figure 5.2.2. We use the subscripts **2d** and *2d* to denote the **d**eparture process from S_2. For instance, $b_{2d}(x;\ s)$ is the density function for the process. Our observer is now sitting just downstream from S_2, watching customers go by. Assuming that C_0 has just left, what can we tell her about customer C_1? Well, either he is at S_2, with probability $1 - d_2(0)$, which from (5.1.9c) equals s, or S_2 is empty, and C_1 is at S_1, already in the process of being served there. The vector $\hat{\mathbf{u}}$ gives her the probability of where in S_1 he is at the moment C_0 left

S_2. (Remember, *she* is the observer, and *he* is C_1.) Thus the startup vector for the interdeparture process is

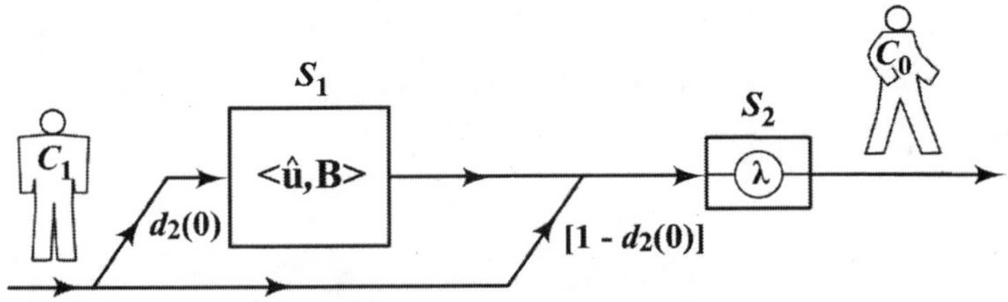

Figure 5.2.2: Pictorial representation of the departure process from S_2, in a G/M/1 open queue. Dependence on the number of customers is implicitly given through the steady-state probabilities at departure times. Given that customer C_0 has just left, C_1 must enter S_2, and be served before leaving $[\lambda]$, or if S_2 is empty, C_1 must finish being served by S_1 $[\langle\, \hat{\mathbf{u}},\, \mathbf{B} \rangle\,]$, and then go to S_2 to be served. The probability that no one is at S_2 at the moment of a departure $d_2(0)$ is given by (5.1.9c).

$$\mathbf{p_{2d}} := [(1-s)\hat{\mathbf{u}},\, s]\,. \tag{5.2.5a}$$

In words, the process starts with C_1 either being at phase i in S_1 with probability $(1-s)[\hat{\mathbf{u}}]_i$, or at S_2 with probability s. Clearly, because $\hat{\mathbf{u}}\boldsymbol{\epsilon}' = 1$, it follows that $\mathbf{p_{2d}}\,\boldsymbol{\epsilon}' = 1$ also. Note that we have changed the ordering of our states from that in Chapter 4, by placing S_1 first. Now the numbering of the states goes from 1 to $m+1$, where the state corresponding to being in S_2 is $m+1$ rather than 0. Figure 5.2.2 is descriptive enough for us to write down the completion rate and transition matrices for the process.

$$\mathbf{M_{2d}} = \begin{bmatrix} \mathbf{M} & \mathbf{o}' \\ \mathbf{o} & \lambda \end{bmatrix}$$

and

$$\mathbf{P_{2d}} = \begin{bmatrix} \mathbf{P} & \mathbf{q}' \\ \mathbf{o} & 0 \end{bmatrix},$$

where $\mathbf{o}(\mathbf{o}')$ is a row (column) vector with the same dimension as $\mathbf{M}$ and $\mathbf{P}$, namely, m. Then in direct analogy with (4.2.17b), we can write down the process rate matrix.

$$\mathbf{B_{2d}} = \mathbf{M_{2d}}(\mathbf{I_{2d}} - \mathbf{P_{2d}}) = \begin{bmatrix} \mathbf{B} & -\mathbf{B}\boldsymbol{\epsilon}' \\ \mathbf{o} & \lambda \end{bmatrix}. \tag{5.2.5b}$$

The process time matrix also follows easily:

$$\mathbf{V_{2d}} = \mathbf{B_{2d}^{-1}} = \begin{bmatrix} \mathbf{V} & \frac{1}{\lambda}\boldsymbol{\epsilon}' \\ \mathbf{o} & \frac{1}{\lambda} \end{bmatrix}. \tag{5.2.5c}$$

We now know enough to state the following theorem concerning interdeparture times.

Theorem 5.2.2 The distribution of times between departures from a steady-state open G/M/1 queue is generated by the vector-matrix pair, $\langle \mathbf{p_{2d}}, \mathbf{B_{2d}} \rangle$, as given by Equations (5.2.5). The following equations must be true (where $\Psi_{2d}[\mathbf{D}] := \mathbf{p_{2d}}\, \mathbf{D}\, \boldsymbol{\epsilon}'_{\mathbf{2d}}$),

$$\mathbb{E}[X_{2d}^n] = n!\Psi_{2d}\left[(\mathbf{V_{2d}})^n\right], \tag{5.2.6a}$$

$$b_{2d}(x) = \Psi_{2d}\left[\mathbf{B_{2d}} \exp(-x\mathbf{B_{2d}})\right], \tag{5.2.6b}$$

and

$$B_{2d}^*(s) = \Psi_{2d}\left[(\mathbf{I} + s\mathbf{V_{2d}})^{-1}\right]. \tag{5.2.6c}$$

The proof follows from Theorem 3.1.1. ■

Before calculating the mean interdeparture time, we use (5.2.5a) and (5.2.5c) to find the following row vector,

$$\mathbf{p_{2d}}\mathbf{V_{2d}} = \left[(1-s)\hat{\mathbf{u}}\mathbf{V},\ \frac{1}{\lambda}\right].$$

Because $\mathbb{E}[X_{2d}] = \mathbf{p_{2d}}\, \mathbf{V_{2d}}\, \boldsymbol{\epsilon}'_{\mathbf{2d}}$, the mean is

$$\mathbb{E}[X_{2d}] = (1-s)\Psi_\omega[\mathbf{V}] + \frac{1}{\lambda} = (1-s)\frac{\rho-1}{(1-s)\lambda} + \frac{1}{\lambda} = \bar{x}_1, \tag{5.2.7a}$$

certainly not a surprising result.

En route to finding the variance, we need $\Psi_{2d}\left[(\mathbf{V_{2d}})^2\right]$, which can be written as $(\mathbf{p_{2d}}\, \mathbf{V_{2d}})\,(\mathbf{V_{2d}}\, \boldsymbol{\epsilon}'_{\mathbf{2d}})$, so first calculate the column vector:

$$\mathbf{V_{2d}}\, \boldsymbol{\epsilon}'_{\mathbf{2d}} = \begin{bmatrix} (\mathbf{V} + \frac{1}{\lambda}\mathbf{I})\, \boldsymbol{\epsilon}' \\ \\ \frac{1}{\lambda} \end{bmatrix}.$$

We can put $\mathbf{p_{2d}}\, \mathbf{V_{2d}}$ and $\mathbf{V_{2d}}\, \boldsymbol{\epsilon}'_{\mathbf{2d}}$ together to get the second moment of $b_{2d}(x;\, s)$, making use of (5.2.2a) and (5.2.3a):

$$\mathbb{E}[X_{2d}^2] = 2\Psi_{2d}\left[(\mathbf{V_{2d}})^2\right] = \frac{2\rho}{\lambda^2} + \mathbb{E}[X_1^2] - \frac{2}{\lambda^2}\frac{\rho-1}{1-s}.$$

We know from (5.2.7a) that $b_{2d}(x)$ and $b_1(x)$ have the same mean, so with some algebraic steps left out,

$$\sigma_{2d}^2 = \mathbb{E}[X_{2d}^2] - (\mathbb{E}[X_1])^2 = \sigma_1^2 + \frac{2(1-\rho\, s)}{\lambda^2(1-s)}. \tag{5.2.7b}$$

We simply divide both sides of the equation by $(\mathbb{E}[X_1])^2$ to find the squared coefficient of variation.

$$C_{2d}^2 = C_1^2 + \frac{2(1-\rho\, s)}{\rho^2(1-s)}. \tag{5.2.7c}$$

It is helpful for the discussion that follows to replace ρ with $1/\varrho$ in (5.2.7c). Then

$$C_{2d}^2 = C_1^2 + \frac{2\varrho(\varrho - s)}{1 - s}. \tag{5.2.7d}$$

We know from Section 5.1.3 that we can view s as a function of ϱ, and as such, when $\varrho = 0$ or 1, $s = 0$ or 1, also. Therefore, when $\varrho = 0$, we get

$$\left(C_{2d}^2\right)_{\varrho=0} = C_1^2.$$

Its value at $\varrho = 1$ is trickier and requires the functional dependence of s with respect to ϱ near 1. From (5.1.22c) and (5.1.23b), we are able to say that $s = 1 - \alpha(1 - \varrho) + \cdots$, with $\alpha = 2/(1 + C_1^2)$. We put this into (5.2.7d), move some things around, and come up with an expected result.

$$\left(C_{2d}^2\right)_{\varrho=1} = 1.$$

Now in general, we see that C_{2d}^2 is greater than (less than) C_1^2 whenever ϱ is greater than (less than) s. We also know that for Erlangian distributions, C_1^2 is less than 1, and s is less than ϱ in the entire range 0 to 1. Furthermore, for hyperexponential distributions, C_1^2 is greater than 1 and s is greater than ϱ. We might thus conclude that C_{2d}^2 always lies between C_1^2 and 1, just as it did for the M/G/1 case in the discussion following (4.2.19d) in Section 4.2.5. But our conclusion would be wrong. In fact, we can find distributions in which s and ϱ switch around several times between 0 and 1. All we can say is that this is true for ϱ sufficiently close to 1.

We continue to follow our procedure in Section 4.2.5 to get the interdeparture distribution itself in terms of $\mathbf{B}, \mathbf{p}$, and $\hat{\mathbf{u}}$. Keep in mind, though, that $\langle \mathbf{p_{2d}} , \mathbf{B_{2d}} \rangle$ can be used directly, in calculating the distribution. We can see that $\mathbf{B_{2d}}$, (5.2.5b), and $\mathbf{B_d}$, (4.2.17b), are quite similar, so we can immediately guess what $(\mathbf{B_{2d}})^n$ is for all n. Its proof can be shown by induction.

$$(\mathbf{B_{2d}})^n = \begin{bmatrix} \mathbf{B}^n & \mathbf{g}'(n) \\ \mathbf{o} & \lambda^n \end{bmatrix}, \tag{5.2.8a}$$

where

$$\mathbf{g}'(n) := -\lambda^{n-1}\mathbf{B}\left[\mathbf{I} + \frac{1}{\lambda}\mathbf{B} + \left(\frac{1}{\lambda}\mathbf{B}\right)^2 + \cdots + \left(\frac{1}{\lambda}\mathbf{B}\right)^{n-1}\right]\boldsymbol{\epsilon}',$$

satisfying the recurrence relation

$$\mathbf{g}'(n+1) = -\lambda^n\mathbf{B}\,\boldsymbol{\epsilon}' + \mathbf{B}\mathbf{g}'(n).^*$$

For the moment let

$$\mathbf{X} := (\mathbf{I} - \lambda\mathbf{V})^{-1}.$$

*The $'$ reminds us that $\mathbf{g}'$ is a column vector of dimension m.

We use the now-familiar summation formula for the finite geometric series, and carry out some further algebra to get the following.

$$\mathbf{g}'(n) = \mathbf{X}(\lambda^n \mathbf{I} - \mathbf{B}^n)\boldsymbol{\epsilon}'. \tag{5.2.8b}$$

We can almost exactly follow the steps leading up to (4.2.21b) to find the reliability matrix for this departure process, giving us

$$\mathbf{R_{2d}}(x) := \exp(-x\mathbf{B_{2d}}) = \begin{bmatrix} \exp(-x\mathbf{B}) & \mathbf{X}[e^{-x\lambda}\mathbf{I} - \exp(-x\mathbf{B})]\boldsymbol{\epsilon}' \\ \mathbf{o} & e^{-x\lambda} \end{bmatrix}$$

$$= \begin{bmatrix} \mathbf{R_1}(x) & \mathbf{X}[e^{-x\lambda}\mathbf{I} - \mathbf{R_1}(x)]\boldsymbol{\epsilon}' \\ \mathbf{o} & e^{-x\lambda} \end{bmatrix}. \tag{5.2.8c}$$

To get $b_{2d}(x;\, s)$, we first must find $\mathbf{B_{2d}}\,\mathbf{R_{2d}}(x)$. This turns out to be

$$\mathbf{B_{2d}}\,\mathbf{R_{2d}}(x) = \begin{bmatrix} \mathbf{R_1}(x) & \mathbf{X}[e^{-x\lambda}\mathbf{I} - \mathbf{B}\,\mathbf{R_1}(x)]\boldsymbol{\epsilon}' \\ \mathbf{o} & e^{-x\lambda} \end{bmatrix}. \tag{5.2.9a}$$

Our next step is to evaluate $\mathbf{B_{2d}}\,\mathbf{R_{2d}}(x)\,\boldsymbol{\epsilon}'_{\mathbf{2d}}$. Because $\mathbf{X}$, $\mathbf{B}$, and $\mathbf{R_1}(x)$ all commute with each other, and $\mathbf{X} - \mathbf{I} = \lambda\mathbf{X}\mathbf{V}$, this turns out to be the following column vector:

$$\mathbf{B_{2d}}\,\mathbf{R_{2d}}(x)\,\boldsymbol{\epsilon}'_{\mathbf{2d}} = \begin{bmatrix} \lambda\mathbf{X}[e^{-x\lambda}\mathbf{I} - \mathbf{B}\,\mathbf{R_1}(x)]\boldsymbol{\epsilon}' \\ \lambda\, e^{-x\lambda} \end{bmatrix}. \tag{5.2.9b}$$

Finally, given that $b_{2d}(x;\, s) = \Psi_{2d}\left[\mathbf{B_{2d}}\,\mathbf{R_{2d}}(x)\right] = \mathbf{p_{2d}}\mathbf{B_{2d}}\mathbf{R_{2d}}(x)\boldsymbol{\epsilon}'\mathbf{_{2d}}$, and $\mathbf{p_{2d}}$ is given by (5.2.5a), we have the density function for the steady-state departure process:

$$b_{2d}(x;\, s) = \lambda e^{-\lambda x}\hat{\mathbf{u}}\mathbf{X}(\mathbf{I} - s\lambda\mathbf{V})\,\boldsymbol{\epsilon}' - (1-s)\lambda\hat{\mathbf{u}}\,\mathbf{X}\,\mathbf{R_1}(x)\,\boldsymbol{\epsilon}'. \tag{5.2.9c}$$

Although this expression looks rather complicated, it is expressed in terms of m-dimensional matrices, whereas the original representation is $(m+1)$-dimensional. It can be used as a practical way to get the pdf for any specific examples, particularly if they are of small dimension. Also, note the striking similarity with its M/G/1 counterpart, $b_{1d}(x)$ [called $b_d(x)$ in (4.2.22a)]. These formulas have not been known until very recently, so not many researchers have worked with them. Therefore, we have no way of knowing if they can be manipulated into simpler or more interesting forms.

Whether $b_{2d}(x)$ can be manipulated into a convenient form or not, we know its generator $\langle\, \mathbf{p_{2d}}\,,\, \mathbf{B_{2d}}\,\rangle$, given by (5.2.5a) and (5.2.5b). Therefore, there is little effort to computing the function once the interarrival time distribution is given.

Example 5.2.2: We have calculated $b_{2d}(x; s)$ for an E_2/M/1 queue, and plotted it in Figure 5.2.3, for several values of ϱ, all less than 1. We already know that when $\varrho \geq 1$ the interdeparture times must look like the service time distribution. Even when ϱ is close to, but less than 1, they look very much like the exponential function. Of course, when ϱ is small, b_{2d} looks like $E_2(x)$, the interarrival time distribution. Notice the rapid change from one to the other when ϱ goes from 0.25 to 0.50. The reader might compare this figure with its M/E_2/1 counterpart in Figure 4.2.3. ▲

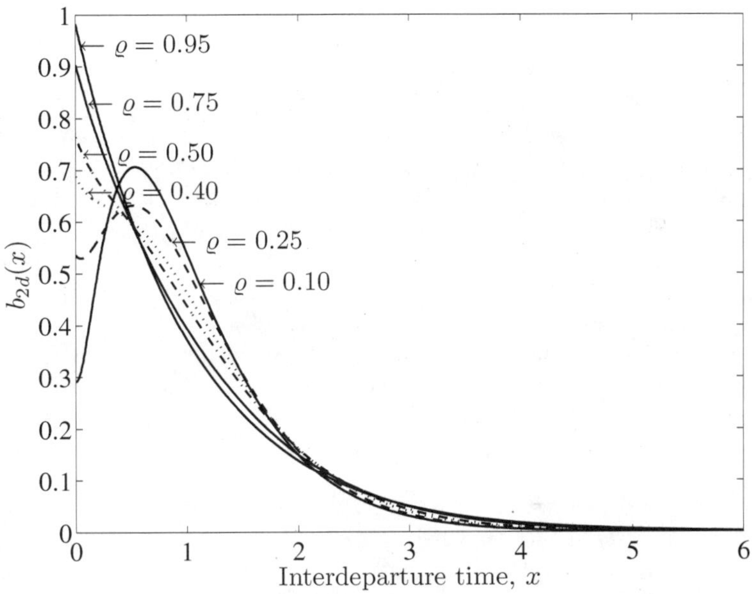

Figure 5.2.3: Distribution of interdeparture times $b_{2d}(x)$ of an E_2/M/1 queue, for ϱ = 0.10, 0.25, 0.40, 0.50, 0.75, and 0.95. When ϱ is small, the interdeparture time distribution looks like the interarrival time distribution $E_2(x)$, and when ϱ is near (or greater than) 1, it looks like the service time distribution $\lambda \exp(-\lambda x)$.

5.3 ME/M/1/N and ME/M/1//N Queues

Now is the time for you to ask again what the difference is between one and two slashes. In Section 2.1.4 we discussed the question in detail for buffer overflow and customer loss in M/M/1-type queues. But in Chapter 4 we brushed the question aside, explaining that in an M/ME/1 queue, they yielded identical results. But for ME/M/1 queues, they do not. For definiteness, let us adhere to the conventions of this chapter. The first position (ME) refers to the service time distribution at S_1, the second (M) refers to S_2, and the third position refers to the maximum number of customers (1) at S_2 who can be active at the same time. The fourth position in this notation refers to the amount of space available at S_2, including the customers in service (finite waiting room, or buffer). If that position has J there, then when J customers are at S_2, new arrivals are turned away (discounted or killed) until someone leaves, at which time there are then only $J-1$ customers there. If that position is blank, it is assumed to be infinite. The fifth position refers to the total number of customers in the system, k of whom are at S_2 and the remaining n are at S_1. If that space is blank, or nonexistent, then we have an open system, (or N is infinite).

Consider the following string, $G_1/G_2/C/J/N$. All systems with $J \geq N$ are equivalent. After all, it does not pay to have more space than there are customers. Similarly, all systems with $C \geq \min[J, N]$ are the same. Somewhat less obvious is the equivalence of all systems with $N > J$. We only need one more customer than there is buffer space, for if a customer is turned away because of a full waiting room, there is no difference between his returning immediately to S_1 or being replaced by another customer. We can say that if the inequality string $C < J < N$ is not satisfied, the violating integer can be replaced by ∞ (or any integer greater than or equal to the next symbol in the sequence).

Although the $G_1/G_2/1/N$ queue is usually classified as an open system, the equivalent (but closed) loop $G_1/G_2/1/N/(N+1)$ may be easier to visualize. In this case, the last customer loops on S_1 until room is made available at S_2. However, even after space becomes available, he must still complete service at S_1 before finally being admitted to S_2. In the $G_1/G_2/1//N$ (or $G_1/G_2/1/N/N$) case, when all N customers are at S_2, S_1 is idle until the customer in service finishes. Only then does S_1 begin processing a customer to generate the next arrival. That is, in the former case S_1 is already processing the next arrival to S_2 when room becomes available, but in the latter case, processing at S_1 begins at the moment a completion occurs at S_2. Only when the residual distribution time for S_1 is the same as the overall distribution time (i.e., when S_1 is exponential) will the customer return to S_2 at the right time to make both systems identical. The algebraic analysis in the next section makes this clear.

5.3.1 Steady-State Solution of the ME/M/1/N Queue

First let us define (the subscript **f** stands for "finite buffer") the steady-state probability vector.

Definition 5.3.1

$\boldsymbol{\pi}_{2f}(k;\, N) :=$ *steady-state probability vector that there are k customers at* S_2 *in an ME/M/1/N system.* There are at least $N+1$ customers in this system. If a customer arrives at S_2 and finds N other customers already there, he immediately returns to S_1. A random observer, with probability $[\boldsymbol{\pi}_{2f}(k;\, N)]_i$, will find the system in state $\{i;\, k;\, N\}$. As usual, $r_{2f}(k;\, N) := \boldsymbol{\pi}_{2f}(k;\, N)\boldsymbol{\epsilon}'$ is the associated scalar probability. □

The more traditional view is that there are an infinite number of customers waiting to be served by S_1. A customer who completes service there and finds

S_2 to be full, immediately self-destructs. The two views are mathematically equivalent, but if nothing else, our view is more humane.

Except when $k = N$, the balance equations for $\boldsymbol{\pi}_{2f}(k; N)$ are identical to those for $\boldsymbol{\pi}_2(k; N)$. Remember to replace the vector $\boldsymbol{\pi}(n; N)$ with $\boldsymbol{\pi}_{2f}(N{-}k; N)$ [see (5.1.1d)] when you examine the equations in Section 4.1.1. The equation for $k = N$ differs from (4.1.3b). Now, even though there are N customers at S_2, S_1 is not idle. Therefore, the vector probability of leaving the state $\{\cdot; N; N\}$ is proportional to $(\lambda\mathbf{I} + \mathbf{M})$; that is, something can happen in either S_1 or S_2. There are three ways to enter state $\{\cdot; N; N\}$. One is to be in some state $\{\cdot; N{-}1; N\}$, $[\boldsymbol{\pi}_{2f}(N{-}1; N)]$, and have a completion $[\mathbf{M}]$ that results in a departure from S_1, $[\mathbf{Mq}']$, while simultaneously the next customer enters S_1, $[\mathbf{p}]$. The second way is for there to be N customers at S_2, $[\boldsymbol{\pi}_{2f}(N; N)]$, with an event again occurring in S_1, $[\mathbf{M}]$, with that customer going to another phase in S_1, $[\mathbf{P}]$. The third way is similar to the second, except that now the customer in S_1 [the lonesome $(N+1)$st customer] leaves $[\mathbf{q}']$, but because the buffer at S_2 is full, he immediately returns to S_1 and starts up again $[\mathbf{p}]$. In total, we have

$$\boldsymbol{\pi}_{2f}(N; N)(\lambda\mathbf{I} + \mathbf{M}) = \boldsymbol{\pi}_{2f}(N{-}1; N)\mathbf{Mq}'\mathbf{p} + \boldsymbol{\pi}_{2f}(N; N)\mathbf{M}(\mathbf{P} + \mathbf{q}'\mathbf{p}).$$

Upon regrouping terms, and recognizing yet once again that $\mathbf{Mq}'\mathbf{p} = \mathbf{BQ}$, we get

$$\boldsymbol{\pi}_{2f}(N; N)(\lambda\mathbf{I} + \mathbf{B} - \mathbf{BQ}) = \boldsymbol{\pi}_{2f}(N{-}1; N)\mathbf{BQ}. \tag{5.3.1a}$$

The equation equivalent to (4.1.3c) gives

$$\boldsymbol{\pi}_{2f}(0; N)\mathbf{B} = \boldsymbol{\pi}_{2f}(1; N)\lambda, \tag{5.3.1b}$$

which in a manner identical to Section 4.1.2 recursively leads to results equivalent to (4.1.5b),

$$\boldsymbol{\pi}_{2f}(k; N)\mathbf{U} = \boldsymbol{\pi}_{2f}(k{-}1; N), \quad 2 \le k \le N. \tag{5.3.1c}$$

But (5.3.1a) is yet to be satisfied. Equation (5.3.1c) with $k = N$ must be made consistent with (5.3.1a). Upon combining the two, we get

$$\boldsymbol{\pi}_{2f}(N; N)(\lambda\mathbf{I} + \mathbf{B} - \mathbf{BQ}) = \boldsymbol{\pi}_{2f}(N; N)\mathbf{UBQ}.$$

But from Lemma 4.1.1, $\mathbf{UBQ} = \lambda\mathbf{Q}$, so we bring everything to the left side of the equation to get

$$\boldsymbol{\pi}_{2f}(N; N)(\lambda\mathbf{I} + \mathbf{B} - \lambda\mathbf{Q} - \mathbf{BQ}) = [\boldsymbol{\pi}_{2f}(N; N)(\lambda\mathbf{I} + \mathbf{B})](\mathbf{I} - \mathbf{Q}) = \mathbf{o}$$

($\mathbf{o}$ is the null row vector). This is an eigenvector equation which says that the vector in brackets is a left eigenvector of $(\mathbf{I} - \mathbf{Q})$ with eigenvalue 0. Can this be satisfied? It had better be. Note that $\mathbf{C} := \mathbf{I} - \mathbf{Q}$ is idempotent, just like $\mathbf{Q}$. That is, $\mathbf{C}^2 = \mathbf{C}$. (See Lemma 3.5.1.) Therefore, all of $\mathbf{C}$'s eigenvalues are either 0 or 1. Now, $\mathbf{Q}$ is of rank 1, so it has only one eigenvalue with value 1. Therefore, $\mathbf{C}$ is of rank $m-1$ and has only one zero eigenvalue. The corresponding left and right eigenvector pair are our old companions $\mathbf{p}$ and $\boldsymbol{\epsilon}'$. The vector in brackets must, then, be proportional to $\mathbf{p}$. Write

$$\boldsymbol{\pi}_{\mathbf{2f}}(N;N)(\lambda\mathbf{I}+\mathbf{B}) = c\mathbf{p},$$

where c is an undetermined constant. Recall from the definition of $\mathbf{A}$ [Equation (4.1.4a)], that $\lambda\mathbf{I}+\mathbf{B} = \lambda(\mathbf{A}+\mathbf{Q})$. Also, multiply both sides of the equation by $\mathbf{U}$ to get

$$\lambda\boldsymbol{\pi}_{\mathbf{2f}}(N;N)(\mathbf{I}+\mathbf{QU}) = c\mathbf{pU},$$

but $\boldsymbol{\pi}_{\mathbf{2f}}(N;N)\mathbf{QU} = \boldsymbol{\pi}_{\mathbf{2f}}(N;N)\boldsymbol{\epsilon}'\,\mathbf{pU} = c'\mathbf{pU}$, where c' is another constant. We regroup, divide by λ, and get

$$\boldsymbol{\pi}_{\mathbf{2f}}(N;N) = g(N)\mathbf{pU}, \tag{5.3.1d}$$

where $g(N)$ is yet another constant, which we *do* evaluate. This time we have noted its dependence on N.

We can now combine (5.3.1b), (5.3.1c), and (5.3.1d) to get the explicit matrix geometric solution to the ME/M/1/N queue:

$$\boldsymbol{\pi}_{\mathbf{2f}}(k;N) = g(N)\mathbf{pU}^{N+1-k} \quad \text{for } 1 \le k \le N,$$

but for $k=0$,

$$\boldsymbol{\pi}_{\mathbf{2f}}(0;N) = g(N)\lambda\mathbf{pU}^{N}\mathbf{V}.$$

The scalar probabilities are, by now, easy to write down. For $k>0$,

$$r_{2f}(k;N) := \boldsymbol{\pi}_{\mathbf{2f}}(k;N)\boldsymbol{\epsilon}' = g(N)\Psi\left[\mathbf{U}^{N+1-k}\right]$$

and the probability that S_2 is idle is given by

$$r_{2f}(0;N) = g(N)\lambda\Psi\left[\mathbf{U}^{N}\mathbf{V}\right].$$

These formulas seem to be very familiar [look at (4.1.6a) and (4.1.6b)], and we relate them to the ME/M/1//$(N+1)$ queue after we have found $g(N)$. We calculate this constant by requiring that the sum of the $r_{2f}(k;N)$s be 1. Then $g(N)$ satisfies the relation

$$\frac{1}{g(N)} = \Psi\left[\lambda\mathbf{U}^{N}\mathbf{V}\right] + \sum_{k=1}^{N}\Psi\left[\mathbf{U}^{N+1-k}\right] = \Psi\left[\mathbf{U}+\mathbf{U}^2+\cdots+\mathbf{U}^{N}+\lambda\mathbf{U}^{N}\mathbf{V}\right].$$

We need only compare this with the definition of $\mathbf{K}(N+1)$ in (4.1.6d) to see that

$$\frac{1}{g(N)} = \Psi\left[\mathbf{UK}(N)\right] = \Psi\left[\mathbf{K}(N+1)\right] - 1. \tag{5.3.2a}$$

We next summarize these equations in the following theorem so that they can all be found in one place.

Theorem 5.3.1 The steady-state vector probabilities of (a random observer) finding k customers in an ME/M/1/N queue are given below.

$$\boldsymbol{\pi_{2f}}(0; N) = \lambda g(N)\mathbf{p}\mathbf{U}^N\mathbf{V} \tag{5.3.2b}$$

and

$$\boldsymbol{\pi_{2f}}(k; N) = g(N)\mathbf{p}\mathbf{U}^{N+1-k} \quad \text{for } 0 < k \le N. \tag{5.3.2c}$$

The associated scalar probabilities are given by the next two formulas.

$$r_{2f}(0; N) = g(N)\Psi\left[\lambda\mathbf{U}^N\mathbf{V}\right] \tag{5.3.2d}$$

and

$$r_{2f}(k; N) = g(N)\Psi\left[\mathbf{U}^{N+1-k}\right] \quad \text{for } 0 < k \le N, \tag{5.3.2e}$$

where $1/g(N) = \Psi\left[\mathbf{UK}(N)\right] = \Psi\left[\mathbf{K}(N+1)\right] - 1$. ■

This theorem is very similar to Theorem 4.1.2 with N replaced by $N+1$, so we can see by inspection, upon invoking (5.1.1c) and (5.1.1d), that the quantities $\boldsymbol{\pi_{2f}}(k; N)$ and $\boldsymbol{\pi_2}(k; N+1)$, together with their scalar counterparts, satisfy the following corollary.

Corollary 5.3.1 The steady-state probabilities of (a random observer) finding k customers in an ME/M/1/N queue are related to the steady-state probabilities of finding k customers in an ME/M/1/ /$(N+1)$ loop by the following formulas.

$$\boldsymbol{\pi_{2f}}(k; N) = c(N)\boldsymbol{\pi_2}(k; N+1) \quad \text{for } 0 \le k \le N \tag{5.3.3a}$$

and

$$r_{2f}(k; N) = c(N)r_2(k; N+1) \quad \text{for } 0 \le k \le N, \tag{5.3.3b}$$

where

$$c(N) := \frac{\Psi\left[\mathbf{K}(N+1)\right]}{\Psi\left[\mathbf{K}(N+1) - \mathbf{I}\right]} = \frac{1}{1 - r_2(N+1; N+1)}. \tag{5.3.3c}$$

The probabilities for the two queues differ only by the fact that $r_2(N+1; N+1)$ exists but $r_{2f}(N+1; N)$ does not. Therefore, they must be multiplied by different constants so that they each sum to 1. If $\varrho < 1$, then as N becomes unboundedly large, the two systems yield identical results. ■

Our view of the ME/M/1/N queue as a closed loop with $N+1$ customers, where a lone customer at S_1 circles until room is made for him at S_2, would seem to be better than we would have expected. Thinking of queues with finite waiting rooms as open systems is certainly not nearly as helpful.

5.3.2 Arrival Probabilities and Customer Loss

Before continuing this section it might be useful for the reader to review Sections 2.1.4 and 4.2.4 first. We have seen that if some loss of customers can be tolerated it might be useful to allow that to happen in order to improve the performance of those who are accepted. This could be tolerable, for instance, when transmitting video streams, or voice. In such cases a small amount of loss will hardly be noticed. It might also be useful to turn away customers if it is (almost) sure that the customers will return later, when the load is lighter. This can be risky, because it can be construed as poor customer service, or customers could try again repeatedly until they are accepted, thus exacerbating the traffic congestion. Before making such decisions it is useful to be able to estimate the probability of a rejection. This is given in the following theorem.

Theorem 5.3.2 The s.s. vector probabilities that an arriving customer will find k $(0 \leq k \leq N)$ customers already in a $G/M/1/N$ queue are:

$$\mathbf{a_{2f}}(k;\, N) = C(N)\mathbf{p}\,\mathbf{U}^{N-k}\mathbf{Q} = C(N)\Psi[\mathbf{U}^{N-k}]\mathbf{p}, \tag{5.3.4a}$$

with scalar probabilities

$$a_{2f}(k;\, N) = C(N)\,\Psi[\mathbf{U}^{N-k}], \tag{5.3.4b}$$

and because $\sum_k a_{2f}(k;\, N) = 1$, it follows that

$$\begin{aligned} 1/C(N) &= \mathbf{p}\left[\mathbf{I} + \mathbf{U} + \mathbf{U}^2 + \cdots \mathbf{U}^N\right]\boldsymbol{\epsilon}' \\ &= \Psi\left[(\mathbf{I} - \mathbf{U}^{N+1})\mathbf{K}\right]. \end{aligned} \tag{5.3.4c}$$

[See Lemma 4.2.2 for properties of $\mathbf{K} = (\mathbf{I} - \mathbf{U})^{-1}$.] The ***customer loss probability*** is

$$P_{2f}(N) = a_{2f}(N;\, N) = C(N). \tag{5.3.4d}$$

As first discussed in the paragraph surrounding (2.1.10b), these equations are valid for all $\varrho < \varrho_m$, where

$$\varrho_m := 1/[1 - P_{2f}(N)].$$

We can also see this directly from (5.3.4c). Clearly, from Equations (5.3.4) and (4.2.3e),

$$P_{2f}(N) < \lim_{N\to\infty} C(N) = \frac{1}{\Psi[\mathbf{K}]} = 1 - \frac{1}{\varrho_m},$$

which upon solving for ϱ yields the above.

Observe from (5.1.1a) that:

$$\mathbf{a_{2f}}(k;\, N) = \mathbf{a_2}(k;\, N+1).$$

Compare these equations with (2.1.9a), where $\mathbf{U} \to \varrho = 1/\rho$. ■

Note that every $\mathbf{a_{2f}}(k; N)$ is proportional to the entrance vector $\mathbf{p}$. This must be so because every arriving customer has just left S_1, and was immediately replaced by another customer (or if he is rejected, he immediately returns to S_1 and re-enters.

Proof: We could simply argue that the previous equation is "obviously true." But it can be proven directly, using techniques previously used. First, exactly as in Section 4.1.3, define $[\mathbf{w_{2f}}(k; N)]_i$ as the s.s. probability that between events in an $G/M/1/N$ system, there are k customers at S_2 and an unboundedly large number of customers (or at least $N-k+1$) at S_1, the active customer there being in state i. Except for $k=N$, $\mathbf{w_{2f}}(k, N)$ satisfies the same balance equations as $\mathbf{w}(n, N)$ in Equations (4.1.9), where $n = N-k$. However,

$$\mathbf{w_{2f}}(N; N) = \mathbf{w_{2f}}(N; N)\left[(\lambda\mathbf{I}+\mathbf{M})^{-1}\mathbf{M}\right](\mathbf{P}+\mathbf{q}'\mathbf{p}) \\ + \mathbf{w_{2f}}(N-1; N)(\lambda\mathbf{I}+\mathbf{M})^{-1}\mathbf{M}\,\mathbf{q}'\mathbf{p}.$$

The terms on the right constitute the three ways that the system can enter a state with a full buffer at S_2. Either the buffer is already full and (1) the active customer in S_1 moves from phase j to i $[(\mathbf{P})_{ji}]$; (2) The customer leaves S_1 $[(\mathbf{q}')_j]$ and, upon finding the buffer full, returns to S_1 and re-enters $[(\mathbf{p})_i]$; or (3) there is one slot left at S_2 and the active customer at S_1 leaves and enters the queue at S_2, while at the same time another customer enters S_1. After the usual manipulations, it follows that

$$\mathbf{w_{2f}}(N; N)(\lambda\mathbf{I}+\mathbf{M})^{-1}[\lambda\mathbf{I}+\mathbf{B}-\mathbf{BQ}] \\ = \mathbf{w_{2f}}(N-1; N)[(\lambda\mathbf{I}+\mathbf{M})^{-1}]\mathbf{BQ}. \tag{5.3.5a}$$

For convenience, let

$$\mathbf{v}(k; N) := \mathbf{w_{2f}}(k; N)(\lambda\mathbf{I}+\mathbf{M})^{-1};$$

then the balance equations imply that for $k > 1$

$$\mathbf{v}(k; N) = \mathbf{v}(k-1; N)\mathbf{A} \quad \text{and} \\ \lambda\mathbf{v}(1; N) = \mathbf{v}(0; N)\mathbf{B}.$$

Using $\mathbf{v}(N-1; N) = \mathbf{v}(N; N)\mathbf{U}$ and $\mathbf{UBQ} = \lambda\mathbf{Q}$, we get after regrouping

$$\mathbf{v}(N; N)\,[\lambda\mathbf{I}+\mathbf{B}-\mathbf{BQ}-\lambda\mathbf{Q}] = \mathbf{v}(N; N)(\lambda\mathbf{I}+\mathbf{B})(\mathbf{I}-\mathbf{Q}) = \mathbf{o}.$$

Using arguments identical to those leading up to (5.3.1d), we get

$$\mathbf{v}(N; N) = c\mathbf{p}(\lambda\mathbf{I}+\mathbf{B})^{-1}. \tag{5.3.5b}$$

It is not hard to show that $\mathbf{p}[\lambda\mathbf{I}+\mathbf{B}]^{-1}\mathbf{A} = \Psi[(\mathbf{I}+\lambda\mathbf{V})^{-1}]\mathbf{p}$. This together with the relation (as taken from (4.1.11) and the surrounding discussion)

$$\mathbf{a_{2f}}(k; N) = \mathbf{w_{2f}}(k; N)(\lambda\mathbf{I}+\mathbf{M})^{-1}\mathbf{Mq}'\mathbf{p}$$

yields Equations (5.3.4), a simple result for such a complicated derivation. **QED**

As a last comment, we mention that the last term of (5.3.4c) is a very efficient expression for computing $P_{2f}(N)$, but only when ϱ is not too close to 1. At $\varrho = 1$, $\mathbf{U}$ has a unit eigenvalue, thus $\mathbf{K}$ does not exist there. It is then more accurate to use the middle expression. Better yet, if the eigenvalues and eigenvectors of $\mathbf{U}$ can be computed easily and accurately, one can perform the sum over scalars. That is, let $m = \text{Dim}[\mathbf{U}]$ and let $\{\nu_i \,|\, 1 \le i \le m\}$ be the eigenvalues of $\mathbf{U}$, with right and left eigenvectors $\{\mathbf{v}'_\mathbf{i}\}$ and $\{\mathbf{u}_\mathbf{i}\}$, respectively. By the spectral decomposition theorem (see Section 1.3.3.1), it follows that

$$\mathbf{S} := \sum_{n=o}^{N} \mathbf{U}^n = \sum_{1=1}^{m} \left[\sum_{n=o}^{N} \nu_i^n \, \mathbf{v}'_\mathbf{i} \, \mathbf{u}_\mathbf{i} \right] = \sum_{i=o}^{m} \left[\frac{1 - \nu_i^{N+1}}{1 - \nu_i} \right] \mathbf{v}'_\mathbf{i} \, \mathbf{u}_\mathbf{i}.$$

If one of the eigenvalues, say ν_1, equals 1, then replace the term for $i = 1$ in large brackets with $N + 1$. That is,

$$\mathbf{S} = (N + 1)\mathbf{v}'_1 \, \mathbf{u}_1 + \sum_{i=2}^{m} \left[\frac{1 - \nu_i^{N+1}}{1 - \nu_i} \right] \mathbf{v}'_\mathbf{i} \, \mathbf{u}_\mathbf{i}.$$

This equation is efficient and stable to roundoff errors, even for very large N. we made use of this in preparing the graphs in the following example.

Example 5.3.1: Using (5.3.4c) and (5.3.4d), we have calculated the smallest value of N for which a $G/M/1/N$ queue will have a $P_{2f} \le .01$ loss rate for seven different interarrival time distributions, and have presented them in Figures 5.3.1 and 5.3.2. Note that this is an integer function of ϱ. Therefore it increases by unit steps, hence the jagged appearance. It begins to look smooth because the graph is in log scale, and the steps thus have step sizes of $\log[1 + 1/(\text{buffer size})] \approx 1/(\text{buffer size})$. Three of the functions chosen were TPTs from Section 3.3.6.2, with $T = 8,\ 16,\ 32$ where $\theta = 0.5$, and $\alpha = 1.4$. The curve labeled M is that for the $M/M/1/N$ queue. The other three curves are for the Erlangian-2 distribution, and two hyperexponential distributions with the same $C_v^2 = 4.75$ as the TPT with $T = 8$. Even though they have the same mean and variance, the three curves differ quite substantially. In fact, the curve for the $H_2/M/1$ system with $p_1 = .0001$ looks a lot more like the one for the $M/M/1$ system until ϱ approaches 1, showing once again that C_v^2 is not necessarily the most important parameter.

Although the buffer size needed for 1% ($P_{2f} = .01$) loss grows very large as ϱ approaches 1 (remember that the buffer size is on a log scale), the inset for Figure 5.3.1 shows that it is finite at $\varrho = 1$ for all the distributions. In general, the curves *do* blow up, but at $\varrho = 1/(1 - P_{2f}) = \varrho_m$, for then the arrival rate of those customers who *are* accepted equals the service rate, finally overwhelming S_2. [See the discussions surrounding (2.1.10b) and (5.3.4).] The blowup is clearly demonstrated in the inset of Figure 5.3.1. In Figure 5.3.2 the buffer size is multiplied by $(\varrho_m - \varrho)$ for the same seven queues, and plotted for $1 \le \varrho \le \varrho_m = 1/.99$. Here we see that the product goes to 0 at $\varrho = \varrho_m$. This tells us that the buffer size blows up as $1/(\varrho_m - \varrho)^a$, where $a < 1$. ▲

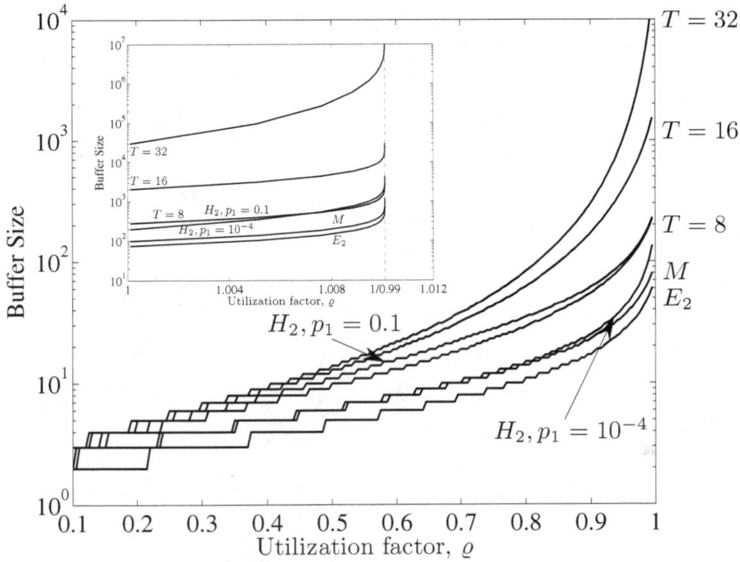

Figure 5.3.1: Buffer size needed for customer loss to be less than 1%, as a function of ϱ, for seven interarrival time distributions with various C_v^2. Three of the curves have TPT interarrival time distributions with $T = 8, 16, 32$ terms. The two curves labeled H_2, $p_1 = \cdots$ have the same $C_v^2 = 4.75$ as the one for $T = 8$, but are very different in shape. All curves are finite at $\varrho = 1$, but they do blow up at $\varrho = 1/(1 - .01)$, as shown by the inset figure, whose x-axis extends beyond the blowup point.

5.4 Steady-State ME/M/C-Type Queues

We are now prepared to give more properties to S_2. It still has a one-dimensional internal representation, but we allow its service rate to vary with its queue length k. This has the obvious application to systems in which several (C) exponential servers are fed by a single queue. Another potentially important application is in the study of complex networks. In this case, one server is singled out to be S_1, the nonexponential server, and the rest of the network is approximated by S_2, with suitably chosen flow rates $\lambda(k)$ to represent customer flow. Thus one can combine the power of the product-form solutions in constructing (maybe) reasonable λ's with the correct representation of one nonexponential server. This technique has been tried but not enough is known as yet to decide under what conditions it will give realistic results.

In Section 2.1.5 we discussed load-dependent exponential servers. We viewed a subsystem in either of two ways. Either there were multiple servers available to handle more than one customer at a time, or a single server worked faster when more customers were present. Because exponential subsystems have only one internal state, the two views are mathematically equivalent. For instance, if there is one customer present, let the probability rate of com-

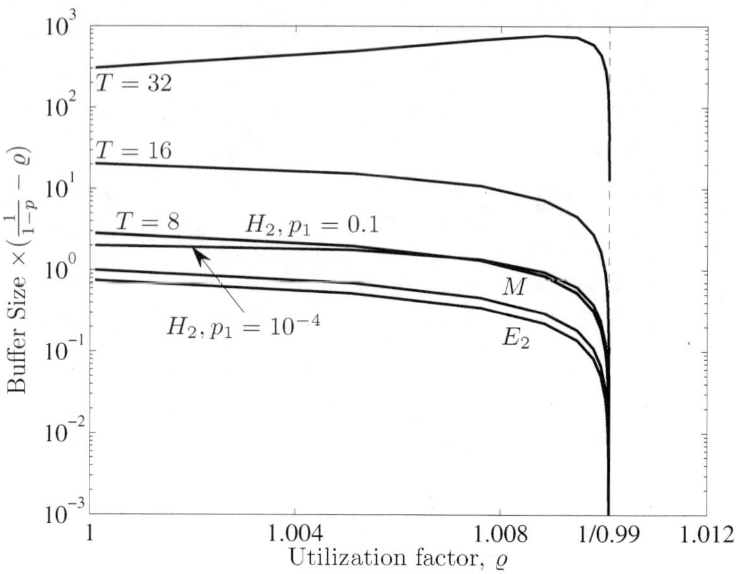

Figure 5.3.2: $(\varrho_m - \varrho)\times$(buffer size) needed For customer loss to be less than 1%, for $1 \le \varrho < \varrho_m$. The interarrival time distributions are the same as those in Figure 5.3.1. Although all the buffer sizes grow unboundedly as ϱ approaches $1/(1 - P_{2f})$, they blow up more slowly than $1/(\varrho_m - \varrho)$. We can deduce this because (buffer size) $\times$ $(\varrho_m - \varrho) \to 0$ at $\varrho_m = \varrho$.

pletion be λ, and if two are present, let the probability rate be 2λ. There is no way to tell if two servers are each processing a customer at the rate of λ, or one server is working twice as fast.

Actually, there is a way to tell the difference: by *marking* the customers. In the first case, if a customer is in service when a second arrives and begins service, there is a distinct possibility that the second will finish before the first (in fact, the probability is 0.5 for exponential servers). In the second case, the FCFS ordering is always maintained. If the customers are marked according to their order of arrival, an observer can tell the difference, because the two-server option will allow customers to leave in a different order from which they arrived. We have been and will continue to take the view that all customers are alike, and unmarkable. To do otherwise would greatly increase the amount of information required, even of exponential subsystems.

In many applications, the customers present share the single server on equal terms. For instance, a customer may be given a small amount of service and whether or not he is finished, the next customer is given an equal amount. After all customers present have been given a share, the first one is given another increment of service, and so on in ***round-robin*** fashion. If the time accorded each in turn is very small compared to the mean service time then we have ***processor sharing***. There is a related queueing discipline known as ***time slicing*** in which each *potential* customer is given an increment of time, whether or not he uses it (e.g., a rotary switch on a multiplexed cable).

Only the processor sharing discipline fits easily into our scheme of things. Conceptually we have multiple servers that are load dependent. If there is one customer present, then he gets the whole server. If two customers are present, then each one gets his own server, but the servers go at half speed. Once again, if the server is exponential then there is no easy way to tell the difference between this and the simple FCFS queue.

5.4.1 Steady-State ME/M/X/ /N Loops

If a subsystem has multiple internal states (i.e., is nonexponential), the three views described in the preceding paragraphs are distinctly different. Modifying the service (actually, completion) rates corresponds to changing $\mathbf{M}$ as a function of queue length but leaving $(\mathbf{I} - \mathbf{P})$ alone. Serving two customers at a time requires keeping track of both customers, for even when one of them leaves, the other is still in some phase of service. The latter view (for ***processor sharing*** as well as ***multiple servers***) is reserved for Chapter 6, because it requires an increase in complexity of our formalism.

Given that S_2 has only one phase, the two views are still equivalent. Also, recall that solution of the M/G/1 and G/M/1 queues depends almost completely on the matrix

$$\mathbf{A} = \mathbf{I} + \frac{1}{\lambda}\mathbf{B} - \mathbf{Q}.$$

We see that λ and $\mathbf{B} = \mathbf{M}(\mathbf{I} - \mathbf{P})$ always appear together. Therefore, changing λ (modifying S_2), or modifying $\mathbf{M}$ by a constant factor, yields the same result. Here we assume that $\mathbf{M}$ is fixed. The difference amounts to deciding whether the load dependence is a function of the number of customers at S_1, $[n]$, or the number of customers at S_2, $[k]$. In a closed loop it does not make any mathematical difference, because $n + k = N$, but if we look at the same system for many values of N, there is an algorithmic difference. There is also a difference from a modeling viewpoint. For instance, if we are interested in the behavior at S_1, and the load factor depends on n, we can think of this as an arrival rate that varies according to the number of customers already at S_1. In the literature this is known as a queue with ***discouraged arrivals*** (although arrivals could also be *encouraged*). For instance, Gupta et al, [GUPTAETAL07], have modelled a multiserver system with join-the-shortest-queue scheduling discipline as an arrival rate that decreases with queue length. On the other hand, stories emanated from the Soviet Union of queues that were joined by passersby because they thought that there must be "something to buy," the longer the queue the more likely that there was merchandise. We do not pursue this view further here.

Let us take the view that S_2 has a service rate which depends on its queue length, and as in Chapter 2, call it $\lambda(k)$. For now, we make no further assumptions concerning the values of $\lambda(k)$. Therefore, following the notational comments at the end of Section 2.1.5, we look at ME/M/$\mathbf{X}$//N loops. The steady-state ***balance equations*** can be taken directly from Equations (4.1.3) by replacing λ with $\lambda(k)$, where k corresponds to the queue number in the matching $\boldsymbol{\pi}_2$. The reader can check this by comparing the steady-state transition diagram in Figure 5.4.1 with Figure 4.1.2. Using the notation of this chapter, we have

$$\lambda(N)\boldsymbol{\pi_2}(N;N) = \boldsymbol{\pi_2}(N-1;N)\mathbf{BQ}, \tag{5.4.1a}$$

$$\boldsymbol{\pi_2}(0;N)\mathbf{M} = \boldsymbol{\pi_2}(1;N)\lambda(1) + \boldsymbol{\pi_2}(0;N)\mathbf{MP}, \tag{5.4.1b}$$

and for $0 < k < N$,

$$\boldsymbol{\pi_2}(k;N)[\mathbf{B} + \lambda(k)\mathbf{I}] = \boldsymbol{\pi_2}(k-1;N)\mathbf{BQ} + \boldsymbol{\pi_2}(k+1;N)\lambda(k+1). \tag{5.4.1c}$$

(Remember that we still maintain the notation $\mathbf{B} = \mathbf{V}^{-1} = \mathbf{M}[\mathbf{I} - \mathbf{P}]$.) $\boldsymbol{\pi_2}(k;N)$ and associated $r_2(k;N)$ retain Definition 5.1.4, including the standard notational assumption that

$$\boldsymbol{\pi_2}(N;N) := r_2(N;N)\mathbf{p}. \tag{5.4.1d}$$

Following the procedure we used in Chapter 4, we would like to solve fo $\boldsymbol{\pi_2}(k;N)$ in terms of $r_2(N;N)$, but (5.4.1a) does not allow us to do that directly because $\mathbf{BQ}$ does not have an inverse. So we must start at the other end. Equation (5.4.1c) can be rewritten as

$$\boldsymbol{\pi_2}(0;N)\mathbf{M}[\mathbf{I} - \mathbf{P}] = \boldsymbol{\pi_2}(1;N)\lambda(1),$$

or

$$\boldsymbol{\pi_2}(0;N) = \boldsymbol{\pi_2}(1;N)\mathbf{U}(0), \tag{5.4.2a}$$

where

$$\mathbf{U}(0) := \lambda(1)\mathbf{V}. \tag{5.4.2b}$$

Next we look at (5.4.1c) for $k = 1$, while making use of (5.4.2a),

$$\begin{aligned}\boldsymbol{\pi_2}(1;N)[\mathbf{B} + \lambda(1)\mathbf{I}] &= \boldsymbol{\pi_2}(0;N)\mathbf{BQ} + \boldsymbol{\pi_2}(2;N)\lambda(2)\\ &= \lambda(1)\boldsymbol{\pi_2}(1;N)\mathbf{Q} + \lambda(2)\boldsymbol{\pi_2}(2;N),\end{aligned}$$

or

$$\boldsymbol{\pi_2}(1;N) = \boldsymbol{\pi_2}(2;N)\mathbf{U}(1), \tag{5.4.2c}$$

where

$$\mathbf{A}(1) := \frac{\lambda(1)}{\lambda(2)}\left[\mathbf{I} + \frac{1}{\lambda(1)}\mathbf{B} - \mathbf{Q}\right] = [\mathbf{U}(1)]^{-1}. \tag{5.4.2d}$$

In preparation for the general solution by induction, first define

$$\mathbf{A}(k) := \frac{\lambda(k)}{\lambda(k+1)}\left[\mathbf{I} + \frac{1}{\lambda(k)}\mathbf{B} - \mathbf{Q}\right] = [\mathbf{U}(k)]^{-1}, \tag{5.4.3}$$

of which (5.4.2d) is a special case. Next observe the following lemma.

Lemma 5.4.1 For matrices $\mathbf{A}(k)$ and $\mathbf{U}(k)$, defined by (5.4.3), the following are matrix identities for all $k \geq 0$,

$$\mathbf{B}\boldsymbol{\epsilon}' = \lambda(k+1)\mathbf{A}(k)\boldsymbol{\epsilon}' \quad \text{and} \quad \mathbf{U}(k)\mathbf{B}\boldsymbol{\epsilon}' = \lambda(k+1)\boldsymbol{\epsilon}', \tag{5.4.4a}$$

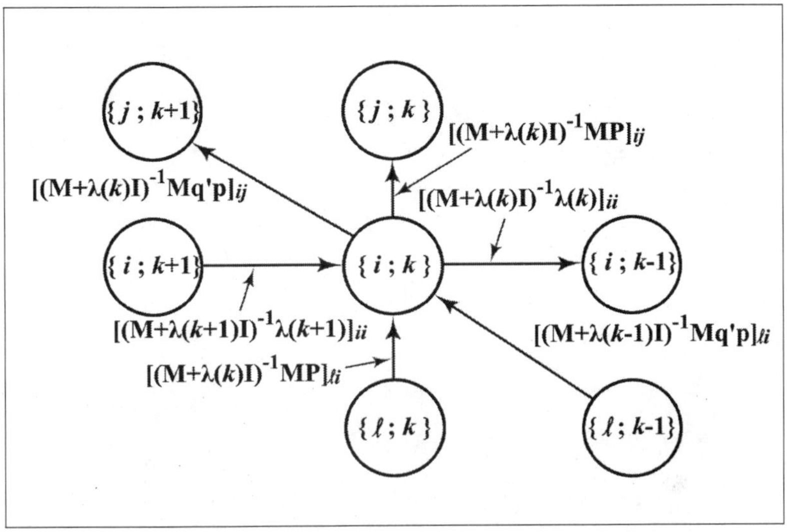

Figure 5.4.1: Steady-state transition diagram for state $\{i; k; N\}$ of an ME/M/$X//N$ closed loop. An arrow pointing diagonally upward to the left represents a customer finishing at phase i in S_1, $\{[(\mathbf{M} + \lambda(k)\mathbf{I})^{-1}\mathbf{M}]_{ii}\}$, and leaving to go to S_2, $[q'_i]$, followed by another customer entering and going to j, $[p_j]$, where j could equal i. A vertical arrow corresponds to a customer finishing at phase i, in S_1 $[(\mathbf{M} + \lambda(k)\mathbf{I})^{-1}\mathbf{M}]$, and going to phase j, $[P_{ij}]$. An arrow to the right (no diagonal arrows allowed) corresponds to a customer finishing at S_2, $[(\lambda(k)\mathbf{I} + \mathbf{M})^{-1}\lambda(k)]$, and immediately going to S_1, without changing the internal state. In all cases, the argument of $\lambda(\cdot)$ matches the value of the queue length of S_2 at the tail of the arrow. Compare with Figure 4.1.2.

and

$$\mathbf{BQ} = \lambda(k+1)\mathbf{A}(k)\mathbf{Q} \quad \text{and} \quad \mathbf{U}(k)\mathbf{BQ} = \lambda(k+1)\mathbf{Q}, \tag{5.4.4b}$$

exactly analogous to Lemma 4.1.1, for which this is a generalization.■

Proof: Given that $\mathbf{I}\boldsymbol{\epsilon}' = \mathbf{Q}\boldsymbol{\epsilon}' = \boldsymbol{\epsilon}'$, all follows directly from the definition of $\mathbf{A}(k)$ and $\mathbf{U}(k)$ in (5.4.3). **QED**

Now assume that (it is certainly true for $j = 0$ and 1)

$$\boldsymbol{\pi}_2(j; N) = \boldsymbol{\pi}_2(j+1; N)\mathbf{U}(j) \quad \text{for } j = 0, 1, \ldots, k-1, \tag{5.4.5}$$

and use it in (5.4.1c) to get

$$\begin{aligned}\boldsymbol{\pi}_2(k; N)[\mathbf{B} + \lambda(k)\mathbf{I}] &= \boldsymbol{\pi}_2(k; N)\mathbf{U}(k-1)\mathbf{BQ} + \boldsymbol{\pi}_2(k+1; N)\lambda(k+1) \\ &= \boldsymbol{\pi}_2(k; N)\lambda(k)\mathbf{Q} + \boldsymbol{\pi}_2(k+1; N)\lambda(k+1),\end{aligned}$$

where we have used (5.4.4b). Solving for $\boldsymbol{\pi}_2(k+1; N)$ yields (5.4.5) for $j = k$, from the definition of $\mathbf{U}(k)$ given in (5.4.3). Thus we have proven our assertion by induction, for all j up to $j = N - 1$. From Lemma 5.4.1, (5.4.1a) is also satisfied.

We are now prepared to put all the above together in the following theorem.

Theorem 5.4.2 The steady-state solution to the ME/M/$X//N$ loop is given by the following formulas, taken from (5.4.2b), (5.4.3), and (5.4.5). For arbitrary $\lambda(k) > 0$, let $\mathbf{U}(0) = \lambda(1)\mathbf{V}$, and for $k > 0$,

$$\mathbf{U}(k) = \frac{\lambda(k+1)}{\lambda(k)}\left[\mathbf{I} + \frac{1}{\lambda(k)}\mathbf{B} - \mathbf{Q}\right]^{-1}.$$

Then

$$\begin{aligned}
\boldsymbol{\pi}_2(N;N) &= r_2(N;N)\mathbf{p}, \\
\boldsymbol{\pi}_2(N-1;N) &= r_2(N;N)\mathbf{p}\mathbf{U}(N-1), \\
\boldsymbol{\pi}_2(N-2;N) &= r_2(N;N)\mathbf{p}\mathbf{U}(N-1)\mathbf{U}(N-2), \\
\cdots & \quad \cdots \\
\boldsymbol{\pi}_2(k;N) &= r_2(N;N)\mathbf{p}\mathbf{U}(N-1)\mathbf{U}(N-2)\cdots\mathbf{U}(k), \\
\cdots & \quad \cdots \\
\boldsymbol{\pi}_2(0;N) &= r_2(N;N)\mathbf{p}\mathbf{U}(N-1)\mathbf{U}(N-2)\cdots\mathbf{U}(k)\cdots\mathbf{U}(0),
\end{aligned}$$

and

$$r_2(k;N) = \boldsymbol{\pi}_2(k;N)\,\boldsymbol{\epsilon}' \quad \text{for all } k.$$

The equivalent recursive formula is given by (5.4.5). $r_2(N;N)$ is evaluated by normalization, or let

$$\begin{aligned}
\mathbf{K}(N) = \mathbf{I} + \mathbf{U}(N-1) + \mathbf{U}(N-1)\mathbf{U}(N-2) + \cdots \\
+\mathbf{U}(N-1)\mathbf{U}(N-2)\cdots\mathbf{U}(N-k) \\
+\mathbf{U}(N-1)\mathbf{U}(N-2)\cdots\mathbf{U}(N-k)\cdots\mathbf{U}(0).
\end{aligned} \tag{5.4.6a}$$

Then, with $\mathbf{K}(1) = \mathbf{I} + \mathbf{U}(0)$, it follows recursively that

$$\mathbf{K}(N) = \mathbf{I} + \mathbf{U}(N-1)\mathbf{K}(N-1) \tag{5.4.6b}$$

and

$$[r_2(N;N)]^{-1} = \Psi\left[\mathbf{K}(N)\right]. \tag{5.4.6c}$$

Compare this with the load-independent case, Theorem 4.1.2, and (4.1.6d), (4.1.6e), and (4.1.6g). ∎

Proof: Note that (5.4.6b) comes from (5.4.6a) by grouping all terms that are left-multiplied by $\mathbf{U}(N-1)$. **QED**

As far as we know, there is no way to take advantage of a simplification such as $\lambda(k) = k\,\lambda$. As long as $\lambda(k) \neq \lambda(k+1)$, we are stuck with this complexity. The same order of complexity occurred for the M/M/$X//N$ loop. Also, the formulas given in Theorem 5.4.2 require families of matrices that require recursive multiplication from both the left and right. This limits our ability to find a recursive procedure that is efficient in both space and time, in studying ME/M/X//N loops for a sequence of values of N.

The algorithm we are about to present is not necessarily the most efficient, but it shows how the matrices fit together. Define the auxiliary matrices for any $n \geq 0$,

$$\mathbf{X}(n,n) := \mathbf{I}, \tag{5.4.7a}$$

and for $k < n$

$$\mathbf{X}(k,n) := \mathbf{U}(n-1)\mathbf{U}(n-2)\cdots\mathbf{U}(k) = \mathbf{U}(n-1)\mathbf{X}(k,n-1). \tag{5.4.7b}$$

This can be helpful in dealing with various objects. For instance, (5.4.6a) can be rewritten as

$$\mathbf{K}(N) = \sum_{k=0}^{N} \mathbf{X}(k,N). \tag{5.4.7c}$$

Then the vector and scalar probabilities, $\boldsymbol{\pi_2}(k;N)$ and $r_2(k;N)$, can be computed in the following way.

Corollary 5.4.2 (Algorithm) To compute the vector and scalar queue-length probabilities of an ME/M/X//N loop for all $N = 1, 2, \cdots, N_{\max}$, do the following.

```
.   X(0,0) = I
.   K(0) = I
.   FOR N = 1 TO N_max
.       X(N,N) = I
.       K(N) = I + U(N−1)K(N−1)
.       r_2(N;N) = 1/Ψ[K(N)]
.       FOR k = 0 TO N − 1
.           X(k,N) = U(N−1)X(k,N−1)
.           π_2(k;N) = r_2(N;N)pX(k,N)
.           r_2(k;N) = π_2(k;N)ε' = r_2(N;N)Ψ[X(k,N)]
.       END FOR(k)
.   END FOR(N)
```

The mean queue length and other performance characteristics can be found by computing them directly. ■

There are no further insights we can gain without becoming more specific about the properties of $\lambda(k)$. Letting $\lambda(k) = k\lambda$ will not tell us much unless we do the calculations. If we let N become infinite, we can say very little unless

$$\lambda_\infty := \lim_{N\to\infty} \lambda(N) < \infty,$$

and $\rho := \bar{x}_1\lambda_\infty < 1$. In that case we would revert back to the steady-state M/ME/1 open queue of Section 4.2, with arrival rate λ_∞. If the inequality is the other way around, (i.e., if $\rho > 1$), we have a problem. We do not even know how to start without more information. However, we can, and in the next section, do solve those systems for which the load-dependent service rates are constant above a certain queue length.

5.4.2 Steady-State ME/M/C Queue

Let us assume that $N > C > 1$, and

$$\lambda(k) = \lambda(C) \quad \text{for } k \geq C. \tag{5.4.8}$$

What the values of $\lambda(1)$, $\lambda(2)$,..., and $\lambda(C)$ actually are does not seem to be helpful for finding simpler solutions, so we leave them unspecified. Then by our own definition at the end of Section 2.1.5, this is an ME/M/$C//N$-type loop, but we do not emphasize that here. However, in Chapter 6, when we examine the M/ME/$C//N$ loop, the generalization is significant, and is examined in detail.

Given our assumption, we see that (5.4.3) becomes

$$\mathbf{A}(k) = \frac{\lambda(C)}{\lambda(C)}\left[\mathbf{I} + \frac{1}{\lambda(C)}\mathbf{B} - \mathbf{Q}\right] = \mathbf{A}(C) \quad \text{for all } k \geq C. \tag{5.4.9a}$$

Then,

$$\mathbf{U}(k) = \mathbf{U}(C) \quad \text{for all } k \geq C. \tag{5.4.9b}$$

This matrix plays a dominant role in this section, therefore we call it by the more concise symbol

$$\mathbf{U_c} := \mathbf{U}(C) \quad \text{and} \quad \mathbf{A_c} := \mathbf{U_c}^{-1}. \tag{5.4.9c}$$

Every formula we derived in Section 5.4.1 is still valid here, but now we can say something more about the various matrices. From assumption (5.4.8), Equations (5.4.7) become

$$\mathbf{X}(k, N) = [\mathbf{U_c}]^{N-k} \quad \text{for } k \geq C \tag{5.4.10a}$$

and for $k < C$,

$$\mathbf{X}(k, N) = [\mathbf{U_c}]^{N-C}\mathbf{U}(C-1)\cdots\mathbf{U}(k) = [\mathbf{U_c}]^{N-C}\mathbf{X}(k, C). \tag{5.4.10b}$$

Also, from (5.4.7c) (remember, $N > C$),

$$\begin{aligned}\mathbf{K}(N) &= \sum_{k=0}^{C}\mathbf{X}(k, N) + \sum_{k=C+1}^{N}\mathbf{X}(k, N) \\ &= \mathbf{U_c}^{N-C}\mathbf{K}(C) + \sum_{k=C+1}^{N}\mathbf{U_c}^{N-k},\end{aligned} \tag{5.4.11a}$$

where $\mathbf{K}(C)$ is the same as it was before, namely

$$\mathbf{K}(C) = \mathbf{I} + \mathbf{U}(C-1) + \mathbf{U}(C-1)\mathbf{U}(C-2) + \cdots + \mathbf{U}(C-1)\cdots\mathbf{U}(0). \tag{5.4.11b}$$

From our knowledge of the partial geometric series, we can rewrite (5.4.11a) as

$$\mathbf{K}(N) = \left(\mathbf{I} - \mathbf{U_c}^{N-C}\right)[\mathbf{I} - \mathbf{U_c}]^{-1} + \mathbf{U_c}^{N-C}\mathbf{K}(C). \tag{5.4.11c}$$

These simplifications are of some help in solving for systems with finite populations, but otherwise they are not particularly enlightening. Their real use comes in solving for the open system, to which we devote the rest of this section. Let $\lambda_c := \lambda(C)$ and $\rho_c := \lambda_c \bar{x}_1$. Then if $\rho_c < 1$, the limit of $\mathbf{K}(N)$, as N goes to infinity exists, and

$$\lim_{N\to\infty} \mathbf{U_c}^N = \mathbf{O} \quad (\text{for } \rho_c < 1).$$

Then from either (5.4.11b) or (5.4.6b), we have

$$\lim_{N\to\infty} \mathbf{K}(N) = [\mathbf{I} - \mathbf{U_c}]^{-1} \quad (\text{for } \rho_c < 1),$$

which is identical to the results in Section 4.2 for the M/ME/1 queue, with λ_c, ρ_c, and $\mathbf{U}_c$ replacing λ, ρ, and $\mathbf{U}$, respectively.

An interesting case occurs when the limit does not exist, presumably when $\rho_c > 1$, so we assume that for the rest of this section. Proceeding in a manner similar to Section 5.1, for which we get similar but not identical results, define s_c to be the smallest eigenvalue in magnitude of $\mathbf{A_c}$, with corresponding eigenvectors $\mathbf{u_c}$, and $\mathbf{v}'_\mathbf{c}$, satisfying $\mathbf{u_c}\mathbf{v}'_\mathbf{c} = 1$. That is,

$$\mathbf{u_c}\mathbf{A_c} = s_c\mathbf{u_c} \quad \text{and} \quad \mathbf{A_c}\mathbf{v}'_\mathbf{c} = s_c\mathbf{v}'_\mathbf{c}, \tag{5.4.12}$$

and $|1/s_c|$ is the largest among all eigenvalues of $\mathbf{U_c}$. Using (5.1.2c), with $\mathbf{U_c}$ replacing $\mathbf{U}$, Equations (5.4.10) become for very large N and $\rho_c > 1$,

$$\lim_{N\to\infty} s_c^N\, \mathbf{X}(k, N) = s_c^k\, \mathbf{v}'_\mathbf{c}\, \mathbf{u_c} \quad \text{for } k \ge C \tag{5.4.13a}$$

and

$$\lim_{N\to\infty} s_c^N\, \mathbf{X}(k, N) = s_c^C\, \mathbf{v}'_\mathbf{c}\, \mathbf{u_c}\, \mathbf{X}(k, C) \quad \text{for } k < C. \tag{5.4.13b}$$

Also, from (5.4.11b) (using $s_c^N\,\mathbf{I} \to \mathbf{0}$), in a manner very similar to that used in deriving (5.1.3a),

$$\begin{aligned}\lim_{N\to\infty} s_c^N\, \mathbf{K}(N) &= [\mathbf{I} - \mathbf{U_c}]^{-1}[\mathbf{0} - s_c^C\mathbf{v}'_\mathbf{c}\,\mathbf{u_c}] + s_c^C\mathbf{v}'_\mathbf{c}\,\mathbf{u_c}\,\mathbf{K}(C) \\ &= \mathbf{v}'_\mathbf{c}\,\mathbf{u_c} s_c^C \left[\mathbf{K}(C) + \frac{s_c}{1 - s_c}\right].\end{aligned} \tag{5.4.13c}$$

Next, take $\Psi[\,\cdot\,]$ of the above to get, in analogy with (5.1.3b),

$$\lim_{N\to\infty} \Psi\left[s_c^N \mathbf{K}(N)\right] = s_c^C(\mathbf{p}\mathbf{v}'_\mathbf{c})(\mathbf{u_c}\boldsymbol{\epsilon}')\left[\frac{s_c}{1 - s_c} + \hat{\mathbf{u}}_\mathbf{c}\,\mathbf{K}(C)\boldsymbol{\epsilon}'\right], \tag{5.4.13d}$$

where we have made the definition analogous to (5.1.4b):

$$\hat{\mathbf{u}}_\mathbf{c} := \frac{\mathbf{u_c}}{\mathbf{u_c}\boldsymbol{\epsilon}'}. \tag{5.4.14}$$

Then we have $\hat{\mathbf{u}}_\mathbf{c}\boldsymbol{\epsilon}' = 1$. Also, note that $\hat{\mathbf{u}}_\mathbf{c}\mathbf{K}(C)\boldsymbol{\epsilon}'$ is a scalar.

Before going on, we must make a slight addition to our notation, so that the symbols we use explicitly reflect their dependence on C. Remember that in Section 5.4.1 there was no C, so we used the same notation as we did in the preceding sections. But now, if one wishes to examine systems that are identical except for differing values of C, the symbols must show it. So, for the rest of this chapter, we use the following.

Definition 5.4.1

$\boldsymbol{\pi_2}(k;\, N \,|\, C)$ = *steady-state vector probability of finding* k *customers at* S_2*, in an ME/M/C//N-type queue. The associated scalar probability is denoted by* $r_2(k;\, N \,|\, C) = \boldsymbol{\pi_2}(k;\, N \,|\, C)\boldsymbol{\epsilon'}$. This change of notation carries over to the open ME/M/C queue as follows:

$$\boldsymbol{\pi_2}(k \,|\, C) := \lim_{N\to\infty} \boldsymbol{\pi_2}(k;\, N \,|\, C)$$

and

$$r_2(k \,|\, C) := \lim_{N\to\infty} r_2(k;\, N \,|\, C).$$

Note the vertical bar, making $r_2(k;\, C)$ very different from $r_2(k \,|\, C)$.□

Now we are ready to calculate the various probabilities from Corollary 5.4.2, Equations (5.4.10), (5.4.13), and (5.4.14).

$$\boldsymbol{\pi_2}(k \,|\, C) = \lim_{N\to\infty} \frac{1}{\Psi\left[\mathbf{K}(N)\right]}\mathbf{p}\mathbf{X}(k, N) = \lim_{N\to\infty} \frac{1}{\Psi\left[s_c^N\,\mathbf{K}(N)\right]}\mathbf{p}s_c^N\mathbf{X}(k, N)$$

$$= \frac{s_c^k(\mathbf{p}\,\mathbf{v_c'})\mathbf{u_c}}{s_c^C(\mathbf{p}\,\mathbf{v_c'})(\mathbf{u_c}\boldsymbol{\epsilon'})\left[\frac{s_c}{1-s_c} + \hat{\mathbf{u}}_\mathbf{c}\,\mathbf{K}(C)\,\boldsymbol{\epsilon'}\right]}$$

and with a slight cleanup, we get

$$\boldsymbol{\pi_2}(k \,|\, C) = \frac{(1-s_c)s_c^{k-C}}{s_c + (1-s_c)\hat{\mathbf{u}}_\mathbf{c}\mathbf{K}(C)\,\boldsymbol{\epsilon'}}\hat{\mathbf{u}}_\mathbf{c} \qquad \text{for} \quad k \geq C.$$

The scalar expression that is in the front of this equation appears often enough to warrant its own symbol. Therefore, define

$$g(C) := \frac{1-s_c}{s_c + (1-s_c)\hat{\mathbf{u}}_\mathbf{c}\mathbf{K}(C)\boldsymbol{\epsilon'}}. \tag{5.4.15}$$

Then

$$\boldsymbol{\pi_2}(k \,|\, C) = g(C)s_c^{k-C}\,\hat{\mathbf{u}}_\mathbf{c} \quad \text{for} \quad k \geq C. \tag{5.4.16a}$$

Also,

$$\boldsymbol{\pi_2}(k \,|\, C) = g(C)\,\hat{\mathbf{u}}_\mathbf{c}\,\mathbf{X}(k,\, C) \quad \text{for} \quad 0 \leq k < C. \tag{5.4.16b}$$

Note that $\hat{\mathbf{u}}_\mathbf{c}\,\mathbf{X}(k, C)$ is a vector that is not usually proportional to $\hat{\mathbf{u}}_\mathbf{c}$. The associated scalar probabilities can then be written as

$$r_2(k \,|\, C) = g(C)s_c^{k-C} \quad \text{for} \quad k \geq C \tag{5.4.17a}$$

and

$$r_2(k|C) = g(C)\hat{\mathbf{u}}_{\mathbf{c}}\mathbf{X}(k,C)\boldsymbol{\epsilon}' \quad \text{for } 0 \le k < C. \tag{5.4.17b}$$

When $C = 1$, these equations reduce to those in Theorem 5.1.2. We summarize the above with the following theorem.

Theorem 5.4.3: The steady-state probability vectors for the ME/M/C queue are given by Equations (5.4.15) to (5.4.17), where s_c is the smallest eigenvalue in magnitude of the matrix from (5.4.9a),

$$\mathbf{A}_{\mathbf{c}} = \mathbf{I} + \frac{1}{\lambda_c}\mathbf{B} - \mathbf{Q},$$

with left eigenvector $\hat{\mathbf{u}}_{\mathbf{c}}$ normalized so that $\hat{\mathbf{u}}_{\mathbf{c}}\,\boldsymbol{\epsilon}' = 1$. It follows that s_c also satisfies the equation

$$s_c = B^*[\lambda_c(1 - s_c)].$$

The matrices $\{\mathbf{A}(k) \,|\, 0 \le k < C\}$ and their inverses $\{\,\mathbf{U}(k)\,\}$, are given by (5.4.3). The matrices $\{\,\mathbf{X}(k,\, C) \,|\, 0 \le k < C\,\}$ are given by (5.4.7b), and $\mathbf{K}(C)$ is defined by (5.4.11b). ■

The geometric parameter s_c has identical properties to the geometric parameter we discussed in Section 5.1.3 in relation to the ME/M/1 queue. The only distinction is using λ_c in the construction of $\mathbf{A}_{\mathbf{c}}$.

The reader should look closely at Equations (5.4.16) and (5.4.17) to see their similarity with Theorem 5.1.2, for $C = 1$. For $k \ge C$, all the probability vectors are proportional to $\hat{\mathbf{u}}_{\mathbf{c}}$, and their magnitudes are geometrically distributed with ratio s_c. However, for $k < C$ they take on a different form, which is easy enough to calculate in specific cases, but about which little can be said in general.

Exercise 5.4.1: Let $C = 2$, and let $\lambda_2 = 2\lambda$. Calculate the steady-state probabilities and the mean queue length of an E_2/M/2 queue, for $\rho_2 = 0.1$, 0.3, 0.5, 0.7, 0.9, and 0.95. Compare the queue lengths with those for the M/M/2 queue for the same ρ_2.

The accomplishments of this section correspond to what a random observer will see when viewing a system that has been in existence for a long time. We must go to the next section to find out what arriving and departing customers would see.

5.4.3 Arrival and Departure Points

What we do here exactly parallels what we did in Section 4.1.3 for load-independent loops. The generalization is direct, but we give new definitions to correspond to our focus on S_2. We deal with ME/M/X//N loops first, and then specialize at the end to look at the ME/M/C queue.

Definition 5.4.2

$\mathbf{w_2}(k; N)$:= *steady-state vector probability of finding k customers at* S_2*, and* $N - k$ *customers at* S_1*, between events.* $[\mathbf{w_2}(k; N)]_i$ is the probability that the ith phase in S_1 is busy (and there are k customers at S_2). $\mathbf{w_2}(N; N)$ is defined to be proportional to $\mathbf{p}$. □

Just as we did with the steady-state balance equations (5.4.1), we can write the balance equations for $\mathbf{w_2}(k;\ N)$ directly, by replacing λ wherever it appears in Equations (4.1.3) by the appropriate $\lambda(k)$. The reader might look again at Figure 5.4.1 before going on. The balance equations can be written directly from a generalization of Equations (4.1.9).

$$\mathbf{w_2}(N;\ N) = \mathbf{w_2}(N-1; N)[\lambda(N-1)\mathbf{I} + \mathbf{M}]^{-1}\,\mathbf{BQ}. \tag{5.4.18a}$$

For $1 \le k \le N-1$,

$$\begin{aligned}\mathbf{w_2}(k;\ N)[\lambda(k)\mathbf{I} + \mathbf{M}]^{-1}[\lambda(k)\mathbf{I} + \mathbf{B}] &= \mathbf{w_2}(k-1; N)[\mathbf{M} + \lambda(k-1)\mathbf{I}]^{-1}\mathbf{BQ}\\ &\quad + \mathbf{w_2}(k+1; N)[\mathbf{M} + \lambda(k+1)\mathbf{I}]^{-1}\lambda(k+1)\mathbf{I}\end{aligned} \tag{5.4.18b}$$

and

$$\mathbf{w_2}(0;\ N)\mathbf{M}^{-1}\mathbf{B} = \mathbf{w_2}(1;\ N)[\lambda(1)\mathbf{I} + \mathbf{M}]^{-1}\lambda(1)\mathbf{I}. \tag{5.4.18c}$$

Notice that if we use the convention that $\lambda(0) := 0$ and $\lambda(k) := 0$ for $k > N$, then (5.4.18a) and (5.4.18c) become special cases of (5.4.18b). But do not get carried away. It is usually the special cases that give us physical insight.

We can easily write down the solutions to the balance equations for $\mathbf{w_2}(k;\ N)$ by comparing them with those for $\boldsymbol{\pi}_2(k;\ N)$, Equations (5.4.1),

Theorem 5.4.4: The steady-state between-event vector probabilities of finding k customers at S_2 in an ME/M/X//N loop are given by the following.

$$\mathbf{w_2}(0;\ N) = c(N)\boldsymbol{\pi}_2(0;\ N)\mathbf{M}, \tag{5.4.19a}$$

for $1 \le k \le N-1$,

$$\mathbf{w_2}(k;\ N) = c(N)\boldsymbol{\pi}_2(k;\ N)[\lambda(k)\mathbf{I} + \mathbf{M}], \tag{5.4.19b}$$

$$\mathbf{w_2}(N;\ N) = c(N)\boldsymbol{\pi}_2(N;\ N)\lambda(N)\mathbf{I}. \tag{5.4.19c}$$

$c(N)$ is a normalization constant to make the $\mathbf{w_2}$s sum to 1, which we do not bother to calculate, and $\boldsymbol{\pi}_2(k;\ N)$ given by Theorem 5.4.2. ■

Proof: By direct substitution. **QED**

As in Chapter 4, six types of events can happen. We repeat Equations (4.1.11), but in the context of this section. $\lambda(k)$ is now load dependent, and k refers to the number of customers at S_2.

$$\begin{aligned}
&(1)\quad \mathbb{P}\mathbf{r}\big[\{\cdot;\ N;\ N\} \to \{i;\ N-1;\ N\}\big] = \mathbf{w_2}(N;\ N);\\
&(2)\quad \mathbb{P}\mathbf{r}\big[\{i;\ k;\ N\} \to \{i;\ k-1;\ N\}\big] = \mathbf{w_2}(k;\ N)[\lambda(k)\mathbf{I} + \mathbf{M}]^{-1}\lambda(k)\mathbf{I};\\
&(3)\quad \mathbb{P}\mathbf{r}\big[\{j;\ k;\ N\} \to \{i;\ k;\ N\}\big] = \mathbf{w_2}(k;\ N)[\lambda(k)\mathbf{I} + \mathbf{M}]^{-1}\mathbf{MP};\\
&(4)\quad \mathbb{P}\mathbf{r}\big[\{j;\ k;\ N\} \to \{i;\ k+1;\ N\}\big] = \mathbf{w_2}(k;\ N)[\lambda(k)\mathbf{I} + \mathbf{M}]^{-1}\mathbf{Mq'p};\\
&(5)\quad \mathbb{P}\mathbf{r}\big[\{j;\ 0;\ N\} \to \{i;\ 0;\ N\}\big] = \mathbf{w_2}(0;\ N)\mathbf{P};\\
&(6)\quad \mathbb{P}\mathbf{r}\big[\{j;\ 0;\ N\} \to \{i;\ 1;\ N\}\big] = \mathbf{w_2}(0;\ N)\mathbf{q'p}.
\end{aligned} \tag{5.4.20}$$

Arrivals at S_2 result in an increase of its queue length, corresponding to (4) and (6) above. Keeping Definitions 5.1.2 to 5.1.4, we have [from term (6)]

$$\mathbf{a_2}(0;\,N) = G(N)\mathbf{w_2}(0;\,N)\mathbf{q}'\mathbf{p}$$

and [from term (4)]

$$\mathbf{a_2}(k;N) = G(N)\mathbf{w_2}(k;N)[\lambda(k)\mathbf{I}+\mathbf{M}]^{-1}\mathbf{BQ} \qquad \text{for } 1 \le k \le N-1.$$

There is no term for $k = N$, because a customer cannot arrive at S_2 and find that everyone (including himself) is already there. The $G(N)$ is the normalizing constant to make the sum of the probabilities add up to 1. Next, using (5.4.19), we replace $\mathbf{w_2}(k;\,N)$ with $\boldsymbol{\pi_2}(k;\,N)$ to get

$$\mathbf{a_2}(0;N) = C(N)G(N)\,\boldsymbol{\pi_2}(0;\,N)\mathbf{BQ}$$

and

$$\mathbf{a_2}(k;\,N) = C(N)G(N)\boldsymbol{\pi_2}(k;\,N)\mathbf{BQ} \quad \text{for } 1 \le k \le N{-}1.$$

These equations look rather uninteresting, being no different than the equivalent ones for load-independent systems. But we are dealing with steady-state phenomena, so $\boldsymbol{\pi_2}\,(k;N) = \boldsymbol{\pi_2}(k{+}1;\,N)\mathbf{U}(k)$ from (5.4.5). Furthermore, from Lemma 5.4.1 $\mathbf{B}\boldsymbol{\epsilon}' = \lambda(k{+}1)\mathbf{A}(k)\boldsymbol{\epsilon}'$, so

$$\boldsymbol{\pi_2}(k;\,N)\mathbf{BQ} = \lambda(k{+}1)\boldsymbol{\pi_2}(k;\,N)\mathbf{A}(k)\mathbf{Q} = \lambda(k{+}1)\boldsymbol{\pi_2}(k{+}1;\,N)\mathbf{Q}.$$

Thus

$$\begin{aligned}\mathbf{a_2}(k;\,N) &= C(N)G(N)\,\lambda(k{+}1)\boldsymbol{\pi_2}(k{+}1;\,N)\mathbf{Q}\\ &= C(N)G(N)\,\lambda(k{+}1)\,r_2(k{+}1;\,N)\mathbf{p}.\end{aligned}$$

Compare with Theorem 5.1.3. and (5.1.1a). The mysterious reason for not counting the arriving customer has to do with steady-state equations. We have

$$\sum_{k=0}^{N-1} \mathbf{a_2}(k;\,N)\boldsymbol{\epsilon}' = C(N)G(N)\sum_{k=1}^{N} \lambda(k)\,r_2(k;\,N) = 1.$$

Now, the sum multiplying $C(N)G(N)$ is the mean rate at which customers leave S_2, which we have already met in Chapter 2, (2.1.14), and labeled $\Lambda(N)$. Therefore,

$$\frac{1}{C(N)G(N)} = \Lambda(N) = \sum_{k=1}^{N} \lambda(k)\,r_2(k;\,N). \tag{5.4.21}$$

Let us next look at the departure probabilities. A departure from S_2 requires that the queue count drop by 1, so we need terms (1), for $\mathbf{d_2}(N{-}1;\,N)$, and (2), for $\mathbf{d_2}(k;\,N)$, from our list in (5.4.20). We use (5.4.19) and go directly to

$$\mathbf{d_2}(k;\,N) = C(N)G(N)\,\lambda(k{+}1)\,\boldsymbol{\pi_2}(k{+}1;\,N) \quad \text{for } 0 \le k \le N{-}1.$$

The sum $\sum_{k=0}^{N-1} \mathbf{d_2}(k;N)\boldsymbol{\epsilon}' = 1$ yields the same result as we got for the arrival; thus we have the following theorem.

Theorem 5.4.5: The steady-state arrival and departure vector probabilities for the ME/M/$X//N$ loop are given by the following equations. For $0 \le k \le N-1$,

$$\mathbf{a_2}(k;\, N) = \frac{\lambda(k+1)}{\Lambda(N)} r_2(k+1;\, N)\mathbf{p}, \tag{5.4.22a}$$

$$\mathbf{d_2}(k;\, N) = \frac{\lambda(k+1)}{\Lambda(N)} \boldsymbol{\pi_2}(k+1;\, N). \tag{5.4.22b}$$

The corresponding scalar probabilities are

$$a_2(k;\, N) = d_2(k;\, N) = \frac{\lambda(k+1)}{\Lambda(N)} r_2(k+1;\, N). \tag{5.4.22c}$$

$\boldsymbol{\pi_2}(k;\, N)$ is given by Theorem 5.4.2 or Corollary 5.4.2, and $\Lambda(N)$ is given by normalization through (5.4.21). Clearly, $\mathbf{a_2}$ and $\mathbf{d_2}$ are related by the formula $\mathbf{a_2}(k;\, N) = \mathbf{d_2}(k;\, N)\,\mathbf{Q}$. ■

These equations are as close to the M/ME/$1//N$ results of Theorem 4.1.4 as one could hope. All the arrival vectors (departure vectors in Chapter 4) are proportional to $\mathbf{p}$ and the scalar arrival and departure probabilities are equal to each other. Even the vector departure probabilities are the same as the load-independent arrival probabilities, but remember that $\mathbf{d_2}(k;N) = \mathbf{a_1}(n-1;N)$ in general. Why, you may ask, did we bother studying the simpler case in the first place? The author would ask in return if you would have had much greater difficulty understanding this section had you not gone through it first in Chapter 4.

Once again we cannot say much more about these equations without providing more information about $\lambda(k)$. We can say this much though: if

$$\lim_{N\to\infty} \lambda(N) > \frac{1}{\bar{x}_1},$$

then S_1 is surely the bottleneck, and the system throughput approaches

$$\lim_{N\to\infty} \Lambda(N) = \frac{1}{\bar{x}_1}. \tag{5.4.23}$$

We turn our attention once again to the ME/M/C queue, and assume that (5.4.8) holds.

Definition 5.4.3

$\mathbf{a_2}(k;N\,|\,C)$ and $\mathbf{d_2}(k;N\,|\,C)$ *are the steady-state vector arrival and departure probabilities for the* ME/M/C//N*-type queue. The associated scalar probabilities are denoted by* $a_2(k;N\,|\,C)$ *and* $d_2(k;N\,|\,C)$. This change of notation carries over to the open ME/M/C queue. For instance,

$$\mathbf{a_2}(k\,|\,C) := \lim_{N\to\infty} \mathbf{a_2}(k;\, N\,|\,C),$$

with similar expressions for $\mathbf{d_2}(k\,|\,C), a_2(k\,|\,C)$, and $d_2(k\,|\,C)$. □

The limiting expressions for these entities are just a little tricky. Let us define

$$\varrho_c := 1/\rho_c$$

and assume that $\varrho_c < 1$. First look at departures. Using (5.4.22a), (5.4.23), and (5.4.16a), we have

$$\mathbf{d_2}(k \,|\, C) = \lim_{N\to\infty} \frac{\lambda_c}{\Lambda(N)} \boldsymbol{\pi_2}(k+1; N \,|\, C)$$
$$= \lambda_c \, \bar{x}_1 \, \boldsymbol{\pi_2}(k+1 \,|\, C) = \frac{1}{\varrho_c} g(C) \, s_c^{k+1-C} \, \hat{\mathbf{u}}_{\mathbf{c}} \quad \text{for } k \geq C-1,$$

where $g(C)$ is defined by (5.4.15). But for $k < C-1$, from (5.4.16b),

$$\mathbf{d_2}(k \,|\, C) = \frac{1}{\varrho_c} g(C) \hat{\mathbf{u}}_{\mathbf{c}} \, \mathbf{X}(k+1,\, C), \quad \text{for } k < C-1.$$

Theorem 5.4.2 tells us that $\mathbf{a_2}(k; N) = \mathbf{d_2}(k; N)\mathbf{Q}$, so the arrival vectors require no further effort. We thus summarize.

Theorem 5.4.6: The steady-state departure and arrival vector probabilities for the ME/M/C queue are given by the following equations. For departures,

$$\mathbf{d_2}(k \,|\, C) = \frac{g(C)}{\varrho_c} s_c^{k+1-C} \, \hat{\mathbf{u}}_{\mathbf{c}} \quad \text{for } k \geq C-1 \tag{5.4.24a}$$

$$\mathbf{d_2}(k \,|\, C) = \frac{g(C)}{\varrho_c} \hat{\mathbf{u}}_{\mathbf{c}} \, \mathbf{X}(k+1,\, C) \quad \text{for } k < C-1. \tag{5.4.24b}$$

For arrivals,

$$\mathbf{a_2}(k \,|\, C) = \frac{g(C)}{\varrho_c} \; s_c^{k+1-C} \, \mathbf{p} \; . \text{ for } k \geq C-1 \tag{5.4.24c}$$

$$\mathbf{a_2}(k \,|\, C) = \frac{g(C)}{\varrho_c} [\hat{\mathbf{u}}_{\mathbf{c}} \mathbf{X}(k+1,\, C) \boldsymbol{\epsilon}'] \mathbf{p} \quad \text{for } k < C-1. \tag{5.4.24d}$$

The associated scalar probabilities are equal to each other, and satisfy

$$a_2(k \,|\, C) = d_2(k \,|\, C) = \frac{1}{\varrho_c} r_2(k+1 \,|\, C) \quad \text{for all } k \geq 0, \tag{5.4.24e}$$

where $r_2(k \,|\, C)$ is given by either (5.4.17a) or (5.4.17b), depending on the value of k. ■

Once again we have a family of geometric distributions. Comparing with Equations (5.4.17), we see that $\mathbf{a_2}(k|\, C)$ and $\mathbf{d_2}(k|\, C)$ for a given k are related to $\boldsymbol{\pi_2}(k+1|\, C)$ (and $r_2(k+1|\, C)$) for $k+1$. Therefore, the geometric form starts at $k = C$ for the steady-state probabilities, but starts at $k = C-1$ for the arrivals and departures. This compares with the ME/M/1 queue, where $\mathbf{a_2}(0)$

and $\mathbf{d_2}(0)$ are part of a general geometric sequence, but $\boldsymbol{\pi}_2(0)$ is not. Remember that by the notation of this section, $\boldsymbol{\pi}_2(k \mid 1)$ is the same as $\boldsymbol{\pi}_2(k)$ of Section 5.1.

It is only fair to ask why one would want to know the vector details of these systems. A perusal of Section 4.5 gives some idea of how they could be useful. For instance, if we wanted to know the mean time for the arrival of the next customer, given that one has just departed from S_2, leaving behind $C-1$ or more customers, one would use $\hat{\mathbf{u}}_\mathbf{c}\,\mathbf{V}\,\boldsymbol{\epsilon}'$. If, however, there were fewer than $C-1$ customers left behind, the mean time until the next arrival would be

$$\frac{\hat{\mathbf{u}}_\mathbf{c}\,[\mathbf{K}(k+1,\,C)\,\mathbf{V}]\,\boldsymbol{\epsilon}'}{\hat{\mathbf{u}}_\mathbf{c}[\,\mathbf{K}(k+1,\,C)]\,\boldsymbol{\epsilon}'}.$$

We could do the same for random observers, or just arrived customers, or more extended combinations. We discuss a little more transient behavior for ME/M/1 queues in the next and final section of this chapter.

5.5 Transient Behavior of G/M/1 Queues

Much of what we do in this section is a copy of what was done in Section 4.5, but from an upside-down point of view. What was there d is $2u$ here, and so on. We should be able to move much more quickly, but there are some new difficulties as well as some new insights. First we examine how the ME/M/1 queue grows with time. Afterward we study how long it takes for a queue to drain, or equivalently, the k-busy period. We need not recommend that you reread Section 4.5, because you will have to do it to retrieve formulas we need here. We note, finally, that all procedures are directly generalizable to the ME/M/X queue.

5.5.1 First-Passage Times for Queue Growth

We have already seen several times that before we can discuss how a queue grows by k we must examine how it grows by 1. And we must see how the state of the system has changed after a unit growth. So we define the equivalent of Definition 4.5.1, which is really the inverse of Definition 4.5.7.

Definition 5.5.1

$\mathbf{H_{2u}}(k)$:=*probability matrix of first passage from k to $k+1$.* $[\mathbf{H_{2u}}(k)]_{ij}$ is the probability that S_1 will be in state j when the queue at S_2 goes from k to $k+1$ for the first time, given that the system started in state $\{i;\, k\}$. The subscript **2u** stands for "S_2 goes up." □

Note that this matrix only has one argument (k), because going up always implies that there is a bottom, namely an empty queue at S_2. We have already derived these in finding $\mathbf{H_d}(n, N)$ in Equations (4.5.10). It was clear, then (in the notation of this chapter), that

$$\mathbf{H_{2u}}(k) = \mathbf{Q} \quad \text{for all } \; k \geq 0. \tag{5.5.1}$$

Why do we bother defining this matrix yet again, when it is of such simple form? We answer that in the next chapter it is not so simple, even though the concept is the same.

First we must define the upside-down version of Definition 4.5.8.

Definition 5.5.2

$\boldsymbol{\tau}'_{\mathbf{2u}}(k)$:= *mean first-passage time vector from* k *to* $k+1$. $[\boldsymbol{\tau}'_{\mathbf{2u}}(k)]_i$ is the mean time for the queue at S_2 to reach $k+1$ for the first time, given that the system started in state $\{i;\, k\}$. □

We can write down the equations for $\boldsymbol{\tau}'_{\mathbf{2u}}(k)$ directly from its equivalent in Chapter 4. Thus (4.5.11a) and (4.5.11b) convert to

$$\boldsymbol{\tau}'_{\mathbf{2u}}(0) = \mathbf{V}\boldsymbol{\epsilon}' \qquad (5.5.2a)$$

and

$$\boldsymbol{\tau}'_{\mathbf{2u}}(k) = \frac{1}{\lambda}\mathbf{U}\boldsymbol{\epsilon}' + \mathbf{U}\boldsymbol{\tau}'_{\mathbf{2u}}(k-1), \qquad (5.5.2b)$$

where $\mathbf{U}$ is defined by (4.1.4). The solution of these equations comes directly from (4.5.12):

$$\boldsymbol{\tau}'_{\mathbf{2u}}(k) = \frac{1}{\lambda}\mathbf{U}\mathbf{K}(k)\,\boldsymbol{\epsilon}' = \frac{1}{\lambda}[\mathbf{K}(k+1) - \mathbf{I}]\boldsymbol{\epsilon}', \qquad (5.5.2c)$$

where $\mathbf{K}(k)$ is the normalization matrix for the M/ME/1//k queue, defined in (4.1.6).

Now we are ready to set up the formulas for time of queue growth, or are we? To do this, we must know the state the system is in originally. That is, we must know the initial vector $\mathbf{p_i}$. If the queue (at S_2) is empty, what does that tell us about the system (i.e., what state is S_1 in)? The initial vector certainly cannot be $\mathbf{p}$, because that would imply that a customer just left S_1, which in turn means that the same customer has just arrived at S_2, contradicting our assumption that S_2 is empty. If ϱ (which you recall is $1/\lambda\bar{x}_1$) is less than 1, there are two possibilities of immediate interest. We could assume that a customer has just departed S_2 in a system that has been running for a long time. This corresponds to

$$\mathbf{p_i} = \frac{\mathbf{d}_2(0)}{d_2(0)} = \hat{\mathbf{u}}.$$

Then the mean time until the first arrival to the empty queue conditioned by a departure (also known as the mean idle time, or time between busy periods), is

$$t_I := \mathbf{p_i}\boldsymbol{\tau}'_{\mathbf{2u}}(0) = \hat{\mathbf{u}}\mathbf{V}\boldsymbol{\epsilon}' = \frac{1-\varrho}{1-s}\bar{x}_1 \qquad (\varrho,\ s < 1). \qquad (5.5.3a)$$

We got the last part from (5.1.5e) and remembered that $\rho = 1/\varrho$. As an aside, this formula gives us some idea of what the difference between s and ϱ means. If we are looking at an M/M/1 queue, then $\varrho = s$, and the mean time until the next arrival is $\bar{x}_1$, as expected. For other systems, we might look at Figure

5.1.1 for insight. If s is greater (less) than ϱ, we would expect to wait longer (less) than $\bar{x}_1$ for the first customer to arrive.

The other possibility is to ask what a random observer would see. This corresponds to

$$\mathbf{p_i} = \frac{\boldsymbol{\pi_2}(0)}{r_2(0)} = \frac{\hat{\mathbf{u}}\mathbf{V}}{\hat{\mathbf{u}}\,\mathbf{V}\,\boldsymbol{\epsilon}'}.$$

Thus the mean time for the first customer to arrive, as seen by a random observer, is [call it $t_r(0)$]

$$t_r(0) := \mathbf{p_i}\boldsymbol{\tau}'_{\mathbf{2u}}(0) = \frac{\hat{\mathbf{u}}\mathbf{V}^2\boldsymbol{\epsilon}'}{\hat{\mathbf{u}}\mathbf{V}\boldsymbol{\epsilon}'}.$$

We can actually get an interesting expression for this by solving for

$$\hat{\mathbf{u}}\mathbf{V} = \frac{1}{\lambda(1-s)}[\lambda\mathbf{p}\mathbf{V} - \hat{\mathbf{u}}] \qquad (\varrho < 1), \tag{5.5.3b}$$

and

$$\frac{\hat{\mathbf{u}}\mathbf{V}}{\hat{\mathbf{u}}\mathbf{V}\,\boldsymbol{\epsilon}'} = \frac{\varrho}{1-\varrho}[\lambda\mathbf{p}\mathbf{V} - \hat{\mathbf{u}}]. \tag{5.5.3c}$$

We put this all together to get

$$t_r(0) = \frac{\Psi\left[\mathbf{V}^2\right]}{(1-\varrho)\bar{x}_1} - \frac{1}{(1-s)\lambda}.$$

It is difficult to see what is going on here, because near $\varrho = 1$ both terms are unboundedly large, so their difference can be anything. Actually, their difference is finite. We leave it as an exercise to show [using (5.1.22b), (5.1.22c), and (5.1.23b)] that (we are 99.44% sure)

$$\lim_{\varrho \to 1_-} t_r(0) = \bar{x}_1 \frac{1 + C_v^2}{2}\left(1 - \frac{s''(1)}{2} \cdot \frac{1 + C_v^2}{2}\right).$$

Even when $\varrho = 1_-$, this expression is not simple, particularly when one notes, from (5.1.24a), that $s''(1)$ is quite complicated. Only when we consider the M/M/1 queue does this simplify, for then $s''(1) = 0$ and $C_v^2 = 1$, so $t_r(0) = \bar{x}_1$. One should compare these results with the ***residual times*** as given in (3.5.12d). There are, of course, any number of other possibilities that one could consider in setting up $\mathbf{p_i}$, all of which would require more information about the history of the system. Now, if $\varrho > 1$, even though (5.5.2a) is still valid, we have nothing to go on for preparing the initial vector. In this case there is no such thing as the steady state, and after a "long period of time," the probability that no one will be at S_2 is 0. Therefore, any initial condition must be based on some transient events. We must be given some special information ("S_1 just woke up," or something).

Once there is someone at S_2 ($k > 0$), we can say something even if $\varrho > 1$. We can talk about the state of the system immediately after a customer arrives, and in fact this is the most important situation. After all, every increase in queue length is the result of an arrival (at S_2), so after the first increase, all subsequent increases begin their epochs with the initial vector $\mathbf{p}$ (at S_1). The other two cases we described for $k = 0$ are still applicable. The initial vector for the time to rise from k to $k+1$, conditioned on a departure, is

$$\mathbf{p_i} = \frac{\mathbf{d_2}(k)}{d_2(k)} = \hat{\mathbf{u}},$$

the same as for the empty queue. Similarly, the random observer, from (5.1.5b) and (5.1.5d), will see the same initial vector as a departing customer! Only when the queue is empty will she see something different. An arriving customer, however, will always see something different. (Speaking from a purely physical point of view, the arriving customer will see nothing special, because the initial vector refers to S_1, the subsystem he left behind.) Thus we see that there are cases when departing customers, arriving customers, and random observers all see different behavior.

We could continue piling variations upon variations, but let us merely consider the mean time for the queue at S_2 to grow to k, given that the first customer has just arrived. Let us call this $t_2(1 \to k)$. Then [using the obvious convention that $t_2(1 \to 1) = 0$]

$$t_2(1 \to k) = \sum_{l=1}^{k-1} \mathbf{p}\boldsymbol{\tau}'_{\mathbf{2u}}(l) = \frac{1}{\lambda} \sum_{l=1}^{k-1} \Psi\left[\mathbf{UK}(l)\right].$$

This formula is easy enough to compute, based on what we know from Chapter 4; however, we indicate how the queue grows for large k. We know that for $\varrho > 1$, $\mathbf{K}(l)$ approaches a limit for large l. Specifically [from (4.2.3)]

$$T := \lim_{l \to \infty} \mathbf{p}\boldsymbol{\tau}'_{\mathbf{2u}}(l) = \frac{1}{\lambda}\Psi\left[\mathbf{UK}\right] = \frac{1}{\lambda}\Psi\left[(\mathbf{I} - \mathbf{U})^{-1} - \mathbf{I}\right]$$

$$= \frac{1}{\lambda}\left[\frac{1}{1 - 1/\varrho} - 1\right] = \frac{1/\lambda}{\varrho - 1} \quad \text{for } \varrho > 1.$$

The expression is independent of everything except ϱ and λ, and tells us that once the queue grows large enough, it will continue to grow linearly with time. Each incremental increase will take the same amount of time (on average, of course). Because T is the mean time for the queue to grow by 1, its reciprocal can be considered to be the rate at which the queue grows. This leads to

$$\frac{1}{T} = \lambda\varrho - \lambda = \frac{1}{\bar{x}_1} - \lambda \quad \text{for } \varrho > 1.$$

We have the perfectly reasonable result that the rate of queue growth is equal to the rate of arrivals minus the rate of departures from S_2. In other words, the queue-length growth curves for all ME/M/1 queues approach straight lines, and have the same slope. You should compare this result with that for the M/M/1 queue [Equation (2.3.2a)] to see that, in fact, the two are asymptotically equal. Keep in mind, however, that this is true only for $\varrho > 1$! When $\varrho < 1$, asymptotic behavior is completely different. We must be very careful when conceptually replacing ***probability flow rates*** with ***physical flow rates***. This is meaningful only in very heavy traffic.

For $\varrho < 1$, the normalization matrix $\mathbf{K}(l)$ does not approach a limit but, rather, grows geometrically as $(1/s)^l$. We saw this in deriving the steady-state solution for the ME/M/1 queue. For large l, and from (5.1.3),

$$\lambda \mathbf{p}\tau'_{\mathbf{2u}}(l) \approx \Psi\,[\mathbf{UF}] \left(\frac{1}{s}\right)^l = \frac{(\mathbf{u}\boldsymbol{\epsilon}')(\mathbf{p}\mathbf{v}')}{\varrho(1-s)} \left(\frac{1}{s}\right)^l \quad (\text{for } \varrho < 1).$$

Now, let us define

$$\mathbf{D}(\sigma) := [\mathbf{I} + \sigma \mathbf{V}]^{-1}.$$

[We have actually used this useful matrix before, in (4.2.8b). It is the generator of the Laplace transform of $b(x)$.] Then it can be shown, when $\sigma = \lambda\,(1-s)$, that

$$\hat{\mathbf{u}} = \lambda \mathbf{p} \mathbf{V}\, \mathbf{D}(\sigma), \tag{5.5.4a}$$

$$\mathbf{v}' = c\lambda \mathbf{V}\, \mathbf{D}(\sigma) \boldsymbol{\epsilon}', \tag{5.5.4b}$$

and

$$c = (\mathbf{u}\boldsymbol{\epsilon}')(\mathbf{p}\mathbf{v}') = \frac{1}{\Psi\,[(\lambda \mathbf{V}\mathbf{D})^2]} = \frac{(1-s)^2}{1 - 2s + \Psi\,[\mathbf{D}^2]}. \tag{5.5.4c}$$

From Equations (4.4.1), c can also be written as

$$\frac{1}{c} = \frac{1}{1-s}\left[1 - \lambda \int_0^\infty x e^{-\sigma x} b(x)\, dx\right]. \tag{5.5.4d}$$

We put this all together, coming up with a form that is valid for G/M/1 queues:

$$\mathbf{p}\tau'_{\mathbf{2u}}(l) \approx \frac{\bar{x}_1}{1 - \lambda \int_0^\infty x e^{-\lambda(1-s)x} b(x) dx} \left(\frac{1}{s}\right)^l, \qquad \varrho < 1.$$

Compare this equation with (2.3.2a) for the M/M/1 queue. Both formulas are of geometric form, therefore we know from the arguments given in deriving (2.3.4a) that the queue length grows logarithmically with time. However, the rates of growth vary enormously, depending on what distribution function is generating the arrival process.

Example 5.5.1: We have combined the data from Figure 4.5.4, for the M/M/1 and M/E_2/1 queues with that for $t_2(1 \to n)$ for the E_2/M/1 queue, and plotted them in Figure 5.5.1. Even without the extra curves, the two figures are different. First of all, the x- and y-axes are interchanged. Second, the Chapter 4 curves give the mean time to grow from 0 to n, but here all curves give the time to go from 1 to n. Looking at this figure, when ρ (or ϱ) is much greater than 1, all three queues give virtually the same growth curve. This agrees with our previous argument that $1/T$, the asymptotic growth rate, depends only on the difference between the arrival and the service rates. However, when ρ (or ϱ) is less than 1, the time for growth is exponential (or

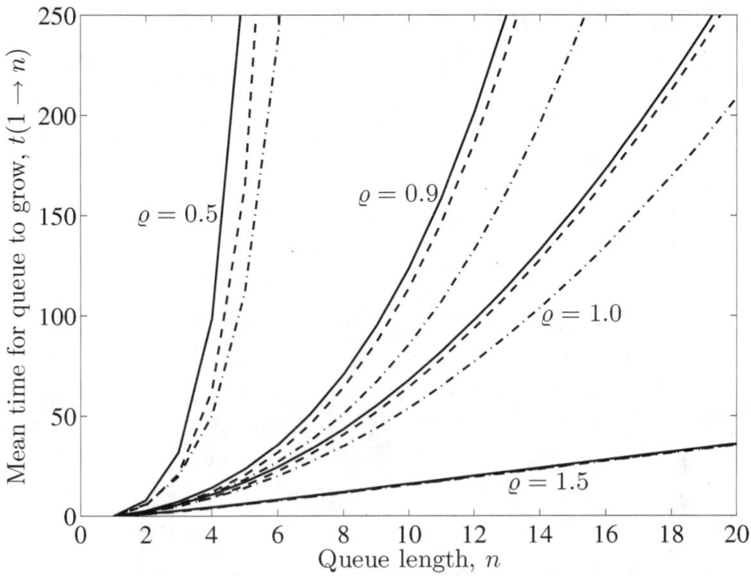

Figure 5.5.1: Mean time for queue growth $t_2(1 \rightarrow n)$ for the E_2/M/1 queue, and the equivalent function $[t(1 \rightarrow n)]$ for the M/M/1 and M/E_2/1 queues, as a function of queue length n. Four values of ρ were used, (0.5, 0.9, 1.0, and 1.5) in calculating the M/ME/1 queues, and the same values for ϱ were used for the ME/M/1 queue. In all cases E_2/M/1 lies above M/E_2/1, which lies above M/M/1.

the growth rate is logarithmic), and all three queues differ from one another. It is somewhat surprising that near saturation, the M/E_2/1 and E_2/M/1 queues are much closer to each other than they are to the M/M/1 queue. ▲

We leave it as an exercise to see how queues with other distributions behave.

Exercise 5.5.1: Calculate $t_2(1 \rightarrow n)$ for the H_2/M/1 and M/H_2/1 queues for the same parameters as those in Example 5.5.1. H_2 is the same hyperexponential distribution as used in previous exercises.

5.5.2 The k-Busy Period

We are now ready to study the draining of an ME/M/1 queue, the final topic of this chapter. As in the preceding section, we can take definitions and formulas directly from their equivalents in Section 4.5 and redress them in the notation of this chapter.

Definition 5.5.3

$\mathbf{H_{2d}}(k; N)$:=*probability matrix of first passage from k to k - 1 in an*

ME/M/1//N *loop.* $[\mathbf{H_{2d}}(k;N)]_{ij}$ is the probability that S_1 will be in state j when the queue at S_2 goes from k to $k-1$ for the first time, given that the system started in state $\{i;\ k;\ N\}$. The subscript **2d** stands for "S_2 goes down." □

This is almost identical to Definition 4.5.7, but is equal to (4.5.2) in value. We can say directly that

$$\mathbf{H_{2d}}(N;N) = \mathbf{Q} \tag{5.5.5a}$$

and

$$\mathbf{H_{2d}}(k;N) = \lambda[\lambda\mathbf{I} + \mathbf{B} - \mathbf{B}\mathbf{Q}\mathbf{H_{2d}}(k+1;N)]^{-1} \quad \text{for } k < N. \tag{5.5.5b}$$

Clearly, $\mathbf{H_{2d}}(k;N)$ is isometric and invertible.

For the open system we need

$$\mathbf{H_{2d}} := \lim_{N\to\infty} \mathbf{H_{2d}}(k;N) = \lambda[\lambda\mathbf{I} + \mathbf{B} - \mathbf{B}\mathbf{Q}\mathbf{H_{2d}}]^{-1}. \tag{5.5.6a}$$

Premultiply both sides with the matrix in square brackets, and get

$$[\lambda\mathbf{I} + \mathbf{B} - \mathbf{B}\mathbf{Q}\mathbf{H_{2d}}]\mathbf{H_{2d}} = \lambda\mathbf{I}$$

which can also be expressed as a matrix quadratic equation,

$$\mathbf{B}\mathbf{Q}[\mathbf{H_{2d}}]^2 - (\lambda\mathbf{I} + \mathbf{B})\mathbf{H_{2d}} + \lambda\mathbf{I} = \mathbf{0}. \tag{5.5.6b}$$

Thus $\mathbf{H_{2d}}$ is independent of k. It would be nice if we had an explicit form for this, but in general, only iterative methods are available to find $\mathbf{H_{2d}}$ or its inverse. For instance, one can start with $\mathbf{H_{2d}} = \mathbf{Q}$, and by brute force, substitute iteratively into (5.5.6a) until convergence is reached. There are other methods available that can find the solution much more efficiently. Interestingly enough, for all ϱ, greater than, as well as less than 1, a physical solution to this equation always exists, because the arguments that created it are physical, and thus each iterate must exist. [Remember, each iterate was really $\mathbf{H_{2d}}(k-1;\infty]$, coming down the recursive ladder, and each one is isometric.)

Definition 5.5.4

$\boldsymbol{\tau}'_{\mathbf{2d}}(k;N)$:= *mean first-passage time vector from k to $k-1$.* $[\boldsymbol{\tau}'_{\mathbf{2d}}(k;N)]_i$ is the mean time for the queue at S_2 to reach $k-1$ for the first time, given that the system started in state $\{i;\ k;\ N\}$. □

Using (4.5.5) directly, we can write $\boldsymbol{\tau}'_{\mathbf{2d}}(N;N) := 1/(\lambda)\,\boldsymbol{\epsilon}'$, and for $1 \le k < N$,

$$\boldsymbol{\tau}'_{\mathbf{2d}}(k;N) = \frac{1}{\lambda}\boldsymbol{\epsilon}' + \frac{1}{\lambda}\mathbf{H_{2d}}(k;N)\,\mathbf{B}\,\mathbf{Q}\,\boldsymbol{\tau}'_{\mathbf{2d}}(k+1;N). \tag{5.5.7a}$$

We find the mean first-passage vector for the open queue by letting N go to infinity, so

$$\boldsymbol{\tau}'_{\mathbf{2d}} := \lim_{N\to\infty} \boldsymbol{\tau}'_{\mathbf{2d}}(k;N) = \frac{1}{\lambda}\boldsymbol{\epsilon}' + \frac{1}{\lambda}\mathbf{H_{2d}}\mathbf{B}\,\mathbf{Q}\,\boldsymbol{\tau}'_{\mathbf{2d}}.$$

This vector is also independent of k, but unlike its first-passage matrix, we can solve for it directly, to get,

$$\boldsymbol{\tau}'_{\mathbf{2d}} := [\lambda \mathbf{I} - \mathbf{H_{2d}}\,\mathbf{B}\,\mathbf{Q}]^{-1}\,\boldsymbol{\epsilon}'. \tag{5.5.7b}$$

This can be rewritten in another form with the use of Lemma 4.2.1:

$$\boldsymbol{\tau}'_{\mathbf{2d}} := \frac{1}{\lambda}\left[\mathbf{I} + \frac{1}{\lambda - \Psi\,[\mathbf{H_{2d}}\,\mathbf{B}]}\mathbf{H_{2d}}\,\mathbf{B}\,\mathbf{Q}\right]\boldsymbol{\epsilon}', \tag{5.5.7c}$$

so if we can find $\mathbf{H_{2d}}$, then we get $\boldsymbol{\tau}'_{\mathbf{2d}}$.

Mean Time for a Busy Period

The mean time for the queue to drop by one, given that a customer has just arrived is, using (5.5.7c),

$$\begin{aligned} t_{2d} := \mathbf{p}\,\boldsymbol{\tau}'_{\mathbf{2d}} &= \frac{1}{\lambda}\left[1 + \frac{\Psi\,[\mathbf{H_{2d}}\,\mathbf{B}]}{\lambda - \Psi\,[\mathbf{H_{2d}}\,\mathbf{B}]}\right] \\ &= \frac{1}{\lambda - \Psi\,[\mathbf{H_{2d}}\,\mathbf{B}]} \quad \text{for } \varrho < 1. \end{aligned} \tag{5.5.7d}$$

This is also the mean time for the ***busy period***, but it is valid only when $\varrho < 1$. Otherwise the busy period may never end. Even though $\mathbf{H_{2d}}$ is meaningful for all ϱ, when $\varrho \geq 1$, the term $\Psi\,[\mathbf{H_{2d}}\,\mathbf{B}] \geq \lambda$, so (5.5.7d) is infinite or negative.

Note that (2.3.7d) gives an alternate expression for the mean busy period. In order for the two to be equal, we must have

$$\Psi\,[\mathbf{H_{2d}}\,\mathbf{B}] = \lambda\, s. \tag{5.5.8a}$$

This leads to the most interesting result that the mean busy period and the mean system time for a G/M/1 queue are equal! Compare (5.5.7d) with (5.1.7c) to get

$$\mathbb{E}[T_2] = t_{2d} = \frac{1/\lambda}{1-s}. \tag{5.5.8b}$$

Equation (5.5.8a) can also be used to simplify (5.5.7c).

Exercise 5.5.2: Prove that (5.5.8) is true by using (2.3.7d), and noting that t_I is given by (5.5.3a). That is, take

$$\lim_{m,N\to\infty} R_b(m) = \frac{t_d}{t_d + t_I}.$$

For single server queues, this limit is the fraction of time the server is busy, which for G/M/1 queues is ϱ. Also, t_d is the mean service time, namely, $1/\lambda$.

To take a closer look at the differences between M/G/1 and G/M/1 queues, we have calculated the mean time for the busy periods for several different distributions and plotted them in Figures 5.5.2 and 5.5.3.

Example 5.5.2: Recall that all M/G/1 queues have the same mean time

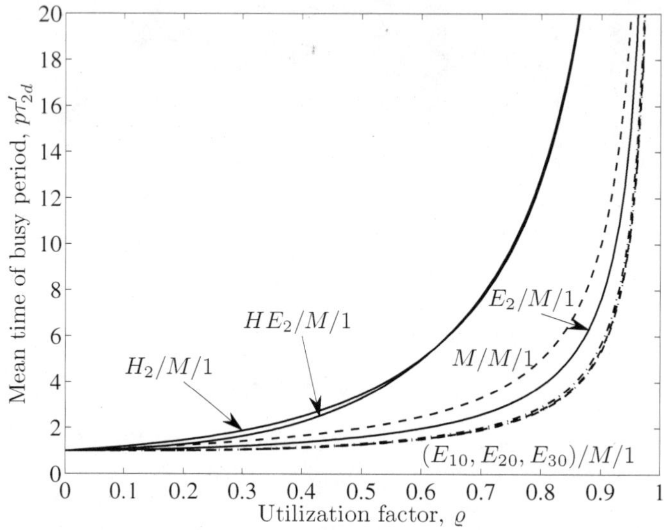

Figure 5.5.2: Mean time of a busy period for various ME/M/1 queues, as a function of ϱ. These curves also represent the mean system times, because the two are equal. All M/G/1 queues have the same mean busy period (but different mean system times), so all are equal to the curve labeled M/M/1. As $\varrho \to 1$, the busy periods rank themselves according to C_v^2. The hyperexponential and the hyper-Erlangian functions have $C_v^2 = 5.0388$, and the Erlangians have $C_v^2 = 1/n$, for $n = 2$, 10, 20, and 30. The D/M/1 queue bounds all these curves from below, and is virtually indistinguishable from the E_{30}/M/1.

for their busy periods, so they are all represented by the same curve, labeled M/M/1 in Figures 5.5.2 and 5.5.3. Yet the figures show that different ME/M/1 queues vary all over the place. There is some order for the examples chosen here. From (5.1.23d), as ϱ approaches 1, bigger C_v^2 for the interarrival time distribution, goes with larger mean system time. This not true for all ϱ. In fact, the hyper-Erlangian function discussed in Section 3.2.3.1 [$E_2(x)$] yields a mean system time that is below that for the M/M/1 queue when ϱ is small, and crosses it as ϱ increases and first crosses and then joins the H_2/M/1 curve with the same C_v^2 as ϱ approaches 1.

The figures certainly show that the arrival pattern is critically important when studying busy periods, and system times. Recall from Theorem 5.1.4 that the behavior of s near $\varrho = 0$ depends on $b^{(\ell)}(0)$, the interarrival time distribution and its derivatives at $x = 0$, and not on its moments. In particular, if $b(0) = 0$ (this includes all Erlangian and hyper-Erlangian

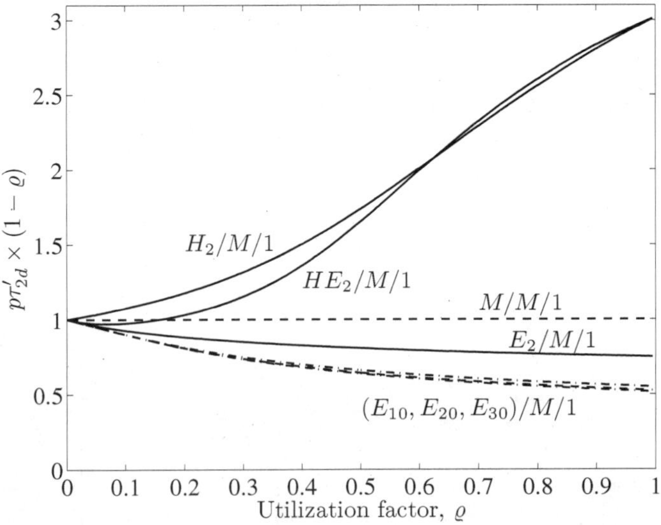

Figure 5.5.3: Mean time of a busy period multiplied by $(1-\varrho)$, for the same ME/M/1 queues as given in Figure 5.5.2. Note that only the M/M/1 queue yields a straight (and horizontal) line. All the E_k/M/1 queues have negative slope at $\varrho = 0$. This is also true of all interarrival time distributions that have $b(0) = 0$, including those with $C_v^2 > 1$, as shown by the curve for the $HE_2(x)$ distribution. Note that only the M/M/1 queue yields a horizontal straight line, and all curves (for interarrival time distributions with $C_v^2 < \infty$) are finite at $\varrho = 1$.

functions) then the mean time for a busy period (and the mean system time) has 0 slope at $\varrho = 0$ (as in Figure 5.5.2). When multiplied by $(1-\varrho)$ (as in figure 5.5.3) the resulting curves have negative slopes at $\varrho = 0$. ▲

As our last subject in this chapter, we discuss the ***k*-busy period**. If we knew the state the system was in at the beginning, the first-passage time for the queue at S_2 to drop by 1 is simply $\mathbf{p_i}\boldsymbol{\tau}'_{\mathbf{2d}}$. At that moment, the system is in state $\mathbf{p_i H_{2d}}$, so the mean first-passage time to drop by one more is simply $\mathbf{p_i H_{2d}}\boldsymbol{\tau}'_{\mathbf{2d}}$, and the time to drop by two is the sum of the two terms. In general, then, the time it takes for an ME/M/1 queue to drop by k is given by the expression

$$\sum_{l=0}^{k-1} \mathbf{p_i}(\mathbf{H_{2d}})^l \boldsymbol{\tau}'_{\mathbf{2d}}.$$

As with the M/G/1 queue, if there were k customers in the queue in the first place, this is the time for the k-busy period, conditioned by $\mathbf{p_i}$. If the queue was longer than k at the start, this would still be the time for the queue to decrease by k for the first time.

It is hoped that the reader is sufficiently skilled by now to be able to set up the equations for the probabilities of queue growth, the $\mathbf{W_x}$, where $\mathbf{x}$ is one of **2u**, **2m**, or **2d**. Therefore, we leave those items as exercises.

Chapter 6

M/G/*C*-TYPE SYSTEMS

Having two bathrooms ruined the capacity to cooperate.
Margaret Mead

The title of this chapter implies that there is more here than M/G/C queues. The straightforward extension of Chapter 4 allows one to have C identical servers serving up to C customers independently and simultaneously. But when we set up those equations we find that they apply to a more general class of systems where the active customers can actually interfere with each other while being served. This can be used as a basis for studying clusters of workstations that must share resources such as a communications channel or central disc. We call such a system a ***generalized* M/G/*C*//*N* *queue***, where N is the total number of customers in the system. Interestingly enough, when $N = C$ then the steady-state soution is the same as for the single class ***Jackson network*** [JACKSON63], but when $N > C$ the well-known ***product form*** solutions are no longer valid, and one must resort to the matrix techniques described here.

6.1 Introduction

In previous chapters when dealing with nonexponential distributions, we always assumed that only one customer was active at a time at S_1. We did look at multiple servers, but only if S_i was exponential, introducing the idea of a load-dependent server (Sections 2.1.5 and 5.4). In doing this, it was not necessary to distinguish between:

1. A subsystem containing a single server that works twice as fast on one customer when a second one is present;
2. A subsystem that has two active servers, one for each customer.

In fact, the only way the two cases can be distinguished is by marking the customers so as to tell if they left in the same order in which they arrived. This has become of interest in recent years, and is called the ***resequencing problem***. LAQT has been used successfully in analyzing the departure process of an M/M/C queue where customers must leave in the same order in which they arrived [DING91]. Because we have made our customers indistinguishable, we have not bothered to consider this at all, nor can we consider it here without expanding our state space.

L. Lipsky, *Queueing Theory*, DOI 10.1007/978-0-387-49706-8_6,

We cannot get away so easily when dealing with nonexponential servers. Case 1 has had few realistic applications, but it can be used in studying queues with, for instance, ***discouraged arrivals*** or ***restricted processor sharing****. It is modeled by multiplying the completion rate matrix **M** by a constant factor when a second customer arrives, leaving the dimension and internal state description of S_1 otherwise unchanged. This turns out to be formally identical to the description of ME/M/$C//N$ loops in Section 4.4, except that the load-dependence factor depends on the number of customers at S_1 instead of the number at S_2. We discuss this further when we look at processor sharing.

The second case is much more complicated. When a second customer arrives, as always, he begins service by going to phase i with probability p_i, but the first customer is already in service and is at some other phase. Furthermore, when one of the customers leaves, the other customer is still in service, in some phase determined by the system's past. Put differently, a departing customer does not leave behind the empty state. We must therefore set up a formalism that keeps track of where both customers are. This is normally done by building a ***direct product space***, the most common convention being the ***Kronecker product***. However, if the service times for the two customers are identically distributed and they are not marked, one can use a ***Reduced-Product* (RP) *space***. The direct product spaces have dimension m^C for C iid customers, but the RP space has dimension

$$D_{RP}(m,\, C) = \begin{pmatrix} C+m-1 \\ C \end{pmatrix}.$$

This amounts to a reduction of dimensions by a factor that approaches $C!$.

We have to introduce new symbols and concepts here, hence it is best to start with the simplest extension possible. Therefore, in the following section we set up the formalism, and find the steady-state solution of a system where S_1 has exactly two identical ME servers (i.e., the M/ME/2//N loop). In doing this, we have selected a three-phase ME server as an example. In Section 6.3 we extend this to C servers, for by then it will be easier for the reader to follow the notation.

After that, we show that the formulas are actually applicable to a more general class of systems, which we call "generalized M/G/$C//N$ systems." With little more than a change of notation and a slight generalization of some parameters, we show that we are suddenly dealing with a network of queues. When $N \leq C$, our generalized network is equivalent to the single-class ***Jackson network***, and we spend some time discussing the connection. We then extend the model further to allow S_2 to be a load-dependent server, as we did in Section 5.4. This is potentially an important extension, because it is the correct treatment of ***timesharing systems*** with ***population-size constraints*** (i.e., when $N > C$).

When doing all this, we find that the equations are still algebraically manipulable but too complex to reduce to simple formulas. Thus we describe in

*This has been done recently by Feng Zhang [ZHANG07] in examining computer systems where a restricted number of jobs can share the CPU

detail algorithms that allow the user to get computational results for particular systems. Our formalism reduces the dimensions of all relevant matrices to their bare minima. (At present, at least, it is impossible to do it with smaller matrices.) Even so, problems can quickly become intractable if C and/or m become too large, so we discuss the computational complexity of the algorithms.

In Section 6.4 we study the open M/G/C system in the usual way by letting N become unboundedly large. The reverse game, which considers systems where S_1, even at full capacity, is slower than S_2 (i.e., the generalization of $\rho > 1$), leads to a ***semi-Markov arrival process*** to S_2. This is treated in Section 6.5.2, but a full discussion of semi-Markov processes is postponed until Chapter 8. In the rest of Section 6.5 we look at some transient phenomena, including those related to the busy periods. Some of these are potentially important in studying the reliability of systems and rush-hour traffic.

Because of time and space limitations, we have foregone the pleasure of fully developing the formulas for departure and arrival times, even though it should prove quite interesting, with several new insights. Its treatment can be found in a series of papers by Ahmed Mohamed and his thesis [MOHAMED04].

We mention that much of this chapter is an outgrowth of material in Aby Tehranipour's PhD thesis [TEHRANIPOUR83] and related publications. Recent applications and extensions have been carried out by Ahmed Mohamed [MOHAMED04] and Feng Zhang [ZHANG07].

6.2 Steady-State M/ME/2//N Loop

Consider the queueing system in Figure 6.2.1. It is identical to Figure 4.1.1 except that now S_1 contains two identical ME servers. Previously, each subsystem contained one ME server, so there was no real distinction between S_1 and a server. Thus the statement, "The subsystem is in state i," meant the same as the statement, "The active customer is at phase i." Now that S_1 contains two servers, and each server is made up of m phases, we must describe where both customers are if there are two or more customers at S_1. Definition 6.2.2 makes this clear.

6.2.1 Definitions

The process is as follows. No more than two customers can be active in subsystem S_1 at any one time, one being in each of the servers. When a customer completes service at either server, he leaves S_1 and joins the queue at S_2 (still exponential), while at the same time another customer (if one is available) takes his place at the momentarily idle server. Any other customer who was active in S_1 at the time the first one finished continues unperturbed. Each of the servers is described by the same objects introduced in Chapter 3: $\mathbf{p}$, $\mathbf{q}'$, $\boldsymbol{\epsilon}'$, $\mathbf{P}$, $\mathbf{M}$, $\mathbf{B}$, and $\mathbf{V}$. As before, N is the number of customers in the system, and n is the number of customers at S_1, including the ones who are being served. Then we have the following definition.

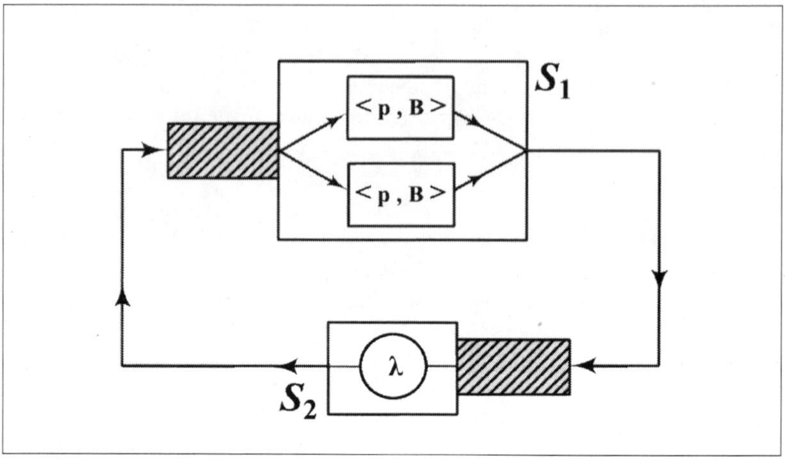

Figure 6.2.1: A two subsystem loop where S_2 is an exponential server, but S_1 is made up of two identical nonexponential ME servers, each made up of m phases, and represented by the vector-matrix pair, $\langle \mathbf{p}, \mathbf{B} \rangle$.

Definition 6.2.1

$\Xi_1 = \{i \mid i = 1, 2, \ldots, m\}$ *is the set of internal states of* S_1 *when* $n = 1$. $D(1) = m$ *is the dimension, or number of elements, of* Ξ_1. The external state of the system is still $\{1; N\}$. Thus we would say that "The system is in internal state $i \in \Xi_1$, and external state, $\{1; N\}$." Alternatively, we could simply say that "The system is in state $\{i; 1; N\}$," with it being understood that $i \in \Xi_1$. □

Definition 6.2.1 is the same as in previous chapters, but with two or more customers at S_1 we must have an extended definition. It would seem that because each of two customers can be in any one of m places, we need m^2 states to describe this. This is actually more than is necessary if we do not care to distinguish one customer from the other or one server from the other. Thus the statement, "Customer 1 is at phase i_1 in server 1, and customer 2 is at phase i_2 in server 2," is more than we want to know. All we need to know is that phase i_1 in one of the servers and i_2 in the other server are busy. This leads to the specification of an internal state by the unordered pair $\{i_1, i_2\}$. Then $\{i_1, i_2\}$ and $\{i_2, i_1\}$ are the same state. Therefore, think of $\{\cdot, \cdot\}$ as a set containing two integers. For the sake of definiteness, we assume that $i_1 \leq i_2$. Then we have

Definition 6.2.2

$\Xi_2 = \{i = \{i_1, i_2\} \mid i_1 \leq i_2 = 1, 2, \ldots, m\}$ *is the set of internal states of* S_1 when $n \geq 2$. $D(2) = m(m+1)/2$ is the number of elements of Ξ_2. The external state of the system is still $\{n; N\}$. Thus we would say that "The system is in internal state $i \in \Xi_2$, and external state, $\{n; N\}$." Alternatively, we could simply say that "The system is in state $\{i;\, n;\, N\}$," with the understanding that $i \in \Xi_2$ if $n \geq 2$ (i.e., $i = \{i_1,\, i_2\}$). □

There is an alternative state space definition that is equivalent to this. Instead of listing the phases that are active, we can enumerate the number of customers at each phase. This requires an m-vector of nonnegative integers whose sum is 2. Although this convention seems more verbose, it proves to be more useful when we consider systems in which $C > 2$ or when we go to the generalized system. For now, we use the definition as given.

Next we define the probability vectors, and their associated scalars, needed for the work of this chapter. We use the obvious notation $\boldsymbol{\epsilon}'_{\mathbf{k}}$ for the $D(k)$-dimension column vector of all 1's. We also use $\mathbf{I_k}$ for the identity matrix of dimension $D(k)$.

Definition 6.2.3

$[\boldsymbol{\pi}_{\mathbf{1}}(1;N)]_i$:= *probability that only one customer is at* S_1 *(with* $N-1$ *at* S_2*), and the system is in internal state* $i \in \Xi_1$ *(i.e., the customer is at phase* i *in either server in* S_1*).* $\boldsymbol{\pi}_{\mathbf{1}}(1;N)$ is a vector with $D(1)$ components.
$r(1;N) = \boldsymbol{\pi}_{\mathbf{1}}(1;N)\,\boldsymbol{\epsilon}'_{\mathbf{1}}$ is the associated scalar probability. □

Definition 6.2.4

$[\boldsymbol{\pi}_{\mathbf{2}}(n;N)]_i$:= *probability that there are* $n \geq 2$ *customers at* S_1 *(with* $N-n$ *at* S_2*), and the system is in internal state* $i = \{i_1,\, i_2\} \in \Xi_2$ *(i.e., the two active customers are at phases* i_1 *and* i_2 *one in each of the two servers in* S_1*).* $\boldsymbol{\pi}_{\mathbf{2}}(n;N)$ is a $D(2)$-vector, and $r(n;N) = \boldsymbol{\pi}_{\mathbf{2}}(n;N)\,\boldsymbol{\epsilon}'_{\mathbf{2}}$ is the associated scalar probability. □

Note that the subscript k on $\boldsymbol{\pi}_{\mathbf{k}}(n;\, N)$ stands for the number of customers active in S_1. Thus our convention differs from the one we used in Chapter 5. Strictly speaking, the subscripts are unnecessary because they correlate with the first integer in the argument ($k = n$ for $n \leq 2$, and $k = 2$ for $n \geq 2$); however, they denote objects of different dimensions, therefore we include them both for emphasis. According to this convention, in this chapter we use the subscript k to denote any object that applies only to space Ξ_k or, if it is an object connecting two spaces (nonsquare matrices), k will correspond to the higher-numbered space.

Although we wish to avoid sounding too abstract, we must say something about the connection between our ***state space*** Ξ_k, and the vector spaces on which our matrices operate. We have defined Ξ_k to be a set with $D(k)$ elements. We could think of each element as being a ***unit vector*** in a $D(k)$-dimensional vector space. Consider the set of row vectors with $D(k)$ components. Then each state $i \in \Xi_k$ corresponds to one such vector with a 1 in one position, and a 0 in all the other positions. These states form a complete basis for the $D(k)$ dimensional vector space, because every vector in that space can be written as a linear combination of the ***basis states***, or ***basis vectors***. This is such a natural correspondence that we can usually get away without having to make a distinction between the set and the vector space its members generate. Remember, though, that i stands for several things itself when $k > 1$.

Consistent with the above, we proceed to rename several of our previously known operators. First, the completion-rate matrix for states in Ξ_1, $\mathbf{M_1} := \mathbf{M}$, is a diagonal matrix whose (ii)th element $[\mathbf{M_1}]_{ii}$, is the probability rate of leaving state $i \in \Xi_1$ by way of a completion inside S_1. The transition matrix for Ξ_1 is $\mathbf{P_1} := \mathbf{P}$, and $\mathbf{V_1} = \mathbf{B_1}^{-1} := \mathbf{V}$. We proved in Section 3.5.4, in the discussion surrounding Lemma 3.5.2, that an exponential server with feedback is equivalent to an exponential server without feedback, but with service rate reduced to $(1-\theta)\mu$, where θ is the feedback probability. This implies that we can assume without loss of generality that $[\mathbf{P_1}]_{ii} = 0$.[†] We do that here, because it simplifies our examples. However, in Section 6.3.2 we allow P_{ii} to be nonzero. There is no need to relabel $\mathbf{Q}$, $\mathbf{p}$, and $\mathbf{q}'$, but we must define a new set of operators that operate on vectors in Ξ_2. First we define the completion rate matrix.

Definition 6.2.5

$\mathbf{M_2}$ *is a diagonal matrix whose* (ii)*th element is the probability rate of leaving the state* $i \in \Xi_2$ *by way of a completion in* S_1. By our definition of this system, $[\mathbf{M_2}]_{ii} = \mu_{i_1} + \mu_{i_2}$. □

The following is another Ξ_2-space object, the transition matrix.

Definition 6.2.6

$[\mathbf{P_2}]_{ij} :=$ *probability of going to state* $j \in \Xi_2$ *upon a completion in* S_1, *given that the system is in internal state* $i \in \Xi_2$. $\mathbf{P_2}$ is a (nonisometric) transition matrix for states in Ξ_2, (i.e., $\mathbf{P_2}\,\boldsymbol{\epsilon}_2' \neq \boldsymbol{\epsilon}_2'$). □

Assume that $[\mathbf{P_1}]_{ii} = 0$, and recall that only one customer can change his phase at a time. Then the elements of $\mathbf{P_1}$ are related to $\mathbf{P_2}$ in the following way.

$$[\mathbf{P_2}]_{ij} = 0 \quad \text{unless} \quad \{i_1, i_2\} \cap \{j_1, j_2\}$$

contains exactly one element.[‡] Let the common element be called h. Call the other member of the i-pair, γ, and the other member of the j-pair, ν. Then, if there is exactly one element in common,

$$[\mathbf{P_2}]_{ij} = [\mathbf{P_1}]_{\gamma\nu} \frac{\mu_\gamma}{[\mathbf{M_2}]_{ii}}, \qquad i_1 \neq i_2,$$

and

$$[\mathbf{P_2}]_{ij} = [\mathbf{P_1}]_{\gamma\nu}, \qquad i_1 = i_2.$$

The reason for this is as follows. If $i_1 \neq i_2$, because only one active customer can move at a time, the probability that it is the customer at phase γ is

[†]Suppose that $\mathbf{P}$ is a transition matrix with $\mathbf{P}_{ii} \neq 0$ for some i. Then construct the new matrix $\bar{\mathbf{P}}$, with $\bar{\mathbf{P}}_{ii} = 0$, $\bar{\mathbf{P}}_{ij} = \mathbf{P}_{ij}/(1-\mathbf{P}_{ii})$, and $\bar{\mathbf{P}}_{kj} = \mathbf{P}_{kj}$ for $j, k \neq i$. Also, replace μ_i with $(1-\mathbf{P}_{ii})\mu_i$ in $\mathbf{M}$. All other components remain the same. See Lemma 3.5.5.

[‡]Note: If we had not assumed that $[\mathbf{P_1}]_{ii} := 0$, we would have had to consider the additional possibility that $i = j$.

$\mu_\gamma/(\mu_\gamma + \mu_\nu)$, and the probability that he will go to ν, given that he is the one who will move is $[\mathbf{P_1}]_{\gamma\nu}$. If $i_1 = i_2$, it makes no difference which one moves.

As an example, let $m = 3$; then

$$\Xi_1 = \{1, 2, 3\},$$

and

$$\Xi_2 = \{\{1,1\},\{1,2\},\{1,3\},\{2,2\},\{2,3\},\{3,3\}\}.$$

The transition matrix is given by the following, where the ordering is the same as that given in the list above.

$$\mathbf{P_2} = \begin{bmatrix} 0 & P_{12} & P_{13} & 0 & 0 & 0 \\ \frac{\mu_2 P_{21}}{\mu_1+\mu_2} & 0 & \frac{\mu_2 P_{23}}{\mu_1+\mu_2} & \frac{\mu_1 P_{12}}{\mu_1+\mu_2} & \frac{\mu_1 P_{13}}{\mu_1+\mu_2} & 0 \\ \frac{\mu_3 P_{31}}{\mu_1+\mu_3} & \frac{\mu_3 P_{32}}{\mu_1+\mu_3} & 0 & 0 & \frac{\mu_1 P_{12}}{\mu_1+\mu_3} & \frac{\mu_1 P_{13}}{\mu_1+\mu_3} \\ 0 & P_{21} & 0 & 0 & P_{23} & 0 \\ 0 & \frac{\mu_3 P_{31}}{\mu_1+\mu_3} & \frac{\mu_2 P_{21}}{\mu_2+\mu_3} & \frac{\mu_3 P_{32}}{\mu_2+\mu_3} & 0 & \frac{\mu_2 P_{23}}{\mu_2+\mu_3} \\ 0 & 0 & P_{31} & 0 & P_{32} & 0 \end{bmatrix}.$$

The Ξ_2-space equivalent of $\mathbf{p}$ is $\mathbf{R_2}$, which we now define.

Definition 6.2.7

$[\mathbf{R_2}]_{ij}$:= *probability that a customer, upon entering* S_1 *will put it in internal state* $j \in \Xi_2$*, given that it was in internal state* $i \in \Xi_1$. This is a $D(1) \times D(2)$-dimensional matrix. □

A matrix element of $\mathbf{R_2}$ is 0 unless either j_1 or $j_2 = i$. As before, let ν be the member of the pair $\{j_1, j_2\}$ that is not i; then

$$[\mathbf{R_2}]_{ij} = p_\nu \quad \text{if } \; j_1 \text{ or } j_2 = i,$$

and

$$[\mathbf{R_2}]_{ij} = 0 \quad \text{otherwise}.$$

The system must end up in some state after a customer enters S_1, therefore we have

$$\mathbf{R_2}\, \boldsymbol{\epsilon}'_{\mathbf{2}} = \boldsymbol{\epsilon}'_{\mathbf{1}}. \tag{6.2.1}$$

For our example with $m = 3$,

$$\mathbf{R_2} = \begin{bmatrix} p_1 & p_2 & p_3 & 0 & 0 & 0 \\ 0 & p_1 & 0 & p_2 & p_3 & 0 \\ 0 & 0 & p_1 & 0 & p_2 & p_3 \end{bmatrix}.$$

This clearly satisfies (6.2.1).

We define the last matrix of this set $\mathbf{Q_2}$ the Ξ_2 equivalent of $\mathbf{q}'$.

Definition 6.2.8

$[\mathbf{Q_2}]_{ij}$:= *probability that upon a completion in S_1 from internal state $i \in \Xi_2$, a customer leaves, putting the system in internal state $j \in \Xi_1$.* This is a $D(2) \times D(1)$-dimensional matrix. This matrix has no direct relation to either $\mathbf{Q} = \boldsymbol{\epsilon}_1' \, \mathbf{p}$, defined in Chapter 3, or $\boldsymbol{Q}$ defined by (1.3.2c), but is the 2-space equivalent of $\mathbf{q}'$. □

Unless $j = i_1$ or i_2, $[\mathbf{Q_2}]_{ij} = 0$. For those matrix elements that are not 0, define ν to be the member of the pair that does not equal j, then

$$[\mathbf{Q_2}]_{ij} = \frac{\mu_\nu q_\nu}{[\mathbf{M_2}]_{ii}} \quad \text{for } i_1 \neq i_2$$

and

$$[\mathbf{Q_2}]_{ij} = q_\nu \quad \text{for } i_1 = i_2.$$

Note that $[\mathbf{Q_2}\, \mathbf{R_2}]_{ij}$ is the probability that upon a completion from internal state $i \in \Xi_2$, one customer leaves and another enters, putting the system in internal state $j \in \Xi_2$. This process can only happen if there are initially $n > 2$ customers at S_1, in which case the system is left in external state $\{n-1; N\}$. Thus we have the equivalent to (3.1.1a), or rather (3.5.11a),

$$(\mathbf{P_2} + \mathbf{Q_2}\, \mathbf{R_2})\boldsymbol{\epsilon}_2' = \boldsymbol{\epsilon}_2'. \tag{6.2.2}$$

So $(\mathbf{P_2} + \mathbf{Q_2}\, \mathbf{R_2})$ is isometric. Given that $\mathbf{R_2}\, \boldsymbol{\epsilon}_2' = \boldsymbol{\epsilon}_1'$ from (6.2.1), we have a relation that compares with $\mathbf{q}' = (\mathbf{I} - \mathbf{P})\, \boldsymbol{\epsilon}'$ from (3.1.1b), namely,

$$\mathbf{Q_2}\, \boldsymbol{\epsilon}_1' = (\mathbf{I_2} - \mathbf{P_2})\boldsymbol{\epsilon}_2'. \tag{6.2.3}$$

We are just beginning to see the problems we will be having. Whereas (3.1.1b) permitted us to express $\mathbf{q}'$ uniquely in terms of $\mathbf{P}$, (6.2.3) only yields a partial relation between $\mathbf{Q_2}$ and $\mathbf{P_2}$.

For our specific example we have

$$\mathbf{Q_2} = \begin{bmatrix} q_1 & 0 & 0 \\ \frac{\mu_2 q_2}{\mu_1+\mu_2} & \frac{\mu_1 q_1}{\mu_1+\mu_3} & 0 \\ \frac{\mu_3 q_3}{\mu_1+\mu_3} & 0 & \frac{\mu_1 q_1}{\mu_1+\mu_3} \\ & q_2 & \\ 0 & \frac{\mu_3 q_3}{\mu_2+\mu_3} & \frac{\mu_2 q_2}{\mu_2+\mu_3} \\ 0 & 0 & q_3 \end{bmatrix}.$$

Exercise 6.2.1: Verify that the example matrices, $\mathbf{P_2}$, $\mathbf{Q_2}$, and $\mathbf{R_2}$ for $m = 3$ do indeed satisfy (6.2.1) to (6.2.3).

6.2.2 Balance Equations

At last we can write the ***balance equations***. The terms on the left-hand side of each equation represent the rate of leaving a given state, and the right-hand side is the rate of entering that state. First let $n = 0$; then there is only one internal state (empty), so we play the same notational game as before, namely,

$$\boldsymbol{\pi}_1(0; N) := r(0; N)\mathbf{p},$$

where $r(0; N)$ is the steady-state probability that there is no one at S_1. The balance equation is identical to (4.1.3a), because there is no way to make use of the second server in S_1. We rewrite it in the notation of this chapter.

$$\lambda\boldsymbol{\pi}_1(0; N) = \boldsymbol{\pi}_1(1; N)\mathbf{B}_1\,\mathbf{Q}. \tag{6.2.4a}$$

Its interpretation should be clear.

The vector equation corresponding to entering and leaving external state $\{1;\, N\}$ provides us with something new.

$$\boldsymbol{\pi}_1(1; N)(\mathbf{M}_1 + \lambda\mathbf{I}_1)$$
$$= \lambda\boldsymbol{\pi}_1(0; N) + \boldsymbol{\pi}_1(1; N)\mathbf{M}_1\mathbf{P}_1 + \boldsymbol{\pi}_2(2; N)\mathbf{M}_2\,\mathbf{Q}_2. \tag{6.2.4b}$$

The interpretation is as follows. The system can leave state $\{i;\, 1;\, N\}$ by being in that state $[\boldsymbol{\pi}_1(1; N)]$, and either have the active customer at S_2 finish $[\lambda\mathbf{I}_1]$, or have the lone customer in S_1 finish at phase i, $[\mathbf{M}_1]$. The system can enter state $\{i;\, 1;\, N\}$ by any of three ways. One path starts with no one initially at S_1, $[r(0; N)]$, a completion occurs at S_2, $[\lambda]$, and that customer immediately goes to S_1 and enters, $[\mathbf{p}]$. Another path starts with one customer already at S_1, $[\boldsymbol{\pi}_1(1; N)]$, a completion occurs in S_1, $[\mathbf{M}_1]$, and that customer moves to another phase, $[\mathbf{P}_1]$. The third path starts with two customers in S_1, $[\boldsymbol{\pi}_2(2; N)]$, one of those two customers has a completion $[\mathbf{M}_2]$, and leaves $[\mathbf{Q}_2]$; thus S_1 remains with one customer, because there is no-one in its queue to replace the customer who just left.

The balance equation for $n = 2$ requires the matrix $\mathbf{R}_2$ for the first time.

$$\boldsymbol{\pi}_2(2; N)(\mathbf{M}_2 + \lambda\mathbf{I}_2)$$
$$= \boldsymbol{\pi}_2(3; N)\mathbf{M}_2\,\mathbf{Q}_2\,\mathbf{R}_2 + \boldsymbol{\pi}_2(2; N)\mathbf{M}_2\mathbf{P}_2 + \lambda\pi_1(1; N)\mathbf{R}_2. \tag{6.2.4c}$$

Two of the terms might require some clarification. When there are at least three customers at S_1, and a departure occurs $[\mathbf{M}_2\,\mathbf{Q}_2]$, a new customer is available in the queue to enter $[\mathbf{R}_2]$, and put the system back into an internal state of Ξ_2. Similarly, if originally there is only one customer at S_1 and a customer arrives $[\lambda\boldsymbol{\pi}_1(1; N)]$, he immediately enters, taking the system from some state $i \in \Xi_1$ to some state $j \in \Xi_2$, $[\mathbf{R}_2]$.

The general vector balance equation for $2 < n < N$ follows.

$$\pi_2(n; N)(\mathbf{M}_2 + \lambda\mathbf{I}_2)$$
$$= \pi_2(n+1; N)\mathbf{M}_2\,\mathbf{Q}_2\,\mathbf{R}_2 + \pi_2(n; N)\mathbf{M}_2\mathbf{P}_2 + \lambda\pi_2(n-1; N). \tag{6.2.4d}$$

The only difference between this equation and the one for $n = 2$ is the missing matrix $\mathbf{R_2}$ in the last term. For $n > 2$, when a customer arrives at S_1, there already are two customers active, so his arrival does not change the internal state of the system.

The final balance equation for external state $\{N;\ N\}$ is

$$\boldsymbol{\pi_2}(N;N)\mathbf{M_2} = \boldsymbol{\pi_2}(N;N)\mathbf{M_2}\mathbf{P_2} + \lambda\boldsymbol{\pi_2}(N-1;N). \qquad (6.2.4e)$$

We next define a new matrix and its inverse

$$\mathbf{B_2} = \mathbf{V_2}^{-1} := \mathbf{M_2}(\mathbf{I_2} - \mathbf{P_2}), \qquad (6.2.5)$$

and combine like terms in the balance equations to get

$$\boldsymbol{\pi_1}(1;N)(\mathbf{B_1} + \lambda\mathbf{I_1}) = \boldsymbol{\pi_2}(2;N)\mathbf{M_2}\,\mathbf{Q_2} + \lambda\boldsymbol{\pi_1}(0;N), \qquad (6.2.6a)$$

$$\boldsymbol{\pi_2}(2;N)(\mathbf{B_2} + \lambda\mathbf{I_2}) = \boldsymbol{\pi_2}(3;N)\mathbf{M_2}\,\mathbf{Q_2}\,\mathbf{R_2} + \lambda\boldsymbol{\pi_1}(1;N)\mathbf{R_2}, \qquad (6.2.6b)$$

$$\boldsymbol{\pi_2}(n;N)(\mathbf{B_2} + \lambda\mathbf{I_2}) = \boldsymbol{\pi_2}(n+1;N)\mathbf{M_2}\,\mathbf{Q_2}\,\mathbf{R_2} + \lambda\boldsymbol{\pi_2}(n-1;N), \qquad (6.2.6c)$$

and

$$\boldsymbol{\pi_2}(N;N)\mathbf{B_2} = \lambda\boldsymbol{\pi_2}(N-1;N). \qquad (6.2.6d)$$

Equation (6.2.5) looks quite familiar, and it should. The matrix $\mathbf{B_2}$ does indeed generate the distribution of the time until one customer leaves S_1, given that it started with two customers in some vector state of Ξ_2. We postpone looking into this until we discuss transient behavior.

6.2.3 Solution of Probability Vectors

The balance equations are quite similar to those for the ME/M/C//N system of Section 5.4, and the solution is also similar. The additional complication we have here is that we are dealing with several different sizes of matrices. As always, we would like to express everything in terms of $r(0;N)\mathbf{p}$, because that depends on only one number. Unfortunately, we cannot start with Equation (6.2.4a) because $\mathbf{B_1}\,\mathbf{Q}$ does not have an inverse. We have already faced this problem in solving for the M/ME/1//N queue in (4.1.2), so we copy that method, and start at the top, at (6.2.6d). Note that if we had attempted to solve the open system directly, we would have no "top" at which to start. Anyway, (6.2.6d) can be rewritten as

$$\boldsymbol{\pi_2}(N;N) = \lambda\boldsymbol{\pi_2}(N-1;N)\mathbf{V_2}. \qquad (6.2.7a)$$

Next we use (6.2.6c) for $n = N-1$, and substitute for $\boldsymbol{\pi_2}(N;N)$ to get

$$\boldsymbol{\pi_2}(N-1;N)(\mathbf{B_2} + \lambda\mathbf{I_2}) = \lambda[\boldsymbol{\pi_2}(N-1;N)\mathbf{V_2}]\mathbf{M_2}\,\mathbf{Q_2}\,\mathbf{R_2} + \lambda\boldsymbol{\pi_2}(N-2;N),$$

or, collecting terms and solving for $\boldsymbol{\pi_2}(N-1;N)$,

$$\boldsymbol{\pi_2}(N-1;N) = \boldsymbol{\pi_2}(N-2;N)\left[\mathbf{I_2} + \frac{1}{\lambda}\mathbf{B_2} - \mathbf{V_2}\,\mathbf{M_2}\,\mathbf{Q_2}\,\mathbf{R_2}\right]^{-1}. \qquad (6.2.7b)$$

This equation is of the form

$$\boldsymbol{\pi_2}(N-1;N) = \boldsymbol{\pi_2}(N-2;N)\,\mathbf{U_2}(1),$$

where

$$\mathbf{U_2}(1) := \left[\mathbf{I_2} + \frac{1}{\lambda}\mathbf{B_2} - \mathbf{V_2}\,\mathbf{M_2}\,\mathbf{Q_2}\,\mathbf{R_2}\right]^{-1}.$$

This matrix, and the family of $\mathbf{U_2}$ matrices we are about to introduce are the direct generalizations of the $\mathbf{U}$ of (4.1.4) and the $\mathbf{U}(k)$ matrices of Section 5.4.

Now suppose that all the $\boldsymbol{\pi_2}$ vectors can be written in the form

$$\boldsymbol{\pi_2}(N-j;N) = \boldsymbol{\pi_2}(N-j-1;N)\mathbf{U_2}(j), \tag{6.2.8}$$

and that $\mathbf{U_2}(j), j = 1, 2, \ldots, n$ are already known. Then put this into (6.2.6c) to get

$$\begin{aligned}&\boldsymbol{\pi_2}(N-n-1;N)\,(\lambda\mathbf{I_2} + \mathbf{B_2})\\ &= \boldsymbol{\pi_2}(N-n;N)\,\mathbf{M_2}\,\mathbf{Q_2}\,\mathbf{R_2} + \lambda\,\boldsymbol{\pi_2}(N-n-2;N)\\ &= \boldsymbol{\pi_2}(N-n-1;N)\mathbf{U_2}(n)\mathbf{M_2}\,\mathbf{Q_2}\,\mathbf{R_2} + \lambda\,\boldsymbol{\pi_2}(N-n-2;N),\end{aligned}$$

leading to

$$\boldsymbol{\pi_2}(N-n-1;N)\,[\mathbf{B_2} + \lambda\mathbf{I_2} - \mathbf{U_2}(n)\mathbf{M_2}\,\mathbf{Q_2}\,\mathbf{R_2}] = \lambda\,\boldsymbol{\pi_2}(N-n-2;N).$$

This implies, starting with $\mathbf{U_2}(0) := \lambda\mathbf{V_2}$, that all the $\mathbf{U_2}$ matrices are recursively defined and can be computed by the following equation.

$$\mathbf{U_2}(n) = \left[\mathbf{I_2} + \frac{1}{\lambda}\mathbf{B_2} - \frac{1}{\lambda}\mathbf{U_2}(n-1)\,\mathbf{M_2}\,\mathbf{Q_2}\,\mathbf{R_2}\right]^{-1} \tag{6.2.9}$$

for $n = 1, 2, \ldots$. Note that the $\mathbf{U_2}(n)$ does not depend on N, and therefore the same set can be used for all N. This point is explored further when we discuss algorithms for evaluating everything. In the meantime, we still have not satisfied (6.2.6a) and (6.2.6b). But with (6.2.8), (6.2.6b) becomes[§]

$$\boldsymbol{\pi_2}(2;N)\left[\mathbf{I_2} + \frac{1}{\lambda}\mathbf{B_2} - \frac{1}{\lambda}\mathbf{U_2}(N-3)\mathbf{M_2}\,\mathbf{Q_2}\,\mathbf{R_2}\right] = \boldsymbol{\pi_1}(1;N)\mathbf{R_2}$$

or

$$\boldsymbol{\pi_2}(2;N) = \boldsymbol{\pi_1}(1;N)\,\mathbf{R_2}\,\mathbf{U_2}(N-2). \tag{6.2.10a}$$

Similarly, (6.2.6a) becomes

$$\boldsymbol{\pi_1}(1;N)\left[\mathbf{I_1} + \frac{1}{\lambda}\mathbf{B_1} - \frac{1}{\lambda}\mathbf{R_2}\,\mathbf{U_2}(N-2)\mathbf{M_2}\,\mathbf{Q_2}\right] = \boldsymbol{\pi_1}(0;N). \tag{6.2.10b}$$

We must show that (6.2.10b) is consistent with (6.2.4a), because they both connect states $\{i;\,1;\,N\}$ with $\{\cdot;\,0;\,N\}$. To do this we must first prove the following, which is analogous to Lemma 4.1.1.

[§]Note that $\mathbf{Q_2}(n)\,\mathbf{X_1}\,\mathbf{R_2}(n)$ is a $D(2)\times D(2)$ matrix, where $\mathbf{X_1}$ is any matrix of dimension $D(1)\times D(1)$. Also, $\mathbf{R_2}(n)\mathbf{X_2}\,\mathbf{Q_2}(n)$ is a $D(1)\times D(1)$ matrix, where $\mathbf{X_2}$ is any matrix of dimension $D(2)\times D(2)$.

Lemma 6.2.1: Let $\mathbf{B_2}$ be defined by (6.2.5), then multiplying (6.2.3) by $\mathbf{M_2}$ yields

$$\mathbf{M_2}\,\mathbf{Q_2}\boldsymbol{\epsilon}'_\mathbf{1} = \mathbf{B_2}\,\boldsymbol{\epsilon}'_\mathbf{2}, \tag{6.2.11a}$$

and given that $\mathbf{R_2}\,\boldsymbol{\epsilon}'_\mathbf{2} = \boldsymbol{\epsilon}'_\mathbf{1}$, we also have

$$\mathbf{M_2}\,\mathbf{Q_2}\,\mathbf{R_2}\,\boldsymbol{\epsilon}'_\mathbf{2} = \mathbf{B_2}\,\boldsymbol{\epsilon}'_\mathbf{2}. \tag{6.2.11b}$$

Furthermore, let $\mathbf{U_2}(0) = \lambda\mathbf{V_2}$, and let $\mathbf{U_2}(n)$ satisfy (6.2.9) for $n \geq 1$. Then

$$\mathbf{U_2}(n)\mathbf{B_2}\,\boldsymbol{\epsilon}'_\mathbf{2} = \lambda\,\boldsymbol{\epsilon}'_\mathbf{2} \quad \text{for all } \ n \geq 0. \tag{6.2.11c}$$

In other words, $[(1/\lambda)\mathbf{U_2}(n)\mathbf{B_2}]$ is isometric. ■

Proof: We actually prove that its inverse is isometric. First, observe [$\mathbf{U_2}(0)$ was defined to be $\lambda\mathbf{V_2}$] that

$$\mathbf{U_2}(0)\,\mathbf{B_2}\,\boldsymbol{\epsilon}'_\mathbf{2} = \lambda\mathbf{V_2}\,\mathbf{B_2}\boldsymbol{\epsilon}'_\mathbf{2} = \lambda\mathbf{I_2}\,\boldsymbol{\epsilon}'_\mathbf{2} = \lambda\boldsymbol{\epsilon}'_\mathbf{2}.$$

Now assume that (6.2.11c) is true for all $k = 0, 1, \ldots, n$, and let

$$\mathbf{A_2}(k) := [\mathbf{U_2}(k)]^{-1};$$

then

$$\begin{aligned}
\left[\frac{1}{\lambda}\mathbf{U_2}(n+1)\,\mathbf{B_2}\right]^{-1} &= \lambda\mathbf{V_2}\,\mathbf{A_2}(n+1) \\
&= \lambda\mathbf{V_2}\left[\mathbf{I_2} + \frac{1}{\lambda}\mathbf{B_2} - \frac{1}{\lambda}\mathbf{U_2}(n)\,\mathbf{M_2}\,\mathbf{Q_2}\,\mathbf{R_2}\right] \\
&= \lambda\mathbf{V_2} + \mathbf{I_2} - \mathbf{V_2}\,\mathbf{U_2}(n)\,\mathbf{M_2}\,\mathbf{Q_2}\,\mathbf{R_2}.
\end{aligned}$$

Next postmultiply both sides of the equation by $\boldsymbol{\epsilon}'_\mathbf{2}$ and get

$$\begin{aligned}
\lambda\mathbf{V_2}\,\mathbf{A_2}(n+1)\,\boldsymbol{\epsilon}'_\mathbf{2} &= \lambda\mathbf{V_2}\,\boldsymbol{\epsilon}'_\mathbf{2} + \boldsymbol{\epsilon}'_\mathbf{2} - \mathbf{V_2}\,\mathbf{U_2}\left[\mathbf{M_2}\,\mathbf{Q_2}\,\mathbf{R_2}\,\boldsymbol{\epsilon}'_\mathbf{2}\right] \\
&= \lambda\mathbf{V_2}\,\boldsymbol{\epsilon}'_\mathbf{2} + \boldsymbol{\epsilon}'_\mathbf{2} - \mathbf{V_2}\left[\mathbf{U_2}(n)\,\mathbf{B_2}\,\boldsymbol{\epsilon}'_\mathbf{2}\right].
\end{aligned}$$

But the expression in the second set of brackets is equal to $\lambda\boldsymbol{\epsilon}'_\mathbf{2}$ by assumption; thus by induction we have

$$\lambda\mathbf{V_2}\,\mathbf{A_2}(n)\,\boldsymbol{\epsilon}'_\mathbf{2} = \boldsymbol{\epsilon}'_\mathbf{2} \quad \text{for all } n.$$

Premultiplying both sides of this equation by $\mathbf{U_2}(n)\mathbf{B_2}$ yields our lemma. **QED**

We now return to (6.2.10b). When we postmultiply both sides by $\boldsymbol{\epsilon}'_\mathbf{1}$, the right-hand side becomes $r(0; N)$, and the left-hand side becomes

$$\frac{1}{\lambda}\boldsymbol{\pi}_\mathbf{1}(1;N)\,\mathbf{B_1}\,\boldsymbol{\epsilon}'_\mathbf{1} + r(1;N) - \boldsymbol{\pi}_\mathbf{1}(1;N)\,\mathbf{R_2}\left[\frac{1}{\lambda}\mathbf{U_2}(N-2)\,\mathbf{M_2}\,\mathbf{Q_2}\,\boldsymbol{\epsilon}'_\mathbf{1}\right]$$

$$= \frac{1}{\lambda}\boldsymbol{\pi}_\mathbf{1}(1;N)\,\mathbf{B_1}\,\boldsymbol{\epsilon}'_\mathbf{1} + r(1;N) - \boldsymbol{\pi}_\mathbf{1}(1;N)\,\mathbf{R_2}\,\boldsymbol{\epsilon}'_\mathbf{2} = \frac{1}{\lambda}\boldsymbol{\pi}_\mathbf{1}(1;N)\,\mathbf{B_1}\,\boldsymbol{\epsilon}'_\mathbf{1}.$$

The two parts together reproduce (6.2.4a), so we have proven our case.

We next define the matrix implied by (6.2.10b),

$$\bar{\mathbf{U}}_1(N) := \left[\frac{1}{\lambda}\mathbf{B}_1 + \mathbf{I}_1 - \mathbf{R}_2\mathbf{U}_2(N-2)\mathbf{M}_2\mathbf{Q}_2\right]^{-1}.$$

This is a Ξ_1-space matrix, and it satisfies the equation

$$\bar{\mathbf{U}}_1(N)\mathbf{B}_1\boldsymbol{\epsilon}_1' = \lambda\boldsymbol{\epsilon}_1'.$$

We now list the solution vectors, which should help the reader make sense of what we have derived so far in this chapter:

$$\boldsymbol{\pi}_1(0;N) = r(0;N)\,\mathbf{p},$$

$$\boldsymbol{\pi}_1(1;N) = r(0;N)\mathbf{p}\,\bar{\mathbf{U}}_1(N),$$
$$\boldsymbol{\pi}_2(2;N) = r(0;N)\mathbf{p}\bar{\mathbf{U}}_1(N)\mathbf{R}_2\mathbf{U}_2(N-2),$$
$$\cdots \qquad \cdots \qquad \cdots$$
$$\boldsymbol{\pi}_2(n;N) = r(0;N)\mathbf{p}\bar{\mathbf{U}}_1(N)\mathbf{R}_2\mathbf{U}_2(N-2)\cdots\mathbf{U}_2(N-n),$$
$$\cdots \qquad \cdots \qquad \cdots$$
$$\boldsymbol{\pi}_2(N;N) = r(0;N)\mathbf{p}\bar{\mathbf{U}}_1(N)\mathbf{R}_2\mathbf{U}_2(N-2)\mathbf{U}_2(N-3)\cdots\mathbf{U}_2(0).$$

We still have to evaluate $r(0;N)$, but that is easy enough to do making the sum of all probabilities add up to 1. That is,

$$\sum_{n=0}^{N} r(n;N) = r(0;N) + \boldsymbol{\pi}_1(1;N)\boldsymbol{\epsilon}_1' + \sum_{n=2}^{N}\boldsymbol{\pi}_2(n;N)\boldsymbol{\epsilon}_2' = 1.$$

We can actually write this in a compact and recursive way, just as we did previously with the matrix $\mathbf{K}(N)$ in (5.4.6b). Recall that $\mathbf{R}_2\,\boldsymbol{\epsilon}_2' = \boldsymbol{\epsilon}_1'$, and define the vector

$$\mathbf{x}_2(N) := \mathbf{p}\bar{\mathbf{U}}_1(N)\mathbf{R}_2;$$

then

$$r(1;N) = r(0;N)\mathbf{x}_2(N)\boldsymbol{\epsilon}_2'.$$

Next define the Ξ_2-space matrix,

$$\begin{aligned}\mathbf{K}_2(N) := \mathbf{I}_2 &+ \mathbf{U}_2(N-2) + \mathbf{U}_2(N-2)\mathbf{U}_2(N-3)\\ &+\cdots+\mathbf{U}_2(N-2)\mathbf{U}_2(N-3)\cdots\mathbf{U}_2(N-n)\\ &+\cdots+\mathbf{U}_2(N-2)\mathbf{U}_2(N-3)\cdots\mathbf{U}_2(0).\end{aligned} \tag{6.2.12a}$$

When we factor the terms right-multiplying $\mathbf{U}_2(N-2)$, we get

$$\mathbf{K}_2(N) = \mathbf{I}_2 + \mathbf{U}_2(N-2)\mathbf{K}_2(N-1), \tag{6.2.12b}$$

and therefore the sum over all states reduces to

$$r(0;N)\left[1 + \mathbf{x}_2(N)\mathbf{K}_2(N)\boldsymbol{\epsilon}_2'\right] = 1$$

or

$$\frac{1}{r(0;N)} = \left[1 + \mathbf{x_2}(N)\mathbf{K_2}(N)\boldsymbol{\epsilon}_2'\right]. \tag{6.2.12c}$$

We discuss an efficient algorithm after we have dealt with the general case, but our accomplishments so far deserve a summary theorem-algorithm.

Theorem 6.2.2: Consider an M/ME/2//N loop with matrices, $\mathbf{M_k}$, $\mathbf{P_k}$, $\mathbf{B_k}$, $\mathbf{V_k}$, $\mathbf{Q_2}$, and $\mathbf{R_2}$, as defined in this section. Given $N > 2$,

BEGIN PROCEDURE
. $\mathbf{U_2}(0;N) = \lambda\mathbf{V_2}$.
∗ Then
. FOR $n = 1$ TO $N-2$:
. $\mathbf{U_2}(n) = \lambda\left[\lambda\mathbf{I_2} + \mathbf{B_2} - \mathbf{U_2}(n-1)\,\mathbf{M_2}\,\mathbf{Q_2}\,\mathbf{R_2}\right]^{-1}$;
. END FOR.
∗ Next evaluate
. $\bar{\mathbf{U}}_\mathbf{1}(N) = \lambda\left[\lambda\mathbf{I_1} + \mathbf{B_1} - \mathbf{R_2}\,\mathbf{U_2}(N-2)\,\mathbf{M_2}\,\mathbf{Q_2}\right]^{-1}$;
. $\mathbf{x_1}(0) = \mathbf{p}$;
. $\mathbf{x_1}(1;N) = \mathbf{x_1}(0)\bar{\mathbf{U}}_\mathbf{1}(N)$;
. $x(1;N) = \mathbf{x_1}(1;N)\boldsymbol{\epsilon}_1'$;
. $\mathbf{x_2}(2;N) = \mathbf{x_1}(1;N)\mathbf{R_2}\mathbf{U_2}(N-2)$;
. $x(2;N) = \mathbf{x_2}(2;N)\boldsymbol{\epsilon}_2'$;
. $sum = 1 + x(1;N) + x(2;N)$.
. FOR $n = 3$ TO N:
. $\mathbf{x_2}(n;N) = \mathbf{x_2}(n-1)\mathbf{U_2}(N-n)$;
. $x(n;N) = \mathbf{x_2}(n;N)\,\boldsymbol{\epsilon}_2'$;
. $sum = sum + x(n;N)$;
. END FOR.
∗ The steady-state probability vectors and their associated scalars are given by the following.
. $r(0;N) = 1/sum$
. $\boldsymbol{\pi}_\mathbf{1}(1;N) = r(0;N)\mathbf{x_1}(1;N)$,
. $r(1;N) = r(0;N)\,x(1;N)$.
. FOR $n = 2$ TO N:
. $\boldsymbol{\pi}_\mathbf{2}(n;N) = r(0;N)\,\mathbf{x_2}(n;N)$;
. $r(n;N) = r(0;N)x(n;N)$;
. END FOR.
∗ The mean throughput is given by
. $\Lambda(N) = \lambda[1 - r(N;N)]$.
END PROCEDURE

All other performance parameters can be calculated from these. ■

It does not pay to go deeply into the significance of this theorem, because derive the solutions for the general system in the next section. We point out though, that as an algorithm, the most computationally intense portion involves finding $\mathbf{U_2}(n)$ in Equation (6.2.9), because that requires taking the inverse of $D(2) \times D(2)$ matrices for (N-1) values of n. In studying closed systems, researchers are usually not interested in just one value of N. Rather, they must look at a whole range of values up to, say, N_{max}. In that case, the matrices required to solve for a system with N_{max} customers can be used to solve for systems with fewer customers. Put differently, if one wishes to solve for a system with $N+1$ customers, after solving for the same system with N customers, only one more inverse need be taken [to find $\mathbf{U_2}(N+1)$].

6.3 Steady-State M/G/C//N-Type Systems

In the preceding section we described the steady-state solution for systems with $C = 2$. The extension to systems in which there are more than two servers in S_1 is straightforward but requires some generalizations of definitions.

6.3.1 Steady-State M/ME/C//N Loop

Let us start with a definition of our state spaces. An alternative, but equivalent, definition is given in Section 6.3.2.

Definition 6.3.1

$\Xi_k := \{i = \{i_1, i_2, \ldots, i_k\} | 1 \le i_1 \le i_2 \le \cdots \le i_k \le m\}^*$ for $1 \le k \le C$. *Ξ_k is the set of all internal states of S_1 when there are k active customers there*. Each k-tuple represents a state in which $k \le C$ customers are active in a subsystem, S_1, which has C identical servers in it. One customer is at phase i_1, another is at phase i_2, and so on, each in a different server. They never get in each other's way, because there are at least as many servers as there are customers. If there are more than C customers at S_1, the excess numbers must queue up outside.□

The number of states in Ξ_k is

$$D(k) = \binom{m+k-1}{k}. \tag{6.3.1}$$

We now make the following generalizations of previous definitions, where $N > C$. First,

$$\boldsymbol{\epsilon}'_{\mathbf{k}} := \textit{the } D(k) - \textit{dimensional column vector of all } 1'\textit{s}.$$

Definition 6.3.2

$[\mathbf{M_k}]$ is a diagonal matrix whose (ii)th component is the probability rate of leaving state $i \in \Xi_k$, for $1 \le k \le C$. Thus if $i = \{i_1, i_2, \ldots, i_k\}$, then $[\mathbf{M_k}]_{ii} = \mu_{i_1} + \mu_{i_2} + \cdots + \mu_{i_k}$. This is the *k-space completion rate matrix*. □

Definition 6.3.3

$\boldsymbol{\pi}_{\mathbf{k}}(n; N) :=$ probability vector of dimension $D(k)$ that there are n customers at S_1, and $N-n$ customers at S_2. The ith component is the

*Note that the i_ls need not be distinct.

probability that the active customers in S_1 are collectively in state $i \in \Xi_k$. We adhere to the notation $k = n$ if $n \leq C$, and $k = C$ otherwise. $r(n; N) = \boldsymbol{\pi_k}(n; N)\, \boldsymbol{\epsilon'_k}$ is the associated scalar probability. □

Note that the relationship between k and n implies that $\boldsymbol{\pi_k}(n; N)$ depends on C as well. So we probably should use the notation $\boldsymbol{\pi_k}(n; N \mid C)$. However, in any application it is assumed that C (the maximum number of customers that can be active at any time), will not change. Therefore, $\boldsymbol{\pi_k}$'s dependence is left implicit. But the reader must keep in mind that $\boldsymbol{\pi_k}(n; N)$ for one value of C is different from the comparable component when applied to a system with a different C.

Definition 6.3.4

$[\mathbf{R_k}]_{ij}$:= *probability that a customer, who upon entering* S_1 *and finding it in internal state* $i \in \Xi_{k-1}$, *will go to the server and phase that puts the system in state* $j \in \Xi_k$. $\mathbf{R_k}$ is a $D(k-1) \times D(k)$-dimensional matrix with the property that $\mathbf{R_k}\, \boldsymbol{\epsilon'_k} = \boldsymbol{\epsilon'_{k-1}}$. We could let $\mathbf{p} = \mathbf{R_1}$ if we so choose. □

For descriptive purposes we think of the index i as representing the set $\{i_1, i_2, \ldots, i_l, \ldots, i_k\}$ (which by Definition 6.3.1 it really is), with the same for j. Then we can say that the matrix element $[\mathbf{R_k}]_{ij}$ is 0 unless

$$i \cap j = i, \quad \text{where} \quad i \in \Xi_{k-1} \ \text{and} \ j \in \Xi_k.$$

Remember, by their definition, the set j has one more member than the set i, so there must be exactly one distinct member of j (possibly appearing more than once in the set) which is not in i in order for $[\mathbf{R_k}]_{ij}$ to have a nonzero value. Then, as a direct generalization of the discussion following Definition 6.2.7, call that one element ν, and

$$[\mathbf{R_k}]_{ij} = p_\nu \quad \text{if} \ \ i \cap j = i. \tag{6.3.2a}$$

Definition 6.3.5

$[\mathbf{Q_k}]_{ij}$:= *probability that a customer, upon leaving* S_1 *when the system was in state* $i \in \Xi_k$, *leaves the system in state* $j \in \Xi_{k-1}$ *after he exits.* This matrix is of dimension $D(k) \times D(k-1)$. If we chose, we could have let $\mathbf{q}' = \mathbf{Q_1}$. □

Here $[\mathbf{Q}_k]_{ij} := 0$, unless $i \cap j = j$. We now have a little generalization problem. Let ν be the left-over element. It is possible that in the set, $i = \{i_1, i_2, \cdots, i_k\}$, $i_l = \nu$ appears more than once; then any one of those customers could complete service and leave. So let α_ν be the number of times ν appears in the set i; then for $i \in \Xi_k$ and $j \in \Xi_{k-1}$,

$$[\mathbf{Q_k}]_{ij} := \frac{\alpha_\nu \mu_\nu \mathbf{q}_\nu}{[\mathbf{M_k}]_{ii}} \quad \text{for} \ \ i \cap j = j. \tag{6.3.2b}$$

Go back to Definition 6.2.8, and verify that this formula actually matches both conditions there, for $k = 2$.

Our last definition of this set is the transition matrix of space Ξ_k.

Definition 6.3.6

$[\mathbf{P_k}]_{ij}$:= *probability that a customer, who upon completing at some phase in S_1, will go to another phase in the same server in S_1, thereby taking the system from state $i \in \Xi_k$ to $j \in \Xi_k$.* $\mathbf{P_k}$ is a nonisometric transition matrix of dimension $D(k) \times D(k)$. □

Exactly as in the case for $k = 2$, $[\mathbf{P_k}]_{ij} := 0$, unless $i \cap j$ is a set with $k - 1$ elements. Let γ be the member of i that is not in $i \cap j$, and let ν be the member of j that is not in $i \cap j$. Also, let α_γ be the number of times γ appears in the set i; then

$$[\mathbf{P_k}]_{ij} := [\mathbf{P_1}]_{\gamma\nu} \frac{\alpha_\gamma \mu_\gamma}{[\mathbf{M_k}]_{ii}}. \tag{6.3.2c}$$

As with $\mathbf{Q_k}$, this matches the discussion following Definition 6.2.6.

If the construction of these matrices seems difficult, rest assured that it can be automated for computer use. We look at the specification problem from a different point of view in Section 6.3.2.

As a direct generalization of (6.2.2) and (6.2.3) we can write

$$[\mathbf{P_k} + \mathbf{Q_k}\mathbf{R_k}]\,\boldsymbol{\epsilon}'_{\mathbf{k}} = \boldsymbol{\epsilon}'_{\mathbf{k}}, \tag{6.3.3a}$$

and given that $\mathbf{R_k}\,\boldsymbol{\epsilon}'_{\mathbf{k}} = \boldsymbol{\epsilon}'_{\mathbf{k-1}}$,

$$\mathbf{Q_k}\,\boldsymbol{\epsilon}'_{\mathbf{k-1}} = [\mathbf{I_k} - \mathbf{P_k}]\,\boldsymbol{\epsilon}'_{\mathbf{k}}. \tag{6.3.3b}$$

We have the natural Ξ_k-space generalizations of (6.2.5)

$$\mathbf{B_k} = \mathbf{V_k}^{-1} := \mathbf{M_k}[\mathbf{I_k} - \mathbf{P_k}], \tag{6.3.4a}$$

which together with (6.3.3b) yields

$$\mathbf{M_k}\,\mathbf{Q_k}\,\boldsymbol{\epsilon}'_{\mathbf{k-1}} = \mathbf{M_k}\,\mathbf{Q_k}\,\mathbf{R_k}\,\boldsymbol{\epsilon}'_{\mathbf{k}} = \mathbf{B_k}\,\boldsymbol{\epsilon}'_{\mathbf{k}}. \tag{6.3.4b}$$

There should be little difficulty in writing down the balance equations directly as generalizations of (6.2.4a) and (6.2.6). They are, for $N > C$ customers:

$$\lambda\boldsymbol{\pi}_{\mathbf{1}}(0; N) = \boldsymbol{\pi}_{\mathbf{1}}(1; N)\mathbf{B_1}\,\mathbf{Q}; \tag{6.3.5a}$$

$$\boldsymbol{\pi}_{\mathbf{1}}(1; N)(\mathbf{B_1} + \lambda\mathbf{I_1}) = \boldsymbol{\pi}_{\mathbf{2}}(2; N)\mathbf{M_2}\,\mathbf{Q_2} + \lambda\boldsymbol{\pi}_{\mathbf{1}}(0; N), \tag{6.3.5b}$$

for $2 \le k < C$,

$$\boldsymbol{\pi}_{\boldsymbol{k}}(k; N)(\mathbf{B_k} + \lambda\mathbf{I_k})$$
$$= \boldsymbol{\pi}_{\mathbf{k+1}}(k+1; N)\mathbf{M_{k+1}}\,\mathbf{Q_{k+1}} + \lambda\boldsymbol{\pi}_{\mathbf{k-1}}(k-1; N)\,\mathbf{R_k}, \tag{6.3.5c}$$

$$\boldsymbol{\pi}_{\mathbf{c}}(C; N)(\mathbf{B_c} + \lambda\mathbf{I_c}) = \boldsymbol{\pi}_{\mathbf{c}}(C{+}1; N)\mathbf{M_c}\,\mathbf{Q_c}\,\mathbf{R_c} + \lambda\boldsymbol{\pi}_{\mathbf{c-1}}(C{-}1; N)\,\mathbf{R_c}; \tag{6.3.5d}$$

and for $C < n < N$,

$$\boldsymbol{\pi}_{\mathbf{c}}(n; N)(\mathbf{B_c} + \lambda\mathbf{I_c}) = \boldsymbol{\pi}_{\mathbf{c}}(n+1; N)\,\mathbf{M_c}\,\mathbf{Q_c}\,\mathbf{R_c} + \lambda\boldsymbol{\pi}_{\mathbf{c}}(n-1; N) \tag{6.3.5e}$$

with

$$\boldsymbol{\pi}_{\mathbf{c}}(N; N)\, \mathbf{B}_{\mathrm{c}} = \lambda \boldsymbol{\pi}_{\mathbf{c}}(N-1; N). \tag{6.3.5f}$$

Again following the usual procedure, let

$$\mathbf{U}_{\mathrm{c}}(0) := \lambda \mathbf{V}_{\mathrm{c}}, \tag{6.3.6a}$$

and assume that the following is true for $n < l \leq N$ [it is certainly true for $l = N$ by (6.3.5f) and (6.3.6a)]:

$$\boldsymbol{\pi}_{\mathbf{c}}(l; N) = \boldsymbol{\pi}_{\mathbf{c}}(l-1; N) \mathbf{U}_{\mathrm{c}}(N-l). \tag{6.3.6b}$$

Be careful. The first index on $\boldsymbol{\pi}_{\mathbf{c}}(\,\cdot\,; N)$ increases with n, but the index on $\mathbf{U}_{\mathrm{c}}(\,\cdot\,)$ decreases. Then combining (6.3.5e) and (6.3.6b) gives

$$\boldsymbol{\pi}_{\mathbf{c}}(n; N)[\mathbf{B}_{\mathrm{c}} + \lambda \mathbf{I}_{\mathrm{c}} - \mathbf{U}_{\mathrm{c}}(N-n-1) \mathbf{M}_{\mathrm{c}}\, \mathbf{Q}_{\mathrm{c}}\, \mathbf{R}_{\mathrm{c}}] = \lambda \boldsymbol{\pi}_{\mathbf{c}}(n-1; N),$$

which implies that [compare with Equations (6.3.6b) and (6.2.8)]

$$\mathbf{U}_{\mathrm{c}}(n) = \lambda [\mathbf{B}_{\mathrm{c}} + \lambda \mathbf{I}_{\mathrm{c}} - \mathbf{U}_{\mathrm{c}}(n-1) \mathbf{M}_{\mathrm{c}}\, \mathbf{Q}_{\mathrm{c}}\, \mathbf{R}_{\mathrm{c}}]^{-1} \quad \text{for } n \geq 1. \tag{6.3.6c}$$

Next, for $n = C$, we have

$$\boldsymbol{\pi}_{\mathbf{c}}(C; N)[\mathbf{B}_{\mathrm{c}} + \lambda \mathbf{I}_{\mathrm{c}} - \mathbf{U}_{\mathrm{c}}(N-C-1) \mathbf{M}_{\mathrm{c}}\, \mathbf{Q}_{\mathrm{c}}\, \mathbf{R}_{\mathrm{c}}] = \lambda \boldsymbol{\pi}_{\mathbf{c-1}}(C-1; N)\, \mathbf{R}_{\mathrm{c}},$$

or

$$\boldsymbol{\pi}_{\mathbf{c}}(C; N) = \boldsymbol{\pi}_{\mathbf{c-1}}(C-1; N)\, \mathbf{R}_{\mathrm{c}}\, \mathbf{U}_{\mathrm{c}}(N-C).$$

Note that the $\mathbf{U}_{\mathbf{c}}(n)$ matrices do not depend on N, in the following sense. Suppose that we were interested in a system with $C = 3$ and $N = 6$. Then to come down the ladder from $n = 6, [N]$, to $n = 2, [C-1]$, we would have to calculate the matrices $\mathbf{U}_{\mathbf{3}}(0)$, $\mathbf{U}_{\mathbf{3}}(1)$, $\mathbf{U}_{\mathbf{3}}(2)$, and $\mathbf{U}_{\mathbf{3}}(3)$. If we then decided that we wanted to study $N = 7$, we would only have to calculate the additional matrix, $\mathbf{U}_{\mathbf{3}}(4)$, because the others are the same. [However, if we wish to study $C = 4$, then everything changes. The matrices $\mathbf{U}_{\mathbf{4}}(k)$ are different.] Now we must consider a class of matrices that depend on N as well as n, in order to deal with the situation for $n < C - 1$. This is a generalization of $\bar{U}_1(N)$ in Theorem 6.2.2. For instance, for $k = C - 1$,

$$\boldsymbol{\pi}_{\mathbf{c-1}}(C-1; N)[\mathbf{B}_{\mathrm{c-1}} + \lambda \mathbf{I}_{\mathrm{c-1}} - \mathbf{R}_{\mathrm{c}}\, \mathbf{U}_{\mathrm{c}}(N-C)\, \mathbf{M}_{\mathrm{c}}\, \mathbf{Q}_{\mathrm{c}}] = \lambda \boldsymbol{\pi}_{\mathbf{c-2}}(C-2; N) \mathbf{R}_{\mathrm{c-1}}.$$

The matrices we are about to define may not be the best selection for efficiency, but they provide a certain elegance that some day may prove to be useful. We define

$$\mathbf{U}_{\mathrm{c}}(N \,|\, C) := \mathbf{U}_{\mathrm{c}}(N-C), \tag{6.3.7a}$$

and

$$\mathbf{U}_{\mathrm{c-1}}(N \,|\, C) := \lambda [\mathbf{B}_{\mathrm{c-1}} + \lambda \mathbf{I}_{\mathrm{c-1}} - \mathbf{R}_{\mathrm{c}}\, \mathbf{U}_{\mathrm{c}}(N \,|\, C) \mathbf{M}_{\mathrm{c}}\, \mathbf{Q}_{\mathrm{c}}]^{-1},$$

which implies that

$$\boldsymbol{\pi}_{\mathbf{c-1}}(C-1; N) = \boldsymbol{\pi}_{\mathbf{c-2}}(C-2; N) \mathbf{R}_{\mathrm{c-1}} \mathbf{U}_{\mathrm{c-1}}(N \,|\, C).$$

In general, we define the $D(k) \times D(k)$-dimensional matrices,

$$\mathbf{U_k}(N \mid C) := \lambda[\mathbf{B_k} + \lambda\mathbf{I_k} - \mathbf{R_{k+1}}\,\mathbf{U_{k+1}}(N \mid C)\,\mathbf{M_{k+1}}\,\mathbf{Q_{k+1}}]^{-1}. \qquad (6.3.7b)$$

Then we can write

$$\boldsymbol{\pi}_\mathbf{k}(k; N) = \boldsymbol{\pi}_\mathbf{k-1}(k-1; N)\mathbf{R_k}\mathbf{U_k}(N \mid C) \quad \text{for } 1 \le k < C. \qquad (6.3.8)$$

Clearly, the matrices $\mathbf{U_k}(N \mid C)$ are very different from the matrices, $\mathbf{U_c}(n)$. Take note of the subtle notational differences. This actually parallels much of Section 5.4.2.

Before collecting the foregoing formulas in a theorem, we wish to state and prove the following lemma concerning the matrices $\mathbf{U_k}(N \mid C)$ and $\mathbf{U_c}(n)$, which is directly related to Lemma 5.4.1.

Lemma 6.3.1: Let $\mathbf{U_c}(n)$ be defined by (6.3.6a) and (6.3.6c). Then

$$\mathbf{U_c}(n)\,\mathbf{B_c}\,\boldsymbol{\epsilon}'_\mathbf{c} = \lambda\boldsymbol{\epsilon}'_\mathbf{c} \quad \text{for } n \ge C. \qquad (6.3.9a)$$

Furthermore, let $\mathbf{U_k}(N \mid C)$ be defined by Equations (6.3.7). Then

$$\mathbf{U_k}(N \mid C)\mathbf{B_k}\,\boldsymbol{\epsilon}'_\mathbf{k} = \lambda\boldsymbol{\epsilon}'_\mathbf{k} \quad \text{for } 1 \le k \le C. \qquad (6.3.9b)$$

■

Proof: First note, by postmultiplying (6.3.6a) with $\mathbf{B_c}\,\boldsymbol{\epsilon}'_\mathbf{c}$, that

$$\mathbf{U_c}(0)\mathbf{B_c}\,\boldsymbol{\epsilon}'_\mathbf{c} = \lambda\boldsymbol{\epsilon}'_\mathbf{c}.$$

Next, define

$$\mathbf{A_c}(n) := [\mathbf{U_c}(n)]^{-1}$$

and assume that (6.3.9a) is true for $0 \le n < l$; then from (6.3.6c),

$$\lambda\mathbf{A_c}(l)\boldsymbol{\epsilon}'_\mathbf{c} = [\mathbf{B_c} + \lambda\mathbf{I_c} - \mathbf{U_c}(l-1)\,\mathbf{M_c}\,\mathbf{Q_c}\,\mathbf{R_c}]\boldsymbol{\epsilon}'_\mathbf{c}.$$

But from (6.3.4b) [for $k = C$], and by assumption,

$$\mathbf{U_c}(l-1)\mathbf{M_c}\,\mathbf{Q_c}\,\mathbf{R_c}\,\boldsymbol{\epsilon}'_\mathbf{c} = \boldsymbol{\epsilon}'_\mathbf{c}.$$

Thus we have

$$\lambda\mathbf{A_c}(l)\,\boldsymbol{\epsilon}'_\mathbf{c} = \mathbf{B_c}\,\boldsymbol{\epsilon}'_\mathbf{c},$$

from which (6.3.9a) follows, for $n = l$. Therefore, by induction, it is true for all n. Next observe that from (6.3.7a) and (6.3.9a), (6.3.9b) must be true for $k = C$. Now, for all relevant k, define

$$\mathbf{A_k}(N \mid C) := [\mathbf{U_k}(N \mid C)]^{-1},$$

assume that (6.3.9b) is true for $k = C, C-1, \ldots, l+1$, and note from (6.3.4b) and Definition 6.3.4 that

$$\mathbf{R_{k+1}}\,\mathbf{U_{k+1}}(N \mid C)\,\mathbf{M_{k+1}}\,\mathbf{Q_{k+1}}\boldsymbol{\epsilon}'_\mathbf{k}$$

$$= \mathbf{R_{k+1}}\mathbf{U_{k+1}}(N \mid C)\mathbf{B_{k+1}}\,\boldsymbol{\epsilon}'_\mathbf{k+1} = \lambda\mathbf{R_{k+1}}\,\boldsymbol{\epsilon}'_\mathbf{k+1} = \lambda\boldsymbol{\epsilon}'_\mathbf{k+1}$$

is true for all $k = C, C-1, \ldots, l$. Then (6.3.9b) must be true for $k = l$, and thus by induction, for all k. **QED**

Compare with Lemma 4.1.1. Also, we see that two new sets of isometric matrices have been created, because $[\lambda \mathbf{V_k}\, \mathbf{A_k}(N\,|\,C)]\boldsymbol{\epsilon}'_{\mathbf{k}} = \boldsymbol{\epsilon}'_{\mathbf{k}}$, and so on. We could have defined the $\mathbf{U}(N\,|\,C)$ matrices to include the $\mathbf{R_k}$, but the new objects would not be square matrices. By defining them the way we did, the matrices $\mathbf{R_k}$ and $\mathbf{Q_k}$, for $1 \le k \le C$, remain as the only matrices that connect objects of different spaces.

At last we can write the solution vectors in terms of the single scalar, $r(0; N)$. We state them in the form of a theoremi. (Compare with the ME/M/C queue in Theorem 5.4.2).

Theorem 6.3.2: The steady-state probability vectors of closed M/ME/$C//N$ loops ($C > 1$) are given below. First define the auxiliary vectors, starting with $\mathbf{x_o}(N\,|\,C) := \mathbf{p}$ and $\mathbf{x_1}(N\,|\,C) := \mathbf{pU_1}(N\,|\,C)$, using (6.3.7b), For $2 \le k \le C$,

$$\begin{aligned}\mathbf{x_k}(N\,|\,C) :=& \mathbf{pU_1}(N\,|\,C)\mathbf{R_2}\,\mathbf{U_2}(N\,|\,C)\cdots \mathbf{R_k}\,\mathbf{U_k}(N\,|\,C)\\ =& \mathbf{x_{k-1}}(N\,|\,C)\mathbf{R_k}\mathbf{U_k}(N\,|\,C).\end{aligned} \tag{6.3.10a}$$

Then starting with $\mathbf{x_c}(C; N) := \mathbf{x_c}(N\,|\,C)$, and using (6.3.6c), define for $C < n \le N$,

$$\begin{aligned}\mathbf{x_c}(n; N) :=& \mathbf{x_c}(N\,|\,C)\,\mathbf{U_c}(N-C-1)\mathbf{U_c}(N-C-2)\cdots \mathbf{U_c}(N-n)\\ =& \mathbf{x_c}(n-1; N)\mathbf{U_c}(N-n).\end{aligned} \tag{6.3.10b}$$

The steady-state probability vectors are given by

$$\boldsymbol{\pi}_{\mathbf{k}}(k; N) = r(0; N)\mathbf{x_k}(N\,|\,C), \quad \text{for } 0 \le k \le C, \tag{6.3.11a}$$

and

$$\boldsymbol{\pi}_{\mathbf{c}}(n; N) = r(0; N)\mathbf{x_c}(n; N) \quad \text{for } C \le n \le N. \tag{6.3.11b}$$

The associated steady-state scalar probabilities are given by

$$r(n; N) = \boldsymbol{\pi}_{\mathbf{k}}(n; N)\,\boldsymbol{\epsilon}'_{\mathbf{k}} \quad \text{for } 0 \le n \le N, \tag{6.3.11c}$$

where $k = n$ for $n < C$, and $k = C$ otherwise. $r(0; N)$ comes from the normalization requirement, therefore,

$$\frac{1}{r(0; N)} = \sum_{k=0}^{C-1} \mathbf{x_k}(N\,|\,C)\boldsymbol{\epsilon}'_{\mathbf{k}} + \sum_{n=C}^{N} \mathbf{x_c}(n; N)\boldsymbol{\epsilon}'_{\mathbf{c}}. \tag{6.3.11d}$$

Given that $\mathbf{x_c}(C; N) := \mathbf{x_c}(N\,|\,C)$, this expression could have been placed in either sum term. The mean queue length (and from Little's formula, the mean system time) can be calculated directly from its definition, $\bar{q} = \sum_{n=1}^{n=N} n\, r(n; N)$. ■

We realize that the contents of this theorem are very difficult to grasp, but we do want the reader to use them computationally at some time in the future. Therefore, let us pause for a moment to look at the equations for some specific values of C and N. Suppose that we let $N = 6$ and $C = 3$; then the solution vectors are given by the following set.

$$\begin{aligned}
\boldsymbol{\pi}_1(0;6) &= r(0;6)\mathbf{p}\\
\boldsymbol{\pi}_1(1;6) &= r(0;6)\mathbf{p}\mathbf{U}_1(6\,|\,3)\\
\boldsymbol{\pi}_2(2;6) &= r(0;6)\mathbf{p}\mathbf{U}_1(6\,|\,3)\mathbf{R}_2\mathbf{U}_2(6\,|\,3)\\
\boldsymbol{\pi}_3(3;6) &= r(0;6)\mathbf{p}\mathbf{U}_1(6\,|\,3)\mathbf{R}_2\mathbf{U}_2(6\,|\,3)\mathbf{R}_3\mathbf{U}_3(3)\\
\boldsymbol{\pi}_3(4;6) &= r(0;6)\mathbf{p}\mathbf{U}_1(6\,|\,3)\mathbf{R}_2\mathbf{U}_2(6\,|\,3)\mathbf{R}_3\mathbf{U}_3(3)\mathbf{U}_3(2)\\
\boldsymbol{\pi}_3(5;6) &= r(0;6)\mathbf{p}\mathbf{U}_1(6\,|\,3)\mathbf{R}_2\mathbf{U}_2(6\,|\,3)\mathbf{R}_3\mathbf{U}_3(3)\mathbf{U}_3(2)\mathbf{U}_3(1)\\
\boldsymbol{\pi}_3(6;6) &= r(0;6)\mathbf{p}\mathbf{U}_1(6\,|\,3)\mathbf{R}_2\mathbf{U}_2(6\,|\,3)\mathbf{R}_3\mathbf{U}_3(3)\mathbf{U}_3(2)\mathbf{U}_3(1)\mathbf{U}_3(0).
\end{aligned}$$

We start with $\mathbf{U}_3(0) = \lambda\mathbf{V}_3$, and then calculate $\mathbf{U}_3(1)$, $\mathbf{U}_3(2)$, and $\mathbf{U}_3(3)$ recursively by (6.3.6c). Next, given that $\mathbf{U}_3(6\,|\,3) = \mathbf{U}_3(3)$, we calculate $\mathbf{U}_2(6\,|\,3)$ and $\mathbf{U}_1(6\,|\,3)$ recursively from (6.3.7b). We can calculate $r(0;6)$ by the procedure mentioned in Theorem 6.3.2, or we can set up a $\mathbf{K}$ matrix, as we did in previous sections. For instance, look at

$$\mathbf{K}_3(6) := \mathbf{I}_3 + \mathbf{U}_3(3) + \mathbf{U}_3(3)\,\mathbf{U}_3(2) + \mathbf{U}_3(3)\,\mathbf{U}_3(2)\,\mathbf{U}_3(1)$$
$$+\mathbf{U}_3(3)\,\mathbf{U}_3(2)\mathbf{U}_3(1)\,\mathbf{U}_3(0) = \mathbf{I}_3 + \mathbf{U}_3(3)[\mathbf{K}_3(5)],$$

where the definition of $\mathbf{K}_3(5)$ should be clear. Next calculate the scalar

$$sum = 1 + \mathbf{p}\mathbf{U}_1(6\,|\,3)\,\boldsymbol{\epsilon}_1'$$

and the vector (which is actually $\mathbf{x}_2(6\,|\,3)\,\mathbf{R}_3$),

$$\mathbf{x}_3 = \mathbf{p}\mathbf{U}_1(6\,|\,3)\,\mathbf{U}_2(6\,|\,3)\,\mathbf{R}_3,$$

then

$$\frac{1}{r(0;6)} = sum + \mathbf{x}_3\,\mathbf{K}_3(6)\,\boldsymbol{\epsilon}_3'.$$

We hope that this has helped. If not, perhaps the reader should give this one more try.

Suppose it is desirable that the probabilities for the same system with $N = 7$ be calculated; then the new set of equations needed is

$$\begin{aligned}
\boldsymbol{\pi}_1(0;7) &= r(0;7)\mathbf{p}\\
\boldsymbol{\pi}_1(1;7) &= r(0;7)\mathbf{p}\mathbf{U}_1(7\,|\,3)\\
\boldsymbol{\pi}_2(2;7) &= r(0;7)\mathbf{p}\mathbf{U}_1(7\,|\,3)\mathbf{R}_2\mathbf{U}_2(7\,|\,3)\\
\boldsymbol{\pi}_3(3;7) &= r(0;7)\mathbf{p}\mathbf{U}_1(7\,|\,3)\mathbf{R}_2\mathbf{U}_2(7\,|\,3)\mathbf{R}_3\mathbf{U}_3(4)\\
\boldsymbol{\pi}_3(4;7) &= r(0;7)\mathbf{p}\mathbf{U}_1(7\,|\,3)\mathbf{R}_2\mathbf{U}_2(7\,|\,3)\mathbf{R}_3\mathbf{U}_3(4)\mathbf{U}_3(3)\\
\boldsymbol{\pi}_3(5;7) &= r(0;7)\mathbf{p}\mathbf{U}_1(7\,|\,3)\mathbf{R}_2\mathbf{U}_2(7\,|\,3)\mathbf{R}_3\mathbf{U}_3(4)\mathbf{U}_3(3)\mathbf{U}_3(2)\\
\boldsymbol{\pi}_3(6;7) &= r(0;7)\mathbf{p}\mathbf{U}_1(7\,|\,3)\mathbf{R}_2\mathbf{U}_2(7\,|\,3)\mathbf{R}_3\mathbf{U}_3(4)\mathbf{U}_3(3)\mathbf{U}_3(2)\mathbf{U}_3(1)\\
\boldsymbol{\pi}_3(7;7) &= r(0;7)\mathbf{p}\mathbf{U}_1(7\,|\,3)\mathbf{R}_2\mathbf{U}_2(7\,|\,3)\mathbf{R}_3\mathbf{U}_3(4)\mathbf{U}_3(3)\mathbf{U}_3(2)\mathbf{U}_3(1)\mathbf{U}_3(0).
\end{aligned}$$

Comparing this to the previous set, we see that only $\mathbf{U}_3(4)$ must be calculated from (6.3.6c), but using this matrix, the matrices $\mathbf{U}_1(7\,|\,3)$ and $\mathbf{U}_2(7\,|\,3)$ must be calculated recursively by (6.3.6c), starting from $\mathbf{U_3}(7\,|\,3) = \mathbf{U_3}(4)$. We must also calculate

$$sum = 1 + \mathbf{p}\mathbf{U_1}(7\,|\,3)\,\boldsymbol{\epsilon}_1',$$

$$\mathbf{x_3} = \mathbf{p}\mathbf{U_1}(7\,|\,3)\,\mathbf{U_2}(7\,|\,3)\,\mathbf{R_3},$$

and

$$\mathbf{K_3}(7) = \mathbf{I_3} + \mathbf{U_3}(4)\,\mathbf{K_3}(6),$$

to get

$$\frac{1}{r(0;7)} = sum + \mathbf{x_3}\,\mathbf{K_3}(7)\,\boldsymbol{\epsilon}_3'.$$

Note that $\boldsymbol{\pi}_2(2;N)$ can be thought of as either the last of the set of vectors which do not use the $\mathbf{R_3}(n-C)$ matrices, or by multiplying it by $\mathbf{R_3}\,\mathbf{I_3}$ (remember that $\mathbf{R_3}\,\boldsymbol{\epsilon}_3' = \boldsymbol{\epsilon}_2'$), the first among those that do. In defining $\mathbf{K_3}(N)$, we have put it in the latter class. That is where the $\mathbf{I_3}$ came from.

It might prove useful for future reference to write down the first few $\boldsymbol{\pi}_\mathbf{k}$ vectors for arbitrary C. Let $N_c := N-C$ and recall that $\mathbf{U_c}(N\,|\,C) = \mathbf{U_c}(N_c)$. Then (with one equation number assigned to the whole collection)

$$\begin{array}{rcl}
\boldsymbol{\pi}_1(0;N) & = & r(0;N)\mathbf{p} \\
\boldsymbol{\pi}_1(1;N) & = & r(0;N)\mathbf{p}\mathbf{U_1}(N\,|\,C) \\
\boldsymbol{\pi}_2(2;N) & = & r(0;N)\mathbf{p}\mathbf{U_1}(N\,|\,C)\mathbf{R_2}\mathbf{U_2}(N\,|\,C) \\
\cdots & . & \cdots \\
\boldsymbol{\pi}_\mathbf{c}(C;N) & = & r(0;N)\mathbf{p}\mathbf{U_1}(N\,|\,C)\mathbf{R_2}\mathbf{U_2}(N\,|\,C)\cdots\mathbf{R_c}\mathbf{U_c}(N_c) \\
\\
\boldsymbol{\pi}_\mathbf{c}(C+1;N) & = & \boldsymbol{\pi}_\mathbf{c}(C;N)\mathbf{U_c}(N_c-1) \\
\boldsymbol{\pi}_\mathbf{c}(C+2;N) & = & \boldsymbol{\pi}_\mathbf{c}(C;N)\mathbf{U_c}(N_c-1)\mathbf{U_c}(N_c-2) \\
\boldsymbol{\pi}_\mathbf{c}(C+3;N) & = & \boldsymbol{\pi}_\mathbf{c}(C;N)\mathbf{U_c}(N_c-1)\mathbf{U_c}(N_c-2)\mathbf{U_c}(N_c-3) \\
\cdots & . & \cdots \\
\boldsymbol{\pi}_\mathbf{c}(C+n;N) & = & \boldsymbol{\pi}_\mathbf{c}(C;N)\mathbf{U_c}(N_c-1)\cdots\mathbf{U_c}(N_c-n).
\end{array} \tag{6.3.12}$$

In general, to calculate the characteristics of any system for one more value of N requires an inversion of one matrix of each of the dimensions $D(1) \times D(1)$, $D(2) \times D(2)$, ..., and $D(C) \times D(C)$. But $D(C)$ is usually much larger than $D(k)$ ($k < C$), so only $\mathbf{U_c}(N-C)$ is computationally significant. For most matrix inversion routines the number of instructional steps required is proportional to the cube of the dimensions of the matrix, which in our case is of order $[D(C)]^3$. Now, matrix multiplication is also of the order $[D(C)]^3$, and it would seem that we need $N-C$ of them (plus other multiplications of lower order). But (6.3.10b) tells us that we can perform our calculations by multiplying matrices on vectors, which is only of order $[D(C)]^2$. In summary, the total computational effort for evaluating an M/ME/C//N network for all customer populations from $N = C+1$ to some maximum $N = N_{mx}$ is

$$\mathrm{O}\left((N_{mx}-C)[D(C)]^3\right) + \mathrm{O}\left([N_{mx}]^2[D(C)]^2\right).$$

The normalization matrix can be calculated recursively by

$$\mathbf{K_c}(C-1) := \mathbf{I_c}, \tag{6.3.13a}$$

and for $N = C, C+1, \ldots, N_{mx}$,

$$\mathbf{K_c}(N) = \mathbf{I_c} + \mathbf{U_c}(N-C)\,\mathbf{K_c}(N-1). \tag{6.3.13b}$$

With this matrix, (6.3.11d) can be rewritten in two forms, depending on whether the term corresponding to $n = C-1$ is included in the first term or the second.

$$\frac{1}{r(0;N)} = \sum_{k=0}^{C-1} \mathbf{x_k}(N \,|\, C)\boldsymbol{\epsilon}'_{\mathbf{k}} + \mathbf{x_c}(C;N)\mathbf{K_c}(N-1)\boldsymbol{\epsilon}'_{\mathbf{c}}, \tag{6.3.13c}$$

or

$$\frac{1}{r(0;N)} = \sum_{k=0}^{C-2} \mathbf{x_k}(N \,|\, C)\boldsymbol{\epsilon}'_{\mathbf{k}} + \mathbf{x_{c-1}}(N \,|\, C)\mathbf{R_c}\,\mathbf{K_c}(N)\boldsymbol{\epsilon}'_{\mathbf{c}}. \tag{6.3.13d}$$

It is yet to be seen which one is ultimately better for algorithmic development. However, only (6.3.13c) reduces directly to the M/ME/1//N loop for $C = 1$.

Clearly [Equation (6.3.1)],

$$D(C) = \binom{m+C-1}{C} = \frac{(m+C-1)!}{C!(m-1)!}$$

is the critical number that determines whether the calculation of a given system is feasible. The inversion of matrices with dimension 300 is a small effort for today's medium-sized computers, even for supermicros, particularly those with array processors or parallel multiprocessors. However, a 10,000-dimensional matrix, although manageable, would be somewhat of a challenge, partly because such a matrix would require 400 megabytes of storage in main memory (remember, N_c matrices are needed, and paging, or swapping, them in and out could make the calculation extremely slow).

Simple manipulation of the binomial coefficients shows that if either m or C is small, the other can be quite large without exceeding these bounds. A subsystem containing four identical servers ($C = 4$) can be solved with relative ease if each server has no more than eight phases ($m = 8$), even with as many as 100 customers ($N_{mx} = 100$), for then $D = 330$. However, a system with $m = 10$ and $C = 5$ ($D = 2002$) would require over 200 times as much computer time. Increasing m by only one to 11 would increase D another 50% to 3003, and over another factor of 3 in computation time. The significance of this is that a small increase in C or m causes a great increase in the time (and space) required to do a calculation. Every year new computers come on the market that are bigger, faster, and cheaper than the previous year's, yet each can boast only a small increase in the soluble problem space. The skeptical reader should try some larger values for C and m, to see how easy it would be to saturate all the computers in existence. The numerical (as opposed to analytical) study of much larger systems must wait until a way is found to decompose the various matrices into smaller parts.

6.3.2 Alternate Representation of M/ME/C//N Systems

We mentioned in the preceding section that an alternative definition of our state spaces was available, and in fact more useful in the long run. The one we gave, however, was more concise and simpler to start with. Observe that if we have $k \leq C$ customers in S_1, where the C servers are identical, and the k customers are indistinguishable, we only have to know how many customers are at each phase. Consider the following set.

Definition 6.3.7

For $1 \leq k \leq C$,

$$\Xi_k := \{i = \langle \alpha_1, \alpha_2, \ldots, \alpha_m \rangle \,|\, 0 \leq \alpha_l \leq k, \text{ and } \sum_{l=1}^{m} \alpha_l = k\}.$$

Ξ_k is the set of all internal states of S_1 when there are k active customers there. Each ordered m-tuple represents a state in which $k \leq C$ customers are active in a subsystem S_1, which has C identical servers in it. There are α_1 customers at phase 1, α_2 customers at phase 2, and so on, each in a different server. They never get in each other's way, because there are at least as many servers as there are customers. If there are more than C customers at S_1, the excess numbers must queue up outside. □

Our claim is that this definition is equivalent to Definition 6.3.1, in that there is a one-to-one mapping of the states in the two sets onto each other. We show this most easily by the following example. Suppose that $m = 5$ and that $k = 4$; then a typical state using Definition 6.3.1 would be

$$\{2, 2, 4, 5\} \qquad (i_1 = i_2 = 2,\ i_3 = 4, \text{ and } i_4 = 5).$$

This means that one of the customers is at phase 2 of one of the servers, another customer is also at phase 2, but in another server, a third customer is at phase 4 in yet another server, and the fourth customer is at phase 5. Therefore, there are no customers at phase 1 ($\alpha_1 = 0$) in any of the servers, there are two customers at phase 2 in two of the servers ($\alpha_2 = 2$), one at phase 4 ($\alpha_4 = 1$), and one at phase 5 ($\alpha_5 = 1$). That is, the following two ordered sequences give us the same information and are therefore equivalent:

$$\{2, 2, 4, 5\} \equiv \langle 0, 2, 0, 1, 1 \rangle.$$

Definitions 6.3.2 to 6.3.6 are all the same, but the various matrix elements can be computed differently. For instance, Definition 6.3.2 can be changed to read: Let $i = \langle \alpha_1, \alpha_2, \ldots, \alpha_m \rangle \in \Xi_k$; then

$$[\mathbf{M_k}]_{ii} = \alpha_1\mu_1 + \alpha_2\mu_2 + \cdots + \alpha_m\mu_m = \sum_{\nu=1}^{m} \alpha_\nu \mu_\nu.$$

Note that each of the objects, $i = \langle \alpha_1, \alpha_2, \ldots, \alpha_m \rangle$ can be thought of as a vector with m components [not to be confused with our row or column vectors of dimension $D(k)$]. Thus subtraction of any two vectors, even from different spaces, is well defined, because they all have the same number of components. But to keep our notation clear, we write the following instead of $(i - j)$. Suppose that we have $i \in \Xi_{k_1}$ with components α_l, and $j \in \Xi_{k_2}$ with components β_l; then we write

$$[\langle i\rangle - \langle j\rangle]_l := \nu_l := \alpha_l - \beta_l,$$

where the following sums are true,

$$\sum_{l=1}^{m} \nu_l = \sum_{l=1}^{m} \alpha_l - \sum_{l=1}^{m} \beta_l = k_1 - k_2.$$

We do not want to get too elaborate with our notation, but we need some definiteness to calculate the other matrix elements.

Look at Definition 6.3.4. $[\mathbf{R_k}]_{ij}$ is zero unless all but one of the components of $[\langle j\rangle - \langle i\rangle]$ is zero, in which case the nonzero element would have the value 1. Let ν be the component that is not 0; then $[\mathbf{R_k}]_{ij}$ is given by (6.3.2a), the same as before.

Next look at Definition 6.3.5. $[\mathbf{Q_k}]_{ij}$ is zero unless all but one of the components of $[\langle i\rangle - \langle j\rangle]$ is zero, in which case the nonzero element would have the value 1. Let ν be the component that is not 0; then $[\mathbf{Q_k}]_{ij}$ is given by (6.3.2b), where α_ν is component ν of $\langle i\rangle$. This is exactly the same as before.

Finally, look at Definition 6.3.6. As with the others, $[\mathbf{P_k}]_{ij} := 0$, unless $[\langle i\rangle - \langle j\rangle]$ has exactly two nonzero elements, one with the value 1 and the other with the value -1. This is nothing more than stating that only one customer can move at a time, and he can only go to one new phase. Let γ be the member of $[\langle i\rangle - \langle j\rangle]$ which is 1 (that is, the phase the customer left), and let ν be the member of $[\langle i\rangle - \langle j\rangle]$ which is -1 (that is the phase to which he went). Also, let α_γ be the γth component of $\langle i\rangle$, then just as we did for the two previous matrices, $[\mathbf{P_k}]_{ij}$ is given by (6.3.2c). Once again this is identical to what we had before, including the meaning of α_ν. We can also include the possibility that $[\mathbf{P}]_{ii} \neq 0$. Let the discussion above be true for $\langle i\rangle \neq \langle j\rangle$. Then for $[\langle i\rangle = \langle j\rangle]$, we have

$$[\mathbf{P_k}]_{ii} = \frac{1}{[\mathbf{M_k}]_{ii}} \sum_{\gamma=1}^{m} [\mathbf{P_1}]_{\gamma\gamma} \alpha_\gamma \, \mu_\gamma.$$

Note that if all the diagonal elements of $\mathbf{P_1}$ are zero, so are all the diagonal elements of $\mathbf{P_k}$.

6.3.3 Generalized M/ME/C//N System

What, you may ask, have we gained by the notational change in the previous section? Well, first of all, it is easier to program. Second, we see that in all expressions for the components of matrix elements, α_ν and μ_ν always appear together as a product. Now let us define load-dependent completion rates for each of the phases in a server.

Definition 6.3.8

$\mu_\nu(l)$ = probability rate that one of the customers at phase ν will complete, given that there are l customers at that phase. Note that there is no distinction between having k identical servers, and only one server whose phases are load dependent. □

How interesting. We can either think of S_1 as a subsystem with C identical servers, each with m phases, or as one server with m phases, where each phase has a completion rate that depends on the number of customers in S_1 who are at that phase.

Now comes the generalization. Why must $\mu_\nu(l)$ be equal to $l \cdot \mu_\nu$, where ν is one of the m phases? If we want to study an M/ME/C//N loop, it must, but if we let $\mu_\nu(l)$ be anything greater than 0, the equations we have derived remain unchanged! Given this new freedom, what have we got? This is described by the following. The word *loop* has such a limited connotation that we are changing to the word *system*, which sounds much broader in scope. Also, the distinction between *server* and *phase* has become confused, so we now use the word *server* or *stage*, and drop *phase*, in order to conform to the terminology associated with Jackson networks. The reader is thus entitled to think of the internal components of S_1 as real things.

Definition 6.3.9

Generalized M/ME/C//N system := a two-subsystem loop in which S_2 is an exponential server (perhaps load dependent), and S_1 is a network of load-dependent exponential servers satisfying the following rules. No more than C customers can be active inside S_1 at a time. If there are more than C customers at S_1 the excess numbers queue up outside. If there are fewer than C customers present, an arriving customer enters immediately. When a customer leaves, a new one, if available, enters. A customer upon entering S_1 goes directly to server ν with probability $[\mathbf{p}]_\nu$. The probability rate of leaving a server is $\mu_\nu(l)$, where l is the number of customers at server ν. If a completion occurs at ν, then with probability $[\mathbf{P_1}]_{\nu\gamma}$ a customer goes to server γ, and with probability $[\mathbf{q}]_\nu$ leaves S_1. □

We summarize this with a theorem.

Theorem 6.3.3: The steady-state vectors for a generalized M/ME/C//N system, with $N > C$, are given by Theorem 6.3.2 with the matrices $\mathbf{M_k}$, $\mathbf{P_k}$, $\mathbf{R_k}$, and $\mathbf{Q_k}$ modified as follows. For $1 \le k \le C$, let

$$\langle i \rangle = \langle \alpha_1, \alpha_2, \ldots, \alpha_\nu, \ldots, \alpha_m \rangle \in \Xi_k,$$

where $\alpha_\nu \ge 0$ and $\sum_{\nu=1}^{m} \alpha_\nu = k$. $\mathbf{M_k}$ is a diagonal matrix with components

$$[\mathbf{M_k}]_{ii} = \sum_{\nu=1}^{m} \mu_\nu(\alpha_\nu). \tag{6.3.14a}$$

$[\mathbf{P_k}]_{ij}$, for $i, j \in \Xi_k$, is zero unless $i = j$ or $[\langle i \rangle - \langle j \rangle]$ has one 1 (at position γ) and one -1 (at position ν), the rest being 0. If this is satisfied, then

$$[\mathbf{P_k}]_{ij} = [\mathbf{P_1}]_{\gamma\nu} \frac{\mu_\gamma(\alpha_\gamma)}{[\mathbf{M_k}]_{ii}} \quad \text{for } i \neq j \tag{6.3.14b}$$

and

$$[\mathbf{P_k}]_{ii} = \frac{1}{[\mathbf{M_k}]_{ii}} \sum_{\gamma=1}^{m} [\mathbf{P_1}]_{\gamma\gamma}\, \mu_\gamma(\alpha_\gamma). \tag{6.3.14c}$$

$[\mathbf{R_k}]_{ij}$, for $i \in \Xi_{k-1}$, $j \in \Xi_k$, is zero unless $[\langle j\rangle - \langle i\rangle]$ has one 1 (at position ν) and the rest are 0. If this is satisfied, then

$$[\mathbf{R_k}]_{ij} = p_\nu. \tag{6.3.14d}$$

$[\mathbf{Q_k}]_{ij}$, for $i \in \Xi_k$, $j \in \Xi_{k-1}$, is zero unless $[\langle i\rangle - \langle j\rangle]$ has one 1 (at position ν) and the rest are all 0. If this is satisfied, then

$$[\mathbf{Q_k}]_{ij} := \frac{\mu_\nu(\alpha_\nu) q_\nu}{[\mathbf{M_k}]_{ii}}. \tag{6.3.14e}$$

If $\mu_\nu(l) = l \cdot \mu_\nu$ for all $0 \le l \le C$ and all $1 \le \nu \le m$, this reduces to an M/ME/C//N loop. ■

Observe that if one or more of the servers is load independent [i.e., if $\mu_\nu(l) = \mu_\nu$ for all l], queueing delays can actually occur inside S_1. The description just given, except for the queueing up outside S_1, is identical to that for Jackson networks. We discuss that in the next section.

With the system described in this way, we can see how ***processor sharing*** queues fit in. Recall from the beginning of Section 5.4 that, using this discipline, some or all the customers at S_1 get equal access to a single server. Suppose there are k customers sharing the server, then each one must be tracked according to his progress in S_1. However, each customer can only get $(1/k)$th the resources. Now if no more than C customers are permitted to share at a time, then we have an M/G/C//N system with the following specifications. The matrices, $\mathbf{M_k}$, $\mathbf{P_k}$, $\mathbf{R_k}$, and $\mathbf{Q_k}$, $k = 1, 2, \ldots, C$, are given by Theorem 6.3.3, where $\mu_\nu(l) = l\,\mu_\nu$, (i.e., the system is not a generalized one). Equations (6.3.6c) and (6.3.7b) are modified by replacing $\mathbf{M_k}$ and $\mathbf{B_k}$, with $(1/k)\mathbf{M_k}$ and $(1/k)\mathbf{B_k}$, respectively. If S_1 is made up of, say, C_1 identical general servers, where $1 \le C_1 < C$, then (6.3.6c) and (6.3.7b) are only modified for $k > C_1$, in which case, use (C_1/k) instead of $(1/k)$.

For $\mathbf{U_c}(n)$, (6.3.6c) tells us that these substitutions are equivalent to replacing λ with $\lambda\, C/C_1$. The same cannot be said for $\mathbf{U_k}(N \mid C)$, because $\mathbf{B_k}$ and $\mathbf{M_{k+1}}$ appear together in (6.3.7b). All this leaves us with a little unsolved mystery. We know that the steady-state solution of an unconstrained network where the general servers use processor sharing is the same as a network with exponential servers. Therefore, if $C \ge N$, our steady-state formulas should collapse to the M/M/C_1//N loop. It would be nice if we could explicitly show that our matrices have this property.

We end this subject with the following summary statement. The *unrestricted* processor sharing queue $[C \geq N]$ is simpler than the M/G/1 queue, but ***restricted processor sharing*** $[C < N]$, is harder, at least for steady state conditions.

6.3.4 Relation to Jackson Networks

It cannot be emphasized too strongly that the generalized M/ME/C//N system can be applied to arbitrarily large networks, limited by their computational difficulty, containing the Jackson networks as a proper subset. In case you are not quite sure what Jackson networks are, you may consider the following theorem as their definition.

Theorem 6.3.4: The steady-state solution of a single-class Jackson network with $m+1$ load-dependent servers and C customers is the same as that for a generalized M/ME/C//C system ($N = C$), where ME has an m-dimensional representation. The $(m+1)$st server is at S_2. Let y_ν be the νth component of $\mathbf{y} := \mathbf{p}(\mathbf{I_1} - \mathbf{P_1})^{-1} = \mathbf{p}\mathbf{V_1}\mathbf{M_1}$, normalized so that $\mathbf{y}\,\boldsymbol{\epsilon}' = 1$. Then, the steady-state solution vectors for both are given by

$$[\pi_{\mathbf{k}}(k;C)]_i = g(C)X_1(\alpha_1)\cdots X_m(\alpha_m)\left(\frac{1}{\lambda}\right)^{C-k}, \tag{6.3.15a}$$

where $\langle i\rangle = \langle \alpha_1, \alpha_2, \ldots, \alpha_\nu, \ldots, \alpha_m\rangle \in \Xi_k$, $X_\nu(0) := 1$, and

$$X_\nu(l) := \frac{y_\nu^l}{\mu_\nu(1)\mu_\nu(2)\cdots\mu_\nu(l)} = X_\nu(l-1)\frac{y_\nu}{\mu_\nu(l)}. \tag{6.3.15b}$$

$g(C)$ is a normalization constant, fixed to make the probabilities sum to 1. As written here, S_2 is load independent. That limitation is not necessary. ■

If ν is a load-independent server, then $X_\nu(l) = (y_\nu/\mu_\nu)^l = [(\mathbf{p}\mathbf{V_1})_\nu]^l$, but if $\mu_\nu(l) = l\,\mu_\nu$, (6.3.15b) becomes

$$X_\nu(l) = \frac{1}{l!}\left(\frac{y_\nu}{\mu_\nu}\right)^l = \frac{1}{l!}\left[(\mathbf{p_1}\mathbf{V_1})_\nu\right]^l.$$

This corresponds to a *delay* stage (discussed below). We used objects similar to $X_\nu(l)$ in discussing load-dependent servers in Section 2.1.5; however, the notation used there was somewhat different.

The ***product-form solution*** for Jackson networks (as given above) is already well known and simpler to set up than our matrix formulation. You can see now why we never bothered to look at algorithms for calculating the solutions in the earlier discussions. However, the product solution *is **not** valid* for systems for which $N > C$, that is, when there are ***constraints*** on the number of customers who can be simultaneously active in S_1. In that case, our procedure cannot be avoided. There is a standard approximation that is used in modeling networks, but it is not known how accurate it is in general. We give an example of this in the next section. For details about applying Jackson networks to computer performance see, e.g., [LAZOWSKAETAL84] or [KANT92].

As a last comment in this section, observe that it is the constraint on population activity that causes our problems to grow to "matrix" proportions. That, in turn, subtly depends on the dimensionality function $D(k)$. Further discussion in this direction is outside the scope of this book, except to note that population constraints are special cases of ***blocking*** (e.g., activity at one node may prevent activity at another node), which also lies outside this book. See, for example, [PERROS94]

6.3.5 Time-Sharing Systems with Population Constraints

The last generalization we can make to our loop without greatly increasing the mathematical complexity of our model was already alluded to in the preceding section. We can make S_2 into a load-dependent server. This slight change turns out to give a potentially powerful tool for studying the behavior of time-sharing systems, as well as other systems with population constraints. Furthermore, the computational complexity is not changed. First we look at the changes that we must make to the formulas, and then we look at an application.

We only need to look at those formulas containing λ, which is now $\lambda(l)$, for $l = 1, 2, \ldots$. Therefore, the matrices $\mathbf{M_k}$, $\mathbf{P_k}$, $\mathbf{R_k}$, and $\mathbf{Q_k}$ are unchanged. Only the matrices $\mathbf{U_k}(N \mid C)$ and $\mathbf{U_c}(n)$ must be modified. What we have to do is combine what we did in Section 5.4.1 with what we have here. The reader may go through the complete derivation alone; we only make some observations. Start with the balance equations (6.3.5) and replace each λ with $\lambda(Ni-n)$, where n is the first argument in $\pi_\mathbf{c}(n;\, N)$, and so on. Remember, n is the number of customers at S_1, but $\lambda(\cdot)$ depends on the number of customers at S_2. This leads to the following modified solutions [compare with (6.3.6a) and (6.3.6c)].

$$\mathbf{U_c}(0) = \lambda(1)\mathbf{V_c}, \tag{6.3.16a}$$

and for $l \geq 1$

$$\mathbf{U_c}(l) = \lambda(l+1)[\mathbf{B_c} + \lambda(l)\mathbf{I_c} - \mathbf{U_c}(l-1)\mathbf{M_c}\,\mathbf{Q_c}\,\mathbf{R_c}]^{-1}. \tag{6.3.16b}$$

Also, (6.3.7a) remains unchanged, and (6.3.7b) changes to

$$\mathbf{U_k}(N \mid C) :=$$

$$\lambda(N-k+1)[\mathbf{B_k} + \lambda(N-k)\mathbf{I_k} - \mathbf{R_{k+1}}\mathbf{U_{k+1}}(N \mid C)\mathbf{M_{k+1}}\mathbf{Q_{k+1}}]^{-1}. \tag{6.3.16c}$$

For $N \leq C$, Theorem 6.3.4 is changed by replacing the λ term in (6.3.15a) with $1/[\lambda(1)\lambda(2)\cdots\lambda(C-k)]$, the λ equivalent of (6.3.15b). That is it. Nothing else changes. A close look at (6.3.6b) shows that $\mathbf{U_c}(l)$ really depends on the number of customers at S_2 (remember, we started at the top), just as $\lambda(l)$ does, so that is all that we have to change. Tehranipour [TEHRANIPOUR83],

[TEHRANIPOURVDLLIP89] was the first one to recognize this. Let us see what that allows us to do. Consider a system with N customers. When a customer is at S_2, he spends some time thinking about what to do, and after a mean time of Z (exponentially distributed) joins the queue at S_1. After a mean time of $R(N)$ he leaves S_1 and returns to S_2, starting the process over again. Z is known as the ***think time***, and $R(N)$ is called the ***response time*** for the process. The probability rate for him to leave S_2, given that he is there thinking, is $1/Z$. If there are ℓ (independently) thinking customers at S_2, the probability rate for any one of them to leave is simply ℓZ. In other words, S_2 is a load-dependent server with service rate

$$\lambda(\ell) = \frac{\ell}{Z}.$$

That is why a server with this kind of behavior is often called a ***think stage***. It also shows up as the description of failures in the ***machine minding model***. Here, any number of machines are running simultaneously and independently of each other, and the rate at which they break down is proportional to the number running. It is also referred to as a ***delay stage***, because customers can pause somewhere (not counting their waiting in a queue) independently of each other.

The view we take here is that of computer users who sit at their terminals and think (no comments, please), or type, and every once in a while hit the "return" key, which sends their prepared ***transactions*** to an external computer network, which they share. It is assumed that they do nothing while they wait for the computer system's response. Drinking coffee or talking to a friend does not count as doing anything, nor does any activity, however productive, that is not related to system usage. This is then a ***time-sharing stage*** (TS) in a ***time-sharing computer system***. Let $L(N)$ be the r.v. denoting the number of customers who are at S_2 at any time, in a network with N customers. From Little's formula (1.1.2) we see that $\mathbb{E}[L(N)]$ is related to the mean rate at which transactions are processed [call it the ***throughput***, with the symbol $\Lambda(N)$] by

$$\mathbb{E}[L(N)] = \Lambda(N)Z,$$

given that Z is the mean time each customer spends at S_2 between transaction submittals. On the other hand, the mean number of transactions that are being processed (or waiting to be processed) at any time must be equal to $N - \mathbb{E}[L(N)]$, and is related to the same throughput by the following version of Little's formula,

$$N - \mathbb{E}[L(N)] = \Lambda(N)R(N),$$

given that $R(N)$ is the mean time a transaction spends at S_1. If we add the two equations above together and solve for $R(N)$, we get the ***fundamental formula for TS systems*** which we state as a theorem.

Theorem 6.3.5: Consider a ***time-sharing system*** as described above. Then the mean response time is given by:

$$R(N) = \frac{N}{\Lambda(N)} - Z. \tag{6.3.17}$$

This equation is as general as Little's formula and tells us some general things about TS systems. (Be careful, though. There are numerous counterexamples that show up just when you least expect.) For instance, when N becomes very large (i.e., when too many users try to access the same computer system simultaneously), S_1 saturates, so the throughput reaches a limiting value,

$$\Lambda := \lim_{N\to\infty} \Lambda(N).$$

Then we see, for large N,

$$R(N) \approx \frac{1}{\Lambda}N - Z.$$

If $\Lambda(N) - \Lambda = O(1/N)$ for large N, then this equation must be modified. See [LipTehrvdLLieu82] for details and examples. ■

In other words, $R(N)$ approaches a straight line whose slope is $1/\Lambda$ and whose y-intercept is $-Z$. At the other extreme, $R(1)$ is the amount of time it should take, on average, for a single transaction to be processed if there is no interference from other tasks. Without too much difficulty, a reasonably good performance modeler should be able to find a satisfactory value for $R(1)$, Λ, and Z. Then all one has to do to get a decent understanding of the performance of the particular time-sharing system is to draw a smooth curve that starts at the point $[1, R(1)]$ and asymptotically approaches the line $x/\Lambda - Z$. Figure 6.3.1 shows several possible ways to do this. Clearly, if we really know what those three parameters are, we know the ballpark we are playing in, but do we know the game we are playing? As you can see, the different curves can differ by a factor of 10 or more in the intermediate region. Clearly, underutilized systems ($N = 1$) almost always perform well (users don't have to compete for resources), and overloaded systems are usually quite unsatisfactory, what planners want to know is: "How many users can a system support in a satisfactory manner?" So the name of the game is finding the right middle.

As long as there are no constraints on the number of transactions that can be processed simultaneously (i.e., when $N \leq C$), Jackson networks can be used quite effectively for performance modeling. However, it is well known that most systems will actually reduce their throughput if too many transactions are present, in a phenomenon known as ***thrashing***. Briefly, if the amount of main memory (or cache memory) is insufficient to hold all active transactions simultaneously, then as each task is given its slice of time to use the central processor (CPU), it must first reclaim its memory space. The more jobs active, the more time is spent reclaiming main memory. To counter this, well-run computer systems will restrict the number of tasks, or transactions (our customers) who can be active simultaneously. That is, they impose a ***population size constraint***, our parameter C.

Common techniques for dealing with constraints of this kind, called ***decomposition***, [Courtois77] or ***aggregation***, or simply the ***natural approximation***, [Lipsky80] effectively "short-circuit" S_1 so that k customers

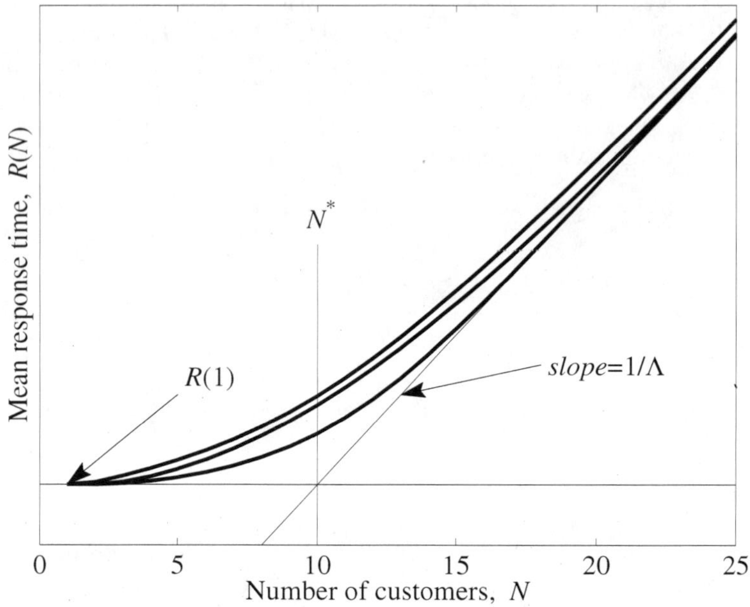

Figure 6.3.1: Response time curves for a family of time-sharing systems with the same value for minimal load $R(1)$, think-time Z, and asymptotic throughput Λ. All are bounded from below by the horizontal line, $y = R(1)$, and the asymptote $y = x/\Lambda - Z$. The intersection of those two lines occurs at $N^* = \Lambda[Z + R(1)]$. N^* is often taken as the number of customers that the TS system can support, but the response times for the different systems can vary enormously at that point.

return as soon as they leave. The rate at which they go around the loop is $\Lambda(k)$, k =1, 2, ... , C. Then S_1 is replaced by a load-dependent server with service rates as follows.

$$\mu(n) = \Lambda(n) \quad \text{for } n \leq C$$

and

$$\mu(n) = \Lambda(C) \quad \text{for } n \geq C.$$

We have seen a simple version of this in Section 4.4.4. The technique is so compelling that many practitioners think it is exact, which it is for those systems where Jackson networks are exact. But it is *not* exact for systems with population constraints! (This is why the author became involved in LAQT in the first place.)

Example 6.3.1: We have calculated response times for an $M/H_2/C//N$ loop, using the exact solution as given by Theorem 6.3.2 or Theorem 6.3.3, and its natural approximation. The calculations of $R(N)$ and $R_a(N)$ (a for approximation) versus N, for C = 1, 2, and 3, are given in Figure 6.3.2. As

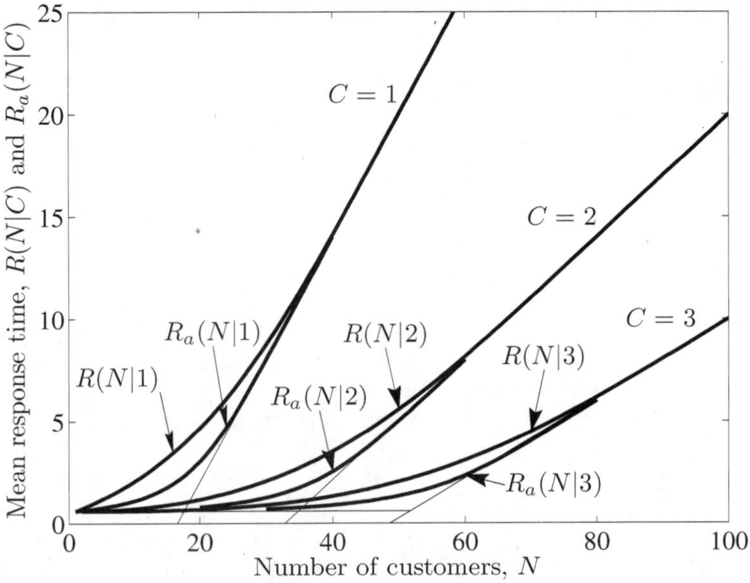

Figure 6.3.2: Response-time curves for a time-sharing system, where the computer subsystem (S_1) is taken to be C identical servers with hyperexponential distributions. The mean service time for each is $R(1) = 0.6$ seconds, with squared coefficient of variation of $C_v^2 = 9.0$. The think time is $Z = 10.0$ seconds. Three different values for C (1, 2, and 3) were used. The curves marked $R(N \mid C)$ are the exact calculations, and the curves marked $R_a(N|C)$ come from the natural, decomposition, aggregation (whatever) approximation. For all C and for all N, the approximation lies below the correct value.

one would expect, the asymptotic slope decreases with increasing C, because $\Lambda(C)$ increases with C. Note that the natural approximation always gives the right asymptotic slope and correct value for $R(1)$ (i.e., it is in the right ballpark), but it can be off by more than a factor of 2 where results are most important, in the intermediate region (it is playing the wrong game). In this case it always yields an overly optimistic result [i.e., $R_a(N) < R(N)$]. We do not really know if this would hold true for all systems. ▲

Although the decomposition method is used regularly, it is not known in general how good (or bad) an approximation it is, partly because system parameters change so rapidly due to technological improvements that most researchers have not had the time to carry out the exact calculations as described here. This is a pity, because LAQT can be used to explore the behavior of even more complicated queueing systems by, for instance, doing an aggregate approximation to S_2, while leaving S_1 as is. In this way one could study the interaction of two arbitrarily complicated subnetworks. Of course, we would not know how accurate that approximation is, but at the moment, we know almost nothing about such systems. Exact solution of such networks exist and fall under the more general name of ***Quasi Birth-Death*** **(QBD)**

processes. However, a full-blown calculation of that magnitude would require using matrices of the size $D_1(C_1) \times D_2(C_2)$. One can see from our discussion on computational complexity at the end of Section 6.3.1 that it could easily become intractable.

6.4 Open Generalized M/G/C Queue

The matrices $\mathbf{M_k}$, $\mathbf{P_k}$, $\mathbf{Q_k}$, $\mathbf{R_k}$, $\mathbf{B_k}$, and $\mathbf{V_k}$, for $k = 1, 2, \ldots, C$, which we tediously described and showed how to build from $\mathbf{M_1}$, $\mathbf{P_1}$, and $\mathbf{p}$ (and the load-dependence factors) in the preceding section, are the only building blocks we need for the rest of this chapter. If that already seems like too much, rest assured that we could not do it with less. We need that much information just to describe such complicated systems.

The procedure for "opening" our loop is the same as always. If the maximal service rate of S_1 is greater than λ, then as N becomes larger, the probability that S_2 will be idle goes to 0. "But what *is* the maximal rate?" you ask. The answer must wait until the next section. For now we assume that the appropriate conditions are satisfied, in which case S_2 behaves as a Poisson source of customers to S_1. It would be expected that the limit as N goes to infinity of $\mathbf{U_c}(N)$ exists, and from (6.3.6c), satisfies the equation

$$\mathbf{U_c} := \lim_{N\to\infty} \mathbf{U_c}(N) = \lambda \left[\lambda \mathbf{I_c} + \mathbf{B_c} - \mathbf{U_c M_c Q_c R_c}\right]^{-1}. \tag{6.4.1}$$

We ran across a formula like this in Equations (5.5.6). There is no known explicit expression for $\mathbf{U_c}$ except when $C = 1$. In that case we are dealing with the M/ME/1 queue, and we know that $\mathbf{U_1}$ is $\mathbf{U}$ of Equations (4.1.4). One way to find the numerical value for a matrix that satisfies the equation is to iterate on $\mathbf{U_c}$. That is, keep calculating $\mathbf{U_c}(C)$, $\mathbf{U_c}(C+1)$, $\mathbf{U_c}(C+2)$, and so on, until no changes are perceived. There are faster methods available if one is not interested in the sequence of finite systems [WALLACE69]. Anyway, suppose that $\mathbf{U_c}$ is known.Then

$$\mathbf{U_c}(\infty \,|\, C) := \lim_{N\to\infty} \mathbf{U_c}(N \,|\, C) = \mathbf{U_c}$$

and calculate $\mathbf{U_1}(\infty \,|\, C)$, $\mathbf{U_2}(\infty \,|\, C), \ldots$, and $\mathbf{U_{c-1}}(\infty \,|\, C)$ using (6.3.7b). That is,

$$\mathbf{U_k}(\infty \,|\, C) := \lim_{N\to\infty} \mathbf{U_k}(N \,|\, C)$$

$$= \lambda \left[\lambda \mathbf{I_k} + \mathbf{B_k} - \mathbf{R_{k+1} U_{k+1}}(\infty \,|\, C)\mathbf{M_{k+1} Q_{k+1}}\right]^{-1}. \tag{6.4.2}$$

All the $\mathbf{U}$ matrices satisfy Lemma 6.3.1. Also, (6.3.10) of Theorem 6.3.2 remains valid with ∞ replacing N. Fortunately, (6.3.11) simplifies to

$$\mathbf{x_c}(C+n) := \lim_{N\to\infty} \mathbf{x_c}(n, N) = \mathbf{x_c}(C)\mathbf{U_c}^n, \tag{6.4.3a}$$

where

$$\mathbf{x_c}(C) := \mathbf{x_c}(\infty \,|\, C). \tag{6.4.3b}$$

Then the steady-state solution vectors are given by the following.

$$\boldsymbol{\pi}_{\mathbf{k}}(k) = r(0)\mathbf{x}_{\mathbf{k}}(\infty \,|\, C) \quad \text{for } 0 \le k \le C \tag{6.4.4a}$$

and

$$\boldsymbol{\pi}_{\mathbf{c}}(n) = r(0)\mathbf{x}_{\mathbf{c}}(n) = r(0)\mathbf{x}_{\mathbf{c}}(C)\mathbf{U}_{\mathbf{c}}{}^{n-c} \quad \text{for } C \le n. \tag{6.4.4b}$$

The associated scalar probabilities are, of course,

$$r(n) = \boldsymbol{\pi}_{\mathbf{k}}(n)\boldsymbol{\epsilon}'_{\mathbf{k}}, \tag{6.4.4c}$$

where $k = n$ for $n \le C$ and $k = C$ otherwise. $r(0)$ comes from the normalization

$$\frac{1}{r(0)} = \sum_{k=0}^{C-1} \mathbf{x}_{\mathbf{k}}(\infty \,|\, C)\boldsymbol{\epsilon}'_{\mathbf{k}} + \sum_{n=C}^{\infty} \mathbf{x}_{\mathbf{c}}(n)\boldsymbol{\epsilon}'_{\mathbf{c}}.$$

We finally get a break. The vectors $\mathbf{x}_{\mathbf{c}}(n)$ are related by matrix geometric formulas, so we can write a closed-form expression for the infinite sum. That is,

$$\frac{1}{r(0)} = \sum_{k=0}^{C-1} \mathbf{x}_{\mathbf{k}}(\infty \,|\, C)\boldsymbol{\epsilon}'_{\mathbf{k}} + \mathbf{x}_{\mathbf{c}}(C)[\mathbf{I}_{\mathbf{c}} - \mathbf{U}_{\mathbf{c}}]^{-1}\boldsymbol{\epsilon}'_{\mathbf{c}}. \tag{6.4.5}$$

The wonderful geometric property, which occurs so often in queueing systems is, almost assuredly, the major reason why researchers have studied open systems more than closed systems. They are easier.

6.5 Transient Generalized M/ME/C Queue

Our final topic for this chapter is, as usual, transient behavior. It is surprising, considering how complex generalized M/ME/C systems are, that what we did in previous chapters extends so easily here. It is also nice to know that everything we can do on this subject depends only on the matrices we have already created, not on their details. However, we do not go into it in such depth, leaving the untouched topics as exercises.

6.5.1 Queue Reduction at S_1 with No New Arrivals

First we must verify the physical meanings of our basic matrices. We were beginning to see in Chapter 5 that it was not always simple to decide what state a system is in initially. We have worse problems here, although sometimes we can come up with interesting answers. For instance, we know that if a system has been running a long time unobserved, we may presume that it is in its steady state. Suppose at some moment there are n customers at S_1, with k customers active. So, $k = C$ if $n \ge C$, and $k = n$ if $n \le C$. We can assume that the system is, at that moment, in state,

$$\mathbf{p}_{\mathbf{ic}} = \frac{1}{r(n; N)}\boldsymbol{\pi}_{\mathbf{c}}(n; N) \quad \text{for } n \ge C, \tag{6.5.1a}$$

and

$$\mathbf{p_{ik}} = \frac{1}{r(k;N)} \boldsymbol{\pi}_\mathbf{k}(k;N) \quad \text{for } n = k \le C. \tag{6.5.1b}$$

The subscript **ik** stands for: **k**-space vector for the **i**nitial composite state. The $\boldsymbol{\pi}$ vectors come from Theorem 6.3.2 for the closed system and (6.4.4) for the open system. Obviously, $\mathbf{p_{ik}}\,\boldsymbol{\epsilon}'_\mathbf{k} = 1$. See Section 4.5.2 for a discussion of what is meant by this vector.

Next define the family of $D(k)$-dimensional row vectors,

$$\mathbf{p_k} := \mathbf{p}\mathbf{R_2}\mathbf{R_3}\cdots\mathbf{R_k} \quad \text{for } 2 \le k \le C.\text{¶} \tag{6.5.2a}$$

Because $\mathbf{R_k}\,\boldsymbol{\epsilon}'_\mathbf{k} = \boldsymbol{\epsilon}'_\mathbf{k-1}$, we see that $\mathbf{p_k}\,\boldsymbol{\epsilon}'_\mathbf{k} = 1$ for all k. Suppose now that the system was initially idle and suddenly n customers showed up en masse. Or suppose that the customers were already there, but S_1 was inoperative and then suddenly started up. The initial vector in this case is given by

$$\mathbf{p_{ik}} = \mathbf{p_k} \quad \text{for } n = k \le C, \tag{6.5.2b}$$

$$\mathbf{p_{ik}} = \mathbf{p_c} \quad \text{for } n \ge C, \tag{6.5.2c}$$

In the latter case there would be $n - C$ customers still waiting outside S_1. Physically, we see that the first customer enters and puts S_1 in composite state $\mathbf{p} \in \Xi_1$. Then the second customer enters and takes the subsystem from that state to $\mathbf{pR_2}$, and so on. How simple.

Next, let us suppose that the subsystem is initially in state $i \in \Xi_k$. How long will it take before someone leaves? Assume that the entryway to the queue at S_1 is shut off so that no new customers can enter. Let us give the symbol a formal definition.

Definition 6.5.1

$[\boldsymbol{\tau}'_\mathbf{k}]_i$:=*mean time until a customer leaves S_1, given that the subsystem was in state $i \in \Xi_k$ $(k \le C)$ and no new customers enter.* $\boldsymbol{\tau}'_\mathbf{k}$ is a $D(k)$-dimensional column vector. This describes a *collective* process, in that any one of the k customers could leave, and we do not know, or care, which. □

The $n = 1$ equivalent was discussed in Section 3.1.1, where we showed in (3.1.2b) that it was equal to $\mathbf{V}\boldsymbol{\epsilon}'$. We give an extension of that derivation here. The vector equation is as follows. If there are k customers in S_1, then

$$\boldsymbol{\tau}'_\mathbf{k} = \mathbf{M}_\mathbf{k}^{-1}\boldsymbol{\epsilon}'_\mathbf{k} + \mathbf{P_k}\,\boldsymbol{\tau}'_\mathbf{k}.$$

In words, the mean time until someone leaves $[\boldsymbol{\tau}'_\mathbf{k}]$ is equal to the sum of two terms; the time until something happens $[1/(\mathbf{M_k})_{ii} = (\mathbf{M}_\mathbf{k}^{-1}\boldsymbol{\epsilon}'_\mathbf{k})_i]$, and if the event did not result in a departure, the system goes to another state $[\mathbf{P_k}]$ and a customer leaves from there. Notice the words we used: "the system goes to another state." We could have said, instead, that "one of the k customers moves from one phase to another, thereby changing the state of S_1."

¶We could have, if we liked, let $\mathbf{R_1} := \mathbf{p_1} := \mathbf{p}$.

We solve for $\boldsymbol{\tau}'_{\mathbf{k}}$, and using (6.3.4a), with the understanding that if $n \geq C$, we are dealing with C-space objects (i.e., replace all subscripts k with C), we get

$$\boldsymbol{\tau}'_{\mathbf{k}} = \mathbf{V_k}\, \boldsymbol{\epsilon}'_{\mathbf{k}}. \tag{6.5.3}$$

Surprised? Of course not. In fact, we can even show that $\mathbf{B_k}$ is the generating matrix for the distribution of the time until someone leaves.

We do have a problem, though. Whereas for a single customer we had a natural candidate for the initial state, namely $\mathbf{p}$, which led to the description of a pdf, now we have many candidates. For instance, if S_1 just opened up and C customers flowed in, we are dealing with (6.5.2) for $\mathbf{p_{ic}}$, so the mean time until the first one leaves will be

$$\mathbf{p}\,\mathbf{R_2}\,\cdots\,\mathbf{R_c}\,\mathbf{V_c}\,\boldsymbol{\epsilon}'_{\mathbf{c}} = \mathbf{p_c}\,\mathbf{V_c}\,\boldsymbol{\epsilon}'_{\mathbf{c}}.$$

Furthermore, the density function (pdf) of the time for that epoch is given by

$$\mathbf{p_c}[\mathbf{B_c}\exp(-x\mathbf{B_c})]\boldsymbol{\epsilon}'_{\mathbf{c}}.$$

Other combinations are equally welcome. This does seem like the appropriate definition of interdeparture times, but when will the second customer leave? We have two possibilities, depending on whether the departed customer is replaced. We have not even begun to look at what happens if a customer enters S_1 before the first customer leaves. Let us postpone consideration of this last possibility, which falls into the category of first-passage times, and answer the intermediate question. "What state will the system be in immediately after the first customer leaves?" We define it as follows.

Definition 6.5.2

$[\mathbf{Y_k}]_{ij}$:=*probability that* S_1 *will be in internal state* $j \in \Xi_{k-1}$ *immediately after a departure, given that the system was initially in state* $i \in \Xi_k$*, and no other customers have entered.* $\mathbf{Y_k}$ is a $D(k) \times D(k-1)$-dimensional matrix, and is isometric, in that $\mathbf{Y_k}\,\boldsymbol{\epsilon}'_{\mathbf{k-1}} = \boldsymbol{\epsilon}'_{\mathbf{k}}$. By definition we are assuming that S_1 has exactly k active customers, thus $1 \leq k \leq C$. $\mathbf{Y_1} = \boldsymbol{\epsilon}'$, because when $k = 1$ a departing customer leaves the empty state behind. □

An equation for $\mathbf{Y_k}$ can be written down directly from the following argument. When an event occurs in S_1, either someone leaves $[\mathbf{Q_k}]$, or the internal state of the subsystem changes $[\mathbf{P_k}]$, and somebody eventually leaves $[\mathbf{Y_k}]$. Mathematically,

$$\mathbf{Y_k} = \mathbf{Q_k} + \mathbf{P_k}\mathbf{Y_k},$$

and solving for $\mathbf{Y_k}$, we get [using (6.3.4a)]

$$\mathbf{Y_k} = [\mathbf{I_k} - \mathbf{P_k}]^{-1}\mathbf{Q_k} = [\mathbf{I_k} - \mathbf{P_k}]^{-1}[\mathbf{M_k}]^{-1}\mathbf{M_k}\mathbf{Q_k} = \mathbf{V_k}\mathbf{M_k}\mathbf{Q_k}. \tag{6.5.4a}$$

[Compare with $\boldsymbol{\epsilon}' = (\mathbf{I} - \mathbf{P})^{-1}\mathbf{q}'$, Equation (3.1.1b), for $k = 1$.] Both the first and third versions of $\mathbf{Y_k}$ may prove useful, and either (6.3.3b) or (6.3.4b) can be used to prove that $\mathbf{Y_k}$ is isometric.

Now we are ready to consider how long it will take for a second customer to leave S_1 after the first one left. Suppose first that no new customer enters; then that time is, for $k \leq C$,

$$\mathbf{p_{ik}}\, \mathbf{Y_k}\, (\mathbf{V_{k-1}}\, \boldsymbol{\epsilon}'_{\mathbf{k-1}}) = \mathbf{p_{ik}}\, \mathbf{Y_k}\, \boldsymbol{\tau}'_{\mathbf{k-1}},$$

where the initial vector depends on the initial conditions. When the observer first looks at the system, it has k customers present, and is in the composite state, $\mathbf{p_{ik}}$. After the first customer leaves, the system is in state $\mathbf{p_{ik}}\, \mathbf{Y_k}$, with $k-1$ customers. The second customer takes time $\boldsymbol{\tau}'_{\mathbf{k-1}}$ to leave next. The time between the second and third departures is

$$\mathbf{p_{ik}}\, \mathbf{Y_k}\, \mathbf{Y_{k-1}}\, \mathbf{V_{k-2}}\, \boldsymbol{\epsilon}'_{\mathbf{k-2}} = \mathbf{p_{ik}}\, \mathbf{Y_k}\, \mathbf{Y_{k-1}}\, \boldsymbol{\tau}'_{\mathbf{k-2}},$$

and so on.

Successive multiplications of the $\mathbf{Y_k}$ matrices occur often, so we provide them with their own symbol and definition.

Definition 6.5.3

$[\mathbf{Y_k}(\ell)]_{ij}$:= *probability that S_1 will be in internal state $j \in \Xi_\ell$ immediately after $k-\ell$ departures, given that the system was initially in state $i \in \Xi_k$, and no other customers have entered.* $\mathbf{Y_k}(\ell)$ is a $D(k) \times D(\ell)$-dimensional matrix and is isometric, in that $\mathbf{Y_k}(\ell)\, \boldsymbol{\epsilon}'_{\boldsymbol{\ell}} = \boldsymbol{\epsilon}'_{\mathbf{k}}$. By definition we are assuming that S_1 starts with exactly k active customers; thus $0 \leq \ell < k \leq C$. Also, $\mathbf{Y_k}(k-1) := \mathbf{Y_k}$. Keep alert to the fact that $\mathbf{Y_k}(\,\cdot\,)$ with an argument is different from $\mathbf{Y_k}$ without an argument. □

These matrices are easy enough to construct because they satisfy the obvious recurrence relation, starting with:

$$\mathbf{Y_k}(k) := \mathbf{I_k},$$

$$\mathbf{Y_k}(\ell - 1) = \mathbf{Y_k}(\ell)\mathbf{Y}_{\boldsymbol{\ell}}, \tag{6.5.4b}$$

or explicitly,

$$\mathbf{Y_k}(\ell - 1) = \mathbf{Y_k}\, \mathbf{Y_{k-1}} \cdots \mathbf{Y}_{\boldsymbol{\ell}+\mathbf{1}}\mathbf{Y}_{\boldsymbol{\ell}}. \tag{6.5.4c}$$

The argument $(\ell-1)$ helps a little, for it tells us that the operator, $\mathbf{Y_k}(\ell-1)$, takes the system from k customers to $\ell - 1$ customers.

ME/C Subsystems and Order Statistics

If S_1 is an ME/C (not generalized) subsystem and $\mathbf{p_{ic}}$ is given by (6.5.2c), we are dealing with the ***order statistics of C iid random variables***. We state this as a theorem after the following formal definition. (See e.g., [TRIVEDI02] for a standard discussion of this.)

Definition 6.5.4

Let $X_1, X_2, \ldots, X_c$ be C identically distributed, mutually independent random variables, whose distribution functions are each generated by $\langle\, \mathbf{p}\,, \mathbf{B} \,\rangle$.

Let $X_{(0)}(C) := 0 \leq X_{(1)}(C) \leq X_{(2)}(C) \leq \cdots \leq X_{(c)}(C)$ be the size place reordering of the (X_k)s. Then the *random variable* $X_{(k)}(C)$ is called the "kth-order statistic." In terms of our ME/C (not generalized) subsystem, $X_{(1)}$ is the time the first customer leaves S_1, leaving behind $C-1$ customers, $X_{(2)}(C)$ is the time the second one leaves, and so on. These are neither independent nor identically distributed, and they even depend on C.

The r.v. of direct interest to us is the ***interdeparture time*** $Z_k(C)$; then

$$Z_k(C) := X_{(k)}(C) - X_{(k-1)}(C), \quad \text{for } 1 \leq k \leq C.$$

These r.v.s denote the time from one departure to the next. □

By constructing the matrices $\mathbf{M_k}$, $\mathbf{P_k}$, $\mathbf{Q_k}$, $\mathbf{R_k}$, $\mathbf{B_k}$, and $\mathbf{V_k}$, for $k = 1, 2, \ldots, C$ according to Equations (6.3.2) [i.e., $\mu_\gamma(l) = l\,\mu_\gamma(1)$ for all l and all $1 \leq \gamma \leq m$] we have made the (X_k)s mutually independent and identically distributed. Also, by selecting $\mathbf{p_{ic}}$ to be equal to $\mathbf{p_c} = \mathbf{p}\mathbf{R_2}\,\mathbf{R_3}\cdots\mathbf{R_c}$ we have started service for all C customers at the same time. We now state the theorem on order statistics.

Theorem 6.5.1: Let $\{Z_k(C)\,|\,1 \leq k \leq C\}$, be given according to Definition 6.5.4. Let S_1 be constructed as an ME/C subsystem. Then

$$\mathbb{E}[Z_1(C)] = \mathbf{p_c}\,\mathbf{V_c}\,\boldsymbol{\epsilon}'_{\mathbf{c}}, \quad \mathbb{E}[Z_2(C)] = \mathbf{p_c}\,\mathbf{Y_c}\,\mathbf{V_{c-1}}\,\boldsymbol{\epsilon}'_{\mathbf{c-1}},$$

and in general (we drop the dependence on C for now)

$$\begin{aligned} \mathbb{E}[Z_k] &= \mathbf{p_c}\,\mathbf{Y_c}\,\mathbf{Y_{c-1}}\cdots\mathbf{Y_{c-k}}\,\mathbf{V_{c-k+1}}\,\boldsymbol{\epsilon}'_{\mathbf{c-k+1}} \\ &= \mathbf{p_c}\,\mathbf{Y_c}(c-k-1)\,\mathbf{V_{c-k+1}}\,\boldsymbol{\epsilon}'_{\mathbf{c-k+1}}. \end{aligned} \tag{6.5.5a}$$

Admittedly, the subscripts can be confusing. The problem is that the first departure occurs when all C customers are still present. With successive departures, fewer customers remain. Thus, the subscript on $Z_k(C)$ plus the subscript on $\mathbf{V_{c-k+1}}$ always add to $C+1$ $[k+C-k+1 = C+1]$.

We can actually say how these variables are distributed.

$$\mathbb{P}\mathbf{r}(Z_1 \geq x) = \mathbf{p_c}\exp(-x\mathbf{B_c})\boldsymbol{\epsilon}'_{\mathbf{c}},$$

$$\mathbb{P}\mathbf{r}(Z_2 \geq x) = \mathbf{p_c}\mathbf{Y_c}\exp(-x\mathbf{B_{c-1}})\boldsymbol{\epsilon}'_{\mathbf{c-1}},$$

and in general,

$$\mathbb{P}\mathbf{r}(Z_{c-k+1} \geq x) = \mathbf{p_c}\,\mathbf{Y_c}(k)\exp(-x\mathbf{B_k})\,\boldsymbol{\epsilon}'_{\mathbf{k}}. \tag{6.5.5b}$$

Note that the r.v.s $[Z_k]$ cover the period immediately after one departure up to and including the next departure, which we call an ***epoch***. $X_{(k)}(C)$ satisfies the following.

$$X_{(k)}(C) = \sum_{\ell=1}^{k} Z_\ell(C) = Z_k(C) + X_{(k-1)}(C),$$

so its pdf can be found from the convolution of the pdfs of the $Z_\ell(C)$s (not so easy). ∎

This may be getting a bit obscure and abstract, so let us interject the simplest of examples. Suppose that ME is exponential (i.e., $m = 1$), and there are exactly C customers at S_1. Then $D(k) = 1$ for all k, $\mathbf{M_k} = \mathbf{B_k} \Rightarrow k\,\mu$, and just about everything else becomes 1. Then

$$\mathbb{E}[Z_1] = \frac{1}{C\,\mu}$$

and in general, we get the well-known formula for the order statistics for exponential distributions, namely

$$\mathbb{E}[Z_k] = \frac{1}{(C-k+1)\mu}.$$

Remember, this is the mean time between departures. The mean time for departures themselves are the partial sums of the interdeparture times. Recall that $\mathbb{E}[X_{(0)}(C)] := 0$; then

$$\mathbb{E}[X_{(k)}(C)] = \mathbb{E}[X_{(k-1)}(C)] + \frac{1}{(C-k+1)\mu} = \frac{1}{\mu}\sum_{\ell=c-k+1}^{c}\frac{1}{\ell}.$$

In particular, the time for the last customer to leave is

$$\mathbb{E}[X_{(c)}(C)] = \frac{1}{\mu}H(C) := \frac{1}{\mu}\sum_{\ell=1}^{c}\frac{1}{\ell},$$

where $H(C)$ is known as the ***harmonic series***. Remember, these last formulas are valid only for the M/M/C queue.

Draining of Generalized ME/C Subsystems

We return to our generalized subsystem, and suppose that $n > C$. Then when a customer leaves, another immediately takes his place, putting the system in the state

$$\mathbf{Y_c R_c} = \mathbf{V_c M_c Q_c R_c}.$$

The element $[\mathbf{Y_c\,R_c}]_{ij}$ can be interpreted in the following way. "Given that the system is in state $i \in \Xi_c$, with more customers in the queue, a customer finally leaves $[\mathbf{Y_c}]$, and immediately thereafter another customer enters $[\mathbf{R_c}]$, putting the system in state $j \in \Xi_c$." This object is a singular, isometric, square matrix of dimension $D(C) \times D(C)$. We first ran across the $C = 1$ version of this in Chapter 3, namely, $\mathbf{Y_1 R_1} = \boldsymbol{\epsilon}'\mathbf{p} = \mathbf{Q}$ (as always, not to be confused with $\mathbf{Q_1} = \mathbf{q}'$, or $\boldsymbol{Q}$).

The formulas for the interdeparture times from a generalized G/C are very similar to those for order statistics, but we must distinguish between $n > C$ and $n < C$, where n is the number of customers remaining. We start with the following.

Definition 6.5.5

Let $Z_\ell(N|C)$ be the r.v. denoting the time between the departures of customers $\ell - 1$ and ℓ. Initially there are N customers at the system, and no more than C customers can be active at one time. The number of customers remaining immediately after departure ℓ (and no new arrivals) is $n = N - \ell$. □

Initially the system is in some composite state $\mathbf{p_{ic}}$ with $N > C$ customers. Then the mean time for the first departure is, using (6.5.3),

$$\mathbb{E}[Z_1(N|C)] = \mathbf{p_{ic}} \mathbf{V_c} \boldsymbol{\epsilon}'_\mathbf{c} = \mathbf{p_{ic}} \boldsymbol{\tau}'_\mathbf{c}.$$

The second customer leaves the following amount of time later,

$$\mathbb{E}[Z_2(N|C)] = \mathbf{p_{ic}} \mathbf{Y_c} \mathbf{R_c} \boldsymbol{\tau}'_\mathbf{c}.$$

In general, as long as $\ell < N - C$ (there are customers still waiting to enter S_1),

$$\mathbb{E}[Z_\ell(N|C)] = \mathbf{p_{ic}} [\mathbf{Y_c} \mathbf{R_c}]^{\ell-1} \boldsymbol{\tau}'_\mathbf{c}. \tag{6.5.6a}$$

When finally $\ell = N - C$ there are C customers remaining. Then (let $j = N - C + k + 1$)

$$\mathbb{E}[Z_j(N|C)] = \mathbf{p_{ic}} [\mathbf{Y_c} \mathbf{R_c}]^{N-C} \mathbf{Y_c}(c-k) \boldsymbol{\tau}'_\mathbf{c-k} \quad 0 \le k < C, \tag{6.5.6b}$$

starting with $k = 0$ (C customers remain),

$$\mathbb{E}[Z_{N-C+1}(N|C)] = \mathbf{p_{ic}} [\mathbf{Y_c} \mathbf{R_c}]^{N-C} \boldsymbol{\tau}'_\mathbf{c},$$

and ending with $k = C - 1$,

$$\mathbb{E}[Z_N(N|C)] = \mathbf{p_{ic}} [\mathbf{Y_c} \mathbf{R_c}]^{N-C} \mathbf{Y_c}(1) \boldsymbol{\tau}'_\mathbf{1}.$$

We see that every interdeparture time depends on the inner product of a "final vector" $[\boldsymbol{\tau}'_\mathbf{k}]$ and an "initial vector" [everything else]. The final vectors depend only on the number of active customers, but the initial vectors (and thus, the interdeparture times themselves) depend on N, C, the number of customers still remaining, and the state the system was in when the whole process began $[\mathbf{p_{ic}}]$. The mean times are all different, but if $N >> C$, then $[\mathbf{Y_c} \mathbf{R_c}]^\ell \to \boldsymbol{\epsilon}'_\mathbf{c} \boldsymbol{\pi}_\mathbf{c}$ [see (6.5.9b) below, and the discussion around it], and the successive interdeparture times approach a constant $[\boldsymbol{\pi}_\mathbf{c} \boldsymbol{\tau}'_\mathbf{c}]$, until there are fewer than C customers remaining. But even so the interdeparture times are correlated. This is discussed fully in Chapter 8.

Let us summarize this with a theorem about the time for a queue to drain.

Theorem 6.5.2: Consider a generalized subsystem S_1 in which a maximum of C customers can be active simultaneously. Suppose that there are N customers at S_1, with no new arrivals possible, and at the moment the process begins, the subsystem is in state $\mathbf{p_{ik}}$. The process ends when all customers are gone. Let T_N be the r.v. denoting the time for the queue to drain. Then from Equations (6.5.6)

$$\mathbb{E}[T_N] = \sum_{\ell=1}^{N} \mathbb{E}[Z_\ell(N|C)]. \tag{6.5.7a}$$

If $N = k \leq C$ this reduces to

$$\mathbb{E}[T_k] = \mathbf{p_{ik}}\, \boldsymbol{\tau}'_{\mathbf{k}} + \mathbf{p_{ik}} \mathbf{Y_k}\, \boldsymbol{\tau}'_{\mathbf{k-1}} + \mathbf{p_{ik}}\, \mathbf{Y_k}(k-2)\, \boldsymbol{\tau}'_{\mathbf{k-2}}$$
$$+ \cdots + \mathbf{p_{ik}} \mathbf{Y_k}(1)\, \boldsymbol{\tau}'_{\mathbf{1}}. \tag{6.5.7b}$$

In general, for $N = l + C, \;\; l > 0$,

$$\mathbb{E}[T_N] = \mathbf{p_{ic}} \left[\sum_{j=0}^{l} (\mathbf{Y_c R_c})^j \right] \boldsymbol{\tau}'_{\mathbf{c}} \tag{6.5.7c}$$

$$+\mathbf{p_{ic}} (\mathbf{Y_c}\, \mathbf{R_c})^l \mathbf{Y_c} \left[\mathbf{Y_c}\, \boldsymbol{\tau}'_{\mathbf{c-1}} + \mathbf{Y_c}(C-2)\, \boldsymbol{\tau}'_{\mathbf{c-2}} + \cdots + \mathbf{Y_c}(1)\, \boldsymbol{\tau}'_{\mathbf{1}} \right].$$

The separate terms are the mean times for each successive customer to leave after the previous one has left. $\boldsymbol{\tau}_{\mathbf{k}}$ is given by (6.5.3) and $\mathbf{Y_k}$ is given by Equations (6.5.4). ■

It is left to the reader to devise a simple recursive algorithm for evaluating Equations (6.5.7). Perhaps we should think of Theorem 6.5.1 as a corollary to Theorem 6.5.2. Some examples where ***time to drain*** can be important are the following. This idea was recently used by Mohamed [MOHAMED04].

1. A multiprogramming computer system has been in operation all day, and everyone except the operator has gone home. The operator cannot go home until all jobs are done, including those in the waiting queue. C is the maximum degree of multiprogramming, and n is the number of jobs in the system. Then $\mathbf{p_{ik}}$ is given by (6.5.1), and T_n is the mean time until the operator can go home.

2. A multiprogramming computer system has been in operation for a long time, and the operating systems people must bring it down for some reason or other. They can shut off the queue of waiting jobs but must let those in progress continue until they finish. C is the maximum degree of multiprogramming, $\mathbf{p_{ik}}$ is given by (6.5.1), and n is the number of jobs in the system when the queue is turned off. If $n = k \leq C$, then T_k is the mean time until they can bring down the system. If $n > C$, then T_c is the mean time, but use (6.5.1a) with n (not C) for $\mathbf{p_{ic}}$.

3. We have $n \geq C$ identical devices, of which we would like C to be running simultaneously (***hot backup***), but we can survive even if all but one are broken. $\mathbf{p_{ic}}$ is given by $\mathbf{p_c}$ (6.5.2a), and $\mathbb{E}[T_n]$ is the mean time until all are broken (MTTF, without repair). There are initially $n - C$ devices in ***cold backup*** and $C - 1$ in hot backup. We can generalize; failure can be defined as occurring when the number still at S_1 drops below a certain value.

4. You are driving cross-country and are in a hurry. Your car has five brand-new tires. You will have time to change, but not to fix, a flat if it occurs. Equation (6.5.2a) for $C = 4$ (unless you are driving a trailer truck) is the initial state, and failure occurs when you are down to three tires (hold the steering wheel steady when this occurs). T is the sum of the first two terms in (6.5.7b).

5. Same as Example 4, but now you are driving a rented car, so the four mounted tires have already been used to an uncertain amount, but the spare is new. What is $\mathbf{p_{ik}}$ now?

Presumably the reader can think up a few more examples.

6.5.2 Markov Renewal (Semi-Markov Departure) Processes

In the second paragraph of Section 6.4 we stated that the maximal service rate of S_1 must be greater than λ for the steady-state M/ME/C queue to exist, without actually determining the maximal rate. We do that now. We also describe the departure process from S_1 (which is, of course, the same as the arrival process at S_2), when its queue is unboundedly large. This is the direct generalization of the renewal processes described in Section 3.5, and is known as a ***Markov Renewal Process*** (MRP). It is also known as a *semi-Markov point process* (SMP). We go into this subject in a more general way, and in more detail in Chapter 8. We are not particularly interested in where names come from, but we give them so that the reader can have a reference point for reading the general literature. Based on our (and everyone else's) definition, this really is not a renewal process, and we hope that by the end of this section, you will see why.

In the preceding section we showed how to calculate the mean time for a customer to leave S_1, given some initial state. We also showed how to calculate the time for the second, third, and all other customers to leave. All these times are different even if the queue is long enough to guarantee that there will always be more than C customers at S_1. Fortunately, this sequence approaches a limit. That is, let (Z_n) be the r.v. for the time interval between the departure of customer n and customer $(n-1)$ for any initial state vector, $\mathbf{p_{ic}}$. Note that the system has up to C customers actively being served, not just the one who ultimately leaves next. Therefore this period should not be identified with the nth customer to arrive. Among other things, the ordering of customers in not preserved. In any case, we call this the ***n*th *epoch***. Then

$$\mathbb{E}[Z_n] = \mathbf{p_{ic}}(\mathbf{Y_c}\,\mathbf{R_c})^{n-1}\mathbf{V_c}\,\boldsymbol{\epsilon}'_{\mathbf{c}}, \tag{6.5.8a}$$

for all n, if the queue is unboundedly large. Let us assume that the following limit exists.

$$\mathbb{E}[Z] := \lim_{n\to\infty} \mathbb{E}[Z_n]. \tag{6.5.8b}$$

For the limit to exist, the matrix $\mathbf{Y_c R_c} = \mathbf{V_c M_c Q_c R_c}$ must satisfy certain properties, some of which we already know to be true. We know, for instance, that this matrix is isometric but not invertible. Thus it has one eigenvalue equal to 1 and multiple occurrences of 0 as an eigenvalue. We know the latter because the matrix $\mathbf{Q_c R_c}$ is of dimension $D(C)$, but $\mathbf{Q_c}$ and $\mathbf{R_c}$ are not square matrices, so $\mathbf{Q_c R_c}$ is at most of rank $D(C-1)$.

We assume that all the other eigenvalues are less than 1 in magnitude. Recall from the definition of isometric that $\boldsymbol{\epsilon}'_{\mathbf{c}}$ is a right eigenvector. Let's take a look. From (6.3.4b)

$$\mathbf{Y_c\, R_c}\, \boldsymbol{\epsilon}'_{\mathbf{c}} = \mathbf{V_c\, M_c\, Q_c\, R_c}\, \boldsymbol{\epsilon}'_{\mathbf{c}} = \mathbf{V_c\, B_c}\, \boldsymbol{\epsilon}'_{\mathbf{c}} = \boldsymbol{\epsilon}'_{\mathbf{c}}.$$

This, as we have seen several times, is an eigenvector equation, with eigenvalue 1. Next, let $\boldsymbol{\pi}_{\mathbf{c}}$ be the left eigenvector of $\mathbf{Y_c\, R_c}$ with eigenvalue 1, normalized so that $\boldsymbol{\pi}_{\mathbf{c}}\, \boldsymbol{\epsilon}'_{\mathbf{c}} = 1$. That is,

$$\boldsymbol{\pi}_{\mathbf{c}}\, \mathbf{Y_c\, R_c} = \boldsymbol{\pi}_{\mathbf{c}}.^{\dagger} \tag{6.5.9a}$$

Now from the spectral decomposition theorem (1.3.8b), we can write

$$(\mathbf{Y_c R_c})^n = \boldsymbol{\epsilon}'_{\mathbf{c}} \boldsymbol{\pi}_{\mathbf{c}} + \sum_{i=2}^{D(C)} \lambda_i^n \mathbf{v}'_{\mathbf{i}}\, \mathbf{u_i},$$

where $\{\lambda_i,\, \mathbf{u_i},\, \mathbf{v}'_{\mathbf{i}}\}$ is the set of eigenvalues and left and right eigenvectors of $\mathbf{Y_c R_c}$, excluding 1, $\boldsymbol{\pi}_{\mathbf{c}}$, and $\boldsymbol{\epsilon}'_{\mathbf{c}}$. Assuming that $|\lambda_i| < 1$ for $i \geq 2$, we can take the limit directly, to get

$$\lim_{n \to \infty} (\mathbf{Y_c R_c})^n = \boldsymbol{\epsilon}'_{\mathbf{c}} \boldsymbol{\pi}_{\mathbf{c}}. \tag{6.5.9b}$$

Then we have

$$\mathbb{E}[Z] = \mathbf{p_{ic}}\, \boldsymbol{\epsilon}'_{\mathbf{c}}\, \boldsymbol{\pi}_{\mathbf{c}}\, \mathbf{V_c}\, \boldsymbol{\epsilon}'_{\mathbf{c}} = \boldsymbol{\pi}_{\mathbf{c}}\, \mathbf{V_c}\, \boldsymbol{\epsilon}'_{\mathbf{c}}, \tag{6.5.10a}$$

given that $\mathbf{p_{ic}}\, \boldsymbol{\epsilon}'_{\mathbf{c}} = 1$. Note that $\mathbb{E}[Z]$ is independent of the state the system was in initially, as all good Markov processes should be. This limit is the correct maximal, mean interdeparture time from S_1, so $1/\mathbb{E}[Z]$ is the maximal service rate of S_1. Therefore, if we define ρ_c as

$$\rho_c := \lambda\, \mathbb{E}[Z] = \lambda\, \left[\boldsymbol{\pi}_{\mathbf{c}}\, \mathbf{V_c}\, \boldsymbol{\epsilon}'_{\mathbf{c}}\right], \tag{6.5.10b}$$

then we can say that the steady-state M/ME/C queue exists as long as $\rho_c < 1$, thus finally completing our thoughts for Section 6.4.

But we have not finished our thoughts for this section. If $\rho_c > 1$, then S_1 becomes an MRP source for S_2. We deal fully with that possibility in Chapter 8, but we do have some items to mention before closing here.

First we would like to give some meaning to the vector $\boldsymbol{\pi}_{\mathbf{c}}$. To do that, look at the isometric matrix [compare with (3.5.11a)]

$$\boldsymbol{P}_{\mathbf{c}} := \mathbf{P_c} + \mathbf{Q_c R_c}. \tag{6.5.11a}$$

This matrix moderates the following process. There are C customers in S_1. The internal transitions are governed by $\mathbf{P_c}$, but when a transition occurs that results in a customer leaving $[\mathbf{Q_c}]$, that customer immediately returns,

†Be careful not to confuse $\boldsymbol{\pi}_{\mathbf{c}}$ with the vector $\boldsymbol{\pi}_{\mathbf{c}}(n)$ in (6.4.4b).

putting the system in a new state of Ξ_c, $[\mathbf{R_c}]$. Therefore, $\boldsymbol{P_c}$ is the transition matrix describing a short-circuited S_1. The left eigenvector $\mathbf{y_c}$, defined by

$$\mathbf{y_c}\,\boldsymbol{P_c} = \mathbf{y_c} \tag{6.5.11b}$$

and $\mathbf{y_c}\,\boldsymbol{\epsilon}'_{\mathbf{c}} = 1$, is interpreted in the following way. $[\mathbf{y_c}]_i$ is the probability that the short-circuited system will be found in state $i \in \Xi_c$ between events. Next rewrite (6.5.11a) and (6.5.11b) in the form

$$\mathbf{y_c Q_c R_c} = \mathbf{y_c}[\mathbf{I_c} - \mathbf{P_c}], \tag{6.5.11c}$$

and compare with the following [from (6.5.9a) using the first part of (6.5.4a)].

$$\boldsymbol{\pi_c} = \boldsymbol{\pi_c}[\mathbf{I_c} - \mathbf{P_c}]^{-1}\mathbf{Q_c R_c}. \tag{6.5.11d}$$

These two equations imply that $\boldsymbol{\pi_c}$ must be proportional to $\mathbf{y_c}[\mathbf{I_c} - \mathbf{P_c}]$; that is,

$$\boldsymbol{\pi_c} \sim \mathbf{y_c}[\mathbf{I_c} - \mathbf{P_c}].$$

Normalize so that $\mathbf{y_c}\,\boldsymbol{\epsilon}'_{\mathbf{c}} = 1$, and let $g := 1/\boldsymbol{\pi_c}[\mathbf{I_c} - \mathbf{P_c}]^{-1}\boldsymbol{\epsilon}'_{\mathbf{c}}$; then

$$\mathbf{y_c} = g\,\boldsymbol{\pi_c}[\mathbf{I_c} - \mathbf{P_c}]^{-1}.$$

Next consider the vector whose ith component is $x_i := y_i\,[\mathbf{M_c}]_{ii}$. Recall that $1/[\mathbf{M_c}]_{ii}$ is the mean time the system spends in state i every time it finds itself there. Therefore, as a direct generalization of the ***mean residual vector*** defined in (3.5.10b),

$$\mathbf{x_c} \sim \mathbf{y_c}[\mathbf{M_c}]^{-1} \tag{6.5.12a}$$

must be proportional to the steady-state probability vector of short-circuited S_1. On the other hand, we have (substituting for $\mathbf{y_c}$)

$$\mathbf{x_c} \sim \pi_\mathbf{c}[\mathbf{I_c} - \mathbf{P_c}]^{-1}[\mathbf{M_c}]^{-1} = \pi_\mathbf{c}\mathbf{V_c}, \tag{6.5.12b}$$

where from (6.5.10a), $\mathbf{x_c}\boldsymbol{\epsilon}'_{\mathbf{c}} = \mathbb{E}[Z]$. Compare this with (3.5.10b) and (6.5.10a). The ith components of the three vectors $\mathbf{y_c}$, $\boldsymbol{\pi_c}$, and $\mathbf{x_c}/\mathbb{E}[Z]$ are, respectively, the steady-state probability of finding S_1 in state $i \in \Xi_c$ between events, the steady-state probability that a leaving–re-entering customer will put S_1 in state i, and the steady-state probability that a random observer will find S_1 in state i.† And then there is $\mathbf{p_c}$ of (6.5.2a). Can anything be clearer?

We have seen that the vector-matrix pair $\langle\, \mathbf{p_{ic}}(\mathbf{Y_c\,R_c})^{n-1}\,,\, \mathbf{B_c}\,\rangle$ generates the interdeparture-time distribution for the nth customer to leave S_1 when there are more than $n + C$ customers in the queue initially. We have also seen that when n is large enough, all the interdeparture distributions are the same and are generated by the pair $\langle\, \boldsymbol{\pi_c}\,,\, \mathbf{B_c}\,\rangle$. Can we not say, then, that this process approaches a renewal process asymptotically? The answer to this is no, but the explanation is very subtle. The manifest property that is missing is *independence*. In renewal processes, interdeparture times for two successive

†Note that $\mathbf{x_c}$ is the same as that given by the product-form solution for Jackson networks.

customers are independent of each other. That is not true here. The physical explanation is as follows. In a renewal process, when a customer leaves S_1, he leaves behind the empty state, no matter how long he was in service himself. That is, the initial state for the next customer is always $\mathbf{p}$. Therefore, the next customer always starts the same way. For our semi-Markov process, the state the subsystem is in immediately after the nth departure is likely to be quite different if the nth interdeparture time were short than if the interdeparture time were long. For instance, suppose that the process has been going on for a long time. Then the nth epoch begins in state $\boldsymbol{\pi}_{\mathbf{c}}$. This is the initial vector averaged over all possible times for all previous departures. If the epoch ends after a short time, the customers remaining have not moved very much, but if the epoch lasts a long time, the other customers may have changed their states quite a bit. So the beginning of epoch number $(n+1)$ depends on the time of the nth departure.

The mathematical explanation is as follows. Suppose that n is very large; then the distribution for Z_n is generated by $\langle \boldsymbol{\pi}_{\mathbf{c}}, \mathbf{B}_{\mathrm{c}} \rangle$. Therefore,

$$\boldsymbol{\pi}_{\mathbf{c}} \exp(-t\mathbf{B}_{\mathrm{c}})$$

is the vector whose ith component is the probability that the nth customer to leave is still in service at time t after the $(n-1)$st customer left, and the system is in state i. The reliability function is

$$\mathbb{P}\mathbf{r}(Z_n > t) := R_{Z_n}(t) = \boldsymbol{\pi}_{\mathbf{c}} \exp(-t\mathbf{B}_{\mathrm{c}})\, \boldsymbol{\epsilon}'_{\mathbf{c}},$$

with density function

$$b_{Z_n}(t) = \boldsymbol{\pi}_{\mathbf{c}} \exp(-t\mathbf{B}_{\mathrm{c}})\, \mathbf{B}_{\mathrm{c}}\, \boldsymbol{\epsilon}'_{\mathbf{c}}.$$

At time t let there be an event in S_1, $[\mathbf{M}_{\mathrm{c}}]$, resulting in a departure $[\mathbf{Q}_{\mathrm{c}}]$, followed immediately by a new entry $[\mathbf{R}_{\mathrm{c}}]$. Then the next departure epoch will have a starting vector of:

$$\boldsymbol{\pi}_{\mathbf{c}}(t) := \frac{1}{b_{Z_n}(t)} \boldsymbol{\pi}_{\mathbf{c}} \exp(-t\mathbf{B}_{\mathrm{c}})\, \mathbf{M}_{\mathrm{c}}\, \mathbf{Q}_{\mathrm{c}}\, \mathbf{R}_{\mathrm{c}},$$

This certainly depends upon t (unless $\mathbf{M}_{\mathrm{c}}\, \mathbf{Q}_{\mathrm{c}}\, \mathbf{R}_{\mathrm{c}}$ is of rank 1, which it is only for $C = 1$).

Observe from (6.5.9a), that

$$\int_0^\infty \boldsymbol{\pi}_{\mathbf{c}}(t)\, b_{Z_n}(t)\, dt = \boldsymbol{\pi}_{\mathbf{c}} \left[\int_0^\infty \exp(-t\mathbf{B}_{\mathrm{c}})\, dt \right] \mathbf{M}_{\mathrm{c}}\, \mathbf{Q}_{\mathrm{c}}\, \mathbf{R}_{\mathrm{c}}$$

$$= \boldsymbol{\pi}_{\mathbf{c}}\, \mathbf{V}_{\mathrm{c}}\, \mathbf{M}_{\mathrm{c}}\, \mathbf{Q}_{\mathrm{c}}\, \mathbf{R}_{\mathrm{c}} = \boldsymbol{\pi}_{\mathbf{c}}\, \mathbf{Y}_{\mathrm{c}}\, \mathbf{R}_{\mathrm{c}} = \boldsymbol{\pi}_{\mathbf{c}}.$$

That is, only if the random observer takes no note of time for the nth epoch, will the $(n+1)$st epoch also start in state $\boldsymbol{\pi}_{\mathbf{c}}$.

The above material is generalized and discussed fully in Chapter 8. But this chapter contains other interesting areas for further study by the reader. We have a few questions of our own.

1. What is the relation between the product-form solution of steady-state Jackson networks and the matrices we had to create for the M/ME/C//C loop? It would seem that the only properties necessary for the two to give the same results is that the dimension of the Ξ_k's be equal to the binomial coefficients as given in (6.3.6b).

2. There is no formal difference between a subsystem with C identical servers and the generalized subsystem. But the former has some special properties, and it would seem that those matrices should be capable of being broken down into smaller parts, so that the difference between the two can be seen explicitly.

3. Do there exist smaller-dimensional matrices that represent these processes equally well? We should be able to study the class of similarity transformations that leave the various equations invariant or the various results unchanged.

6.5.3 A Little Bit of Up and Down, with Arrivals

The work we did in Chapters 4 and 5 on first-passage matrices and times, as well as the various **W** matrices and other properties of the busy period, can be generalized to the networks we are treating in this chapter. We must be more careful though, because the operators, both in size and content, change from one queue length to the next. We give a sampling of how this can be done in just two areas, first-passage times up and first-passage times down. These two topics have increasingly important applicability to real-world problems. "Up" is easier, so we do that first.

6.5.3.1 First-Passage Processes for Queue Growth

What we are about to do is taken directly from Section 4.5.1 with the added problem that dimensions and operators change as we go up the ladder. We also have the problem of setting up new notation. As in previous chapters, we use the symbol **H** for our isometric first-passage matrices. We also need an auxiliary matrix for definition purposes. So, for our first definition,

Definition 6.5.6

$\mathbf{X_k}$:= *probability matrix of first passage from* k *to* $k+1$ *where* $k < C$. That is, $[\mathbf{X_k}]_{ij}$ is the probability that S_1 will be in state $j \in \Xi_{k+1}$ when its queue goes from k to $k+1$ for the first time, given that it started in state $i \in \Xi_k$. This is a $D(k) \times D(k+1)$-dimensional matrix and is isometric, because $\mathbf{X_k}\boldsymbol{\epsilon'}_{\mathbf{k+1}} := \boldsymbol{\epsilon}'_{\mathbf{k}}$. $\mathbf{X_k}$ will soon be replaced by $\mathbf{H_k}$ so we are not bothering to use **u** for *up* Note that this matrix is only defined for $k < C$. □

To be consistent with previous notation, **X** should have been subscripted as $\mathbf{k+1}$, because that matches the higher dimension of this rectangular matrix. However, we soon after define the related matrix **H**, which is the one we actually use in our final formulas.

Look at the time-dependent state diagram in Figure 6.5.1. There are five different types of equations we must look at for queue growth, namely $0 < 1 < k < C < n$. N is relevant only for queue decrease. Let us start with no-one at S_1. Then all that can happen is for a customer to arrive, putting S_1 into state $\mathbf{p}$. Therefore,

$$\mathbf{X}_o = \mathbf{p}.$$

Next consider one customer in S_1. Three things can happen.

1. A second customer arrives directly, with probability $\lambda[\mathbf{M_1} + \lambda\mathbf{I_1}]^{-1}$, and enters, thereby changing the state of the subsystem $[\mathbf{R_2}]$.

2. A transition occurs in S_1, $[\mathbf{M_1}(\mathbf{M_1} + \lambda\mathbf{I_1})^{-1}]$, resulting in a customer changing phase $[\mathbf{P_1}]$, and then eventually the queue gets to length 2, $[\mathbf{X_1}]$.

3. A transition occurs in S_1, $[\mathbf{M_1}(\mathbf{M_1} + \lambda\mathbf{I_1})^{-1}]$, resulting in a customer leaving $[\mathbf{Q_1} = \mathbf{q}']$, and then the queue eventually grows from 0 to 1 to 2, $[\mathbf{X}_o\,\mathbf{X_1}]$.

The equation for this is [where $\mathbf{M_1}(\mathbf{M_1} + \lambda\mathbf{I_1})^{-1} = (\mathbf{M_1} + \lambda\mathbf{I_1})^{-1}\,\mathbf{M_1}$]

$$\mathbf{X_1} = \lambda[\mathbf{M_1} + \lambda\mathbf{I_1}]^{-1}\mathbf{R_2} + \mathbf{M_1}[\mathbf{M_1} + \lambda\mathbf{I_1}]^{-1}\mathbf{P_1}\mathbf{X_1}$$

$$+\mathbf{M_1}[\mathbf{M_1} + \lambda\mathbf{I_1}]^{-1}\mathbf{Q_1}\,\mathbf{X}_o\,\mathbf{X_1}.$$

Premultiply both sides by $[\mathbf{M_1} + \lambda\mathbf{I_1}]$, collect all terms multiplying $\mathbf{X_1}$, and get

$$[\mathbf{M_1} + \lambda\mathbf{I_1} - \mathbf{M_1}\,\mathbf{P_1} - \mathbf{M_1}\,\mathbf{Q_1}\,\mathbf{R_1}]\,\mathbf{X_1} = \lambda\mathbf{R_2}.$$

We have deliberately used $\mathbf{Q_1}$ and $\mathbf{R_1}$ for $\mathbf{q}'$ and $\mathbf{p}$, respectively. Now solve for $\mathbf{X_1}$, using $\mathbf{B_1} = \mathbf{M_1}(\mathbf{I_1} - \mathbf{P_1})$,

$$\mathbf{X_1} = \lambda[\lambda\mathbf{I_1} + \mathbf{B_1} - \mathbf{M_1}\mathbf{Q_1}\mathbf{R_1}]^{-1}\mathbf{R_2}. \tag{6.5.13a}$$

Let us make some simplifying definitions. Let $\mathbf{H_{uo}} := 1$ [a one-dimensional matrix, given that $D(0) = 1$], and let

$$\mathbf{H_{u1}} := \lambda[\lambda\mathbf{I_1} + \mathbf{B_1} - \mathbf{M_1}\mathbf{Q_1}\mathbf{H_{uo}}\mathbf{R_1}]^{-1}; \tag{6.5.13b}$$

then $\mathbf{X_1} = \mathbf{H_{u1}}\mathbf{R_2}$. What is nice is that $\mathbf{H_{u1}}$ is an isometric, invertible, square matrix. We prove the isometric property by multiplying (6.5.13b) from the right with the expression in brackets [notice that we could not do this in (6.5.13a), because $\mathbf{R_2}$ is in the way] and then right-multiply by $\boldsymbol{\epsilon}_1'$ to get

$$\mathbf{H_{u1}}[\lambda\mathbf{I_1} + \mathbf{B_1} - \mathbf{M_1}\mathbf{Q_1}\mathbf{R_1}]\boldsymbol{\epsilon}_1' = \lambda\boldsymbol{\epsilon}_1'.$$

We know from (6.3.4b) that $\mathbf{M_1}\,\mathbf{Q_1}\,\mathbf{R_1}\,\boldsymbol{\epsilon}_1' = \mathbf{B_1}\,\boldsymbol{\epsilon}_1'$, so we are indeed left with

$$\mathbf{H_{u1}}\,\boldsymbol{\epsilon}_1' = \boldsymbol{\epsilon}_1'.$$

Only then does it follow that

$$\mathbf{X_2}\,\boldsymbol{\epsilon}_2' = \boldsymbol{\epsilon}_1'.$$

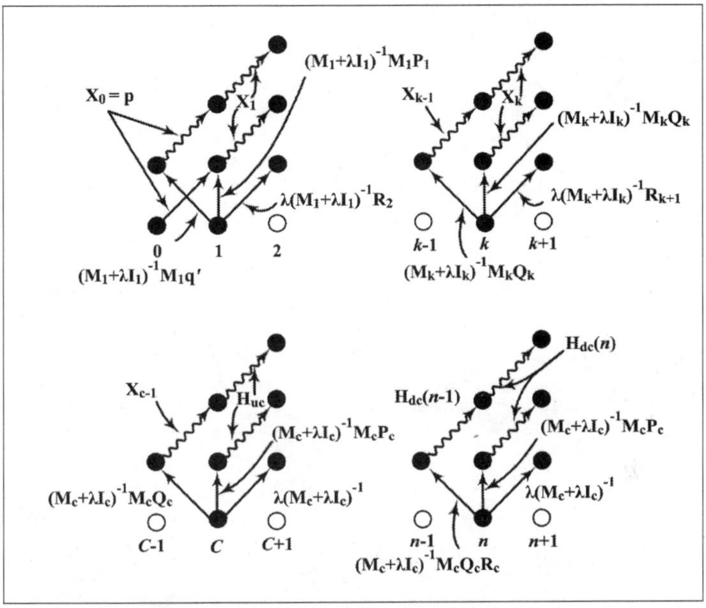

Figure 6.5.1: Time-dependent state transition diagram for *up* processes for M/ME/$C//N$ queues, where $C < N$. This is also applicable to open systems where $N \to \infty$. There are five different sets of transition types, one each for $n = 0$, $n = 1$, $n = k < C, n = C, N > n > C$. $n = N$ is only relevant for *down* processes.

We can do the very same thing for $1 < k < C$, so

$$\mathbf{X_k} = \lambda[\mathbf{M_k} + \lambda\mathbf{I_k}]^{-1}\mathbf{R_{k+1}} + \mathbf{M_k}[\mathbf{M_k} + \lambda\mathbf{I_k}]^{-1}\,\mathbf{X_k}$$

$$+\mathbf{M_k}[\mathbf{M_k} + \lambda\mathbf{I_k}]^{-1}\,\mathbf{Q_k}\mathbf{X_{k-1}}\mathbf{X_k}.$$

Doing the usual maneuverings, we come up with

$$\mathbf{X_k} = \lambda[\lambda\mathbf{I_k} + \mathbf{B_k} - \mathbf{M_k}\mathbf{Q_k}\mathbf{X_{k-1}}]^{-1}\mathbf{R_{k+1}}.$$

Next we let

$$\mathbf{X_k} = \mathbf{H_{uk}}\mathbf{R_{k+1}}; \tag{6.5.14}$$

then we have

$$\mathbf{H_{uk}} = \lambda[\lambda\mathbf{I_k} + \mathbf{B_k} - \mathbf{M_k}\mathbf{Q_k}\mathbf{H_{uk-1}}\mathbf{R_k}]^{-1}. \tag{6.5.15a}$$

We prove that $\mathbf{H_{uk}}$ is isometric, by induction. We know that $\mathbf{H_{u1}}\,\boldsymbol{\epsilon}'_\mathbf{1} = \boldsymbol{\epsilon}'_\mathbf{1}$, and assume that it is true for $1 \le l < k$; then

$$\mathbf{H_{uk}}[\lambda\mathbf{I_k} + \mathbf{B_k} - \mathbf{M_k}\mathbf{Q_k}\mathbf{H_{uk-1}}\mathbf{R_k}]\boldsymbol{\epsilon}'_\mathbf{k} = \mathbf{H_{uk}}\,\boldsymbol{\epsilon}'_\mathbf{k} = \lambda\,\boldsymbol{\epsilon}'_\mathbf{k}.$$

It follows from this that $\mathbf{X_k}$ is isometric. Note that $\mathbf{H_{uk}}$ does not depend on C as long as k is less than C. We can interpret $[\mathbf{H_{uk}}]_{ij}$ as given in the following.

Definition 6.5.7

$[\mathbf{H_{uk}}]_{ij}$:= *probability that* S_1 *will be in state* $j \in \Xi_k$ *just before a customer arrives and enters* [$\mathbf{R_{k+1}}$] *to raise the queue length from* k *to* $k+1$ *for the first time, given that* S_1 *started in state* $i \in \Xi_k$. $\mathbf{H_{uk}}$ and $\mathbf{X_k}$ are related by (6.5.14). □

Now we must look at the system when there are C or more customers at S_1. To do that we must first define a set of matrices for $n \geq C$.

Definition 6.5.8

$\mathbf{H_{uc}}(n)$:= *probability matrix of first passage from* n *to* $n+1$ *where* $n \geq C$. Thus $[\mathbf{H_{uc}}(n)]_{ij}$ is the probability that S_1 will be in state $j \in \Xi_c$ just after a customer arrives to raise the queue length from n to $n+1$ for the first time, given that the process started with the system in state $i \in \Xi_c$. □

We do not need the auxiliary $\mathbf{X}$ matrices, because the first-passage matrices of Definition 6.5.8 are already square and isometric. Put another way, from what we know of their meanings, they must be equal. After all, if the queue length at S_1 is greater than or equal to C, the system will be in the same internal state immediately before and immediately after an arrival.

Let us start with $n = C$. The first-passage matrix satisfies

$$\mathbf{H_{uc}}(C) = \lambda[\mathbf{M_c} + \lambda\mathbf{I_c}]^{-1} + \mathbf{M_c}[\mathbf{M_c} + \lambda\mathbf{I_c}]^{-1}\mathbf{P_c}\,\mathbf{H_{uc}}(C)$$
$$+ \mathbf{M_c}[\mathbf{M_c} + \lambda\mathbf{I_c}]^{-1}\mathbf{Q_c}\,\mathbf{H_{u(c-1)}}\,\mathbf{R_c}\,\mathbf{H_{uc}}(C).$$

When we solve explicitly for $\mathbf{H_{uc}}(C)$ we get

$$\mathbf{H_{uc}}(C) = \lambda[\lambda\,\mathbf{I_c} + \mathbf{B_c} - \mathbf{M_k}\mathbf{Q_c}\mathbf{H_{u(c-1)}}\mathbf{R_c}]^{-1}.$$

This is in exactly the same form as (6.5.15a), so we can say that

$$\mathbf{H_{uc}}(C) = \mathbf{H_{uc}},$$

but things are a little different from now on. The defining equation when $n > C$ is the following.

$$mathbf{H}_{uc}(n) = \lambda[\mathbf{M_c} + \lambda\mathbf{I_c}]^{-1} + \mathbf{M_c}[\mathbf{M_c} + \lambda\mathbf{I_c}]^{-1}\mathbf{P_c}\mathbf{H_{uc}}(n)$$
$$+ \mathbf{M_c}[\mathbf{M_c} + \lambda\mathbf{I_c}]^{-1}\mathbf{Q_c}\mathbf{R_c}\mathbf{H_{uc}}(n-1)\mathbf{H_{uc}}(n).$$

Notice the subtle change. In the last term, $\mathbf{R_c}$ is now to the left of $\mathbf{H_{uc}}(n-1)$ and $\mathbf{H_{uc}}(n)$ instead of between them. The reason is simple. When there are more than C customers at the subsystem, a departing customer can immediately be replaced [$\mathbf{R_c}$], and eventually a customer comes to raise the queue to $n+1$ for the first time [$\mathbf{H_{uc}}(n)$]. If there are C or fewer customers at S_1, then eventually the subsystem has $k-1$ customers when a new one arrives, [$\mathbf{H_{u(k-1)}}$], and imediately enters [$\mathbf{R_k}$]. This, by the way, shows us the significance of having matrices that do not commute ($\mathbf{H_{u(c-1)}}\mathbf{R_c} \neq \mathbf{R_c}\mathbf{H_{u(c-1)}}$). This slight difference yields a somewhat different recursive equation:

$$\mathbf{H_{uc}}(n) = \lambda[\lambda\mathbf{I_c} + \mathbf{B_c} - \mathbf{M_c}\,\mathbf{Q_c}\,\mathbf{R_c}\,\mathbf{H_{uc}}(n-1)]^{-1}. \tag{6.5.15b}$$

We leave it as an exercise to prove that these matrices are isometric.

Recall that $\mathbf{p_k}$ from Equations (6.5.2) is the state probability vector for S_1 if k customers entered the empty subsystem simultaneously. If the customers arrived randomly, the state S_1 would be in when there are finally k customers there for the first time is defined by (compare with Definition 4.5.4) the following.

Definition 6.5.9

$\mathbf{p_{uk}}(n)$:= *probability vector of first passage from 0 to n.* $[\mathbf{p_{uk}}(n)]_i$ is the probability that S_1 will be in state $i \in \Xi_k$ when there are n customers there for the first time. Two conventions go with this. First, $k = n$ when $n \le C$, and $k = C$ when $n \ge C$. Second, when $k = n \le C$, we drop the argument:

$$\mathbf{p_{uk}} := \mathbf{p_{uk}}(k) \quad \text{for } k \le C.$$

The process starts with the arrival of the first customer and ends when the queue (including the customers in service) reaches n. The queue could have gone back to 0 any number of times before the process ends.

□

It is plain to see that

$$\mathbf{p_{uk}} := \mathbf{p}\mathbf{H_{u1}}\mathbf{R_2}\mathbf{H_{u2}}\mathbf{R_3}\cdots\mathbf{H_{uk-1}}\mathbf{R_k} \quad \text{for } n = k \le C \tag{6.5.16a}$$

and for $n > C$

$$\begin{aligned}\mathbf{p_{uc}}(n) :&= \mathbf{p}\mathbf{H_{u1}}\mathbf{R_2}\mathbf{H_{u2}}\mathbf{R_3}\cdots\mathbf{H_{uc\text{-}1}}\mathbf{R_c}\mathbf{H_{uc}}\mathbf{H_{uc}}(C+1)\cdots\mathbf{H_{uc}}(n-1)\\ &= \mathbf{p_{uc}}\,\mathbf{H_{uc}}\,\mathbf{H_{uc}}(C+1)\cdots\mathbf{H_{uc}}(n-1).\end{aligned} \tag{6.5.16b}$$

We can read these formulas physically. A first customer arrives $[\mathbf{p}]$. There is one customer at S_1 when a second one arrives $[\mathbf{H_{u1}}]$, and enters $[\mathbf{R_2}]$. Eventually, there are two customers at S_1 when a third one arrives $[\mathbf{H_{u2}}]$, and enters $[\mathbf{R_3}]$, and so on. Once there are C or more customers in the subsystem $[\mathbf{H_c}(n)]$, the arriving customer does not enter (no $\mathbf{R}$). The $\mathbf{p_u}$ vectors satisfy a natural recursive equation.

$$\mathbf{p_{u(k+1)}} = \mathbf{p_{uk}}\mathbf{H_{uk}}\mathbf{R_{k+1}} \quad \text{for } k < C, \tag{6.5.16c}$$

$$\mathbf{p_{uc}}(n+1) = \mathbf{p_{uc}}(n)\mathbf{H_{uc}}(n) \quad \text{for } n \ge C. \tag{6.5.16d}$$

Without belaboring the point, note the difference between $\mathbf{p_c}$ and $\mathbf{p_{uc}}(n)$. In the former, even if more than C customers arrive simultaneously, only C of them will enter, so the vector is the same for all $n \ge C$. In the latter case, when that special customer who will raise the queue to $n+1$ for the first time, arrives, even though he does not enter S_1, the system is in a special state. That special state $\mathbf{p_{uc}}(n)$ is different for all n.

After the following definition, we are finally ready to set up equations for the first-passage times, after which we summarize everything in a theorem.

Definition 6.5.10

$[\boldsymbol{\tau}'_{\mathbf{uk}}(n)]$:= *mean first-passage time vector for an M/ME/C//N loop to go from n to n + 1.* Component i is the mean time until the queue at S_1 (as usual, including the ones in service) reaches $n+1$ customers for the first time, given that the process started in state $\{i\,;\,n\}$. The conventions are the same as in Definition 6.5.9, namely, $k = n$ for $n \le C$ and $k = C$ when $n \ge C$. Also,

$$\boldsymbol{\tau}'_{\mathbf{uk}} := \boldsymbol{\tau}'_{\mathbf{uk}}(k) \quad \text{for } k \le C.$$

This is a $D(k)$-dimensional column vector. □

Clearly, when no one is at S_1, the mean time until someone arrives is $1/\lambda$, so

$$\boldsymbol{\tau}'_{\mathbf{uo}}{}^{\dagger} = \frac{1}{\lambda}. \tag{6.5.17a}$$

The mean time to go from 1 to 2 for the first time is governed by the equation

$$\begin{aligned}\boldsymbol{\tau}'_{\mathbf{u1}} &= [\lambda\mathbf{I}_1 + \mathbf{M}_1]^{-1}\boldsymbol{\epsilon}'_1 + [\lambda I_1 + \mathbf{M}_1]^{-1}\mathbf{M}_1\,\mathbf{P}_1\,\boldsymbol{\tau}'_{\mathbf{u1}} \\ &\quad + [\lambda\mathbf{I}_1 + \mathbf{M}_1]^{-1}\mathbf{M}_1\mathbf{q}'[\boldsymbol{\tau}'_{\mathbf{o}} + \mathbf{p}\,\boldsymbol{\tau}'_{\mathbf{u1}}].\end{aligned}$$

Solve for $\boldsymbol{\tau}'_{\mathbf{u1}}$ to get

$$[\mathbf{M}_1 + \lambda\mathbf{I}_1 - \mathbf{M}_1\,\mathbf{P}_1 - \mathbf{M}_1\,\mathbf{q}'\,\mathbf{p}]\boldsymbol{\tau}'_{\mathbf{u1}} = \boldsymbol{\epsilon}'_1 + \mathbf{M}_1\,\mathbf{q}'\,\boldsymbol{\tau}'_{\mathbf{o}}$$

or

$$[\lambda\mathbf{I}_1 + \mathbf{B}_1 - \mathbf{M}_1\,\mathbf{Q}_1\,\mathbf{R}_1]\boldsymbol{\tau}'_{\mathbf{u1}} = \boldsymbol{\epsilon}'_1 + \frac{1}{\lambda}\mathbf{M}_1\,\mathbf{q}'.$$

Identifying the object in brackets with (6.5.13b), we get

$$\begin{aligned}\lambda\,\boldsymbol{\tau}'_{\mathbf{u1}} &= \mathbf{H}_{\mathrm{u1}}\left[\boldsymbol{\epsilon}'_1 + \frac{1}{\lambda}\mathbf{M}_1\mathbf{q}'\right] = \mathbf{H}_{\mathrm{u1}}\left[\boldsymbol{\epsilon}'_1 + \frac{1}{\lambda}\mathbf{B}_1\,\boldsymbol{\epsilon}'_1\right] \\ &= \mathbf{H}_{\mathrm{u1}}\left[\mathbf{I}_1 + \frac{1}{\lambda}\mathbf{B}_1\right]\boldsymbol{\epsilon}'_1.\end{aligned} \tag{6.5.17b}$$

Compare this with (4.5.5) for $n = 1$. Next, for k up to C,

$$\begin{aligned}\boldsymbol{\tau}'_{\mathbf{uk}} &= [\mathbf{M}_{\mathrm{k}} + \lambda\mathbf{I}_{\mathrm{k}}]^{-1}\boldsymbol{\epsilon}'\mathbf{k} + [\mathbf{M}_{\mathrm{k}} + \lambda\mathbf{I}_{\mathrm{k}}]^{-1}\mathbf{M}_{\mathrm{k}}\mathbf{P}_{\mathrm{k}}\,\boldsymbol{\tau}'_{\mathbf{uk}} \\ &\quad + [\mathbf{M}_{\mathrm{k}} + \lambda\mathbf{I}_{\mathrm{k}}]^{-1}\mathbf{M}_{\mathrm{k}}\mathbf{Q}_{\mathrm{k}}[\boldsymbol{\tau}'_{\mathbf{uk-1}} + \mathbf{H}_{\mathrm{uk-1}}\mathbf{R}_{\mathrm{k}}\boldsymbol{\tau}'_{\mathbf{uk}}],\end{aligned}$$

which when solved in the usual fashion, noting (6.5.15a), yields

$$\lambda\boldsymbol{\tau}'_{\mathbf{uk}} = \mathbf{H}_{\mathrm{uk}}[\boldsymbol{\epsilon}'\mathbf{k} + \mathbf{M}_{\mathrm{k}}\,\mathbf{Q}_{\mathrm{k}}\,\boldsymbol{\tau}'_{\mathbf{uk-1}}] \quad \text{for } 1 < k \le C. \tag{6.5.17c}$$

We merely give the final result for queue lengths above C.

$$\lambda\,\boldsymbol{\tau}'_{\mathbf{uc}}(n) = \mathbf{H}_{\mathrm{uc}}(n)[\boldsymbol{\epsilon}'_{\mathbf{c}} + \mathbf{M}_{\mathrm{c}}\,\mathbf{Q}_{\mathrm{c}}\,\mathbf{R}_{\mathrm{c}}\,\boldsymbol{\tau}'_{\mathbf{uc}}(n-1)] \quad \text{for } n > C. \tag{6.5.17d}$$

Well, we finally got to the end, so we can now present our summary theorem.

---

† We have used boldface even though this is a one-dimensional object.

Theorem 6.5.3: Given a generalized M/ME/C-type queue, the mean first-passage time vectors for the queue at S_1 to grow by 1, and associated matrices, can be constructed in the following way.

(a) Probability matrices of first passage from n to $n+1$, $\mathbf{H_{uk}}, \mathbf{H_{uc}}(n)$, as defined by Definitions 6.5.5 through 6.5.7 and Equation (6.5.14), are given by the following.

$$\mathbf{H_{u0}} = 1 \qquad \mathbf{Q_1} = \mathbf{q}, \ \mathbf{R_1} = \mathbf{p}$$

[from (6.5.15a)]

$$\mathbf{H_{uk}} = \lambda[\lambda\mathbf{I_k} + \mathbf{B_k} - \mathbf{M_k Q_k H_{uk-1} R_k}]^{-1}, \qquad k = 1, 2, \ldots, C,$$

and from (6.5.15b), with $\mathbf{H_{uc}}(C) = \mathbf{H_{uc}}$,

$$\mathbf{H_{uc}}(n) = \lambda[\lambda\mathbf{I_c} + \mathbf{B_c} - \mathbf{M_c}\,\mathbf{Q_c}\,\mathbf{R_c}\,\mathbf{H_{uc}}(n-1)]^{-1}, \qquad n > C.$$

Every $\mathbf{H_u}$ is isometric.

(b) The first-passage time vectors, as defined by Definition 6.5.10, are given by the following [(6.5.17a) and (6.5.17b)].

$$\boldsymbol{\tau}'_{\mathbf{u0}} = \frac{1}{\lambda} \quad \text{and} \quad \boldsymbol{\tau}'_{\mathbf{u1}} = \frac{1}{\lambda}\mathbf{H_{u1}}\left[\mathbf{I_1} + \frac{1}{\lambda}\mathbf{B_1}\right]\boldsymbol{\epsilon}'_1$$

[from (6.5.17c)],

$$\boldsymbol{\tau}'_{\mathbf{uk}}(n) = \frac{1}{\lambda}\mathbf{H_{uk}}[\boldsymbol{\epsilon}'\mathbf{k} + \mathbf{M_k Q_k}\,\boldsymbol{\tau}'_{\mathbf{uk-1}}], \qquad 1 < k \le C,$$

and [from (6.5.17d)], with $\boldsymbol{\tau}'_{\mathbf{uc}}(C) = \boldsymbol{\tau}'_{\mathbf{uc}}$,

$$\boldsymbol{\tau}'_{\mathbf{uc}}(n) = \frac{1}{\lambda}\mathbf{H_c}(n)[\boldsymbol{\epsilon}'_{\mathbf{c}} + \mathbf{M_c}\,\mathbf{Q_c}\,\mathbf{R_c}\,\boldsymbol{\tau}'_{\mathbf{uc}}(n-1)], \qquad n > C.$$

(c) The probability vectors of first passage from 0 to n, as defined in Definition 6.5.9, are given by the following.

$$\mathbf{p_{u1}} = \mathbf{p}$$

[from (6.5.16)]

$$\mathbf{p_{u(k+1)}} = \mathbf{p_{uk} H_{uk} R_{k+1}} \qquad k = 1,\ 2, \ldots,\ C-1,$$
$$\mathbf{p_{uc}}(n+1) = \mathbf{p_{uc}}(n)\mathbf{H_{uc}}(n) \qquad n = C,\ C+1, \ldots.$$

These equations are equally applicable to closed M/ME/C//N loops, as long as n does not exceed N. ∎

Remember that these processes include the possibility that the queue could drop to zero one or more times before rising to the given length.

Many things can be calculated from these objects. We enumerate several types below.

1. Given that S_1 is initially empty:

(a) Mean time for the queue to rise by 1:

$$t_u(k) = \mathbf{p_{uk}}\, \boldsymbol{\tau}'_{\mathbf{uk}}, \quad \text{for } 1 \le k \le C, \tag{6.5.18a}$$
$$t_u(n) = \mathbf{p_{uc}}(n) \boldsymbol{\tau}'_{\mathbf{uc}}(n), \quad n = C+1, \ldots. \tag{6.5.18b}$$

(b) Mean time for the queue to rise from 0 to n

$$t(0 \to n) = \frac{1}{\lambda} + \sum_{j=1}^{n-1} t_u(j). \tag{6.5.18c}$$

2. Given that there are n customers at S_1 who initially start up simultaneously [see discussion surrounding Equations (6.5.2)]:

(a) For k initially less than C, $(1 \le k < C)$ mean time for the queue to rise by 1:

$$t_u(k) = \mathbf{p_k}\, \boldsymbol{\tau}'_{\mathbf{uk}}, \tag{6.5.19a}$$
$$t_u(k{+}1) = \mathbf{p_k}\, \mathbf{H_{uk}}\, \mathbf{R_{k+1}}\, \boldsymbol{\tau}'_{\mathbf{u(k+1)}}, \tag{6.5.19b}$$
$$t_u(k{+}2) = \mathbf{p_k}\, \mathbf{H_{uk}}\, \mathbf{R_{k+1}}\, \mathbf{H_{u(k+1)}}\, \mathbf{R_{k+2}}\, \boldsymbol{\tau}'_{\mathbf{u(k+2)}}, \tag{6.5.19c}$$

and so on, as long as $k + l \le C$. After that, continue on without $\mathbf{R_k}$, and use $\mathbf{H_c}(n)$ instead of $\mathbf{H_{uk}}$.

(b) For initial $n \ge C$, mean time for the queue to rise by 1:

$$t_u(n) = \mathbf{p_c}\, \boldsymbol{\tau}'_{\mathbf{uc}}(n), \tag{6.5.20a}$$
$$t_u(n+1) = \mathbf{p_c}\, \mathbf{H_{uc}}(n)\, \boldsymbol{\tau}'_{\mathbf{uc}}(n+1), \tag{6.5.20b}$$
$$t_u(n+2) = \mathbf{p_c} \mathbf{H_{uc}}(n) \mathbf{H_{uc}}(n+1) \boldsymbol{\tau}'_{\mathbf{uc}}(n+2), \tag{6.5.20c}$$

and so on, taking care not to exceed N if this is a closed loop.

(c) Mean time for the queue to rise from n to $n + l + 1$;

$$t(n \to n+l+1) = \sum_{j=n}^{n+l} t_u(j). \tag{6.5.20d}$$

3. Given that the system has been running for a long time (it is in its steady state), but it is observed that there are n (or k) customers in the queue, the mean time for the queue to grow thereafter is the same as type 2 above, except use as initial vectors Equations (6.5.1) instead of the $\mathbf{p_k}$ vectors of Equations (6.5.2).

Variation 1, of course, can give us some idea of how long it takes for the M/ME/C queue to reach its steady-state queue length, which is a reasonable estimate of how long it might take for such a system to reach its steady state.

Variation 2 is a model of a system that starts up in the morning with n jobs left over from the night before. Comparison with variation 1 could give an idea of what the impact is for allowing carryover.

Variation 3 can give an idea of how bad things might get for the rest of the day. For instance, the afternoon arrival rate may be different from that which was used to calculate Equations (6.5.1). Presumably, other variations and interpretations can be thought up.

6.5.3.2 First Passages for Queue Decrease

What we do here is very similar to that which we did in the preceding section, with one extra complication (there always is one more). In going *up* there is always the natural floor, namely, the queue can never be less than 0. Here, unfortunately, the top can be anywhere, so we must carry N along in all our notation. Of course, when we go to the open system, N disappears, but in reliability theory, one seldom has an infinite number of backups, so the closed loop is important in its own right. Therefore, in what follows, we are looking at the M/ME/C//N loop.

Let us start, as usual, with the definition of a first-passage matrix.

Definition 6.5.11

$\mathbf{H_{dc}}(n;N) :=$ *probability matrix of first passage from* n *to* $n-1$*, where* $N \geq n > C$. $[\mathbf{H_{dc}}(n;N)]_{ij}$ is the probability that S_1 will be in state $j \in \Xi_c$ when its queue drops to $n-1$ for the first time, given that it started in state $i \in \Xi_c$ with n customers in the queue (including the C customers in service). This is a square isometric matrix of dimension $D(C)$, but it has no inverse. □

For queue lengths less than, or equal to C we need slightly different matrices, which we define now.

Definition 6.5.12

$\mathbf{H_{dk}}(N \mid C) :=$ *probability matrix of first passage from* k *to* $k-1$*, where* $C \geq k > 0$. $[\mathbf{H_{dk}}(N \mid C)]_{ij}$ is the probability that S_1 will be in state $j \in \Xi_{k-1}$ when its queue drops to $k-1$ for the first time, given that it started in state $i \in \Xi_k$ with k customers in the queue (all k customers are in service). This is an isometrix, $D(k) \times D(k-1)$-dimensional matrix (proven below). □

In a moment we introduce a set of matrices that are invertible, although their interpretation is more difficult to grasp than these, but prove to be more convenient for our purposes. First let us set up the equation for the $\mathbf{H_{dc}}$ matrices. When all customers are at S_1 (refer to Figure 6.5.2), there can be no arrivals, so

$$\mathbf{H_{dc}}(N;N) = \mathbf{Q_c R_c} + \mathbf{P_c H_{dc}}(N;N),$$

which yields

$$\mathbf{H_{dc}}(N;N) = \mathbf{V_c M_c Q_c R_c}. \tag{6.5.21a}$$

We already proved that this matrix is isometric in Section 6.5.2. Next, let us look at any other n greater than C. Figure 6.5.2 shows that now three different types of events can occur, leading to *

$$\mathbf{H_{dc}}(n;N) = (\lambda\mathbf{I_c} + \mathbf{M_c})^{-1}\mathbf{M_c Q_c R_c} + (\lambda\mathbf{I_c} + \mathbf{M_c})^{-1}\mathbf{M_c P_c H_{dc}}(n;N)$$
$$+\lambda(\lambda\mathbf{I_c} + \mathbf{M_c})^{-1}\mathbf{H_{dc}}(n+1;N)\mathbf{H_{dc}}(n;N),$$

which yields

$$\mathbf{H_{dc}}(n;N) = [\lambda\mathbf{I_c} + \mathbf{B_c} - \lambda\mathbf{H_{dc}}(n+1;N)]^{-1}\,\mathbf{M_c}\,\mathbf{Q_c}\,\mathbf{R_c}. \qquad (6.5.21b)$$

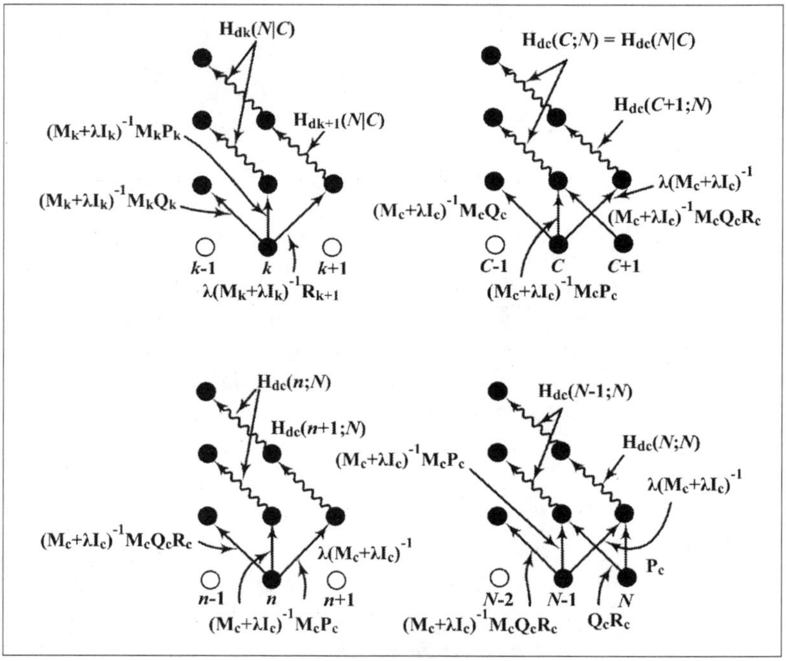

Figure 6.5.2: Time-dependent state transition diagram for *down* processes. This is applicable to the closed M/ME/$C//N$ queue, where $C < N$. There are five different sets of transition types, one each for $0 < n = k < C$, $n = C$, $N-1 > n > C$, $n = N-1$, and $n = N$. $n = 0$ is only relevant for *up* processes.

We can see why the $(\mathbf{H_{dc}})$ matrices are not invertible from the presence of the term, $\mathbf{Q_c R_c}$. Let us now define the set of auxiliary matrices suggested by this equation:

$$\mathbf{X_c}(n;N) := [\lambda\mathbf{I_c} + \mathbf{B_c} - \lambda\mathbf{H_{dc}}(n+1;N)]^{-1}. \qquad (6.5.22a)$$

Then clearly,

$$\mathbf{H_{dc}}(n;N) = \mathbf{X_c}(n;N)\mathbf{M_c Q_c R_c}. \qquad (6.5.22b)$$

*Notice the subtle difference between $\mathbf{H_{dc}}$ and its *up* counterpart in (6.5.15b).

We add to that the initial definition,

$$\mathbf{X_c}(N;N) := \mathbf{V_c}, \tag{6.5.22c}$$

and substitute (6.5.22b) back into (6.5.22a) to get for $C < n < N$,

$$\mathbf{X_c}(n;N) = [\lambda\mathbf{I_c} + \mathbf{B_c} - \lambda\mathbf{X_c}(n+1;N)\mathbf{M_c Q_c R_c}]^{-1}. \tag{6.5.22d}$$

Then (6.5.22c) and (6.5.22d) completely define the $(\mathbf{X_c})$ matrices and (6.5.22b) gives all the $(\mathbf{H_{dc}})$s from N down to $C+1$.

When there are exactly C customers at S_1, everything is as before, except that when the queue finally drops, there is no new customer waiting to enter, so there is no need for $\mathbf{R_c}$. Thus the first-passage equation comes to

$$\mathbf{H_{dc}}(N \,|\, C) = [\lambda\mathbf{I_c} + \mathbf{B_c} - \lambda\mathbf{H_{dc}}(C+1;N)]^{-1}\,\mathbf{M_c Q_c}. \tag{6.5.23a}$$

This equation is almost identical in form to (6.5.21b), but as already mentioned, it is missing $\mathbf{R_c}$. But if we let (6.5.22a) be valid for $n = C$ (up to now we only made it true down to $C+1$), then we have

$$\mathbf{H_{dc}}(N \,|\, C) = \mathbf{X_c}(C;N)\mathbf{M_c Q_c}. \tag{6.5.23b}$$

With fewer than C customers at S_1, a new arrival immediately enters, but a departure leaves one less customer in service. This leads to the last set of equations:

$$\mathbf{H_{dk}}(N \,|\, C) = [\lambda\mathbf{I_c} + \mathbf{B_c} - \lambda\mathbf{R_{k+1}H_{dk+1}}(N \,|\, C)]^{-1}\,\mathbf{M_c Q_c}. \tag{6.5.23c}$$

We define our last set of $\mathbf{X}$ matrices, starting with

$$\mathbf{X_c}(N \,|\, C) := \mathbf{X_c}(C;N), \tag{6.5.24a}$$

and for all other k, $1 \le k < C$,

$$\mathbf{X_k}(N \,|\, C) := [\lambda\mathbf{I_c} + \mathbf{B_c} - \lambda\mathbf{R_{k+1}X_{k+1}}(N \,|\, C)\mathbf{M_{k+1}Q_{k+1}}]^{-1}. \tag{6.5.24b}$$

This lets us write

$$\mathbf{H_{dk}}(N \,|\, C) := \mathbf{X_k}(N \,|\, C)\mathbf{M_c Q_c} \qquad 1 \le k \le C, \tag{6.5.24c}$$

where we have incorporated (6.5.23b).

STOP! Surely we have seen this all before. Of course, they all look alike, but exactly alike? In this case they are just like the equations governing the steady-state matrices. Compare the following sets of equations: (6.5.22c) with (6.3.6a), (6.5.22d) with (6.3.6c), (6.5.24a) with (6.3.7a), and (6.5.24b) with (6.3.7b).

Clearly, $\lambda\mathbf{X_c}(n;N)$ satisfies exactly the same recursive equation as $\mathbf{U_c}(N-n)$, and just as important, with the same initial condition [(6.5.22c) versus (6.3.6a)]. Therefore, we have discovered that

$$\mathbf{X_c}(n;N) = \frac{1}{\lambda}\mathbf{U_c}(N-n) \quad \text{for } C \le n \le N \tag{6.5.25a}$$

and

$$\mathbf{X_k}(N \mid C) = \frac{1}{\lambda}\mathbf{U_k}(N \mid C) \quad \text{for } 1 \le k \le C. \tag{6.5.25b}$$

We now have everything we want to know about the $\mathbf{H_d}$ matrices.

Lemma 6.5.4: The matrices described in Definitions 6.5.10 and 6.5.11 are isometric and are related to the steady-state matrices by the following equations.

$$\mathbf{H_{dc}}(n; N) = \frac{1}{\lambda}\mathbf{U_c}(N-n)\mathbf{M_c Q_c R_c} \quad \text{for } C < n \le N \tag{6.5.26a}$$

and

$$\mathbf{H_{dk}}(N \mid C) = \frac{1}{\lambda}\mathbf{U_k}(N \mid C)\mathbf{M_k Q_k} \quad \text{for } 1 \le k \le C. \tag{6.5.26b}$$

The $\mathbf{U}$ matrices are given by Equations (6.3.6) and (6.3.7). ▲

Proof: The isometric property follows directly from (6.3.4b). **QED**

We saw something like this in Section 4.5.3, but $\mathbf{H_d}(n; N)$ [the $C = 1$ equivalent to $\mathbf{H_{dc}}(n; N)$] turned out to be the matrix $\mathbf{Q}$, so the relation equivalent to (6.5.26a) is trivial.

Note from (6.3.9) that it is $[(1/\lambda)\mathbf{U_c}(N-n)\mathbf{B_c}]$ that is isometric, and not $\mathbf{U_c}(N-n)$ itself. Indeed, it is this product that has the physical interpretation, for we can rewrite (6.5.26a) as

$$\mathbf{H_{dc}}(n; N) = \frac{1}{\lambda}\mathbf{U_c}(N-n)\mathbf{B_c V_c M_c Q_c R_c} = \left[\frac{1}{\lambda}\mathbf{U_c}(N-n)\mathbf{B_c}\right]\mathbf{Y_c R_c},$$

where $\mathbf{Y_c}$ comes from Definition 6.5.2 and (6.5.4a). From their definitions we see that the $[\mathbf{Y_c R_c}]$ portion carries a process to a departure and subsequent entry without any intervening arrivals. Therefore, the (ij)th component of the portion in brackets must be the probability that S_1 is in state $j \in \Xi_c$, with n customers, immediately after the last arrival but before the departure that finally lowers the queue to $n-1$ for the first time (given that the system was originally in state $i \in \Xi_c$ with n customers). This is a rather complicated interpretation, but it need not be understood for the development of our formulas. Perhaps we should have given a special symbol to the isometric product and used it in our exposition, and maybe we will in the future. From now on we stop using the $\mathbf{X}$ matrices and express the first-passage times in terms of the already familiar $\mathbf{H}$ matrices. First we give the *down* equivalent of $\boldsymbol{\tau}'_{\mathbf{uk}}(n)$ in Definition 6.5.10.

Definition 6.5.13

$[\boldsymbol{\tau}'_{\mathbf{dk}}(n; N \mid C)]$:= *mean first-passage time vector for a generalized M/ME/C//N loop to go from n to n − 1. The ith component is the mean time until the queue at S_1 (as usual, including the ones in service) reaches n − 1 customers for the first time, given that the process* *started in state* $\{i;\, n\}$. The conventions are the same as in Definition 6.5.10; namely, $k = n$ for $n \le C$ and $k = C$ when $n \ge C$. Also,

$$\boldsymbol{\tau}'_{\mathbf{dk}}(N|C) := \boldsymbol{\tau}'_{\mathbf{dk}}(k; N\,|\,C) \quad \text{for } k \le C, \quad \text{and}$$

$$\boldsymbol{\tau}'_{\mathbf{dc}}(n; N) := \boldsymbol{\tau}'_{\mathbf{uc}}(n; N|C) \quad \text{for } C < n \le N.$$

These are $D(k)$-dimensional column vectors, and they depend on N.□

When all customers are at S_1, there are no arrivals, so the mean time to drop is simply

$$\boldsymbol{\tau}'_{\mathbf{dc}}(N; N) = \mathbf{V}_{\mathbf{c}}\, \boldsymbol{\epsilon}'_{\mathbf{c}}. \tag{6.5.27a}$$

Otherwise, we must go down, across, and up, giving

$$\boldsymbol{\tau}'_{\mathbf{dc}}(n; N) = (\lambda \mathbf{I_c} + \mathbf{M_c})^{-1}\, \boldsymbol{\epsilon}'_{\mathbf{c}} + (\lambda \mathbf{I_c} + \mathbf{M_c})^{-1}\, \mathbf{M_c P_c}\, \boldsymbol{\tau}'_{\mathbf{dc}}(n;\; N)$$
$$+\lambda\, (\lambda \mathbf{I_c} + \mathbf{M_c})^{-1}\, [\boldsymbol{\tau}'_{\mathbf{dc}}(n+1; N) + \mathbf{H_{dc}}(n+1;\; N)\boldsymbol{\tau}'_{\mathbf{dc}}(n; N)],$$

which rearranges to yield

$$[\lambda \mathbf{I_c} + \mathbf{M_c} - \mathbf{M_c P_c} - \lambda \mathbf{H_{dc}}(n+1; N)]\boldsymbol{\tau}'_{\mathbf{dc}}(n; N) = \boldsymbol{\epsilon}'_{\mathbf{c}} + \lambda \boldsymbol{\tau}'_{\mathbf{dc}}(n+1; N).$$

Use (6.5.26a) for $\mathbf{H_{dc}}(n+1; N)$ and compare with (6.3.6c) to get for $C \le n < N$,

$$\lambda \boldsymbol{\tau}'_{\mathbf{dc}}(n; N) = \mathbf{U_c}(N-n)\boldsymbol{\epsilon}'_{\mathbf{c}} + \lambda \mathbf{U_c}(N-n)\boldsymbol{\tau}'_{\mathbf{dc}}(n+1; N). \tag{6.5.27b}$$

This equation (as noted) is valid for $n = C$. There is another expression that is more useful, which we include in the theorem below.

For $k < C$ we have a somewhat different set of equations.

$$\boldsymbol{\tau}'_{\mathbf{dk}}(N\,|\,C) = (\lambda \mathbf{I_k} + \mathbf{M_k})^{-1}\boldsymbol{\epsilon}'_{\mathbf{k}} + (\lambda \mathbf{I_k} + \mathbf{M_k})^{-1}\mathbf{M_k}\, \mathbf{P_k}\, \boldsymbol{\tau}'_{\mathbf{dk}}(N\,|\,C)$$
$$+\lambda(\lambda \mathbf{I_k} + \mathbf{M_k})^{-1}\mathbf{R_{k+1}}[\boldsymbol{\tau}'_{\mathbf{d(k+1)}}(N\,|\,C) + \mathbf{H_{d(k+1)}}(N\,|\,C)\boldsymbol{\tau}'_{\mathbf{dk}}(N\,|\,C)].$$

Just as we did above, regroup terms, use (6.5.26b), compare with (6.3.7b), and get for $1 \le k < C$,

$$\lambda \boldsymbol{\tau}'_{\mathbf{dk}}(N\,|\,C) = \mathbf{U_k}(N\,|\,C)\, \boldsymbol{\epsilon}'_{\mathbf{k}} + \lambda \mathbf{U_k}(N\,|\,C)\mathbf{R_{k+1}}\, \boldsymbol{\tau}'_{\mathbf{d(k+1)}}(N\,|\,C). \tag{6.5.27c}$$

The summary theorem now follows.

Theorem 6.5.5: Given a generalized M/ME/C//N loop, the first-passage matrices and vectors for decreasing length, as given in Definitions 6.5.10 to 6.5.12, satisfy the following formulas.

(a) The first-passage matrices are given by [Equations (6.5.26)]

$$\mathbf{H_{dc}}(n; N) = \frac{1}{\lambda}\mathbf{U_c}(N-n)\mathbf{M_c Q_c R_c} \quad \text{for } C \le n \le N,$$

$$\mathbf{H_{dk}}(N\,|\,C) = \frac{1}{\lambda}\mathbf{U_k}(N\,|\,C)\mathbf{M_k Q_k} \quad \text{for } 1 \le k \le C.$$

(b) The first-passage vectors are given by [Equations (6.5.27)]

$$\boldsymbol{\tau}'_{\mathbf{dc}}(N;N) = \mathbf{V}_{\mathrm{c}}\,\boldsymbol{\epsilon}'_{\mathbf{c}};$$

for $C \le n < N$,

$$\boldsymbol{\tau}'_{\mathbf{dc}}(n;N) = \frac{1}{\lambda}\mathbf{U}_{\mathrm{c}}(N-n)\boldsymbol{\epsilon}'_{\mathbf{c}} + \mathbf{U}_{\mathrm{c}}(N-n)\boldsymbol{\tau}'_{\mathbf{dc}}(n+1;N);$$

and for $1 \le k < C$,

$$\boldsymbol{\tau}'_{\mathbf{dk}}(N \mid C) = \frac{1}{\lambda}\mathbf{U}_{\mathrm{k}}(N \mid C)\boldsymbol{\epsilon}'_{\mathbf{k}} + \mathbf{U}_{\mathrm{k}}(N \mid C)\mathbf{R}_{\mathrm{k+1}}\,\boldsymbol{\tau}'_{\mathbf{dk+1}}(N \mid C).$$

(c) The formula (6.5.27b) can be written in another form. Let l be the number of customers at S_2. Then for $0 < l \le N - C$,

$$\lambda\,\boldsymbol{\tau}'_{\mathbf{dc}}(N-l;N) = \mathbf{U}_{\mathrm{c}}(l)\mathbf{K}_{\mathrm{c}}(C+l-1)\boldsymbol{\epsilon}'_{\mathbf{c}}$$
$$= [\mathbf{K}_{\mathrm{c}}(C+l) - \mathbf{I}_{\mathrm{c}}]\boldsymbol{\epsilon}'_{\mathbf{c}} \qquad (6.5.28a)$$

or, replacing l with n (where $l = N - n$)

$$\lambda\boldsymbol{\tau}'_{\mathbf{dc}}(n;N) = \mathbf{U}_{\mathrm{c}}(N-n)\mathbf{K}_{\mathrm{c}}(N-n+C-1)\boldsymbol{\epsilon}'_{\mathbf{c}}$$
$$= [\mathbf{K}_{\mathrm{c}}(N-n+C) - \mathbf{I}_{\mathrm{c}}]\boldsymbol{\epsilon}'_{\mathbf{c}} \quad \text{for } C \le n < N. \qquad (6.5.28b)$$

$\mathbf{K}_{\mathrm{c}}(n)$ is the steady-state normalization matrix defined by (6.3.13). The middle form of both versions is also valid for $l = 0$ (or $n = C$). The right-hand side of (6.5.28a) does not contain N explicitly. Therefore, $\boldsymbol{\tau}'_{\mathbf{dc}}(N-l;N)$ depends only on l, the number of customers at S_2. ■

Proof: Substitute (6.5.28b) directly into (6.5.27b), and use (6.3.13). **QED**

Equations (6.5.28) reduce to (4.5.14a) for $C = 1$, the result for the generalized M/ME/1//N loop, except that things change once the queue length drops below C. After all, $\mathbf{K}_{\mathrm{c}}(\mathbf{n})$ is only defined for $n \ge C - 1$. This theorem is quite interesting, because it lets us find out about transient behavior using no more information than is needed for the steady-state solution.

What can we do with these? Well, first of all, by definition

$\mathbf{p}\,\boldsymbol{\tau}'_{\mathbf{d1}}(N \mid C) =$ *mean busy-period time of a generalized* M/ME/C//N *system.*

For anything else, we require more information. Let us suppose for definiteness that there are $N > C$ customers at S_1, and that the system is in some internal state represented by $\mathbf{p}_{\mathbf{ic}}$, the same initial vectors we discussed in Equations (6.5.1), (6.5.2), and (6.5.16). Then the mean time for the queue to drop by 1 is given by

$$t_d(n;1;N) := \mathbf{p}_{\mathbf{ic}}\boldsymbol{\tau}'_{\mathbf{dc}}(n;N).$$

The time it takes to drop by one more is

$$t_d(n;2;N) := \mathbf{p}_{\mathbf{ic}}\mathbf{H}_{\mathrm{dc}}(n;N)\boldsymbol{\tau}'_{\mathbf{dc}}(n-1;\ N).$$

In general, the state the system will be in after the queue has dropped by $l \geq 1$ customers is

$$\mathbf{p_{dc}}(n; l; N) = \mathbf{p_{ic}}\mathbf{H_{dc}}(n; N)\mathbf{H_{dc}}(n-1; N)\cdots\mathbf{H_{dc}}(n-l+1; N), \quad (6.5.29a)$$

and if we let, by definition,

$$\mathbf{p_{dc}}(n; 0; N) := \mathbf{p_{ic}}, \quad (6.5.29b)$$

then

$$\mathbf{p_{dc}}(n; l+1; N) := \mathbf{p_{dc}}(n; l; N)\mathbf{H_{dc}}(n-l; N) \quad \text{for } l > 0. \quad (6.5.29c)$$

This is (more or less) the *down* equivalent of Definition 6.5.9, except that we can start with any length and in any initial state. We do not have an official name for it, so we do not give it an official definition designation. In any case, the mean time to drop from l to $l-1$, given the constraints above, is

$$t_d(n; l+1; N) = \mathbf{p_{dc}}(n; l; N)\boldsymbol{\tau}'_{\mathbf{dc}}(n-l; N). \quad (6.5.30)$$

In all of the above, if the queue should drop below C, use (6.5.26b) instead of (6.5.26a). That is, if $n - l < C$, then replace **dc** with **dk**.

Remember, these objects are the times to drop by one more customer. The total time it takes to drop from n to $n - l$ is the sum,

$$t_d(n \to n-l; N) := \sum_{j=0}^{l-1} t_d(n; j; N). \quad (6.5.31)$$

Now, this object has a name, several names, in fact. If, for instance, we have $l = n$, we have the ***n-busy period***, starting with initial condition $\mathbf{p_{ic}}$. Potentially, the most important interpretation of this is the MTTF, with backup and repair. It is important enough to give it a definition.

6.5.3.3 MTTF with Backup and Repair

An important subject for study in ***reliability theory*** concerns the time until a failure occurs. We have already found a relevant formula concerning this subject, so we discuss it here.

Definition 6.5.14

MTTF for a C-parallel, $(N-C)$-backup system, with exponential repair times is an M/ME/C//N loop with the initial state given by (6.5.2) for $k = N$. The system starts with N brand new identical devices. Their individual failure times are generated by $\langle \mathbf{p}, \mathbf{B} \rangle$. C devices are started simultaneously and the rest are kept in ***cold backup***. When one device breaks, it is immediately replaced by one of the backups and is sent to a single "repairman" who takes exponential time (with mean $1/\lambda$) to pick up, repair, and return a device that is as good as new. Failure occurs when the number of devices that are functional (including the number that are running) drops to a prespecified number, say, $\phi \geq 0$. The mean time for this process is given by $t_d(N \to \phi; N)$. □

Consider some of the variations we can perform.

1. The system has been running for a long time, and presently there are n functional devices (and $N-n$ devices in repair). The initial vector is given by (6.5.1) for $k=n$, and MTTF is given by $t_d(n \to \phi; N)$.

2. We are starting with new devices, but only n are available at the moment, with $N-n$ still awaiting single delivery at rate λ. If a device fails, an order is made for a new one. The initial vector is given by (6.5.2) for $k=n$, and MTTF is $t_d(n \to \phi; N)$.

3. The system was originally as given in Definition 6.5.13, but two devices have already failed and one has been repaired. The initial vector is given by (assuming that $N \geq C$)

$$\mathbf{p_{ic}} = \mathbf{p_c H_{dc}}(N;N)\mathbf{H_{dc}}(N-1;N)\mathbf{H_{uc}}(N-2),$$

and MTTF is given by $t_d(N-1 \to \phi; N)$. Notice the *up* first-passage matrix.

The last example can be very useful for ***dynamically updating*** the MTTF. Every time a device fails, postmultiply the initial vector by the appropriate $\mathbf{H_{dk}}$ to create an updated initial vector for the MTTF starting now. Similarly, every time a device is returned from repair, postmultiply by the appropriate $\mathbf{H_{uk}}$. The MTTFs change accordingly. By virtue of the fact that the $\mathbf{H}$ matrices do not commute, we see that the sequence "two failures followed by one repair" gives different results from "one failure followed by one repair and then another failure." Dynamic updating can help us even if we do not know the initial state. Pick any initial vector; then update it regularly. Eventually, your poor guess will be forgotten, and the updated vector will converge to the correct updated initial vector.

We could go on indefinitely enumerating systems that can be described this way, but we do only one more analysis before giving up on this chapter. Consider what happens when $N \to \infty$. Ah yes, of course, the open system. We have actually done this already, because the $\mathbf{H_{dk}}$ matrices are known in terms of the $\mathbf{U_k}$ matrices. Remember, though, that the limit exists only if ρ_c given by (6.5.10b) is less than 1. From (6.4.1),

$$\mathbf{H_{dc}} := \lim_{N\to\infty} \mathbf{H_{dc}}(n;N) := \frac{1}{\lambda}\mathbf{U_c M_c Q_c R_c} \quad \text{for } n \geq C \tag{6.5.32a}$$

and

$$\mathbf{H_{dk}}(\infty \,|\, C) := \lim_{N\to\infty} \mathbf{H_{dk}}(N \,|\, C) = \frac{1}{\lambda}\mathbf{U_k}(\infty \,|\, C)\mathbf{M_c Q_c}. \tag{6.5.32b}$$

So we do not have to cascade the $\mathbf{H_d}$ matrices down from infinity to find out what they are. In fact, they are all the same for $n \geq C$. All we have to do is solve for $\mathbf{U_c}$ in (6.4.1). Similarly, we can find the first-passage times,

$$\boldsymbol{\tau}'_{\mathbf{dc}} := \lim_{N\to\infty} \boldsymbol{\tau}'_{\mathbf{dc}}(n;N) = \frac{1}{\lambda}[\mathbf{K_c}(\infty) - \mathbf{I_c}]\boldsymbol{\epsilon}'_{\mathbf{c}}.$$

But from its recursive definition, (6.3.13b), $\mathbf{K_c}(\infty)$ can be shown to be

$$\mathbf{K_c} := \mathbf{K_c}(\infty) = [\mathbf{I_c} - \mathbf{U_c}]^{-1} \tag{6.5.33}$$

[compare with (4.2.2a)]. Therefore,

$$\boldsymbol{\tau}'_{\mathbf{dc}} := \frac{1}{\lambda}\mathbf{U_c}[\mathbf{I_c} - \mathbf{U_c}]^{-1}\boldsymbol{\epsilon}'_{\mathbf{c}}. \tag{6.5.34}$$

How interesting (we think lots of things are interesting). These vectors are independent of n, just like the M/ME/1 queue in (4.5.16a). Some thought would lead us to believe that this is reasonable. Does this mean that the time for the queue to drop by n is simply n multiplied by the time it takes to drop by 1, just as it is for the M/G/1 queue, based on (4.5.16b)? The answer is NO, because the departing customer leaves the system in a different state from that which it was in at the previous departure. Because of (6.5.32a), (6.5.29a) still holds true, and becomes

$$\mathbf{p_{dc}}(n;\, l) := \lim_{N\to\infty} \mathbf{p_{dc}}(n;\, l;\, N) = \mathbf{p_{ic}}\mathbf{H}^{l}_{\mathbf{dc}}. \tag{6.5.35a}$$

Also,

$$t_d(n;\, l+1) := \lim_{N\to\infty} t_d(n; l+1; N) = \mathbf{p_{dc}}(n-l)\boldsymbol{\tau}'_{\mathbf{dc}} = \mathbf{p_{ic}}\mathbf{H}^{l}_{\mathbf{dc}}\boldsymbol{\tau}'_{\mathbf{dc}}. \tag{6.5.35b}$$

Each step takes a different amount of time from the previous one, but they are independent of n as long as the queue length at S_1 (including those in service) is greater than C. That is,

$$\mathbf{p_{dc}}(n_1; l) = \mathbf{p_{dc}}(n_2;\, l) \quad \forall\ n_1,\, n_2, \ \text{ such that } \ n_i - l > C.$$

There are many useful applications of this set of equations. Here are some that come to mind. Let $\bar{q}$ be the mean number of customers at S_1 in a steady-state system.

1. A computer system has been in operation for a long time, when suddenly n_b jobs arrive in a bunch, while the Poisson arrivals continue at the same rate. How long will it take before the system settles back down to its steady state? Use (6.5.1) as the initial vector, with $k = \bar{q}$, but use n for $n-l+1$ in (6.5.35b). We call this the ***rush-hour traffic*** approximation.

2. A computer system has been running for a long time, with an arrival rate of λ_1. After 5 P.M., the arrival rate drops to λ_2. How long will it take to reach its new steady state? When can a part of the subsystem be taken offline (reduce C)?

3. The system has been down for a while, and when it starts up there are $n > \bar{q}$ jobs in the queue. How long will it take for the system to settle down?

6.6 Conclusions

We have seen that there are innumerable problems that can be explored using M/ME/C queues. They are more general than single-class Jackson networks. In fact, the formulas as derived here apply to more general systems than the ones we called "generalized M/ME/C//N systems." The equations depend on the defined properties of the input matrices (i.e., $\mathbf{M_k}$, $\mathbf{Q_k}$, $\mathbf{R_k}$, and $\mathbf{P_k}$) and not how they were constructed. Although we did describe how to construct them, we did not make use of those properties. In other words, almost any QBD process may be analyzed in this way. We have seen that our formalism covers a larger class of problems than we had intended. Therefore we wonder whether the matrices can be given more detailed properties that can be incorporated to yield more specific results.

Most of the material laid out here remains unexplored, even though it is now computationally manageable. It is hoped that this chapter, in particular, will help stimulate such activity.

The two groups who this author feels would be most interested in this material are researchers in computer performance and systems reliability. Yet their interests tend to be at opposite ends of the ρ scale. That is, performance modelers usually assume that the system can handle the load ($\rho_c < 1$). Otherwise, throw away the system. Therefore, they are interested in steady-state solutions (probably overly so), and even open systems, particularly because systems with millions of customers now exist (e.g., packets on the internet). On the other hand, reliability researchers usually assume that it takes less time to fix an object than it took to break it ($\rho_c > 1$). Therefore, except for questions of *inventory*, open systems are uninteresting. Furthermore, the steady state tells us nothing about MTTF. Yet the underlying formalism is identical for both groups. So it is important that the queueing theory practitioners in each camp understand clearly the difference of their goals when they communicate with each other.

Chapter 7

G/G/1/ /N LOOP

Those who cannot remember the past are condemned to repeat it.
George Santayana

We are finally facing up to giving structure to S_2. In many ways, this is the hardest queueing system for which analytic results are known. The mathematics required at present to describe such systems is too complicated for one to get reasonable insight from the formulas themselves. Furthermore, we must now specify two nonexponential functions, finding that the system behavior depends not merely on ρ, the ratio of their mean service times, and their second moments, or variances, but to a great extent on the parameter $C(x)$, which is the probability that the customer in service at S_1 will finish before the customer at S_2. This parameter, in turn, depends on x, the difference between the times when the two customers started service.

As long as S_2 was exponentially distributed, $C(x)$ (for $x \geq 0$) reduced to the Laplace transform of $b_1(t)$, and everything came out to be reasonably manageable, as described in previous chapters. For the G/G/1//N queue, things get messy (messier?). In matrix representations, this shows up in the difficulty one has in describing two different servers that are simultaneously active. This involves taking the direct product of two independent vector spaces. Presently, we discuss one such way to do this, the Kronecker product, and then go on to find the steady-state solution of the ME/ME/1/ /N loop. We do not continue on to the open queue, because we have not found how to get an explicit solution for that case. We do, however, discuss how this might be done eventually. In the final section we discuss some transient behavior, by looking at the mean time to failure for a system with small N.

This material is taken in large part from the PhD thesis by Appie van de Liefvoort [LIEFVOORT82], most of which was also published in [LIEF-LIP86]. But first we look at $C(x \geq 0)$, without relying on any direct-product representation.

7.1 Basis-Free Expression for $\mathbb{P}\mathbf{r}[X_1 < X_2]$

Let us consider two subsystems, S_i, $i = 1, 2$, each represented by $\langle \mathbf{p_i}, \mathbf{B_i} \rangle$ with dimension m_i. Let X_i be the random variables for the service times of the two servers. Now suppose that S_2 started service x units of time before

L. Lipsky, *Queueing Theory*, DOI 10.1007/978-0-387-49706-8_7,

S_1, but has not finished when S_1 begins. Then $C(x)$ is defined to be the probability that S_1 will finish before S_2. That is,

$$C(x) = \mathbb{P}\mathbf{r}[X_1 < X_2 + x] \tag{7.1.1a}$$

From elementary probability theory we can write, for $x \geq 0$,

$$C(x) = \frac{\int_0^\infty R_2(x+t)\, b_1(t)\, dt}{R_2(x)}. \tag{7.1.1b}$$

We now naively try to find an operator expression for $C(x)$, without first explicitly defining what the product of two operators from different spaces looks like, component by component. We do know, however, that because $\mathbf{B_1}$ operates only on vectors describing S_1, and $\mathbf{B_2}$ operates only on vectors describing S_2, they cannot have any affect on each other. After all, S_1 and S_2 are completely independent of each other (i.e., what happens in one subsystem cannot directly affect what happens in the other). We thus assert the ***independence principle***, which states: "all operations on S_1 vectors commute with all operations on S_2 vectors." In particular, this means that

$$\mathbf{B_1 B_2} = \mathbf{B_2 B_1}, \quad \mathbf{p_1 p_2} = \mathbf{p_2 p_1}, \quad \boldsymbol{\epsilon}'_\mathbf{1}\boldsymbol{\epsilon}'_\mathbf{2} = \boldsymbol{\epsilon}'_\mathbf{2}\boldsymbol{\epsilon}'_\mathbf{1},$$

and so on. We refer to the vector space made up of all linear combinations of the vectors that describe the internal state of S_i as *space* i, or i*-space*.

Before going on, we mention that the behavior of customers in S_1 and that of customers in S_2 eventually becomes correlated to each other as the two subsystems exchange customers, despite the independence principle. We show later that the exchange of customers requires that operators from the different spaces be added together, and through these, the commutativity property is lost. For instance, let $\mathbf{X_i}$ and $\mathbf{Y_i}$ be operators on vectors in space i. Then, of course, $\mathbf{X_1X_2} = \mathbf{X_2X_1}$, $\mathbf{X_1Y_2} = \mathbf{Y_2X_1}$, and so on. But suppose that $\mathbf{Y_i}$ does not commute with $\mathbf{X_i}$. Then the operator

$$\mathbf{Z} := \mathbf{Y_1} + \mathbf{X_1} + \mathbf{Y_2} + \mathbf{X_2}$$

does not commute with any of them.

Let us replace $R_i(\cdot)$ and $b_i(\cdot)$ in (7.1.1b) with their matrix equivalents, and then see what happens.

$$\mathbf{p_2}\,[\exp(-x\mathbf{B_2})]\,\boldsymbol{\epsilon}'_\mathbf{2}\, C(x)$$

$$= \int_0^\infty \mathbf{p_2}\,[\exp\{-(x+t)\mathbf{B_2}\}]\,\boldsymbol{\epsilon}'_\mathbf{2}\boldsymbol{p}_\mathbf{1}\,[\mathbf{B_1}\exp(-t\mathbf{B_1})]\,\boldsymbol{\epsilon}_\mathbf{1}\, dt.$$

Next recognize that $\exp[-(x+t)\mathbf{B_2}] = \exp(-x\mathbf{B_2})\exp(-t\mathbf{B_2})$, and apply the commutativity rule as many times as necessary to get

$$\mathbf{p_2}\,[\exp(-x\mathbf{B_2})]\,\boldsymbol{\epsilon}'_\mathbf{2} C(x)$$

$$= \mathbf{p_1p_2B_1}\exp(-x\mathbf{B_2}) \int_0^\infty [\exp(-t\mathbf{B_2})\exp(-t\mathbf{B_1})dt]\,\boldsymbol{\epsilon}_\mathbf{1}\boldsymbol{\epsilon}'_\mathbf{2}.$$

Given that $\mathbf{B_1}$ and $\mathbf{B_2}$ commute, we have

$$\exp[-t(\mathbf{B_1}+\mathbf{B_2})] = \exp(-t\mathbf{B_1})\exp(-t\mathbf{B_2}),$$

so

$$\begin{aligned}&\mathbf{p_2}\left[\exp(-x\mathbf{B_2})\right]\boldsymbol{\epsilon}_2' C(x)\\ &= \mathbf{p_1}\mathbf{p_2}\mathbf{B_1}\exp(-x\mathbf{B_2})\left[\int_0^\infty \exp[-t(\mathbf{B_1}+\mathbf{B_2})]dt\right]\boldsymbol{\epsilon}_1'\boldsymbol{\epsilon}_2'\\ &= \mathbf{p_1}\,\mathbf{p_2}\left[\exp(-x\mathbf{B_2})\,\mathbf{B_1}(\mathbf{B_1}+\mathbf{B_2})^{-1}\right]\boldsymbol{\epsilon}_1'\,\boldsymbol{\epsilon}_2'.\end{aligned}$$

We have made use of the fact that for any invertible matrix,

$$\int_0^\infty \exp(-t\mathbf{X})\,dt = \mathbf{X}^{-1}.$$

Last, define the following vectors (without asking until the next section what their components look like, or even their dimensions),

$$\mathbf{p} := \mathbf{p_1}\,\mathbf{p_2} \quad \text{and} \quad \boldsymbol{\epsilon}' := \boldsymbol{\epsilon}_1'\,\boldsymbol{\epsilon}_2';$$

then the original definition of Ψ is the same as it was before; namely

$$\Psi\left[\mathbf{X}\right] = \mathbf{p}\left[\mathbf{X}\right]\boldsymbol{\epsilon}' = \mathbf{p_1}\mathbf{p_2}\left[\mathbf{X}\right]\boldsymbol{\epsilon}_1'\boldsymbol{\epsilon}_2', \tag{7.1.2a}$$

where $\mathbf{X}$ can be anything like $\mathbf{B_1}$, $\mathbf{B_2}$, $\mathbf{B_1B_2}$, $\mathbf{B_1}+\mathbf{B_2}$, or any combination of such things. For instance,

$$\Psi\left[\mathbf{B_1}\right] = \mathbf{p_1}\mathbf{p_2}\left[\mathbf{B_1}\right]\boldsymbol{\epsilon}_1'\,\boldsymbol{\epsilon}_2' = \mathbf{p_1}\left[\mathbf{B_1}\right]\boldsymbol{\epsilon}_1'\,\mathbf{p_2}\,\boldsymbol{\epsilon}_2' = \mathbf{p_1}\left[\mathbf{B_1}\right]\boldsymbol{\epsilon}_1' \tag{7.1.2b}$$

(just as before),

$$\Psi\left[\mathbf{B_1B_2}\right] = \mathbf{p_1}\left[\mathbf{B_1}\right]\boldsymbol{\epsilon}_1'\,\mathbf{p_2}\left[\mathbf{B_2}\right]\boldsymbol{\epsilon}_2' = \Psi\left[\mathbf{B_1}\right]\Psi\left[\mathbf{B_2}\right], \tag{7.1.2c}$$

and

$$\Psi\left[\mathbf{B_1}+\mathbf{B_2}\right] = \Psi\left[\mathbf{B_1}\right]+\Psi\left[\mathbf{B_2}\right]. \tag{7.1.2d}$$

Then we can write (remembering that $\mathbf{V_i}$ is still $\mathbf{B_i}^{-1}$)

$$C(x) = \frac{\Psi\left[\exp(-x\mathbf{B_2})(\mathbf{I}+\mathbf{V_1B_2})^{-1}\right]}{\Psi\left[\exp(-x\mathbf{B_2})\right]}. \tag{7.1.3a}$$

In particular, the probability that the customer in S_1 will finish before the one in S_2, given that they started at the same time, is

$$\begin{aligned}C(0) &= \int_0^\infty R_2(t)\,b_1(t)\,dt = \Psi\left[\mathbf{B_1}(\mathbf{B_1}+\mathbf{B_2})^{-1}\right]\\ &= \Psi\left[(\mathbf{I}+\mathbf{V_1B_2})^{-1}\right].\end{aligned} \tag{7.1.3b}$$

Note that when S_2 is exponential (i.e., one-dimensional), $\mathbf{B_2}=\lambda$ and $C(0) = \Psi\left[(\mathbf{I}+\lambda\mathbf{V_1})^{-1}\right]$, which from (3.1.10) and Theorem 3.1.1 is indeed the Laplace transform, $[B_1^*(\lambda)]$ of $b_1(x)$, as stated in the second paragraph of this chapter. Some authors have used the symbolic notation for $C(0)$ in general,

$$C(0) = B_1^*(\mathbf{B_2}),$$

although it is not clear what it means, except in terms of (7.1.3b). The reader should be wary of this notation, because different authors assign different meanings to the same expression.

Now, you are dying to ask, "What can $(\mathbf{B_1} + \mathbf{B_2})$ [or $(\mathbf{I} + \mathbf{V_1 B_2})$] mean? How can one add two matrices from two different spaces together? After all, they may not even have the same dimensions. Why, that is like adding apples and oranges!" (and indeed it is). We can still delay giving the full answer if we avoid having to use $(\mathbf{B_1} + \mathbf{B_2})$ directly. For instance, we can formally expand the expression for $C(0)$ in a Maclaurin series, as follows.

$$C(0) = \Psi \left[\mathbf{I} + \sum_{k=1}^{\infty} (-1)^k \, \mathbf{V_1}^k \, \mathbf{B_2}^k \right] = 1 + \sum_{k=1}^{\infty} (-1)^k \, \Psi \left[\mathbf{V_1}^k \right] \, \Psi \left[\mathbf{B_2}^k \right].$$

[Remember that if two operators, $\mathbf{A}$ and $\mathbf{B}$, commute, then $(\mathbf{AB})^k = \mathbf{A}^k \, \mathbf{B}^k$.] We know what $\Psi \left[\mathbf{V_1}^k \right]$ and $\Psi \left[\mathbf{B_2}^k \right]$ are from (3.1.8b) and (3.1.9). Therefore, if the series converges, we can write

$$C(0) = \sum_{k=o}^{\infty} \frac{\mathbf{E}[X_1^k]}{k!} R_2^{(k)}(0). \tag{7.1.3c}$$

We could get this expression directly from the integral form for $C(0)$ in (7.1.3b), but still, it does show that the matrix forms in that equation have real meaning. The power of our formalism is utilized only when we can use $(\mathbf{B_1} + \mathbf{B_2})^{-1}$ directly. So, without further delay, we finally show how this is done.

7.2 Direct Products of Vector Spaces

Equations involving matrices that operate on vectors in different spaces are not uncommon, although they are usually restricted to combinations of square matrices of order m with matrices of order 1, the scalars. In this case, no problems arise, given that there is a natural embedding of the scalars into the matrices of order m: The scalars are isomorphic to the diagonal matrices whose nonzero elements are all equal. Because of this embedding, one does not hesitate to write $a = a \cdot \mathbf{I}$, even though this equality does not make any sense technically. In this chapter we are dealing with two sets of matrices of order greater than 1. Before equations containing these objects can be evaluated, the matrices must be replaced by their images under an embedding into a *direct-product space*, much as the scalar a is replaced by $a \cdot \mathbf{I}$ before the expression $\mathbf{A} + a \cdot \mathbf{I}$ can be evaluated.

7.2.1 Kronecker Products

The ***Kronecker product*** is one way to represent the ***direct product space*** from combining two disjoint operator spaces. (For a standard exposition of the subject see e.g., [GRAHAM81].) In particular, if $\mathbf{K_1}$ is an $m_1 \times n_1$ matrix operating on objects in space 1, and $\mathbf{K_2}$ is an $m_2 \times n_2$ matrix of space 2, the Kronecker product of $\mathbf{K_1}$ and $\mathbf{K_2}$, denoted by $\mathbf{K_1} \otimes \mathbf{K_2}$, is the matrix of size $(m_1 m_2) \times (n_1 n_2)$ that is obtained by multiplying each element of $\mathbf{K_1}$ [designated as $(\mathbf{K_1})_{ij}$] by the full matrix, $\mathbf{K_2}$. Observe that $\mathbf{K_1} \otimes \mathbf{K_2}$ can be regarded as an $m_1 \times n_1$ matrix whose elements are themselves matrices of size $m_2 \times n_2$. For instance, let $\mathbf{K_1}$ be 2×3; then

$$\mathbf{K} := \mathbf{K_1} \otimes \mathbf{K_2} = \begin{bmatrix} (\mathbf{K_1})_{11}\mathbf{K_2} & (\mathbf{K_1})_{12}\mathbf{K_2} & (\mathbf{K_1})_{13}\mathbf{K_2} \\ (\mathbf{K_1})_{21}\mathbf{K_2} & (\mathbf{K_1})_{22}\mathbf{K_2} & (\mathbf{K_1})_{23}\mathbf{K_2} \end{bmatrix}. \tag{7.2.1}$$

Note that the Kronecker product is neither commutative nor symmetric. That is, $\mathbf{K_1} \bigotimes \mathbf{K_2} \neq \mathbf{K_2} \bigotimes \mathbf{K_1}$, although the two representations are equivalent. What we are doing, in essence, is creating a supermatrix $\mathbf{K}$, with elements $K_{\underline{kl}}$, where $\underline{k}$ and $\underline{l}$ are themselves ordered pairs. That is,

$$\underline{k} = (k_1, k_2) \in \{(k_1, k_2) |\ k_1 \in \Xi,\ k_2 \in \Xi_2\},$$

where Ξ_i is the set of internal states of S_i. In order to write down $\mathbf{K}$ in a rectangular array, it is necessary to give a linear ordering to the pairs (k_1, k_2). Equation (7.2.1) implies one such ordering; $\bar{\mathbf{K}} := \mathbf{K_2} \otimes \mathbf{K_1}$ would give a different ordering. $\mathbf{K}$ and $\bar{\mathbf{K}}$ are the same size and have the same elements, but they are arranged differently. With this definition, the following multiplication rule is valid. Let $\mathbf{K_i}$ and $\mathbf{L_i}$ be any two arrays in space i for which $\mathbf{K_i}\,\mathbf{L_i}$ is defined; then

$$\mathbf{K}\,\mathbf{L} = [\mathbf{K_1} \otimes \mathbf{K_2}] \cdot [\mathbf{L_1} \otimes \mathbf{L_2}] = \mathbf{K_1 L_1} \otimes \mathbf{K_2 L_2}. \tag{7.2.2}$$

Note that $\mathbf{K}\,\mathbf{L} = \mathbf{L}\,\mathbf{K}$ if and only if $\mathbf{K_1}\,\mathbf{L_1} = \mathbf{L_1}\,\mathbf{K_1}$ and $\mathbf{K_2}\,\mathbf{L_2} = \mathbf{L_2}\,\mathbf{K_2}$.

To keep our ordering of elements consistent, we adhere to the following conventions. What we must do is embed the row vectors, column vectors, and square matrices of each space (e.g., $\mathbf{p_i}$, $\mathbf{B_i}$, and $\boldsymbol{\epsilon}'$) into the product space. As implied by the nonequality of $\mathbf{K}$ and $\bar{\mathbf{K}}$, this cannot be done in a symmetric manner. We use the single symbol, $\hat{}$ (called a *caret* or *hat*), to designate this mapping. Thus

$$\hat{\mathbf{A}}_\mathbf{1} := \mathbf{A_1} \otimes \mathbf{I_2}$$

$$\hat{\mathbf{A}}_\mathbf{2} := \mathbf{I_1} \otimes \mathbf{A_2},$$

where $\mathbf{I_i}$ is the identity matrix of dimensions $m_i \times m_i$, and $\mathbf{A_i}$ is any matrix of that dimension. Both $\hat{\mathbf{A}}_\mathbf{1}$ and $\hat{\mathbf{A}}_\mathbf{2}$ are of dimension $(m_1 m_2) \times (m_1 m_2)$. The subscripts 1 or 2 on all matrices and vectors denote the space they come from, even after the embedding. Matrices without any subscript are assumed to be in the product space already. The special matrix

$$\mathbf{I} := \mathbf{I_1} \otimes \mathbf{I_2}$$

is the identity matrix of the product space. From (7.2.2) we have the nice property that

$$\hat{\mathbf{A}}_1 \cdot \hat{\mathbf{A}}_2 = \mathbf{A}_1 \otimes \mathbf{A}_2 = \hat{\mathbf{A}}_2 \cdot \hat{\mathbf{A}}_1.$$

This is just the property we needed to satisfy our independence principle. The embedded matrices commute, even though the Kronecker product of the two matrices does not. We also can see that the *hat* and *inverse* operators commute. Let $\mathbf{R}_1 := \mathbf{A}_1^{-1}$; then

$$\hat{\mathbf{R}}_1 = \mathbf{R}_1 \otimes \mathbf{I}_2 = \mathbf{A}_1{}^{-1} \otimes \mathbf{I}_2 - (\mathbf{A}_1 \otimes \mathbf{I}_2)^{-1} = (\hat{\mathbf{A}}_1)^{-1}.$$

Our next project is to embed the various vectors into the product space. Let $\mathbf{a}_i$ be any row vector in space i, and $\mathbf{b}'_i$ be any column vector. Then

$$\hat{\mathbf{a}}_1 := \mathbf{a}_1 \otimes \mathbf{I}_2, \qquad \hat{\mathbf{b}}'_1 := \mathbf{b}'_1 \otimes \mathbf{I}_2, \tag{7.2.3a}$$

and

$$\hat{\mathbf{a}}_2 := \mathbf{I}_1 \otimes \mathbf{a}_2, \qquad \hat{\mathbf{b}}'_2 := \mathbf{I}_1 \otimes \mathbf{b}'_2. \tag{7.2.3b}$$

This seems simple enough, but these objects are not vectors in the product space. They are, in fact, rectangular matrices of the following dimensions (read "dimensions of ·" for "Dim [·]"):

$$\mathrm{Dim}[\,\hat{\mathbf{a}}_1\,] = (m_2) \times (m_1 m_2),$$

$$\mathrm{Dim}[\,\hat{\mathbf{b}}'_1\,] = (m_1 m_2) \times (m_2),$$

$$\mathrm{Dim}[\,\hat{\mathbf{a}}_2\,] = (m_1) \times (m_1 m_2),$$

and

$$\mathrm{Dim}[\,\hat{\mathbf{b}}'_2\,] = (m_1 m_2) \times (m_1).$$

We know that the simple dot product $\mathbf{a}_2\,\mathbf{b}'_2$ is a scalar; call it c. But

$$\hat{\mathbf{a}}_2\,\hat{\mathbf{b}}'_2 = [\mathbf{I}_1 \otimes \mathbf{a}_2] \cdot [\mathbf{I}_1 \otimes \mathbf{b}'_2] = \mathbf{I}_1\,\mathbf{I}_1 \otimes \mathbf{a}_2\,\mathbf{b}'_2 = c\mathbf{I}_1 \otimes 1 = c\mathbf{I}_1. \tag{7.2.3c}$$

What, then, are the appropriate vectors for the product space? Just as we found that the Kronecker product of two square matrices is a square matrix, we can see that the Kronecker product of two row vectors is a row vector with $(m_1 m_2)$ components (i.e., $\mathbf{a}_1 \otimes \mathbf{a}_2$ is a row vector), and similarly for column vectors. In particular, we define the two special vectors

$$\mathbf{p} := \mathbf{p}_1 \otimes \mathbf{p}_2 \tag{7.2.4a}$$

and

$$\boldsymbol{\epsilon}' := \boldsymbol{\epsilon}'_1 \otimes \boldsymbol{\epsilon}'_2. \tag{7.2.4b}$$

Yes, $\boldsymbol{\epsilon}'$ is an $(m_1 m_2)$-dimensional column vector of all 1's. Also,

$$\mathbf{p} \cdot \boldsymbol{\epsilon}' = [\mathbf{p}_1 \otimes \mathbf{p}_2] \cdot [\boldsymbol{\epsilon}'_1 \otimes \boldsymbol{\epsilon}'_2] = \mathbf{p}_1\,\boldsymbol{\epsilon}'_1 \otimes \mathbf{p}_2\,\boldsymbol{\epsilon}'_2 = 1 \otimes 1 = 1. \tag{7.2.4c}$$

Well, strictly speaking, $1 \otimes 1$ is not exactly the same as "1," but they have the same effect on everything. After all, what is a 1 by 1 matrix whose only element is 1?

The embedded vectors $\hat{\mathbf{a}}_\mathbf{i}$ and $\hat{\mathbf{b}}'_\mathbf{i}$ are needed, but we must be careful how they are used. For instance,

$$\hat{\mathbf{p}}_1 \cdot \hat{\mathbf{p}}_2 \neq \mathbf{p}.$$

In fact, it is not defined, because the object $\mathbf{I_2}\,\mathbf{p_2}$ has no meaning. What we must use, instead, is

$$\mathbf{p} = \mathbf{p}_1\,\hat{\mathbf{p}}_2 = \mathbf{p}_2\,\hat{\mathbf{p}}_1.$$

In general, we have the following lemma.

Lemma 7.2.1: Let $\mathbf{a_i}$, $\mathbf{b}'_\mathbf{i}$, and $\mathbf{A_i}$ be objects from space i $(i = 1, 2)$. Then the following are all vectors in the product space.

Row vectors:†

$$\mathbf{a}_1\,\hat{\mathbf{a}}_2 = \mathbf{a}_2\,\hat{\mathbf{a}}_1 = \mathbf{a}_1 \otimes \mathbf{a}_2 \neq \mathbf{a}_2 \otimes \mathbf{a}_1;$$

$$\mathbf{a}_2\,\hat{\mathbf{a}}_1\,\hat{\mathbf{A}}_2 = \mathbf{a}_1\,\hat{\mathbf{a}}_2\,\hat{\mathbf{A}}_2 = \mathbf{a}_2\,\mathbf{A}_2\,\hat{\mathbf{a}}_1;$$

$$\mathbf{a}_1\,\mathbf{A}_1\,\hat{\mathbf{a}}_2 = \mathbf{a}_1\,\hat{\mathbf{a}}_2\,\hat{\mathbf{A}}_1 = \mathbf{a}_2\,\hat{\mathbf{a}}_1\,\hat{\mathbf{A}}_1.$$

Column vectors:†

$$\hat{\mathbf{b}}'_1\,\mathbf{b}'_2 = \hat{\mathbf{b}}'_2\,\mathbf{b}'_1 = \mathbf{b}'_1 \otimes \mathbf{b}'_2 \neq \mathbf{b}'_2 \otimes \mathbf{b}'_1;$$

$$\hat{\mathbf{b}}'_1\,\mathbf{A}_2\,\mathbf{b}'_2 = \hat{\mathbf{A}}_2\,\hat{\mathbf{b}}'_1\,\mathbf{b}'_2 = \hat{\mathbf{A}}_2\,\hat{\mathbf{b}}'_2\,\mathbf{b}'_1;$$

$$\hat{\mathbf{A}}_1\,\hat{\mathbf{b}}'_2\,\mathbf{b}'_1 = \hat{\mathbf{b}}'_2\,\mathbf{A}_1\,\mathbf{b}'_1 = \hat{\mathbf{A}}_1\,\hat{\mathbf{b}}'_1\,\mathbf{b}'_2.$$

Mixed vectors:

$$\hat{\mathbf{a}}_1 \cdot \hat{\mathbf{b}}'_1 = [\mathbf{a}_1 \cdot \mathbf{b}'_1]\,\mathbf{I}_2$$

$$\hat{\mathbf{a}}_2 \cdot \hat{\mathbf{b}}'_2 = [\mathbf{a}_2 \cdot \mathbf{b}'_2]\,\mathbf{I}_1,$$

where $[\mathbf{a_i} \cdot \mathbf{b_i}]$ is a scalar. The first and third sets of these equations come close to satisfying our commutativity property, so with some care we can assume that our independence principle applies. ■

7.2.2 Ψ Projections onto Subspaces

We next deal with ***projections***, or ***deflations***. Here we *project* or *deflate* a square matrix in the product space to one in space i. We already deflated matrices to scalars by use of the $\Psi\,[\cdot]$ operators. We generalize that here. First define (or rather define again)

$$\Psi\,[\mathbf{X}] := \mathbf{p}\mathbf{X}\,\boldsymbol{\epsilon}'$$

where $\mathbf{X}$ is any square matrix in the product space and $\mathbf{p}$ and $\boldsymbol{\epsilon}'$ are given by (7.2.4). This is clearly a scalar, with the same properties that we wanted it to

†For embedded row vectors, the *hatted* object must be on the right, whereas for embedded column vectors, the *hatted* object must be on the left.

have in (7.1.2a). The two new projections are those that deflate $\mathbf{X}$ to space i. Define the following operations on any $\mathbf{X}$.

$$\Psi_2[\mathbf{X}] := \hat{\mathbf{p}}_1[\mathbf{X}]\hat{\boldsymbol{\epsilon}}'_1, \tag{7.2.5a}$$

$$\Psi_1[\mathbf{X}] := \hat{\mathbf{p}}_2[\mathbf{X}]\hat{\boldsymbol{\epsilon}}'_2. \tag{7.2.5b}$$

Note the apparent mismatch between the subscripts on Ψ_i and on the vectors. This is correct, for $\Psi_2[\mathbf{X}]$ is a matrix in space 2. In a sense, the vectors $\mathbf{p}_1$ and $\boldsymbol{\epsilon}'_1$ have deflated the dependence of $\mathbf{X}$ on space 1 to a scalar. This is quite clear if $\mathbf{X}$ is itself an embedding of an operator in space 2. Suppose that $\mathbf{X} = \hat{\mathbf{X}}_2 = \mathbf{I}_1 \otimes \mathbf{X}_2$. Then

$$\begin{aligned}\Psi_2[\mathbf{X}] &= \hat{\mathbf{p}}_1[\mathbf{I}_1 \otimes \mathbf{X}_2]\hat{\boldsymbol{\epsilon}}'_1 = (\mathbf{p}_1 \otimes \mathbf{I}_2)\cdot[\mathbf{I}_1 \otimes \mathbf{X}_2]\cdot(\boldsymbol{\epsilon}'_1 \otimes \mathbf{I}_2)\\ &= \left[\mathbf{p}_1\mathbf{I}_1\,\boldsymbol{\epsilon}'_1\right] \otimes (\mathbf{I}_2\mathbf{X}_2\mathbf{I}_2) = 1 \otimes \mathbf{X}_2 = \mathbf{X}_2.\end{aligned}$$

Thus we see that the projections $\Psi_i[\mathbf{X}]$ are inverses of the embeddings $\hat{\mathbf{X}}_\mathbf{i}$, in an operator sense, and in fact satisfy the idempotent properties,

$$\hat{\Psi}_i\left[\hat{\Psi}_i[\mathbf{X}]\right] = \hat{\Psi}_i[\mathbf{X}], \tag{7.2.5c}$$

which can be proven after some effort by direct substitution. The most important single property of projection operators is that they are idempotent. That is, successive operations yield the same result, which indeed is shown by (7.2.5c). We look further at $\Psi_1[\mathbf{X}]$, with the intention of reducing it to a scalar. Then

$$\mathbf{p}_1\Psi_1[\mathbf{X}]\boldsymbol{\epsilon}'_1 = \boldsymbol{p}_1\hat{\mathbf{p}}_2[\mathbf{X}]\hat{\boldsymbol{\epsilon}}'_2\boldsymbol{\epsilon}'_1 = \mathbf{p}[\mathbf{X}]\boldsymbol{\epsilon}' = \Psi[\mathbf{X}]. \tag{7.2.6a}$$

Similarly,

$$\mathbf{p}_2\Psi_2[\mathbf{X}]\boldsymbol{\epsilon}'_2 = \Psi[\mathbf{X}]. \tag{7.2.6b}$$

Thus the order in which one deflates $\mathbf{X}$ is immaterial. Now, we could have written $\Psi_2[\Psi_1[\mathbf{X}]] = \Psi_1[\Psi_2[\mathbf{X}]]$, but the outer Ψ_2 (or Ψ_1) implies that this is an object in 2-space (or 1-space), when in fact it is a scalar. Therefore, we use the notation

$$\Psi[\Psi_1[\mathbf{X}]] = \Psi[\Psi_2[\mathbf{X}]] = \Psi[\mathbf{X}], \tag{7.2.6c}$$

because it unambiguously says that whatever is inside the brackets is reduced to a scalar.

Before going on to the ME/ME/1//N queue, we conclude this section with three important lemmas.

Lemma 7.2.2: [***Eigenvalues and eigenvectors of*** $(\mathbf{A}_1 \otimes \mathbf{B}_2)$ ***and*** $(\hat{\mathbf{A}}_1 + \hat{\mathbf{B}}_2)$]. Let

$$\alpha_1,\ \alpha_2,\ \ldots,\ \alpha_{m_1}$$

be the eigenvalues of $\mathbf{A}_1$, with corresponding left eigenvectors

$$\mathbf{a}_1,\ \mathbf{a}_2,\ \ldots,\ \mathbf{a}_{m_1}.$$

Furthermore, let

$$\beta_1, \beta_2, \ldots, \beta_{m_2}$$

be the eigenvalues of $\mathbf{B_2}$, with corresponding left eigenvectors

$$\mathbf{b_1}, \mathbf{b_2}, \ldots, \mathbf{b_{m_2}}.$$

Then the eigenvalues of $\mathbf{A_1} \otimes \mathbf{B_2}$ ($= \hat{\mathbf{A}}_1 \hat{\mathbf{B}}_2$) are the $(m_1 \cdot m_2)$ products,

$$\alpha_k \, \beta_l$$

(i.e., any eigenvalue of $\mathbf{A_1}$ times any eigenvalue of $\mathbf{B_2}$ is an eigenvalue of their Kronecker product). The corresponding left eigenvector is

$$\mathbf{a_k} \otimes \mathbf{b_l}.$$

Similarly, the eigenvalues of $\hat{\mathbf{A}}_1 + \hat{\mathbf{B}}_2$ are the $(m_1 \cdot m_2)$ sums,

$$\alpha_k + \beta_l,$$

with the same eigenvector, $\mathbf{a_k} \otimes \mathbf{b_l}$. The right eigenvectors are similarly constructed from the right eigenvectors of $\hat{\mathbf{A}}_1$ and $\hat{\mathbf{B}}_2$. ■

We do not make any use of this lemma in this book, but it may be significant in future research, perhaps in conjunction with the next lemma.

Lemma 7.2.3: Remember that $\mathbf{Q_i} = \boldsymbol{\epsilon}'_i \boldsymbol{p}_i$. Thus

$$\hat{\mathbf{Q}}_1 = [\boldsymbol{\epsilon}'_1 \boldsymbol{p}_1] \otimes \mathbf{I_2} = [\boldsymbol{\epsilon}'_1 \otimes \mathbf{I_2}] \cdot [\mathbf{p_1} \otimes \mathbf{I_2}] = \hat{\boldsymbol{\epsilon}}'_1 \hat{\boldsymbol{p}}_1$$

and

$$\hat{\mathbf{Q}}_2 = \mathbf{I_1} \otimes [\boldsymbol{\epsilon}'_2 \boldsymbol{p}_2] = \hat{\boldsymbol{\epsilon}}'_2 \hat{\boldsymbol{p}}_2.$$

The product space $\mathbf{Q}$ is idempotent [i.e., $\mathbf{Q^2} = \mathbf{Q}$] and of rank 1,[‡] and satisfies the following:

$$\mathbf{Q} := \boldsymbol{\epsilon}' \boldsymbol{p} = [\boldsymbol{\epsilon}'_1 \otimes \boldsymbol{\epsilon}'_2] \cdot [\mathbf{p_1} \otimes \mathbf{p_2}] = \boldsymbol{\epsilon}'_1 \, \mathbf{p_1} \otimes \boldsymbol{\epsilon}'_2 \, \mathbf{p_2} = \mathbf{Q_1} \otimes \mathbf{Q_2} = \hat{\mathbf{Q}}_1 \, \hat{\mathbf{Q}}_2.$$

Both $\hat{\mathbf{Q}}_1$ and $\hat{\mathbf{Q}}_2$ are also idempotent but they are not of rank 1. Instead, $\hat{\mathbf{Q}}_1$ is of rank m_2, and $\hat{\mathbf{Q}}_2$ is of rank m_1. Furthermore, there exist m_2 (left and right) eigenvectors of $\hat{\mathbf{Q}}_1$ with eigenvalue 1, and $m_2(m_1 - 1)$ (left and right) eigenvectors with eigenvalue 0. Furthermore, the matrix $(\mathbf{I} - \hat{\mathbf{Q}}_1)$ is also idempotent, with rank $m_2(m_1 - 1)$, satisfying the *null* or *orthogonality* equation,

$$(\mathbf{I} - \hat{\mathbf{Q}}_1)\hat{\mathbf{Q}}_1 = \mathbf{O},$$

[‡]Recall that the *rank* of a finite dimensional matrix is equal to the number of its nonzero eigenvalues. $\mathbf{Q}$ has one eigenvalue equal to 1, and all the rest are equal to 0; thus it is of rank 1.

with an identical result for $\hat{\mathbf{Q}}_2$. In fact, every idempotent matrix satisfies the null equation. It follows directly that the following are true:

$$\hat{\mathbf{Q}}_1 \hat{\boldsymbol{\epsilon}}'_1 = \hat{\boldsymbol{\epsilon}}'_1, \quad \hat{\mathbf{Q}}_1 \boldsymbol{\epsilon}' = \boldsymbol{\epsilon}', \quad \hat{\mathbf{p}}_1 \hat{\mathbf{Q}}_1 = \hat{\mathbf{p}}_1, \quad \mathbf{p}\,\hat{\mathbf{Q}}_1 = \mathbf{p}.$$

Recall that $\hat{\boldsymbol{\epsilon}}'_1$ is not a vector, but the first of the equations above tells us that each of its m_2 columns is a right eigenvector of $\hat{\mathbf{Q}}_1$ with eigenvalue 1. Given that $\hat{\mathbf{Q}}_1$ is of rank m_2, there are no other unit eigenvectors. The equivalent can be said of the m_2 rows of $\hat{\mathbf{p}}_1$. The duals of all these statements are valid for $\hat{\mathbf{Q}}_2$. ∎

Also, from (7.2.3c) we know that $\hat{\mathbf{p}}_1 \hat{\boldsymbol{\epsilon}}'_1 = \mathbf{I}_2$ and $\hat{\mathbf{p}}_2 \hat{\boldsymbol{\epsilon}}'_2 = \mathbf{I}_1$.

Lemma 7.2.4: Let $\mathbf{F}$ and $\mathbf{G}$ be any matrices in the product space, and let $\Psi_2[\mathbf{I} - \mathbf{GF}]$ be nonsingular. Then the matrix $\mathbf{I} - \mathbf{F}\hat{\mathbf{Q}}_1\mathbf{G}$ is nonsingular, and its inverse is

$$(\mathbf{I} - \mathbf{F}\hat{\mathbf{Q}}_1\mathbf{G})^{-1} = \mathbf{I} + \mathbf{F}\left(\hat{\Psi}_2[\mathbf{I} - \mathbf{GF}]\right)^{-1} \hat{\mathbf{Q}}_1\mathbf{G}. \tag{7.2.7}$$

Interchanging the indices 1 and 2 gives the dual result. We have used the notation

$$\hat{\Psi}_2[\mathbf{X}] := \mathbf{I}_1 \otimes \Psi_2[\mathbf{X}].$$

The proof, although tedious, is by direct multiplication. ∎

Note that this lemma is a direct generalization of Lemma 4.2.1, and Equations (4.2.2).

Before going on, the reader should be sure that the material of this section is fairly familiar. However, a specific example of embedded matrices is deferred until we have the explicit solution for the ME/ME/1/ /N loop. Perhaps the best strategy would be to read everything, up through the example, as best one can, and then go back to the beginning of this section.

7.3 Steady-State ME/ME/1/ /N Loop

We have set up a rather elaborate mathematical apparatus and present a considerable number of formulas before this chapter is completed. If the reader feels that the concrete results we give appear small in comparison, be encouraged. We are presenting more formulas than necessary in the hope that they will help some reader to discover further significant results. We touch on this at the end of the chapter.

7.3.1 Balance Equations

Let us consider the usual two-server loop as given in Figure 7.3.1. Each subsystem S_i, $i = 1, 2$, can only have one active customer at a time, and the queueing discipline is FCFS. Both S_1 and S_2 are nonexponential and represented by $\langle \mathbf{p_i}, \mathbf{B_i} \rangle$, with dimension $m_i > 1$, and with associated objects, $\mathbf{M_i}$, $\mathbf{V_i}$, ϵ_i', $\mathbf{Q_i}$, $\mathbf{P_i}$, and $\mathbf{q_i'} = (\mathbf{I_i} - \mathbf{P_i})\epsilon_i'$. As before, the diagonal elements of $\mathbf{M_1}$ are denoted by μ_k ($k = 1$ to m_1), and as a generalization of previous chapters, the diagonal elements of $\mathbf{M_2}$ are denoted by λ_k ($k = 1$ to m_2). N is the number of customers in the system, and n is the number at S_1 (with $N - n$ customers at S_2). If neither subsystem is empty, we must know where both of the active customers are to specify the system completely. Let Ξ_i be the set of phases associated with S_i, where $|\Xi_i| = m_i$. We extend the notation further.

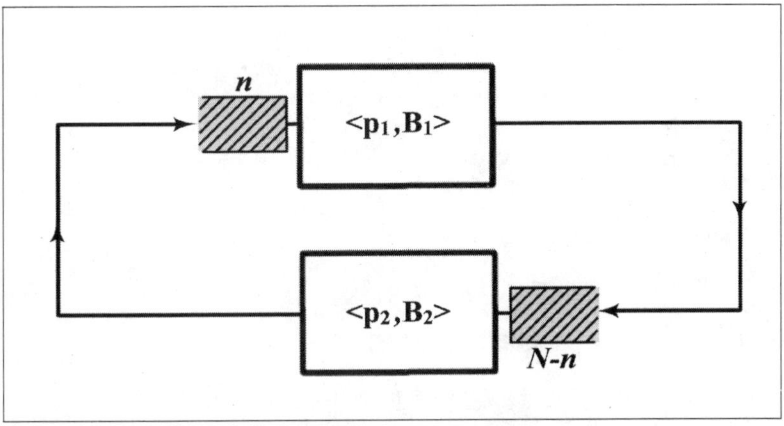

Figure 7.3.1: Closed loop of two matrix exponential servers. There are n customers at S_1, and the one being served is at phase $k_1 \in \Xi$. $N - n$ customers are at S_2, with the active one being at phase $k_2 \in \Xi_2$. Thus the system is in state $\{\underline{k};\, n;\, N\}$, where $\underline{k} = (k_1, k_2) \in \Xi$.

Definition 7.3.1

$\{\underline{k};\, n;\, N\}$ *corresponds to one possible state of an ME/ME/1//N loop, for* $0 < n < N$. N *is the total number of customers in the system,* n *is the number of customers at* S_1*, including the one in service, and* $\underline{k}$ *stands for the ordered pair* (k_1, k_2)*,where* $k_i \in \Xi_i$. We say that the system is in the state $\{\underline{k};\, n;\, N\}$. $\Xi := \Xi_1 \otimes \Xi_2 := \{(k_1, k_2) | k_i \in \Xi_i, i = 1, 2\}$. Given that only one customer can be active at a time in S_i, Ξ is the set of all internal states of the system as a whole. As long as neither queue is empty, we can say that the system is in internal state $\underline{k} \in \Xi$, or that the active customers are at phases k_1 and k_2 in their respective subsystems. □

Clearly, $|\Xi| = (m_1 \cdot m_2)$, but this full space is relevant only if $n \neq 0$ and $n \neq N$. In those two cases, the state space collapses to Ξ_2 or Ξ_1, respectively. With this understanding, we define the steady-state probability vectors.

Definition 7.3.2

$[\mathbf{\Pi}(n;\, N)]_{\underline{k}}$:= *steady-state probability that there are* n $(0 < n < N)$

customers at S_1 *and* $N-n$ *customers at* S_2, *where* $\underline{k} = (k_1, k_2) \in \Xi$ (i.e., the active customer at S_i is at phase k_i). $[\mathbf{\Pi}(n;\ N)]$ is an $(m_1 \cdot m_2)$-dimensional row vector whose components are ordered according to the Kronecker product convention implied in (7.2.1), which also corresponds to the lexicographical ordering

$$\mathbf{\Pi}(n;\ N) = [\Pi_{(1,1)}, \Pi_{(1,2)}, \ldots, \Pi_{(1,m_2)}, \Pi_{(2,1)}, \ldots, \Pi_{(m_1,m_2)}].$$

[We have suppressed the components' dependence on $(n; N)$.] The associated scalar probability is denoted by

$$r(n; N) = \mathbf{\Pi}(n;\ N)\boldsymbol{\epsilon}'. \tag{7.3.1}$$

The steady-state probability vector for $n = 0$ is a vector in 2-space, because no one is at S_1, and is denoted by $\boldsymbol{\pi}_2(0; N)$. Similarly, the probability vector for $n = N$ is denoted by $\boldsymbol{\pi}_1(N; N)$. For convenience [in analogy with what we did in (4.1.1)], we define

$$\mathbf{\Pi}(0;\ N) := \mathbf{p_1} \otimes \boldsymbol{\pi}_2(0; N) \tag{7.3.2a}$$

and

$$\mathbf{\Pi}(N;\ N) := \boldsymbol{\pi}_1(N; N) \otimes \mathbf{p_2}. \tag{7.3.2b}$$

With these definitions, (7.3.1) is valid for all n. □

We are now ready to set up the balance equations. The process is a straightforward extension of Section 4.1.1. The complications arise in rewriting the equations as matrix equations of objects in the product space. Recall that the balance equations are derived from the fact that the sum of probability rates of arrows entering a given state is equal to the sum of those leaving. The arrows are shown in Figure 7.3.2 for an arbitrary state $\{(k, s);\ n;\ N\}$, where $(k, s) \in \Xi$ (i.e., $k \in \Xi_1$ and $s \in \Xi_2$) and $0 < n < N$. The probability rate of an arrow is, in turn, equal to the steady-state probability that the system is in the state designated by its tail, times the probability rate of leaving that state, times the probability that an arrow will occur, given that the system is in the state of the tail. For instance, the probability rate of the arrow going from $\{(k, s);\ n;\ N\}$ to $\{(k, t);\ n+1;\ N\}$ is

$$\left[[\mathbf{\Pi}(n;\ N)]_{(k,s)}\right] \times [\mu_k + \lambda_s] \times \left[\frac{\lambda_s}{\lambda_s + \mu_k}(\mathbf{q}_2')_s(\mathbf{p_2})_t\right]$$

$$= [\mathbf{\Pi}(n;\ N)]_{(k,s)}\lambda_s(\mathbf{q}_2')_s(\mathbf{p_2})_t.$$

This particular arrow corresponds to the following process. The customer at phase s in S_2 finishes there and leaves $[(\mathbf{q}_2')_s]$, going to S_1 and raising its queue length to $n+1$. Simultaneously, the next customer in the queue enters S_2, and goes to phase t, $[(\mathbf{p_2})_t]$. There is one arrow for each phase in S_2, so we must sum over t.

When doing the same for the other seven types of arrows, we get the balance equations for $0 < n < N$. Given that the sum of the probabilities of

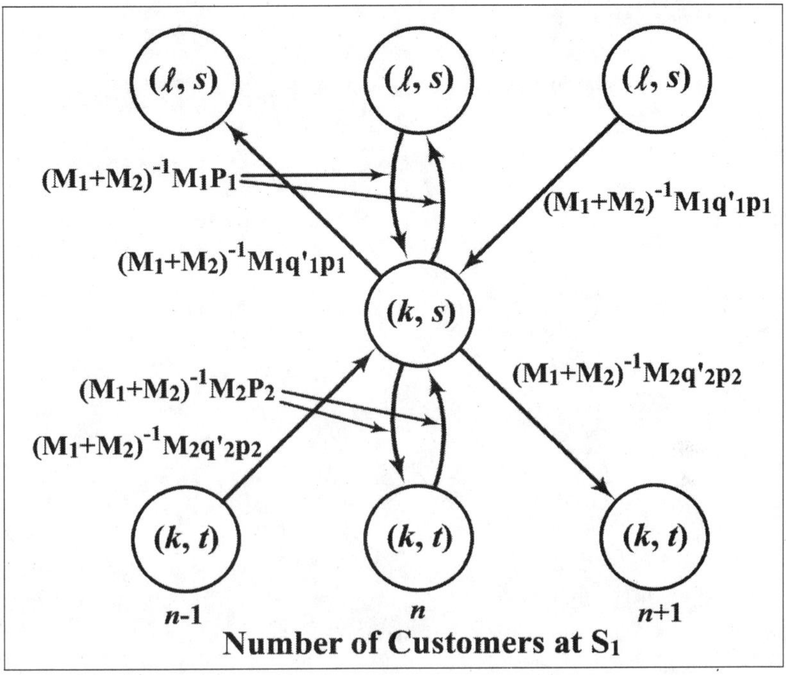

Figure 7.3.2: Steady-state transition diagram for state $\{(k,s);\, n;\, N\}$ of an ME/ME/1//N closed loop. Arrows coming from or going to (k,s) from above correspond to events that occurred in S_1, and arrows below (k,s) correspond to events that occurred in S_2. Vertical lines are internal transitions. There are no horizontal arrows, because exactly one internal state must change [transitions such as $(\mathbf{P_1})_{kk}$ and $(\mathbf{q}'_1)_k(\mathbf{p_1})_k$ are to be visualized as changes]. The expression next to each arrow is the probability that the corresponding event will occur, given that the system is in the state designated by the node at the arrow's tail. Thus the sum of all arrows leaving node $\{(k,s);\, n;\, N\}$ equals 1. (This includes the sum over all $l \in \Xi_1$ for *up* arrows, and the sum over all $t \in \Xi_2$ for *down* arrows.)

the four arrows leaving the state sum to 1, the left-hand side of this equation is simple.

$$[\mathbf{\Pi}(n;\, N)]_{(k,s)}\,(\lambda_s + \mu_k)$$

$$= \sum_{l\in\Xi_1} [\mathbf{\Pi}(n+1;\, N)]_{(l,s)}\,\mu_l(\mathbf{q}'_1)_l(\mathbf{p_1})_k + \sum_{l\in\Xi_1} [\mathbf{\Pi}(n;\, N)]_{(l,s)}\,\mu_l(\mathbf{P_1})_{lk}$$
$$+ \sum_{t\in\Xi_2} [\mathbf{\Pi}(n;\, N)]_{(k,t)}\,\lambda_t(\mathbf{P_2})_{ts} + \sum_{t\in\Xi_2} [\mathbf{\Pi}(n-1;\, N)]_{(k,t)}\,\lambda_t(\mathbf{q}'_2)_s(\mathbf{p_2})_t.$$

Let us clean this up. By our definitions, $(\mathbf{M_1})_{kk} = \mu_k$ and $(\mathbf{M_2})_{ss} = \lambda_s$. Therefore, we have $\mu_l\,(\mathbf{P_1})_{lk} = [\mathbf{M_1}\,\mathbf{P_1}]_{lk}$ and $\mu_l\,(\mathbf{q}'_1)_l(\mathbf{p_1})_k = [\mathbf{M_1}\mathbf{q}'_1\mathbf{p_1}]_{lk}$, with comparable expressions for objects with subscript 2. Next, from (4.1.3a), we know that

$$\mathbf{M_i}\mathbf{q}'_i = \mathbf{B_i}\,\boldsymbol{\epsilon}'_i \quad \text{and} \quad \mathbf{M_i}\mathbf{q}'_i = \mathbf{B_i}\mathbf{Q_i}.$$

Last, the reader should verify that

$$\mu_k + \lambda_s = \left[\hat{\mathbf{M}}_{\mathbf{1}} + \hat{\mathbf{M}}_{\mathbf{2}}\right]_{(k,s)(k,s)}.$$

The last problem is to convert the summations in one space to a sum over indices in the product space. We can do this here because each term is made up of some $\mathbf{\Pi}$ times an object that is in only one of the subspaces. For instance, for any matrix $\mathbf{X}$ we can do the following.

$$\sum_{l\in\Xi_1} \Pi_{(l,s)}(\mathbf{X_1})_{lk} = \sum_{l\in\Xi_1}\sum_{t\in\Xi_2} \Pi_{(l,t)}(\mathbf{X_1})_{lk}(\mathbf{I_2})_{ts} = \sum_{\underline{l}\in\Xi} \Pi_{\underline{l}}(\hat{\mathbf{X}}_{\mathbf{1}})_{\underline{lk}} = [\mathbf{\Pi}\hat{\mathbf{X}}_{\mathbf{1}}]_{\underline{k}},$$

where

$$\underline{l} := (l,t) \in \Xi \quad \text{and} \quad \underline{k} := (k,s) \in \Xi.$$

After some practice, the reader can become comfortable with this. Given that the balance equations are valid for all $\underline{k} \in \Xi$, we can put all the pieces together and write the following vector balance equation.

$$\mathbf{\Pi}(n;\, N)\left[\hat{\mathbf{M}}_{\mathbf{1}} + \hat{\mathbf{M}}_{\mathbf{2}}\right]$$

$$= \mathbf{\Pi}(n+1;\, N)\hat{\mathbf{B}}_{\mathbf{1}}\hat{\mathbf{Q}}_{\mathbf{1}} + \mathbf{\Pi}(n;\, N)\hat{\mathbf{M}}_{\mathbf{1}}\hat{\mathbf{P}}_{\mathbf{1}} + \mathbf{\Pi}(n;\, N)\hat{\mathbf{M}}_{\mathbf{2}}\hat{\mathbf{P}}_{\mathbf{2}} + \mathbf{\Pi}(n-1;\, N)\hat{\mathbf{B}}_{\mathbf{2}}\hat{\mathbf{Q}}_{\mathbf{2}}.$$

Now we take all the terms with $\mathbf{\Pi}(n;\, N)$ to the left side, and recognize that $\hat{\mathbf{M}}_{\mathbf{i}} - \hat{\mathbf{M}}_{\mathbf{i}}\hat{\mathbf{P}}_{\mathbf{i}} = \hat{\mathbf{B}}_{\mathbf{i}}$, and get, finally,

$$\mathbf{\Pi}(n;\, N)\left[\hat{\mathbf{B}}_{\mathbf{1}} + \hat{\mathbf{B}}_{\mathbf{2}}\right] = \mathbf{\Pi}(n+1;\, N)\hat{\mathbf{B}}_{\mathbf{1}}\hat{\mathbf{Q}}_{\mathbf{1}} + \mathbf{\Pi}(n-1;\, N)\hat{\mathbf{B}}_{\mathbf{2}}\hat{\mathbf{Q}}_{\mathbf{2}}. \qquad (7.3.3a)$$

With similar but simpler procedures, we can find the balance equations for $n = 0$ and $n = N$. We summarize these equations with the next theorem.

Theorem 7.3.1: The steady-state balance equations for an ME/ME/1//N loop are given by (7.3.3a) for $n = 1, 2, \ldots, N-1$, and

$$\mathbf{\Pi}(0;\, N)\hat{\mathbf{B}}_{\mathbf{2}} = \mathbf{\Pi}(1;\, N)\hat{\mathbf{B}}_{\mathbf{1}}\hat{\mathbf{Q}}_{\mathbf{1}} \qquad (7.3.3b)$$

and

$$\mathbf{\Pi}(N;\, N)\hat{\mathbf{B}}_{\mathbf{1}} = \mathbf{\Pi}(N-1;\, N)\hat{\mathbf{B}}_{\mathbf{2}}\hat{\mathbf{Q}}_{\mathbf{2}}. \qquad (7.3.3c)$$

Because S_1 and S_2 now play symmetric roles, these equations are invariant to the interchanges $n \Leftrightarrow N - n$, together with $(\cdot)_1 \Leftrightarrow (\cdot)_2$. ■

Observe the similarity between these equations and the balance equations of Equations (4.1.3) for the M/ME/1//N queue.

7.3.2 Steady-State Solution

Setting up the balance equations, even in such an elegant form as given in Theorem 7.3.1, in no way guarantees that an explicit solution can be found. As we saw in Chapter 6, often one must be satisfied with a recursive algebraic solution. In attempting to solve finite difference equations, of which this is an example, one is almost always denied even a recursive solution, and as with the solution of differential equations, one must settle for a brute force numerical solution. We know this much in general: that if by luck, ingenuity, or stroke of genius one could find a formula that satisfied all the balance equations, it would be the unique nontrivial solution. Appie van de Liefvoort did just that. We now present the solution and outline the proof that it is correct.

The formula has not been used very much, and no one knows just which of the several forms that it can take will ultimately prove to be the most useful. Thus we present several expressions for the same variables. We start with the usual set of definitions. We begin with an operator we used in Section 7.1. Let

$$\mathbf{D} := \left[\hat{\mathbf{B}}_1 + \hat{\mathbf{B}}_2\right]^{-1}. \tag{7.3.4}$$

Recall that this operator is the generator of first-finishing probabilities, and in simpler days (when one of the $\mathbf{B}$ matrices was exponential) was the generator of the Laplace transform. We next introduce two matrices that look suspiciously like the $\mathbf{A}$ matrix of (4.1.4a) but are not.

$$\mathbf{S}^+ := \hat{\mathbf{B}}_1 + \hat{\mathbf{B}}_2 - \hat{\mathbf{B}}_2\hat{\mathbf{Q}}_1 = \mathbf{D}^{-1}\left[\mathbf{I} - \mathbf{D}\hat{\mathbf{B}}_2\hat{\mathbf{Q}}_1\right], \tag{7.3.5a}$$

$$\begin{aligned}\mathbf{S}^- &:= \hat{\mathbf{B}}_1 + \hat{\mathbf{B}}_2 - \hat{\mathbf{B}}_1\hat{\mathbf{Q}}_2 = \mathbf{D}^{-1}\left[\mathbf{I} - \mathbf{D}\hat{\mathbf{B}}_1\hat{\mathbf{Q}}_2\right] \\ &= \left[\mathbf{I} - \hat{\mathbf{B}}_1\hat{\mathbf{Q}}_2 D\right]\mathbf{D}^{-1}.\end{aligned} \tag{7.3.5b}$$

Note that these matrices cannot be decomposed into a product of matrices from the two separate spaces. Also, they do not commute with each other if both S_1 and S_2 are nontrivial (i.e., have dimension greater than 1). If S_2 is one-dimensional, $\hat{\mathbf{B}}_2 \Rightarrow \lambda\mathbf{I}$, $\hat{\mathbf{Q}}_2 \Rightarrow \mathbf{I}$, and $\mathbf{S}^-$ reduces to $\lambda\mathbf{I}$, whereas while $\mathbf{S}^+ \Rightarrow \lambda\mathbf{A}$.

We next collect several formulas that $\mathbf{S}^\pm$ satisfy in relation to $\boldsymbol{\epsilon}_1'$ and $\boldsymbol{\epsilon}_2'$.

Lemma 7.3.2: The following relations hold:

$$\mathbf{S}^+\,\hat{\boldsymbol{\epsilon}}_1' = \hat{\mathbf{B}}_1\,\hat{\boldsymbol{\epsilon}}_1' \quad \text{and} \quad \mathbf{S}^-\,\hat{\boldsymbol{\epsilon}}_2' = \hat{\mathbf{B}}_2\,\hat{\boldsymbol{\epsilon}}_2', \tag{7.3.6a}$$

or equivalently [see (7.2.4b) and Lemma 7.2.3],

$$\mathbf{S}^+\hat{\mathbf{Q}}_1 = \hat{\mathbf{B}}_1\hat{\mathbf{Q}}_1 \quad \text{and} \quad \mathbf{S}^-\hat{\mathbf{Q}}_2 = \hat{\mathbf{B}}_2\hat{\mathbf{Q}}_2. \tag{7.3.6b}$$

We can also see that

$$\mathbf{S}^+\boldsymbol{\epsilon}' = \hat{\mathbf{B}}_1\boldsymbol{\epsilon}' \quad \text{and} \quad \mathbf{S}^-\boldsymbol{\epsilon}' = \hat{\mathbf{B}}_2\boldsymbol{\epsilon}', \tag{7.3.6c}$$

or equivalently,

$$\mathbf{S}^{+}\mathbf{Q} = \hat{\mathbf{B}}_1\mathbf{Q} \quad \text{and} \quad \mathbf{S}^{-}\mathbf{Q} = \hat{\mathbf{B}}_2\mathbf{Q}. \tag{7.3.6d}$$

The proofs follow directly just by carrying out the algebra. ■

Keep in mind that whereas Equations (7.3.6c) are vector equations, Equations (7.3.6a) are not, because $\boldsymbol{\epsilon}'$ is a vector in the product space, but $\hat{\boldsymbol{\epsilon}}_1'$ and $\hat{\boldsymbol{\epsilon}}_2'$ are rectangular matrices of dimensions $(m_1 \cdot m_2) \times (m_2)$ and $(m_1 \cdot m_2) \times (m_1)$, respectively.

Given that $\hat{\mathbf{Q}}_1$ commutes with $\hat{\mathbf{B}}_2$, and so on, there is an equivalent set of equations for $\hat{\mathbf{p}}_\mathbf{i}$, and so on, namely as follows.

Lemma 7.3.3: The following relations hold:

$$\hat{\mathbf{p}}_1\mathbf{S}^{+} = \hat{\mathbf{p}}_1\hat{\mathbf{B}}_1 \quad \text{and} \quad \hat{\mathbf{p}}_2\mathbf{S}^{-} = \hat{\mathbf{p}}_2\hat{\mathbf{B}}_2, \tag{7.3.7a}$$

or equivalently [see (7.2.4a) and Lemma 7.2.3],

$$\hat{\mathbf{Q}}_1\mathbf{S}^{+} = \hat{\mathbf{Q}}_1\hat{\mathbf{B}}_1 \quad \text{and} \quad \hat{\mathbf{Q}}_2\mathbf{S}^{-} = \hat{\mathbf{Q}}_2\hat{\mathbf{B}}_2. \tag{7.3.7b}$$

We can also see that

$$\mathbf{p}\mathbf{S}^{+} = \mathbf{p}\hat{\mathbf{B}}_1 \quad \text{and} \quad \mathbf{p}\mathbf{S}^{-} = \mathbf{p}\hat{\mathbf{B}}_2, \tag{7.3.7c}$$

or equivalently,

$$\mathbf{Q}\mathbf{S}^{+} = \mathbf{Q}\hat{\mathbf{B}}_1 \quad \text{and} \quad \mathbf{Q}\mathbf{S}^{-} = \mathbf{Q}\hat{\mathbf{B}}_2. \tag{7.3.7d}$$

The proofs are identical to those in Lemma 7.3.2. As in the previous lemma, Equations (7.3.7c) are vector equations, but Equations (7.3.7a) are not. ■

We need the inverses of $\mathbf{S}^{\pm}$, which if they exist, we call $\mathbf{T}^{\pm}$. Therefore, by Lemma 7.2.4 and (7.3.5a),

$$\begin{aligned} \mathbf{T}^{+} :&= (\mathbf{S}^{+})^{-1} := \left(\mathbf{I} - \mathbf{D}\hat{\mathbf{B}}_2\hat{\mathbf{Q}}_1\right)^{-1}\mathbf{D} \\ &= \left(\mathbf{I} + \mathbf{D}\hat{\mathbf{B}}_2\hat{\mathbf{Q}}_1\hat{\Psi}_2^{-1}\left[\mathbf{D}\hat{\mathbf{B}}_1\right]\right)\mathbf{D}, \end{aligned} \tag{7.3.8a}$$

where we have used $\hat{\Psi}_1^{-1}[\cdot]$* for $\left(\hat{\Psi}_1[\cdot]\right)^{-1}$. Similarly, we have

$$\begin{aligned} \mathbf{T}^{-} :&= (\mathbf{S}^{-})^{-1} := \left(\mathbf{I} - \mathbf{D}\hat{\mathbf{B}}_1\hat{\mathbf{Q}}_2\right)^{-1}\mathbf{D} \\ &= \left(\mathbf{I} + \mathbf{D}\hat{\mathbf{B}}_1\hat{\mathbf{Q}}_2\hat{\Psi}_1^{-1}\left[\mathbf{D}\hat{\mathbf{B}}_2\right]\right)\mathbf{D}. \end{aligned} \tag{7.3.8b}$$

*This is as good a place as any to caution the reader that, in general, $\Psi_i\left[\mathbf{F}^{-1}\right]$ does not equal $\Psi_i^{-1}[\mathbf{F}]$.

These equations are rather complicated, but it seems clear that $\mathbf{T}^+$ and $\mathbf{T}^-$ exist as long as $\Psi_2\left[\mathbf{D}\hat{\mathbf{B}}_1\right]$ and $\Psi_1\left[\mathbf{D}\hat{\mathbf{B}}_2\right]$ are nonsingular. We assume this to be true. To assume otherwise would end our exploration instantly. We now introduce the pivotal matrix of this chapter, the one that is the true generalization of the $\mathbf{U}$ in Equations (4.1.4), and the one that provides the geometric solution to the ME/ME/1//N loop. We use the same symbol for it.

$$\mathbf{U} := \mathbf{T}^+\mathbf{S}^- = \left[\mathbf{I} - \mathbf{D}\hat{\mathbf{B}}_2\hat{\mathbf{Q}}_1\right]^{-1}\left[\mathbf{I} - \mathbf{D}\hat{\mathbf{B}}_1\hat{\mathbf{Q}}_2\right]. \tag{7.3.9a}$$

Using (7.3.8a) and (7.3.5b), $\mathbf{U}$ can also be expressed as

$$\mathbf{U} = \left(\mathbf{I} + \mathbf{D}\hat{\mathbf{B}}_2\hat{\mathbf{Q}}_1\hat{\Psi}_2^{-1}\left[\mathbf{D}\hat{\mathbf{B}}_1\right]\right)\left[\mathbf{I} - \mathbf{D}\hat{\mathbf{B}}_1\hat{\mathbf{Q}}_2\right]. \tag{7.3.9b}$$

From Equations (7.3.5) and the discussion following them, we see that $\mathbf{U}$ reduces precisely to (4.1.4b) when S_2 is one-dimensional, and

$$\mathbf{U}^{-1} = \mathbf{T}^-\mathbf{S}^+ = \left[\mathbf{I} - \mathbf{D}\hat{\mathbf{B}}_1\hat{\mathbf{Q}}_2\right]^{-1}\left[\mathbf{I} - \mathbf{D}\hat{\mathbf{B}}_2\hat{\mathbf{Q}}_1\right] \tag{7.3.9c}$$

reduces to $\mathbf{A}$ in (4.1.4a). Actually, another matrix, defined by

$$\mathbf{R} := \mathbf{S}^-\mathbf{T}^+ = \left[\mathbf{I} - \hat{\mathbf{B}}_1\hat{\mathbf{Q}}_2\mathbf{D}\right]\left[\mathbf{I} - \hat{\mathbf{B}}_2\hat{\mathbf{Q}}_1\mathbf{D}\right]^{-1}, \tag{7.3.9d}$$

could equally be the pivotal matrix.

We need one final set of equations before presenting the major goal of this chapter, which as usual we precede with a definition:

$$\mathbf{E} := (\mathbf{I} - \hat{\mathbf{Q}}_1)(\mathbf{I} - \hat{\mathbf{Q}}_2) = (\mathbf{I} - \hat{\mathbf{Q}}_2)(\mathbf{I} - \hat{\mathbf{Q}}_1). \tag{7.3.10a}$$

$\mathbf{E}$ is idempotent, with rank $(m_1-1)\cdot(m_2-1)$. As with all idempotent matrices, $(\mathbf{I} - \mathbf{E})$ is also idempotent, with rank $m_1 + m_2 - 1$. Clearly, $[m_1 + m_2 - 1] + [(m_1 - 1) \cdot (m_2 - 1)] = m_1 \cdot m_2$.

Lemma 7.3.4: For any matrix $\mathbf{X}$ in the product space,

$$(\mathbf{I} - \mathbf{X}\hat{\mathbf{Q}}_\mathbf{i})(\mathbf{I} - \hat{\mathbf{Q}}_\mathbf{i}) = (\mathbf{I} - \hat{\mathbf{Q}}_\mathbf{i}). \tag{7.3.10b}$$

Therefore, given that $\hat{\mathbf{Q}}_1$ and $\hat{\mathbf{Q}}_2$ commute,

$$\mathbf{S}^+\mathbf{E} = (\hat{\mathbf{B}}_1 + \hat{\mathbf{B}}_2)\mathbf{E} = \mathbf{S}^-\mathbf{E}$$

and (7.3.10c)

$$\mathbf{E}\mathbf{S}^+ = \mathbf{E}(\hat{\mathbf{B}}_1 + \hat{\mathbf{B}}_2) = \mathbf{E}\mathbf{S}^-,$$

so the following identities hold,

$$\mathbf{U}\mathbf{E} = \mathbf{E} \quad \text{or} \quad (\mathbf{I} - \mathbf{U})\mathbf{E} = \mathbf{O}, \tag{7.3.10d}$$

$$\mathbf{E}\mathbf{R} = \mathbf{E} \quad \text{or} \quad \mathbf{E}(\mathbf{I} - \mathbf{R}) = \mathbf{O}, \tag{7.3.10e}$$

$$\mathbf{T}^{\pm}(\hat{\mathbf{B}}_1 + \hat{\mathbf{B}}_2)\mathbf{E} = \mathbf{E} = \mathbf{E}(\hat{\mathbf{B}}_1 + \hat{\mathbf{B}}_2)\mathbf{T}^{\pm}. \tag{7.3.10f}$$

Also,

$$\mathbf{S}^{-}\,\hat{\mathbf{Q}}_1 + \mathbf{S}^{+}\,\hat{\mathbf{Q}}_2 = [\hat{\mathbf{B}}_1 + \hat{\mathbf{B}}_2][\mathbf{I} - \mathbf{E}] \tag{7.3.10g}$$

and

$$\hat{\mathbf{Q}}_1\mathbf{S}^{-} + \hat{\mathbf{Q}}_2\mathbf{S}^{+} = [\mathbf{I} - \mathbf{E}][\hat{\mathbf{B}}_1 + \hat{\mathbf{B}}_2]. \tag{7.3.10h}$$

The proofs are by direct substitution for $\mathbf{U}$, $\mathbf{R}$, $\mathbf{S}^{\pm}$, and $\mathbf{T}^{\pm}$. ■

Equations (7.3.10) are used to prove our theorem, and they contain information that may be of critical importance for future research. Equations (7.3.10d) and (7.3.10e) look like eigenvalue equations, and in fact, imply that there are as many eigenvectors of $\mathbf{U}$ (and $\mathbf{R}$) with eigenvalue 1 as the rank of $\mathbf{E}$. Therefore, $(\mathbf{I} - \mathbf{U})$ has at most $m_1 + m_2 - 1$ nonzero eigenvalues. In the previous chapters, $m_2 = 1$, so $(\mathbf{I} - \mathbf{U})$ had m_1 nonzero eigenvalues, which was all of them, and so was invertible. But now that $m_2 > 1$, this is no longer true. The same statement can be made for $\mathbf{R}$. This inhibits our ability to find an explicit solution to the open ME/ME/1 queue.

The main theorem is now stated and proved.

Theorem 7.3.5: Given a closed ME/ME/1//N loop, with $N > 1$, the steady-state vector and scalar probabilities are described by

$$\mathbf{\Pi}(n;\, N) = \mathbf{\Pi}(0;\, N)\hat{\mathbf{B}}_2\mathbf{U}^{n}\mathbf{T}^{-}, \qquad n = 1,\, 2,\, \ldots,\, N-1\,, \tag{7.3.11a}$$

and

$$\mathbf{\Pi}(N;\, N) = \mathbf{\Pi}(0;\, N)\hat{\mathbf{B}}_2\mathbf{U}^{N-1}\hat{\mathbf{V}}_1. \tag{7.3.11b}$$

Equation (7.3.11a) can also be written in the form

$$\mathbf{\Pi}(n;\, N) = \mathbf{\Pi}(0;\, N)\hat{\mathbf{B}}_2\mathbf{T}^{-}\,\mathbf{R}^{n-1}. \tag{7.3.11c}$$

This form would seem to be preferred, because the geometric factor appears at the right of the expression, allowing one to use

$$\mathbf{\Pi}(n;\, N) = \mathbf{\Pi}(n-1;\, N)\mathbf{R}, \qquad n = 1,\, 2,\, \ldots,\, N-1$$

(which we actually do in the algorithm below). It remains to be seen which is more significant in the long run. ■

Proof: First we show that Equations (7.3.11) are symmetric in S_1 and S_2. We do this by expressing everything in terms of $\mathbf{\Pi}(N;\, N)$ and interchanging 1 and 2. The interchange, in turn, causes + and − to interchange; thus $\mathbf{U}$ goes to $\mathbf{U}^{-1}$, which we call $\mathbf{A}$. From (7.3.11b) we get

$$\mathbf{\Pi}(0;\, N) = \mathbf{\Pi}(N;\, N)\hat{\mathbf{B}}_1\mathbf{A}^{N-1}\hat{\mathbf{V}}_2.$$

Similarly, from (7.3.11a) and the above, we get

$$\mathbf{\Pi}(n;\, N) = \mathbf{\Pi}(N;\, N)\hat{\mathbf{B}}_1\mathbf{A}^{N-1}\hat{\mathbf{V}}_2\hat{\mathbf{B}}_2\mathbf{U}^{n}\mathbf{T}^{-}$$

$$= \mathbf{\Pi}(N;\, N)\hat{\mathbf{B}}_1 \mathbf{A}^{N-1} \mathbf{U}^n \mathbf{T}^- = \mathbf{\Pi}(N;\, N)\hat{\mathbf{B}}_1 \mathbf{A}^{N-n} \mathbf{U}\mathbf{T}^-$$

or by expressing the first argument in terms of the number of customers at S_2, namely, $k = N - n$, and observing that $\mathbf{UT}^- = \mathbf{T}^+$, we obtain

$$\mathbf{\Pi}(N-k;\, N) = \mathbf{\Pi}(N-0;\, N)\hat{\mathbf{B}}_1 \mathbf{A}^{k} \mathbf{T}^+.$$

Clearly, these equations look just like the original ones after one makes the required interchanges. This means, then, that if we satisfy (7.3.3b), by duality we automatically satisfy (7.3.3c).

To satisfy (7.3.3b), take (7.3.11a) for $n = 1$, recall again that $\mathbf{UT}^- = \mathbf{T}^+$, and manipulate to get

$$\mathbf{\Pi}(1;\, N)\mathbf{S}^+ = \mathbf{\Pi}(0;\, N)\hat{\mathbf{B}}_2.$$

Now multiply both sides by $\hat{\mathbf{Q}}_1$; use (7.3.2), (7.3.6b), and Lemma 7.2.1 to get

$$\mathbf{\Pi}(1;\, N)\hat{\mathbf{B}}_1\hat{\mathbf{Q}}_1 = [\mathbf{p}_1 \otimes (\boldsymbol{\pi}_2(0; N)\mathbf{B}_2)] \cdot [\mathbf{Q}_1 \otimes \mathbf{I}_2] = \mathbf{\Pi}(0;\, N)\hat{\mathbf{B}}_2.$$

In the last step we used (7.2.2) and the fact that $\mathbf{p}_1\mathbf{Q}_1 = \mathbf{p}_1$. This is indeed the same as (7.3.3b).

Last, we substitute (7.3.6b) and (7.3.11c) into the right-hand side of (7.3.3a) and get

$$\mathbf{\Pi}(n;\, N)[\mathbf{S}^-\, \mathbf{T}^+\, \mathbf{S}^+\, \hat{\mathbf{Q}}_1 + \mathbf{S}^+\, \mathbf{T}^-\, \mathbf{S}^-\, \hat{\mathbf{Q}}_2] = \mathbf{\Pi}(n;\, N)[\mathbf{S}^-\, \hat{\mathbf{Q}}_1 + \mathbf{S}^+\, \hat{\mathbf{Q}}_2]$$

$$= \mathbf{\Pi}(n;\, N)[\hat{\mathbf{B}}_1 + \hat{\mathbf{B}}_2] - \mathbf{\Pi}(n;\, N)[\hat{\mathbf{B}}_1 + \hat{\mathbf{B}}_2]\mathbf{E},$$

where we used (7.3.10d). But from (7.3.10b) and (7.3.10c), we see that the last term vanishes. That is,

$$\mathbf{\Pi}(n;\, N)[\hat{\mathbf{B}}_1 + \hat{\mathbf{B}}_2]\mathbf{E} = \mathbf{\Pi}(0;\, N)\hat{\mathbf{B}}_2\mathbf{U}^n\mathbf{T}^-[\hat{\mathbf{B}}_1 + \hat{\mathbf{B}}_2]\mathbf{E}$$

$$= \mathbf{\Pi}(0;\, N)\hat{\mathbf{B}}_2\mathbf{U}^{\mathbf{n}}\mathbf{E} = \mathbf{p}_1 \otimes [\boldsymbol{\pi}_2(0; N)\mathbf{B}_2]\mathbf{E} = [\boldsymbol{\pi}_2(0; N)\mathbf{B}_2][\hat{\mathbf{p}}_1\mathbf{E}] = \mathbf{o},$$

because $[\hat{\mathbf{p}}_1\, \mathbf{E}] = \mathbf{o}$. The term that remains is equal to the left-hand side of (7.3.3a). **QED**

This was surely a tedious proof, but we are not yet finished. Note that the solution is given in terms of $\boldsymbol{\pi}_2(0; N)$ [or $\boldsymbol{\pi}_1(N; N)$]. This is an m_2 (or m_1) component object, and we can only fix one constant with the normalization requirement that the sum of all probabilities be 1. Naturally, when m_2 was 1 there was no problem, but now there is. Equation (7.3.11b) is a matrix equation with $(m_1 \cdot m_2)$ components, but only $(m_1 + m_2)$ unknowns. Therefore, these unknowns must be related in some way. We rewrite the equation using (7.3.2).

$$\boldsymbol{\pi}_1(N; N)\mathbf{B}_1 \otimes \mathbf{p}_2 = \mathbf{p}_1 \otimes \boldsymbol{\pi}_2(0; N)\mathbf{B}_2\mathbf{U}^{N-1}.$$

Next rewrite this equation using Lemma 7.2.1 (and momentarily drop the dependence of $\boldsymbol{\pi}_\mathbf{i}$ on n and N),

$$\mathbf{p_2}\hat{\boldsymbol{\pi}}_\mathbf{1}\hat{\boldsymbol{B}}_\mathbf{1} = \boldsymbol{\pi}_\mathbf{2}\,\mathbf{B_2}\,\hat{\mathbf{p}}_\mathbf{1}\mathbf{U}^{N-1}.$$

Next postmultiply both sides with $\hat{\boldsymbol{\epsilon}}'_\mathbf{1}$ to get

$$\mathbf{p_2}\cdot\left(\hat{\boldsymbol{\pi}}_\mathbf{1}\,\hat{\mathbf{B}}_\mathbf{1}\hat{\boldsymbol{\epsilon}}'_\mathbf{1}\right) = \boldsymbol{\pi}_\mathbf{2}\,\mathbf{B_2}\hat{\Psi}_2\left[\mathbf{U}^{N-1}\right]. \tag{7.3.12a}$$

The expression in parentheses is the inner product of two 1-space hatted vectors and is therefore equal to a scalar times $\mathbf{I_2}$ (see Lemma 7.2.1). Define that scalar to be

$$\beta(N) := \boldsymbol{\pi}_\mathbf{1}\,\mathbf{B}_\mathbf{1}\,\boldsymbol{\epsilon}'_\mathbf{1}.$$

Observe that the right-hand expression of (7.3.12a), just like the other side, depends only on 2-space objects; therefore, we can remove the *hats*, and the equation becomes

$$\beta(N)\mathbf{p_2} = \boldsymbol{\pi}_\mathbf{2}\,\mathbf{B_2}\Psi_2\left[\mathbf{U}^{N-1}\right].$$

Solving for $\boldsymbol{\pi}_\mathbf{2}$, we get

$$\boldsymbol{\pi}_\mathbf{2}(0;N) = \beta(N)\mathbf{p_2}\Psi_2^{-1}\left[\mathbf{U}^{N-1}\right]\mathbf{V_2}. \tag{7.3.12b}$$

By similar manipulations, it can be shown that $\boldsymbol{\pi}_\mathbf{2}$ also satisfies the following eigenvector equation.

$$\boldsymbol{\pi}_\mathbf{2} = \boldsymbol{\pi}_\mathbf{2}\,\mathbf{B_2}\Psi_2\left[\mathbf{U}^{N-1}\hat{\mathbf{Q}}_\mathbf{2}\mathbf{A}^{N-1}\right]\mathbf{V_2}. \tag{7.3.12c}$$

Either of these last two equations can be used to find $\boldsymbol{\pi}_\mathbf{2}$.

It is not understood what the significance is to having two defining equations for $\boldsymbol{\pi}_\mathbf{2}$. Clearly, both must yield the same vector, to within a constant [which we can take to be $\beta(N)$]. This constant can be determined by normalization as follows:

$$1 = \sum_{n=o}^{N} r(n;N) = \sum_{n=o}^{N}\boldsymbol{\Pi}(n;\,N)\,\boldsymbol{\epsilon}'$$

$$= \boldsymbol{\Pi}(0;\,N)\boldsymbol{\epsilon}' + \boldsymbol{\Pi}(0;\,N)\hat{\mathbf{B}}_\mathbf{2}[\mathbf{U}+\mathbf{U}^2+\cdots+\mathbf{U}^{N-1}]\mathbf{T}^{-}\boldsymbol{\epsilon}' + \boldsymbol{\Pi}(0;\,N)\hat{\mathbf{B}}_\mathbf{2}\mathbf{U}^{N-1}\hat{\mathbf{V}}_\mathbf{1}\boldsymbol{\epsilon}'.$$

These expressions are so cumbersome to work with that one can get discouraged from going on. But only with continued use will we be able to find simpler formulas. For now, we follow what we did for the M/G/1//N queue in (4.1.6d), and define

$$\mathbf{K}(N) := \mathbf{I} + [\mathbf{U}+\mathbf{U}^2+\cdots+\mathbf{U}^{N-1}]\mathbf{T}^{-}\hat{\mathbf{B}}_\mathbf{2} + \mathbf{U}^{N-1}\hat{\mathbf{V}}_\mathbf{1}\hat{\mathbf{B}}_\mathbf{2}.$$

Then

$$1 = \boldsymbol{\Pi}(0;\,N)\hat{\mathbf{B}}_\mathbf{2}\,\mathbf{K}(N)\hat{\mathbf{V}}_\mathbf{2}\boldsymbol{\epsilon}' = \boldsymbol{\pi}_\mathbf{2}(0;N)\mathbf{B_2}\hat{\mathbf{p}}_\mathbf{1}\,\mathbf{K}(N)\hat{\boldsymbol{\epsilon}}'_\mathbf{1}\,\mathbf{V_2}\,\boldsymbol{\epsilon}'_\mathbf{2},$$

and using (7.3.12b), we obtain

$$\begin{aligned} 1 &= \beta(N)\mathbf{p_2}\Psi_2^{-1}\left[\mathbf{U}^{N-1}\right]\mathbf{V_2}\,\mathbf{B_2}\Psi_2\left[\mathbf{K}(N)\right]\mathbf{V_2}\,\boldsymbol{\epsilon}_2' \\ &= \beta(N)\Psi\left[\Psi_2^{-1}\left[\mathbf{U}^{N-1}\right]\Psi_2\left[\mathbf{K}(N)\right]\mathbf{V_2}\right]. \end{aligned} \tag{7.3.13}$$

We summarize this maze of formulas with the following theorem.

Theorem 7.3.6: Explicit expressions for the steady-state vector probabilities for a closed ME/ME/1//N loop, with $N > 1$ and $0 < n < N$, are

$$\mathbf{K}(N) = \mathbf{I} + [\mathbf{U} + \mathbf{U}^2 + \cdots + \mathbf{U}^{N-1}]\mathbf{T}^-\,\hat{\mathbf{B}}_2 + \mathbf{U}^{N-1}\,\hat{\mathbf{V}}_1\,\hat{\mathbf{B}}_2. \tag{7.3.14a}$$

$$\beta(N)^{-1} = \Psi\left[\Psi_2^{-1}\left[\mathbf{U}^{N-1}\right]\Psi_2\left[\mathbf{K}(N)\right]\mathbf{V_2}\right], \tag{7.3.14b}$$

$$\boldsymbol{\pi}_2(0; N) = \beta(N)\mathbf{p_2}\Psi_2^{-1}\left[\mathbf{U}^{N-1}\right]\mathbf{V_2}, \tag{7.3.14c}$$

$$\boldsymbol{\Pi}(n;\, N) = \beta(N)\mathbf{p_2}\Psi_2^{-1}\left[\mathbf{U}^{N-1}\right]\hat{\mathbf{p}}_1\mathbf{U}^{n-1}\mathbf{T}^+, \tag{7.3.14d}$$

$$\boldsymbol{\Pi}(N;\, N) = \beta(N)\mathbf{p_2}\Psi_2^{-1}\left[\mathbf{U}^{N-1}\right]\hat{\mathbf{p}}_1\mathbf{U}^{N-1}\hat{\mathbf{V}}_1. \tag{7.3.14e}$$

The associated scalar probabilities are given by

$$r(0; N) = \boldsymbol{\pi}_2(0; N)\cdot\boldsymbol{\epsilon}_2' = \beta(N)\Psi\left[\Psi_2^{-1}\left[\mathbf{U}^{N-1}\right]\mathbf{V_2}\right], \tag{7.3.14f}$$

$$\begin{aligned} r(n; N) &= \boldsymbol{\Pi}(n;\, N)\cdot\boldsymbol{\epsilon}' \\ &= \beta(N)\Psi\left[\Psi_2^{-1}\left[\mathbf{U}^{N-1}\right]\cdot\Psi_2\left[\mathbf{U}^{n-1}\mathbf{T}^+\right]\right], \end{aligned} \tag{7.3.14g}$$

$$\begin{aligned} r(N; N) &= \boldsymbol{\Pi}(N;\, N)\cdot\boldsymbol{\epsilon}' \\ &= \beta(N)\Psi\left[\Psi_2^{-1}\left[\mathbf{U}^{N-1}\right]\cdot\Psi_2\left[\mathbf{U}^{N-1}\hat{\mathbf{V}}_1\right]\right]. \end{aligned} \tag{7.3.14h}$$

Surely we will find something better someday. ■

7.3.3 Outline of an Efficient Algorithm

The formulas we have derived for the ME/ME/1//N queue appear rather intimidating, but they actually can be calculated systematically and efficiently. We aid the reader in recognizing the relative ease with which this can be done by giving an algorithm for the calculation of the steady-state scalar probabilities, the mean queue length, and the throughput, parametrically on N, the number of customers in the system. We make no claims that this is the most efficient possible, but it could be worse.

We state without proof that $(\boldsymbol{\Pi}(n;\, N)\hat{\mathbf{B}}_1\,\boldsymbol{\epsilon}')$ is the equilibrium flow from external state n to $n+1$. Therefore [see (1.1.1), (2.1.5a), and (4.1.8)],

$$\Lambda(N) = \sum_{n=1}^{N}\boldsymbol{\Pi}(n;\, N)\hat{\mathbf{B}}_1\,\boldsymbol{\epsilon}'. \tag{7.3.15}$$

In general, computational costs can be greatly reduced by working with matrix-vector products rather than matrix-matrix products. Therefore, we introduce the vector $\mathbf{k}'(N)$ of dimension $(m_1 \cdot m_2)$:

$$\mathbf{k}'(N) := \mathbf{K}(N)\hat{\mathbf{V}}_\mathbf{2}\,\boldsymbol{\epsilon}',$$

which has the following properties.

$$\mathbf{k}'(1) = (\hat{\mathbf{V}}_\mathbf{1} + \hat{\mathbf{V}}_\mathbf{2}) \cdot \boldsymbol{\epsilon}' = [\mathbf{V}_\mathbf{1}\,\boldsymbol{\epsilon}'_\mathbf{1}] \otimes \boldsymbol{\epsilon}'_\mathbf{2} + \boldsymbol{\epsilon}'_\mathbf{1} \otimes [\mathbf{V}_\mathbf{2}\,\boldsymbol{\epsilon}'_\mathbf{2}],$$
$$\mathbf{k}'(N) = T_2\boldsymbol{\epsilon}' + \mathbf{U} \cdot \mathbf{k}'(N-1) \quad \text{for } N > 1,$$

and

$$\hat{\mathbf{p}}_\mathbf{1} \cdot \mathbf{k}'(N) = \Psi_2\left[\mathbf{K}(N)\right] \cdot \mathbf{V}_\mathbf{2} \cdot \boldsymbol{\epsilon}',$$

where $T_2 = \Psi\left[\mathbf{V}_\mathbf{2}\right]$ is the mean service time of S_2 and $\hat{\mathbf{p}}_\mathbf{1} \cdot \mathbf{k}'(N)$ is a column vector in 2-space. Next, the ***block vectors*** of dimension $(m_1 \cdot m_2) \times m_2$, defined by

$$\mathbf{u}'(N) := \mathbf{U}^N \hat{\boldsymbol{\epsilon}}'_\mathbf{1}$$

satisfy the recursive relations, starting with $\mathbf{u}'(0) = \hat{\boldsymbol{\epsilon}}'_\mathbf{1}$,

$$\mathbf{u}'(N) := \mathbf{U} \cdot \mathbf{u}'(N-1) \quad \text{for } N > 0.$$

Finally, to avoid needless repetitions (and perhaps to clarify), the symbols $\hat{\mathbf{y}}_\mathbf{1}$, $\mathbf{X}$, $\mathbf{x}'$, and $\mathbf{z}_\mathbf{2}$ are used to keep intermediate results for $\hat{\mathbf{p}}_\mathbf{1}\mathbf{T}^+$, $\mathbf{S}^-\hat{\mathbf{V}}_\mathbf{1}$, $\hat{\mathbf{B}}_\mathbf{1}\,\boldsymbol{\epsilon}'$, and $\mathbf{p}_\mathbf{2}\Psi_2^{-1}\left[\mathbf{U}^N\right]$, respectively. It is important in understanding the equations, as well as in coding the algorithms, to keep track of the dimensions of each of these objects. Therefore, we have given them symbols that match their dimensions. But be warned that the subscripts on these temporary variables in no way imply that they commute with objects from the other space. Their dimensions are

$$\mathrm{Dim}[\hat{\mathbf{y}}_\mathbf{1}] = \mathrm{Dim}[\hat{\mathbf{p}}_\mathbf{1}\mathbf{T}^+] = \mathrm{Dim}[\hat{\mathbf{p}}_\mathbf{1}] = \mathrm{m}_2 \times (\mathrm{m}_1 \cdot \mathrm{m}_2),$$

$$\mathrm{Dim}[\mathbf{X}] = \mathrm{Dim}[\mathbf{S}^-\hat{\mathbf{V}}_\mathbf{1}] = \mathrm{Dim}[\mathbf{S}^-] = (\mathrm{m}_1 \cdot \mathrm{m}_2) \times (\mathrm{m}_1 \cdot \mathrm{m}_2),$$

$$\mathrm{Dim}[\hat{\mathbf{B}}_\mathbf{1}\,\boldsymbol{\epsilon}'] = \mathrm{Dim}[\mathbf{x}'] = \mathrm{Dim}[\boldsymbol{\epsilon}'] = (\mathrm{m}_1 \cdot \mathrm{m}_2) \times 1,$$

$$\mathrm{Dim}\left[\mathbf{p}_\mathbf{2}\Psi_2^{-1}\left[\mathbf{U}^\mathrm{n}\right]\right] = \mathrm{Dim}[\mathbf{z}_\mathbf{2}] = \mathrm{Dim}[\mathbf{p}_\mathbf{2}] = 1 \times \mathrm{m}_2.$$

Algorithm for Calculating Properties of ME/ME/1/ /N Loops

∗ *Initialization*
∗ *Assume that* $\mathbf{p}_\mathbf{1}, \mathbf{P}_\mathbf{1}, \mathbf{M}_\mathbf{1}$, $\mathbf{p}_\mathbf{2}, \mathbf{P}_\mathbf{2}$, *and* $\mathbf{M}_\mathbf{2}$ *are given, then*:
BEGIN PROCEDURE
. FOR $i = 1$ TO 2, DO
. $\quad\mathbf{B}_\mathrm{i} \leftarrow \mathbf{M}_\mathrm{i}(\mathbf{I}_\mathrm{i} - \mathbf{P}_\mathrm{i})$
. $\quad\mathbf{V}_\mathrm{i} \leftarrow inverse[\mathbf{B}_\mathrm{i}]$
. $\quad T_i \leftarrow \mathbf{p}_\mathrm{i}\,\mathbf{V}_\mathrm{i}\,\boldsymbol{\epsilon}'_i$
. END FOR
. $\mathbf{S}^- \leftarrow \hat{\mathbf{B}}_\mathbf{1} + \hat{\mathbf{B}}_\mathbf{2} - \hat{\mathbf{B}}_\mathbf{1}\hat{\mathbf{Q}}_\mathbf{2}$

. $\mathbf{S}^+ \leftarrow \hat{\mathbf{B}}_1 + \hat{\mathbf{B}}_2 - \hat{\mathbf{B}}_2\hat{\mathbf{Q}}_1$
. $\mathbf{T}^+ \leftarrow inverse[\mathbf{S}^+]$
. $\mathbf{U} \leftarrow \mathbf{T}^+\,\mathbf{S}^-$
. $\mathbf{R} \leftarrow \mathbf{S}^-\,\mathbf{T}^+$
. $\mathbf{k}'(1) \leftarrow [\mathbf{V}_1\,\boldsymbol{\epsilon}_1'] \otimes \boldsymbol{\epsilon}_2' + \boldsymbol{\epsilon}_1' \otimes [\mathbf{V}_2\,\boldsymbol{\epsilon}_2']$
. $\mathbf{u}'(0) \leftarrow \hat{\boldsymbol{\epsilon}}_1'$
. $\hat{\mathbf{y}}_1 \leftarrow \hat{\mathbf{p}}_1\,\mathbf{T}^+$
. $\mathbf{X} \leftarrow \hat{\mathbf{V}}_1\,\hat{\mathbf{B}}_2 + \mathbf{I} - \hat{\mathbf{Q}}_2 \left(= \mathbf{S}^-\,\hat{\mathbf{V}}_1 = \hat{\mathbf{V}}_1\,\mathbf{S}^-\right)$
. $\mathbf{x}' \leftarrow \hat{\mathbf{B}}_1\boldsymbol{\epsilon}'$
**For a parametric study, where the number of customers N varies from 2*
. ** to a certain limit N_m the normalization constant and the initial vector*
. ** need to be calculated. Also, the vector $\mathbf{\Pi}(1;\,N)$ can be calculated, and*
. ** initial values for mean queue length and throughput must be set.*
FOR $N = 2$ TO N_m, DO
. $\mathbf{k}'(N) \leftarrow T_2\boldsymbol{\epsilon}' + \mathbf{U}\,\mathbf{k}'(N-1)$
. $\mathbf{u}'(N-1) \leftarrow \mathbf{U}\,\mathbf{u}'(N-2)$
. $\mathbf{z_2} \leftarrow \mathbf{p_2} \cdot inverse[\hat{\mathbf{u}}_1\,\mathbf{u}'(N-1)]$
. $[\beta(N)]^{-1} \leftarrow \mathbf{z_2}\hat{\mathbf{p}}_1\,\mathbf{k}'(N)$
. $\boldsymbol{\pi}_2(0;N) \leftarrow \beta(N)\mathbf{z_2}\mathbf{V_2}$
. $r(0;N) \leftarrow \boldsymbol{\pi}_2(0;N)\boldsymbol{\epsilon}_2'$
. $\mathbf{\Pi}(1;\,N) \leftarrow \beta(N)\mathbf{z_2} \cdot \hat{\mathbf{y}}_1$
. $r(1;N) \leftarrow \mathbf{\Pi}(1;\,N)\boldsymbol{\epsilon}'$
. $\bar{q} \leftarrow r(1;N)$
. $\Lambda \leftarrow \mathbf{\Pi}(1;\,N) \cdot \mathbf{x}'$

* *Each steady-state probability vector can now be calculated iteratively.*
. FOR $i = 2$ TO $N-1$, DO
. $\mathbf{\Pi}(i;\,N) \leftarrow \mathbf{\Pi}(i-1;\,N) \cdot \mathbf{R}$
. $r(i;N) \leftarrow \mathbf{\Pi}(i;\,N) \cdot \boldsymbol{\epsilon}'$
. $\bar{q} \leftarrow \bar{q} + i \cdot r(i;N)$
. $\Lambda \leftarrow \Lambda + \mathbf{\Pi}(i;\,N) \cdot \mathbf{x}'$
. END FOR

. * *The last terms need to be calculated separately.*
. $\mathbf{\Pi}(N;\,N) \leftarrow \mathbf{\Pi}(N-1;\,N) \cdot \mathbf{X}$
. $r(N;N) \leftarrow \mathbf{\Pi}(N;\,N) \cdot \boldsymbol{\epsilon}'$
. $\bar{q} \leftarrow \bar{q} + N \cdot r(N;N)$
. $\Lambda \leftarrow \Lambda + \mathbf{\Pi}(N;\,N) \cdot \mathbf{x}'$
END FOR
END PROCEDURE

It is worth discussing the computational complexity of this algorithm. Let $T(N_m)$ be the number of multiplications and divisions for this procedure. Then

$$T(N_m) = 3m_1^\alpha \cdot m_2^\alpha + m_1^2 \cdot m_2^2 + m_1^\alpha + m_2^\alpha + 2m_1^2 + m_2^2 + m_1 \cdot m_2$$

$$+(N_m-1)\cdot(m_1^2 \cdot m_2^\alpha \cdot 2m_1^2 \cdot m_2^2 + 2m_1 \cdot m_2^2 + m_2^\alpha + m_2^2 + 4m_1 \cdot m_2 + 2m_2 + 1)$$

$$+\frac{1}{2}(N_m-1)\cdot(N_m-2)\cdot(m_1^2\cdot m_2^2+m_1\cdot m_2+1)$$
$$=\mathrm{O}\left(3m_1^\alpha\cdot m_2^\alpha+N_m\cdot m_1^2\cdot m_2^\alpha+\frac{1}{2}N_m^2\cdot m_1^2\cdot m_2^2\right),$$

where m^α is the complexity for multiplying two $m\times m$ matrices. For the special case where $\alpha=3$, the order of complexity reduces to

$$T(N_m)=\mathrm{O}\left(3m_1^3\cdot m_2^3+N_m\cdot m_1^2\cdot m_2^3+\frac{1}{2}N_m^2\cdot m_1^2\cdot m_2^2\right).$$

In most cases, the complexity is likely to be dominated by the N_m^2 term. Suppose one is interested in $\bar{q}$ and Λ but not in $r(n;N)$. Then $\bar{q}$ and Λ can be calculated in a way analogous to the way β is calculated [using $\mathbf{k}'(N)$], thereby eliminating the inner loop on i, and consequently, reducing the complexity by an order of N_m. In such a case, it would take no more to compute the performance for all N from 1 to N_m than it would to calculate the performance for N_m alone.

7.3.4 An Example

We now present an example of the simplest nontrivial loop, just to see what the specific matrices look like. Let both S_1 and S_2 be Erlangian-2 servers, with parameters μ and λ, respectively. Then $\rho=\lambda/\mu$ and

$$\mathbf{p_i}=[1\ 0],\qquad \mathbf{M_1}=\mu\mathbf{I_1},\qquad \mathbf{M_2}=\lambda\mathbf{I_2},$$

$$\mathbf{q_i'}=\begin{bmatrix}0\\1\end{bmatrix},\qquad \mathbf{P_i}=\begin{bmatrix}0&1\\0&0\end{bmatrix},\qquad \mathbf{Q_i}=\begin{bmatrix}1&0\\1&0\end{bmatrix},$$

$$\mathbf{B_1}=\mu\begin{bmatrix}1&-1\\0&1\end{bmatrix},\qquad \mathbf{B_2}=\lambda\begin{bmatrix}1&-1\\0&1\end{bmatrix},$$

$$\mathbf{V_1}=\frac{1}{\mu}\begin{bmatrix}1&1\\0&1\end{bmatrix},\qquad \mathbf{V_2}=\frac{1}{\lambda}\begin{bmatrix}1&1\\0&1\end{bmatrix}.$$

The embedded matrices [from (7.2.1)] are given by

$$\hat{\mathbf{p}}_1=\begin{bmatrix}1&0&0&0\\0&1&0&0\end{bmatrix},\qquad \hat{\mathbf{p}}_2=\begin{bmatrix}1&0&0&0\\0&0&1&0\end{bmatrix},$$

$$\mathbf{p}=\mathbf{p_1}\otimes\mathbf{p_2}=\mathbf{p_1}\hat{\mathbf{p}}_2=\mathbf{p_2}\hat{\mathbf{p}}_1=[1\,0\,0\,0],$$

$$\hat{\mathbf{Q}}_1=\begin{bmatrix}1&0&0&0\\0&1&0&0\\1&0&0&0\\0&1&0&0\end{bmatrix},\qquad \hat{\mathbf{Q}}_2=\begin{bmatrix}1&0&0&0\\1&0&0&0\\0&0&1&0\\0&0&1&0\end{bmatrix},$$

$$\mathbf{Q}=\boldsymbol{\epsilon}'\boldsymbol{p}=\begin{bmatrix}1&0&0&0\\1&0&0&0\\1&0&0&0\\1&0&0&0\end{bmatrix},$$

where $\mathbf{Q} = \hat{\mathbf{Q}}_1\hat{\mathbf{Q}}_2 = \mathbf{Q}_1 \otimes \mathbf{Q}_2$, and

$$\mathbf{E} = (\mathbf{I} - \hat{\mathbf{Q}}_1)(\mathbf{I} - \hat{\mathbf{Q}}_2) = \begin{bmatrix} 0 & 0 & 0 & 0 \\ 0 & 0 & 0 & 0 \\ 0 & 0 & 0 & 0 \\ 1 & -1 & -1 & 1 \end{bmatrix}.$$

Note that both $\hat{\mathbf{Q}}_1$ and $\hat{\mathbf{Q}}_2$ are of rank 2, $[m_i]$, because they each have two linearly independent rows when considered as vectors. On the other hand, $\mathbf{Q}$ is of rank 1, as it should be, because all four of its rows are the same. $\mathbf{E}$ is also of rank 1 $[(m_1 - 1) \cdot (m_2 - 1) = 1]$, because all of its columns are proportional to each other.

$$\hat{\mathbf{B}}_1 = \mu \begin{bmatrix} 1 & 0 & -1 & 0 \\ 0 & 1 & 0 & -1 \\ 0 & 0 & 1 & 0 \\ 0 & 0 & 0 & 1 \end{bmatrix}, \qquad \hat{\mathbf{B}}_2 = \lambda \begin{bmatrix} 1 & -1 & 0 & 0 \\ 0 & 1 & 0 & 0 \\ 0 & 0 & 1 & -1 \\ 0 & 0 & 0 & 1 \end{bmatrix},$$

$$\hat{\mathbf{V}}_1 = \frac{1}{\mu} \begin{bmatrix} 1 & 0 & 1 & 0 \\ 0 & 1 & 0 & 1 \\ 0 & 0 & 1 & 0 \\ 0 & 0 & 0 & 1 \end{bmatrix}, \qquad \hat{\mathbf{V}}_2 = \frac{1}{\lambda} \begin{bmatrix} 1 & 1 & 0 & 0 \\ 0 & 1 & 0 & 0 \\ 0 & 0 & 1 & 1 \\ 0 & 0 & 0 & 1 \end{bmatrix}.$$

Some composite matrices in the product space follow.

$$\mathbf{D}^{-1} = \hat{\mathbf{B}}_1 + \hat{\mathbf{B}}_2 = \mu \begin{bmatrix} 1+\rho & -\rho & -1 & 0 \\ 0 & 1+\rho & 0 & -1 \\ 0 & 0 & 1+\rho & -\rho \\ 0 & 0 & 0 & 1+\rho \end{bmatrix},$$

$$\mu\mathbf{D} = \frac{1}{(1+\rho)^3} \begin{bmatrix} (1+\rho)^2 & \rho(1+\rho) & (1+\rho) & 2\rho \\ 0 & (1+\rho)^2 & 0 & (1+\rho) \\ 0 & 0 & (1+\rho)^2 & \rho(1+\rho) \\ 0 & 0 & 0 & (1+\rho)^2 \end{bmatrix}.$$

Recall that in Section 7.1 we used this operator to find the expression for $C(0)$, the probability that S_1 would finish before S_2, given that they started at the same time. In our example, this turns out to be [using (7.1.3b)]

$$C(0) = \Psi\left[\hat{\mathbf{B}}_1\mathbf{D}\right] = \frac{1+3\rho}{(1+\rho)^3}. \qquad (7.3.16)$$

Exercise 7.3.1: You are to compare $C(0)$ for three different cases as a function of ρ. The cases are (a) exponential-exponential, from Equation (2.1.1b) (call it C_{11}); (b) exponential-Erlangian-2 [C_{12}, see (3.1.10) and recall the interpretion of $B^*(s)$]; and (c) Equation (7.3.16) (call it C_{22}). First verify that

$$\Psi_2\left[\hat{\mathbf{B}}_1\,\mathbf{D}\right] = \frac{1}{(1+\rho)^3}\begin{bmatrix} 1+\rho & 2\rho \\ 0 & 1+\rho \end{bmatrix}.$$

Then verify that C_{22} is correct [use (7.2.6)], and find similar expressions for the other two. Prove that the following inequalities hold.

$$C_{12} < C_{11} < C_{22} \quad \text{for } \rho < 1,$$

$$C_{12} < C_{22} < C_{11} \quad \text{for } 1 < \rho < \frac{1+\sqrt{17}}{2},$$

$$C_{22} < C_{12} < C_{11} \quad \text{for } \frac{1+\sqrt{17}}{2} < \rho.$$

Remember that $\rho = \bar{x}_1/\bar{x}_2$, which for C_{12} is not λ/μ.

Continuing with matrices in the product space,

$$\mathbf{S}^+ = \mu\begin{bmatrix} 1 & 0 & -1 & 0 \\ 0 & 1 & 0 & -1 \\ -\rho & \rho & 1+\rho & -\rho \\ 0 & -\rho & 0 & 1+\rho \end{bmatrix}, \quad \mathbf{S}^- = \mu\begin{bmatrix} \rho & -\rho & 0 & 0 \\ -1 & 1+\rho & 1 & -1 \\ 0 & 0 & \rho & -\rho \\ 0 & 0 & -1 & 1+\rho \end{bmatrix}.$$

The determinants of $S^{\pm}$ are μ^4 and λ^4, respectively, so these matrices are nonsingular. Their inverses are

$$\mathbf{T}^+ = \frac{1}{\mu}\begin{bmatrix} 1+\rho & -\rho & 1 & 0 \\ 0 & 1+\rho & 0 & 1 \\ \rho & -\rho & 1 & 0 \\ 0 & \rho & 0 & 1 \end{bmatrix}, \quad \mathbf{T}^- = \frac{1}{\mu\,\rho^2}\begin{bmatrix} 1+\rho & \rho & -1 & 0 \\ 1 & \rho & -1 & 0 \\ 0 & 0 & 1+\rho & \rho \\ 0 & 0 & 1 & \rho \end{bmatrix}.$$

The most important matrix, $\mathbf{U}$, is not so simple looking:

$$\mathbf{U} = \mathbf{T}^+\mathbf{S}^- = \begin{bmatrix} \rho(2+\rho) & -2\rho(1+\rho) & 0 & 0 \\ -(1+\rho) & (1+\rho)^2 & \rho & 0 \\ \rho(1+\rho) & -\rho(1+2\rho) & 0 & 0 \\ -\rho & \rho(1+\rho) & \rho-1 & 1 \end{bmatrix},$$

from which we can get

$$\Psi_2\left[\mathbf{U}\right] = \begin{bmatrix} \rho(2+\rho) & -2\rho(1+\rho) \\ -1 & (1+\rho)^2 \end{bmatrix}.$$

From either of these equations one can calculate $\Psi\left[\mathbf{U}\right] = \Psi\left[\Psi_2\left[\mathbf{U}\right]\right] = -\rho^2$. The characteristic equation for $\mathbf{U}$ is

$$\phi(\alpha) = |\mathbf{U} - \alpha\mathbf{I}| = (\alpha - 1)\left(\alpha - \rho^2\right)\left(\alpha^2 - [1 + 4\rho + \rho^2]\alpha + \rho^2\right).$$

Therefore, the eigenvalues of $\mathbf{U}$ are

$$\alpha_1 = 1, \qquad \alpha_2 = \rho^2, \qquad \alpha_3 = \frac{(\rho^2 + 4\rho + 1) + Z(1+\rho)}{2}$$

and

$$\alpha_4 = \frac{(\rho^2 + 4\rho + 1) - Z(1+\rho)}{2},$$

where $Z^2 = \rho^2 + 6\rho + 1$. Sadly, we see that one of the eigenvalues is 1. Therefore, $\mathbf{I} - \mathbf{U}$ has no inverse. We knew this would happen from Lemma 7.3.2 and the discussion following it. We said that there are at most $m_1 + m_2 - 1$ roots, which do not equal 1. In our case, $m_1 = m_2 = 2$, so there are at most three. In fact, there are exactly three if $\rho \neq 1$. The other difficulty we have is that α_3 is greater than 1 for all ρ. Therefore, some matrix elements of $\mathbf{U}^n$ must become unboundedly large as n increases. For what it is worth, the four eigenvalues satisfy the following inequality.

$$\alpha_4 < \alpha_2 < \alpha_1 = 1 < \alpha_3 \quad \text{for} \;\; \rho < 1$$

and

$$\alpha_4 < \alpha_1 = 1 < \alpha_2 < \alpha_3 \quad \text{for} \;\; \rho > 1.$$

The matrix $\mathbf{R}$, having a unit eigenvalue, can do no better. It presumably also has an eigenvalue greater than 1. We leave it as an exercise for the reader to analyze $\mathbf{R}$ in the way that we just analyzed $\mathbf{U}$.

Where do we go from here? Despite all these formulas, we cannot go to the open system. In Section 4.2.1 we successfully took the limit of $\mathbf{K}(N)$ as N went to infinity because $(\mathbf{I} - \mathbf{U})^{-1}$ existed. It does not here. In Section 5.1.1 we were able to take the limit because we were able to isolate a unique eigenvalue and its associated left and right eigenvectors. So far we have not been successful in finding an appropriate generalization of this. We know this much: Victor Wallace proved that all open QBD processes of a certain type (of which the ME/ME/1 queue is a special case) must have a matrix geometric solution [WALLACE69]. It is just that neither $\mathbf{U}$ nor $\mathbf{R}$ appears to be that matrix. But an isometric transformation of $\mathbf{U}$ or $\mathbf{R}$ in the product space may well yield the correct matrix. We do not go into detail here, but it should be possible to find a transformation that yields a matrix for which the eigenvectors belonging to the eigenvalue 1 drop out of the solution. The solution, whatever it turns out to be, almost surely will reflect the characteristics of both the M/ME/1 and ME/M/1 queues, given that the ME/ME/1 queue is the generalization of both. (See, however, [LATOUCHE-RAM99] for an iterative solution.) We have presented far more formulas than are necessary, in the hope that they will help some reader to discover how this can be done.

We close out the chapter with a short look at mean first-passage times for the queue at S_1 to drop. Extensions to other transient properties are left to the reader's ingenuity.

7.4 A Modicum of Transient Behavior

We do not go into too much detail of transient behavior for two nonexponential servers, not so much because it is so hard, but because it looks so much like what we already did in Section 4.5. All objects are in the product space, so should be wearing hats. To make things simple for us, we revert to the naive approach of Section 7.1. We only cover the first-passage processes to drop by 1, and thereby reproduce (4.5.29a) for this more general case. The reader should review Section 4.5 before continuing.

First recall Definition 4.5.7. The matrix $[\mathbf{H_d}(n;N)]_{\underline{kl}}$ is identical in meaning, except that now

$$\underline{l},\ \underline{k} \in \Xi = \Xi_1 \otimes \Xi_2.$$

As in Chapter 4, after a single event occurs, the queue at S_1 can grow by one, decrease by one, or stay the same. The difference now is that there are two ways that it can stay the same, either by a transition in S_1, $[\mathbf{P_1}]$, or a transition in S_2, $[\mathbf{P_2}]$. Thus $\mathbf{H_d}$ satisfies the following.

$$\begin{aligned}\mathbf{H_d}(n;N) &= [\mathbf{M_1}+\mathbf{M_2}]^{-1}[\mathbf{M_1}\,\mathbf{P_1}+\mathbf{M_2}\,\mathbf{P_2}]\,\mathbf{H_d}(n;N)\\ &\quad+[\mathbf{M_1}+\mathbf{M_2}]^{-1}\mathbf{M_1}\,\mathbf{q_1'}\,\mathbf{p_1}\\ &\quad+[\mathbf{M_1}+\mathbf{M_2}]^{-1}\,\mathbf{M_2}\,\mathbf{q_2'}\,\mathbf{p_2}\,\mathbf{H_d}(n+1;N)\,\mathbf{H_d}(n;N).\end{aligned}$$

The quantity

$$[(\mathbf{M_1}+\mathbf{M_2})^{-1}\,\mathbf{M_1}]_{\underline{kk}} = \frac{\mu_{k_1}}{\mu_{k_1}+\lambda_{k_2}}$$

is the probability that the next event, when it occurs, will be in S_1, given that the system is in state $\underline{k} = (k_1, k_2) \in \Xi$. Therefore, the first term $[\mathbf{P_1}]$ corresponds to an internal transition in S_1, with the eventual drop $[\mathbf{H_d}(n;N)]$ to $n-1$.

Similarly, the second term $[\mathbf{P_2}\,\mathbf{H_d}(n;N)]$ is an internal transition in S_2. The third term corresponds to a transition in S_1 that results in a departure $[\mathbf{q_1'}]$, followed immediately by the entry of the next customer $[\mathbf{p_1}]$ at S_1. In this process, nothing more need happen because S_1 now has $n-1$ customers. The last term corresponds to a departure from S_2, $[\mathbf{q_2'}]$, immediately followed by the entry of the next customer $[\mathbf{p_2}]$ and then the eventual drop from $n+1$ to n, $[\mathbf{H_d}(n+1;N)]$, followed eventually by a drop to $n-1$, $[\mathbf{H_d}(n;N)]$.

Recall the following, which we have seen so many times: $\mathbf{B_i} = \mathbf{M_i}\,(\mathbf{I}-\mathbf{P_i})$ and $\mathbf{M_i}\,\mathbf{q_i'} = \mathbf{B_i}\,\mathbf{Q_i}$, for $i = 1, 2$.† Then multiply both sides of the equation by $[\mathbf{M_1}+\mathbf{M_2}]$, regroup terms, and for $0 < n < N$, come up with

$$\mathbf{H_d}(n;N) = [\mathbf{B_1}+\mathbf{B_2}-\mathbf{B_2}\,\mathbf{Q_2}\,\mathbf{H_d}(n+1;N)]^{-1}\mathbf{B_1}\,\mathbf{Q_1}. \tag{7.4.1a}$$

We must still get an equation for $\mathbf{H_d}(N;N)$, because there is no way to go up. There is one other difficulty with this state. Because there is no customer

†Keep in mind that $\mathbf{I}$ is the identity matrix of the product space and that $\mathbf{M_1}$, $\mathbf{B_2}$, and so on, are already embedded (*hatted*) onto that space.

at S_2, $[\mathbf{H_d}(N;N)]_{\underline{i}\underline{l}}$ generates a transition from $i \in \Xi_1$ to $\underline{l} \in \Xi$, (i.e., it is not a square matrix). Thus

$$\mathbf{H_d}(N;N) = \mathbf{P_1}\,\mathbf{H_d}(N;N) + \mathbf{q}_1'\,\mathbf{p_1}\,\mathbf{p_2}$$

(the customer who leaves S_1 immediately enters S_2, $[\mathbf{p_2}]$, because there was no one there before his arrival), or

$$\mathbf{H_d}(N;N) = [\mathbf{I} - \mathbf{P_1}]^{-1}\mathbf{q}_1'\,\mathbf{p_1}\,\mathbf{p_2} = \mathbf{Q_1}\,\mathbf{p_2}, \tag{7.4.1b}$$

which folows from $[\mathbf{I} - \mathbf{P_1}]^{-1}\mathbf{q_1} = \boldsymbol{\epsilon}_1'$. Alternatively (as we have been doing all along), we can make believe that when S_2 is empty, it is in state $\mathbf{p_2}$, but cannot do anything. Then we must wipe out that state $[\boldsymbol{\epsilon}_2']$ before reentering it $[\mathbf{p_2}]$. This leads to the simpler formula,

$$\mathbf{H_d}(N;N) = \mathbf{Q_1}\,\mathbf{Q_2} = \mathbf{Q}. \tag{7.4.1c}$$

In either case, (7.4.1a) leads to

$$\mathbf{H_d}(N-1;N) = [\mathbf{B_1} + \mathbf{B_2} - \mathbf{B_2}\,\mathbf{Q}]^{-1}\mathbf{B_1}\,\mathbf{Q_1}.$$

Next we define $[\boldsymbol{\tau}_d'(n;N)]_{\underline{k}}$ in the way we did in Definition 4.5.8 where now $\underline{k} \in \Xi$. This means that the time for the queue at S_1 to drop by 1 depends on the internal state of S_2 as well as S_1. First, let all the customers be at S_1,

$$\boldsymbol{\tau}_d'(N;N) = \mathbf{M}_1^{-1}\boldsymbol{\epsilon}_1' + \mathbf{P_1}\boldsymbol{\tau}_d'(N;N),$$

leading to

$$\boldsymbol{\tau}_d'(N;N) = \mathbf{V_1}\,\boldsymbol{\epsilon}', \tag{7.4.2a}$$

which is identical to (4.5.11a), as it should be, given that S_2 plays no role in the process. For $n < N$,

$$\begin{aligned}\boldsymbol{\tau}_d'(n;N) = {} & (\mathbf{M_1} + \mathbf{M_2})^{-1}\boldsymbol{\epsilon}' \\ & + (\mathbf{M_1} + \mathbf{M_2})^{-1}(\mathbf{M_1}\mathbf{P_1} + \mathbf{M_2}\mathbf{P_2})\boldsymbol{\tau}_d'(n;N) \\ & + (\mathbf{M_1} + \mathbf{M_2})^{-1}\mathbf{M_2}\,\mathbf{q}_2'\,\mathbf{p_2}[\boldsymbol{\tau}_d'(n+1;N) \\ & + \mathbf{H_d}(n+1;N)\boldsymbol{\tau}_d'(n;N)],\end{aligned}$$

which regroups, and rearranges to

$$\boldsymbol{\tau}_d'(n;N)$$

$$= [\mathbf{B_1} + \mathbf{B_2} - \mathbf{B_2}\,\mathbf{Q_2}\,\mathbf{H_d}(n+1,N)]^{-1}[\boldsymbol{\epsilon}' + \mathbf{B_2}\,\mathbf{Q_2}\,\boldsymbol{\tau}_d'(n+1;N)] \tag{7.4.2b}$$

[compare with (4.5.11b)]. Equations (7.4.1) and (7.4.2) are sufficient for finding all times recursively, by following the discussion in Section 4.5.3.

Let us look in particular at the special case $N = 2$. We have discussed its significance in Section 4.5.4, but now we generalize to two nonexponential servers. First,

$$t_d(2;2) = \mathbf{p}\,\boldsymbol{\tau}_d'(2;2) = T_1 = \Psi\,[\mathbf{V_1}]$$

and

$$\tau'_d(1;2) = [\mathbf{B}_1 + \mathbf{B}_2 - \mathbf{B}_2\mathbf{Q}]^{-1}[\epsilon' + \mathbf{B}_2\,\mathbf{Q}_2\,\mathbf{V}_1\,\epsilon'].$$

Given that $\mathbf{V}_1$ commutes with $\mathbf{Q}_2$, $\mathbf{Q}_2\,\epsilon' = \epsilon'$, the expression in the second set of brackets becomes

$$[\mathbf{I} + \mathbf{B}_2\mathbf{V}_1]\epsilon' = [\mathbf{B}_1 + \mathbf{B}_2]\mathbf{V}_1\,\epsilon' = \mathbf{D}^{-1}\,\mathbf{V}_1\,\epsilon',$$

where we have used (7.3.4) as the definition for $\mathbf{D}$. Lemma 4.2.1 can be applied to the expression in the first set of brackets (not Lemma 7.2.4) because $\mathbf{Q}$ itself appears rather than $\mathbf{Q}_\mathbf{i}$. We get

$$[\mathbf{B}_1 + \mathbf{B}_2 - \mathbf{B}_2\mathbf{Q}]^{-1} = [\mathbf{D}^{-1}(\mathbf{I} - \mathbf{D}\mathbf{B}_2\mathbf{Q})]^{-1}$$

$$= [\mathbf{I} - \mathbf{D}\mathbf{B}_2\mathbf{Q}]^{-1}\mathbf{D} = \left(\mathbf{I} + \frac{1}{1 - \Psi\,[\mathbf{D}\mathbf{B}_2]}\mathbf{D}\mathbf{B}_2\mathbf{Q}\right)\mathbf{D}.$$

Therefore,

$$\tau'_d(1;2) = \left(\mathbf{I} + \frac{1}{1 - \Psi\,[\mathbf{D}\mathbf{B}_2]}\mathbf{D}\,\mathbf{B}_2\,\mathbf{Q}\right)\mathbf{D}\,\mathbf{D}^{-1}\,\mathbf{V}_1\,\epsilon'$$

$$= \mathbf{V}_1\,\epsilon' + \frac{T_1}{1 - \Psi\,[\mathbf{D}\,\mathbf{B}_2]}\mathbf{D}\,\mathbf{B}_2\,\epsilon'.$$

Finally,

$$t_d(1;2) = \mathbf{p}\,\tau'_d(1;2) = T_1 + \frac{T_1\Psi\,[\mathbf{D}\,\mathbf{B}_2]}{1 - \Psi\,[\mathbf{D}\,\mathbf{B}_2]} = \frac{T_1}{\Psi\,[\mathbf{D}\,\mathbf{B}_1]}$$

because $1 - \Psi\,[\mathbf{D}\,\mathbf{B}_2] = \Psi\left[\mathbf{I} - (\mathbf{B}_1 + \mathbf{B}_2)^{-1}\mathbf{B}_2\right] = \Psi\,[\mathbf{D}\,\mathbf{B}_1]$. Then, following Section 4.5.4,

$$MTTF(2) = t_d(2;2) + t_d(1;2) = T_1\left(1 + \frac{1}{\Psi\,[\mathbf{D}\mathbf{B}_1]}\right). \qquad (7.4.3)$$

This equation is identical to (4.5.29a) when one takes into account the slight difference of notation. In Chapter 4 we used $\mathbf{D} = (\mathbf{I} + \lambda\mathbf{V})^{-1}$, and because $\lambda \Rightarrow \mathbf{B}_2$ in this chapter, we have $\mathbf{D}$ (Chapter 4) $\Rightarrow \mathbf{B}_1\mathbf{D}$ (Chapter 7). We have already shown that $\Psi\,[\mathbf{D}\mathbf{B}_1] = C(0)$ [(7.1.3b)] is the probability that the customer in S_1 will finish before the customer in S_2, given that they started at the same time. In the context of MTTF, this is the probability that the second device will break before the first is fixed, and is true for any pair of distributions. See Section 4.5.4 for a more thorough discussion.

We hope that the reader will be able to solve for other transient properties using the material expounded upon in previous chapters. We have seen by this example that certain transient events can be computed more easily than can the steady-state solution for the same system, particularly if N is small. This should become a useful and practical tool.

Exercise 7.4.1: Take the results you got from Exercise 7.3.1 (C_{11}, C_{12}, and C_{22}), and use (7.4.3) to calculate MTTF as a function of ρ for all three systems. Assume that $T_1 = 1$ and let ρ take on the values, 0_+, 0.1, 0.5, 0.8, 1.0, 1.25, 2.0, 10.0, 100, and 1000.

Chapter 8

SEMI-MARKOV PROCESS

Prediction is difficult, particularly about the future.
Niels Bohr
(also attributed to Mark Twain,
but falsely attributed to Yogi Berra).

We can chart our future clearly and wisely only when we know the path which has led to the present.
Adlai Stevenson.

In many (if not most) real-world applications, the arrival of customers to a service center is not well described by renewal processses. Quite often, the times between successive arrivals are correlated, whereas renewal processes have independent interarrival times. A natural generalization is the class of ***semi-Markov processes*** (SMP), which when specifically applied to the arrival of customers are called ***Markov Renewal Processes*** (MRP) or ***Markov Arrival Processes*** (MAP). Of course arrivals to one station correspond to departures from some other station. So, to avoid confusion, we use the terms SMP or MRP here.

In this chapter we set up a general procedure for creating a sequence of random variables $\{X_i\}$ which may be thought of as the interarrival times of successive customers for some arrival process. The $\{X_i\}$ has PDFs $\{F_i(x_i)\}$ which are generated by a sequence of representations with the same $\mathcal{B}$ but different entrance vectors, namely $\{\langle\, \wp_{\mathbf{i}}\, , \mathcal{B}\, \rangle\}$. Interval i we call the $\boldsymbol{i}$*thepoch*. Recall that for a renewal process the X_i r.v.s are iid. In this chapter they are not independent, but they are asymptotically identically distributed. That is, for i large enough, $\{F_i(x_i)\}$ approaches a limit. Hence, some researchers retain the word, renewal in describing M**R**Ps.

The set of formulas for the joint interdeparture distributions and correlation lag-k number are then set up, thereby showing that, indeed, the X_i and X_j are in most cases, correlated. We then show how they can be used to solve for various performance properties of SMP/M/1 queues. One of the first papers to try to formalize this was by Ramaswami [RAMASWAMI80]. The particular formulation presented here stems from the PhD thesis by Pierre Fiorini [FIORINI98] and other works [FIORINILIPVDLHSIN95].

L. Lipsky, *Queueing Theory*, DOI 10.1007/978-0-387-49706-8_8,

8.1 Introduction

Because the formulas presented here are abstract, it may be unclear how they are to be applied to specific systems. Therefore, after presenting the general formalism, we supply explicit formulas for a wide variety of processes, each having a different state-space structure from the others. The following processes are considered.

(1) Departures from a general server that has an infinite queue (renewal process);

(2) Markov regulated departure processes (direct-sum space);

(3) Markov Modulated Poisson processes (MMPP);

(4) *ON-OFF* Models, or the *N-BURST* Process;

(5) Merging of two renewal streams (direct-product space);

(6) Departures from overloaded generalized X/G/C queues (reduced-product space);

(7) Departures from open G/G/1 queues (infinite direct-product space) with reduction to G/M/1 and M/G/1 queues.

The method can be applied to closed (finite number of customers) systems as easily as, or more easily than, to open ones.

Finally, we show (yet again) that departures from an open M/M/1 queue approach Poisson as the system approaches its steady state. The formulas make it very clear that this is a special property that does not carry over to other arrival or service distributions or to closed systems.

8.1.1 Matrix Representations of Subsystems

The equations of the previous chapters can be extended to any Markov-like subsystem with a countable state space. Let $\wp_o$ be the probability vector of the state of the subsystem at the time $x = 0$ with $\wp_o \boldsymbol{\varepsilon}' = 1$ ($\boldsymbol{\varepsilon}'$ is the subsystem vector equivalent to $\boldsymbol{\epsilon}'$), and $\boldsymbol{\mathcal{B}}$ is the infinitesimal generator matrix of the process. Then, as in (3.1.7d), $\wp_o \exp(-x\boldsymbol{\mathcal{B}})\boldsymbol{\varepsilon}'$ has the interpretation of the probability that the process has not ended by time x. Furthermore, the ith component of the vector $\wp_o \exp(-x\boldsymbol{\mathcal{B}})$ has the following meaning.

Given that the subsystem was in vector state $\wp_o$ *at time* $x = 0$, $[\wp_o \exp(-x\boldsymbol{\mathcal{B}})]_i$ *is the probability that the process has not yet completed by time* x*, and the subsystem is in state* i.

Usually, $\boldsymbol{\mathcal{B}}$ can be constructed from the underlying Markov chain using the relation

$$\boldsymbol{\mathcal{B}} = \boldsymbol{\mathcal{M}}(\boldsymbol{\mathcal{I}} - \boldsymbol{\mathcal{P}}), \tag{8.1.1}$$

where $\boldsymbol{\mathcal{M}}$ is a diagonal matrix whose (ii)th component is the probability rate of leaving state i, and $\boldsymbol{\mathcal{P}}$ is a ***substochastic matrix*** whose ij^{th} component is the probability that the subsystem will transfer to state j after leaving state i. At least one of the row sums of $\boldsymbol{\mathcal{P}}$ (i.e., $\boldsymbol{\mathcal{P}\mathcal{E}'}$) is strictly less than 1. Thus, there exist state sequences that result in a departure from the subsystem (often visualized as passage to an ***absorbing state***). The requirement that $[\boldsymbol{\mathcal{I}} - \boldsymbol{\mathcal{P}}]$ be invertible is equivalent to there being an exit path from every state.

As we show in the next section, the following theorem about functions of matrices lets us easily calculate many integrals that are otherwise very difficult.

Theorem 8.1.1: Let $\boldsymbol{\mathcal{B}}$ be an invertible finite matrix with $\boldsymbol{\mathcal{V}} = \boldsymbol{\mathcal{B}}^{-1}$ and eigenvalues $\beta_1, \beta_2, \ldots, \beta_m$. Furthermore, let $\Re(\beta_i) > 0$ for all i. Then

$$\int_0^\infty x^n \exp(-x\boldsymbol{\mathcal{B}})\boldsymbol{\mathcal{B}}\, dx = n!\, \boldsymbol{\mathcal{V}}^n. \tag{8.1.2a}$$

(Compare with Theorem 3.1.1.) It is also true that:

$$\int_0^\infty e^{-sx} \exp(-x\boldsymbol{\mathcal{B}})\boldsymbol{\mathcal{B}}\, dx = \int_0^\infty \exp[-x(s\boldsymbol{\mathcal{I}} + \boldsymbol{\mathcal{B}})]\boldsymbol{\mathcal{B}}\, dx$$

$$= [s\boldsymbol{\mathcal{I}} + \boldsymbol{\mathcal{B}}]^{-1}\boldsymbol{\mathcal{B}} = [\boldsymbol{\mathcal{I}} + s\boldsymbol{\mathcal{V}}]^{-1}. \tag{8.1.2b}$$

(Again compare with Theorem 3.1.1.) ■

We remind the reader that although the integration is over a scalar $[x]$, both sides of these equations are square matrices. With appropriate constraints, this theorem is valid even if $\boldsymbol{\mathcal{B}}$ is infinite-dimensional.

8.2 Markov Renewal Processes

In this section we consider the end of a process to coincide with the departure of a customer from a subsystem. As in previous chapters we refer to the periods between departures as ***epochs***. The formulas given in the previous section, with generator $\langle\, \wp_o\,, \boldsymbol{\mathcal{B}}\, \rangle$, yield the distribution of the departure time of the first customer. We need the following material to describe the departure of the second, and succeeding, customers.

8.2.1 Interdeparture Time Distributions

Let $\{\, X_n |\, n \geq 1\}$ be a set of random variables where X_n denotes the time for the nth epoch, or interdeparture time of the nth customer. Consider the following matrix.

Definition 8.2.1

$[\boldsymbol{\mathcal{L}}]$: Given that the subsystem is in state i $[\boldsymbol{\mathcal{L}}]_{ij}\Delta$ is the probability that a departure will occur within the small time interval, Δ, and the subsystem will be in state j immediately afterwards. In other words, $[\boldsymbol{\mathcal{L}}]_{ij}$ is the subsystem instantaneous departure rate from state i that leaves behind state j. □

From this definition, it follows that $\sum_j \mathcal{L}_{ij} = [\mathcal{L}\varepsilon']_i$ is the subsystem instantaneous departure rate from state i. But that is what $[\mathcal{B}\varepsilon']_i$ is. Therefore

$$\mathcal{L}\varepsilon' = \mathcal{B}\varepsilon'. \tag{8.2.1}$$

Although $\mathcal{L}$ and $\mathcal{B}$ are related by this relation, they describe different parts of the process of interest. $\mathcal{B}$ generates what happens during the epoch, and $\mathcal{L}$ tells what happens immediately after the departure. (8.2.1) states that they agree about the rate of departure.

Given that $\mathcal{V} := \mathcal{B}^{-1}$, we have

$$\mathcal{V}\mathcal{L}\varepsilon' = \varepsilon'.$$

Because of its importance, we define

$$\mathcal{Y} := \mathcal{V}\mathcal{L}, \quad \text{with the property } \mathcal{Y}\varepsilon' = \varepsilon' \tag{8.2.2}$$

(i.e., $\mathcal{Y}$ is *isometric*;ε' is a right eigenvector of $\mathcal{Y}$ with eigenvalue 1).

We can now observe that the jth component of the vector, $[\wp_o \exp(-x\mathcal{B})\,\mathcal{L}]$ is the instantaneous probability rate for service to end at time x, and for the subsystem to be in state j immediately after the departure. The sum over all post-departure states must yield the pdf for the process, and indeed it does. After all, from (8.2.1),

$$f_{X_1}(x) := \wp_o\,[\exp(-x\mathcal{B})\,\mathcal{L}]\varepsilon' = \wp_o\,[\exp(-x\mathcal{B})\,\mathcal{B}]\varepsilon' \tag{8.2.3}$$

(compare with Theorem 3.1.1.) Note that although $f_{X_1}(x)$ is a scalar function of x, the objects in square brackets are square matrices.

The initial state for the second customer, given that $X_1 = x$, is

$$\wp_1(x) = \frac{1}{f_{X_1}(x)}\wp_o \exp(-x\mathcal{B})\,\mathcal{L}. \tag{8.2.4}$$

The initial state for the second customer, averaged over all first-process times is given by

$$\begin{aligned}\wp_1 &= \int_o^\infty f_{X_1}(x)\,\wp_1(x)\,dx = \int_o^\infty \wp_o \exp(-x\mathcal{B})\,\mathcal{L}\,dx \\ &= \wp_o\left[\int_o^\infty \exp(-x\mathcal{B})\,dx\right]\mathcal{L} = \wp_o\,\mathcal{V}\mathcal{L} = \wp_o\,\mathcal{Y},\end{aligned} \tag{8.2.5}$$

where (8.1.2a) for $n = 0$ was used. One can immediately generalize that the probability state of the system immediately after the nth departure (and the starting vector for the $(n+1)$st epoch) is

$$\wp_n = \wp_{n-1}\,\mathcal{Y} = \wp_o\,\mathcal{Y}^n. \tag{8.2.6}$$

Observe that the state the subsystem is in immediately after customer number (n-1) departs is the beginning state of the subsystem for generating the nth departure. We can then say that the (unconditional) distribution function for X_n is generated by $\langle \wp_{n-1}, \boldsymbol{\mathcal{B}} \rangle$.

The steady-state start-up vector must satisfy the equation

$$\wp := \lim_{n\to\infty} \wp_n = \lim_{n\to\infty} \wp_o \boldsymbol{\mathcal{Y}}^n = (\lim_{n\to\infty} \wp_{n-1})\boldsymbol{\mathcal{Y}} = \wp\boldsymbol{\mathcal{Y}}; \tag{8.2.7}$$

that is, $\wp$ must be a left eigenvector of $\boldsymbol{\mathcal{Y}}$ with eigenvalue 1. That such a vector exists is guaranteed by the fact that $\boldsymbol{\mathcal{Y}}$ is isometric ($\boldsymbol{\mathcal{Y}}\boldsymbol{\varepsilon}' = \boldsymbol{\varepsilon}'$). More precisely, this limit exists if 1 is the largest eigenvalue in magnitude of $\boldsymbol{\mathcal{Y}}$. In this case, $\boldsymbol{\mathcal{Y}}^n \to \boldsymbol{\varepsilon}'\wp$. Then, as n approaches infinity, the X_n's approach the common distribution generated by $\langle \wp, \boldsymbol{\mathcal{B}} \rangle$. But they are almost always correlated, as shown in the next subsection.

Although $\boldsymbol{\mathcal{L}}$ and $\boldsymbol{\mathcal{B}}$ describe the same departure rate, their difference is also a useful matrix. Define the ***generator of the underlying Markov process*** as

$$\boldsymbol{\mathcal{Q}} := \boldsymbol{\mathcal{B}} - \boldsymbol{\mathcal{L}}. \tag{8.2.8a}$$

Clearly, $\boldsymbol{\mathcal{Q}}\boldsymbol{\varepsilon}' = 0$ from (8.2.1), so there must exist a vector $\boldsymbol{\pi}$ such that $\boldsymbol{\pi}\boldsymbol{\mathcal{Q}} = \mathrm{o}'$ and $\boldsymbol{\pi}\,\boldsymbol{\varepsilon}' = 1$. In fact it can be shown by direct substitution that

$$\boldsymbol{\pi} = \frac{\wp\boldsymbol{\mathcal{V}}}{\wp\boldsymbol{\mathcal{V}}\boldsymbol{\varepsilon}'}. \tag{8.2.8b}$$

If we multiply $\boldsymbol{\pi}$ by either $\boldsymbol{\mathcal{L}}$ or $\boldsymbol{\mathcal{B}}$, we can get $\wp$ in terms of $\boldsymbol{\pi}$, that is,

$$(\wp\boldsymbol{\mathcal{V}}\boldsymbol{\varepsilon}')\boldsymbol{\pi}\boldsymbol{\mathcal{L}} = \wp\boldsymbol{\mathcal{V}}\boldsymbol{\mathcal{L}} = \wp\boldsymbol{\mathcal{Y}} = \wp$$

and given that $\wp\boldsymbol{\varepsilon}' = 1$, we have

$$(\wp\boldsymbol{\mathcal{V}}\boldsymbol{\varepsilon}')(\boldsymbol{\pi}\boldsymbol{\mathcal{L}}\boldsymbol{\varepsilon}') = 1. \tag{8.2.8c}$$

This provides us with an interesting relation. $(\wp\boldsymbol{\mathcal{V}}\boldsymbol{\varepsilon}')$ is the mean interdeparture time, and thus its reciprocal $(\boldsymbol{\pi}\boldsymbol{\mathcal{L}}\boldsymbol{\varepsilon}')$, must be the long-term departure rate. This makes sense, because $(\boldsymbol{\pi})_i$ is the fraction of time the generating system is in state i, and $(\boldsymbol{\mathcal{L}}\boldsymbol{\varepsilon}')_i$ is the rate of departure when the system is in state i. Their dot product averages over all states. For emphasis, we restate this now:

$$\begin{aligned} \mathbf{E}[X] &= \wp\boldsymbol{\mathcal{V}}\boldsymbol{\varepsilon}' = \text{mean interdeparture time}, \\ \kappa &:= \boldsymbol{\pi}\boldsymbol{\mathcal{L}}\boldsymbol{\varepsilon}' = \text{long} - \text{term departure rate}. \end{aligned} \tag{8.2.8d}$$

In (8.2.8b) we expressed $\boldsymbol{\pi}$ in terms of $\wp$. We now reverse the relation and express $\wp$ in terms of $\boldsymbol{\pi}$. The equations above and the fact that $\boldsymbol{\pi}\boldsymbol{\mathcal{B}} = \boldsymbol{\pi}\boldsymbol{\mathcal{L}}$ lead to

$$\wp = (\wp\boldsymbol{\mathcal{V}}\boldsymbol{\varepsilon}')\boldsymbol{\pi}\boldsymbol{\mathcal{L}} = \frac{\boldsymbol{\pi}\boldsymbol{\mathcal{L}}}{\boldsymbol{\pi}\boldsymbol{\mathcal{L}}\boldsymbol{\varepsilon}'} = \frac{\boldsymbol{\pi}\boldsymbol{\mathcal{B}}}{\boldsymbol{\pi}\boldsymbol{\mathcal{B}}\boldsymbol{\varepsilon}'}. \tag{8.2.8e}$$

The three matrices, $\boldsymbol{\mathcal{Q}}$, $\boldsymbol{\mathcal{L}}$, and $\boldsymbol{\mathcal{B}}$, play equally important roles in SM processes, and given any two, the third follows directly. Depending on the application it may be easier to construct $\mathcal{Q}$ than one of the other two. We note that $\mathcal{B}$ always has an inverse (namely, $\mathcal{V}$), $\mathcal{Q}$ never has an inverse ($\mathcal{Q}\varepsilon' = \mathrm{o}'$ implies that $\mathcal{Q}$ has a 0 eigenvalue), and $\mathcal{L}$ may or may not have an inverse (but we wouldn't know what to do with it anyway).

As mentioned earlier, $\mathcal{B}$ controls the subsystem during an epoch and $\mathcal{L}$ connects each epoch to the next. We show in some of the applications below that $\mathcal{Q}$ controls the subsystem irrespective of departures. This is a direct generalization of the discussion surrounding Figure 3.5.3, leading to $\boldsymbol{\pi}_r$ the mean residual vector. $\mathcal{Q}$ can also be thought of as thc ***rate matrix***, or *generator of a continuous Markov chain* as given in the discussion surrounding (1.3.2c) in Chapter 1. So if $\wp$ describes the state of the subsystem at the beginning of an arbitrary epoch, then $\boldsymbol{\pi}$ describes the state of the system as seen by a random observer who has no idea when the epoch began. This is discussed further in Section 8.3.1.

Before going on, we describe how our approach differs from that of other researchers. The matrix distribution function $Q_{ij}(x)$, as defined in many books (e.g.,[COOPER81]), in our case denotes the probability that "a departure will occur by time x and the system will find itself in state j, given that the system was in state i at time $x = 0$." We, on the other hand, use the matrix density function, $\exp(-x\mathcal{B})\mathcal{L}$, which when integrated from $0 \to x$ yields $[\mathbf{I} - \exp(-x\mathcal{B})]\mathcal{Y}$, the equivalent to $Q_{ij}(x)$, except that, like [NEUTS81], the matrix elements themselves can be matrices. Also, our $\mathcal{Y}$ corresponds to their $P_{ij} := \lim_{x\to\infty} Q_{ij}(x)$. For the applications given here, because of Theorem 8.1.1, the actual values of the components of $\exp(-x\mathcal{B})$ are not usually needed to get useful results.

8.2.2 Correlation of Departures

Based on the material of the previous section, we can write down the joint probability distributions for the interdeparture times. The joint density function for the departure of the first $n + k$ customers is given by

$$f_{X_1\,X_2\cdots X_n\ldots X_{n+k}}(x_1,\, x_2, \ldots,\, x_n, \cdots,\, x_{n+k})$$
$$= \wp_{\mathrm{o}}[\exp(-x_1\mathcal{B})\mathcal{L} \cdots \exp(-x_n\mathcal{B})\mathcal{L} \cdots \exp(-x_{n+k}\mathcal{B})\mathcal{L}]\varepsilon'. \qquad (8.2.9)$$

The joint distribution has the appearance of being separable, but the separate epochs are connected by $\mathcal{L}$. Only if $\mathcal{L}$ is of rank 1 (i.e., only if $\mathcal{L} = \mathcal{B}\varepsilon'\wp$), are the interdeparure times independent of each other. For instance, let us examine the relation between two variables, say X_n and X_{n+k}. To do this, we integrate over all the other variables, and for convenience replace x_n with x and x_{n+k} with t. Then the joint density function for X_n and X_{n+k} is

$$f_{nk}(x,\, t) := \wp_{\mathrm{o}}\,[\mathcal{Y}^{n-1}\exp(-x\mathcal{B})\mathcal{L}\,\mathcal{Y}^{k-1}\exp(-t\mathcal{B})\mathcal{L}]\varepsilon'. \qquad (8.2.10a)$$

We can prove the following from this.

Theorem 8.2.1: Let X_n and X_{n+k} $(n,\, k > 0)$ be random variables denoting the nth and $(n + k)$th interdeparture times. Then X_n and

X_{n+k} are ***independent variables*** if and only if $\mathcal{L}$ is of rank 1, or equivalently, $\mathcal{Y} = \varepsilon' \wp$. By *independent* we mean:

$$f_{nk}(x, t) = f_n(x)\, f_{n+k}(t).$$

Furthermore, except perhaps, for $n = 1$, they are identically distributed, and $\{X_n\}$ is a renewal process. ■

Proof: By definition, $\mathcal{L} = \mathcal{B}\mathcal{Y}$ and if $\mathcal{L}$ is of rank 1, then $\mathcal{Y}$ must also be of rank 1. Therefore, $\mathcal{Y} = \varepsilon' \wp$. Assume this is so, then $\mathcal{Y}^n = \varepsilon' \wp$ and from (8.2.10a),

$$f_{nk}(x, t) = \wp_{\text{o}} [\varepsilon' \wp \exp(-x\mathcal{B})\, \mathcal{B}\varepsilon' \wp \exp(-t\mathcal{B})\mathcal{L}]\varepsilon'$$

$$= [\wp \exp(-x\mathcal{B})\, \mathcal{B}\varepsilon'] \, [\wp \exp(-t\mathcal{B})\mathcal{B}\varepsilon'] = f(x)\, f(t),$$

where we have used the properties: $\mathcal{L}\varepsilon' = \mathcal{B}\varepsilon'$ and $\wp_{\text{o}}\, \varepsilon' = 1$.

The converse is more complicated, but note that (8.2.10a) can be written as

$$f_{nk}(x, t) = \mathbf{a_n}(x) \cdot \mathbf{b'_k}(t),$$

where the $\mathbf{a_n}$ and $\mathbf{b'_k}$ are vector functions of x and t, respectively, namely:

$$\mathbf{a_n}(x) = \wp_{\text{o}} [\mathcal{Y}^{n-1} \exp(-x\mathcal{B})\mathcal{L}]$$

and

$$\mathbf{b'_k}(t) = [\mathcal{Y}^{k-1} \exp(-t\mathcal{B})\mathcal{L}]\varepsilon'.$$

f_{nk} is a function of the form: $a_1(x)b_1(t) + a_2(x)b_2(t) + \cdots$. The only way this can be separated into a single function of x times a single function of t is if the $a_i(x)$s are proportional to each other. Similarly for the $b_i(t)$s. This means that $\mathbf{a_n}(x)$ equals a scalar function of x times a constant vector, which in turn forces $\mathcal{L}$ to be of the form $\mathbf{b'} \cdot \mathbf{a}$, that is, a matrix of rank 1. It must follow that $\mathcal{L} = \mathcal{B}\varepsilon' \wp$. **QED**

We now move on to get expressions for covariance and autocorrelation coefficients. From its definition, again using (8.1.2a), we can evaluate the mean time for the nth epoch:

$$\mathbb{E}[X_n] = \int_{\text{o}}^{\infty} \int_{\text{o}}^{\infty} x\, f_{nk}(x, t)\, dx\, dt = \wp_{\text{o}} [\mathcal{Y}^{n-1} \mathcal{V}^2 \mathcal{L}\mathcal{Y}^{k-1} \mathcal{V}\mathcal{L}]\varepsilon'$$

$$= \wp_{\text{o}} [\mathcal{Y}^{n-1} \mathcal{V}\mathcal{Y}^{k+1}]\varepsilon' = \wp_{\text{o}} [\mathcal{Y}^{n-1} \mathcal{V}]\varepsilon' = \wp_{\mathbf{n-1}}[\mathcal{V}]\varepsilon', \tag{8.2.10b}$$

because $\mathcal{V}\mathcal{L} = \mathcal{Y}$ and $\mathcal{Y}\varepsilon' = \varepsilon'$. Similarly,

$$\mathbb{E}[X_{n+k}] = \wp_{\text{o}} [\mathcal{Y}^{n-1} \mathcal{V}\mathcal{L}\mathcal{Y}^{k-1} \mathcal{V}^2\mathcal{L}]\varepsilon'$$

$$= \wp_{\text{o}} [\mathcal{Y}^{n+k-1} \mathcal{V}]\varepsilon' = \wp_{\mathbf{n+k-1}}[\mathcal{V}]\varepsilon'. \tag{8.2.10c}$$

We see that the mean time for successive epochs is not constant. But, for n very large [because of (8.2.7)],

$$\lim_{n\to\infty} \mathbb{E}[X_n] = \lim_{n\to\infty} \mathbb{E}[X_{n+k}] = \wp\,[\mathcal{V}\,]\boldsymbol{\varepsilon}'. \tag{8.2.10d}$$

The covariance of two random variables is given by

$$\mathrm{Cov}(X, Y) := \mathbb{E}[(X - \mathbb{E}[X])\,(Y - \mathbb{E}[Y])] = \mathbb{E}[X\,Y] - \mathbb{E}[X]\,\mathbb{E}[Y]. \tag{8.2.11a}$$

The normalized ***correlation coefficient*** is defined by:

$$\varrho(X, Y) := \frac{\mathrm{Cov}(X, Y)}{\sqrt{\sigma_X^2\,\sigma_Y^2}} \tag{8.2.11b}$$

satisfies the inequality, $-1 \le \varrho(X, Y) \le 1$.

If X and Y are two members of a sequence, as is the case here, then $\mathrm{Cov}(X_n, X_{n+k})$ is called the ***autocovariance n lag-k*** of the interdeparture times, and ϱ is called the ***autocorrelation coefficient n lag-k***. The first term on the right of (8.2.11a) evaluates to

$$\mathbb{E}[X_n\,X_{n+k}] = \int_o^\infty \int_o^\infty x\,t\,f_{nk}(x, t)\,dx\,dt = \wp_o\,[\mathcal{Y}^{n-1}\,\mathcal{V}\,\mathcal{Y}^k\,\mathcal{V}\,]\boldsymbol{\varepsilon}', \tag{8.2.11c}$$

giving

$$\mathrm{Cov}(X_n, X_{n+k}) = \wp_{n-1}\mathcal{V}\,\mathcal{Y}^k\,\mathcal{V}\,\boldsymbol{\varepsilon}' - (\wp_{n-1}\mathcal{V}\boldsymbol{\varepsilon}')(\wp_{n+k-1}\mathcal{V}\boldsymbol{\varepsilon}'). \tag{8.2.11d}$$

It is virtually impossible to measure these parameters. Instead, one must average over n, which is the same as using $\wp$ as the initial vector ($\wp_o \to \wp$), making the covariance independent of n (but not of k). That is, when the subsystem is already in its steady state (or averaged over very large n), (8.2.11c) can be written as

$$\mathbb{E}(X, X_{+k}) := \lim_{n\to\infty} \mathbb{E}(X_n, X_{n+k}) = \wp\,\left[\mathcal{V}[\mathcal{Y}^k]\mathcal{V}\right]\boldsymbol{\varepsilon}'$$

$$= [\wp\mathcal{V}]\,\mathcal{Y}^k\,[\mathcal{V}\boldsymbol{\varepsilon}'], \tag{8.2.12a}$$

leading to the ***autocovariance lag-k***:

$$\mathrm{Cov}(X, X_{+k}) = [\wp\mathcal{V}]\,\mathcal{Y}^k\,[\mathcal{V}\boldsymbol{\varepsilon}'] - (\wp\mathcal{V}\boldsymbol{\varepsilon}')(\wp\mathcal{V}\boldsymbol{\varepsilon}'). \tag{8.2.12b}$$

Thus (8.2.11b) becomes the ***autocorrelation coefficient lag-k*** :

$$\hat{r}(k) := \lim_{n\to\infty} \varrho(X_n, X_{n+k}) = \frac{\wp\,\left[\mathcal{V}[\mathcal{Y}^k - \boldsymbol{\varepsilon}'\,\wp]\mathcal{V}\right]\boldsymbol{\varepsilon}'}{2\wp\mathcal{V}^2\boldsymbol{\varepsilon}' - (\wp\mathcal{V}\boldsymbol{\varepsilon}')^2}. \tag{8.2.12c}$$

In this form, the following theorem is clearly valid.

Theorem 8.2.2: If 1 is larger in magnitude than all other eigenvalues of $\mathcal{Y}$, then

$$\lim_{k\to\infty} \mathcal{Y}^k = \varepsilon' \wp$$

and

$$\lim_{k\to\infty} \mathrm{Cov}(X,\, X_{+k}) = \lim_{k\to\infty} \hat{r}(k) = 0.$$

On the other hand, if $\mathcal{Y}$ has at least one other eigenvalue of magnitude 1 (e.g., the subsystem is periodic), then the above limits are not valid. (See Example 8.3.1 below for such a case.) But even if all other eigenvalues are less than 1 in magnitude, it is possible for the ***autocorrelation lag-k*** numbers to be significant for arbitrarily large k. This will not happen for a finite state-space, but with one caveat. The rate at which $\hat{r}(k)$ goes to 0 depends on the difference between 1 and the next largest eigenvalue. Therefore, for some systems, k may have to be very large indeed before the covariance can be considered to be negligible. If the state-space is infinite, and 1 is an accumulation point for the set of eigenvalues (there are an infinite number of eigenvalues arbitrarily close to 1), then one must worry about this point. An important instance of this occurs in telecommunications traffic, where ***long-range dependence*** or ***self-similar traffic*** is regularly observed. We present an example of this below, where PT functions are involved. ■

Equations (8.2.12b) and (8.2.12c) can be computed as given, if k is small enough. But as k increases it can become numerically unstable. However, it can be evaluated by replacing $\mathcal{Y}$ with its spectral decomposition over its eigenvalues and eigenvectors. Let $\mathbf{u}_i$ and $\mathbf{v}_i'$ be the left and right eigenvectors of $\mathcal{Y}$ with eigenvalue λ_i such that $\mathbf{u}_i\, \mathbf{v}_i' = 1$ (remember that $\wp$ and ε' are the left and right eigenvectors with eigenvalue 1). Then

$$\mathcal{Y} = \varepsilon' \wp + \sum_{i*} \lambda_i\, \mathbf{v}_i'\, \mathbf{u}_i,$$

where the $*$ denotes a sum over all terms excluding eigenvalue 1. Given that $\mathbf{u_i}\, \mathbf{v_j}' = \delta_{ij}$, it follows that

$$\mathcal{Y}^k = \varepsilon' \wp + \sum_{i*} \lambda_i^k\, \mathbf{v}_i'\, \mathbf{u}_i.$$

Although this is stable, it requires knowing all the eigenvectors and eigenvalues. However, it can also be written in a form where only $\wp$ has to be known. Let

$$\bar{\mathcal{Y}} := \mathcal{Y} - \varepsilon' \wp,$$

where $\bar{\mathcal{Y}}$ has no unit eigenvalues and $\bar{\mathcal{Y}}\varepsilon' = \mathbf{o}'$. Then

$$\mathcal{Y}^k - \varepsilon' \wp = \bar{\mathcal{Y}}^k := (\mathcal{Y} - \varepsilon' \wp)^k$$

and (8.2.12a) can be written as

$$\mathrm{Cov}(X,\, X_{+k}) = \wp \left[\mathcal{V} \bar{\mathcal{Y}}^k \mathcal{V}\right] \varepsilon'. \tag{8.2.13a}$$

Either of these two formulas can be used to evaluate $\mathrm{Cov}(X,\, X_{+k})$.

An interesting parameter sometimes evaluated in studying correlations is their sum over all k. This cannot be done directly, because $\sum_k \mathcal{Y}^k$ diverges. But when either of the two formulas above is put into (8.2.12a), one gets

$$\sum_{k=1}^{\infty} \mathrm{Cov}(X,\, X_{+k}) = \sum_{i^*} \frac{\lambda_i}{1-\lambda_i} [\wp \mathcal{V}\, \mathbf{v}_i'] \, [\mathbf{u}_i \, \mathcal{V} \boldsymbol{\varepsilon}']$$

$$= \wp \mathcal{V} \bar{\mathcal{Y}} [\mathcal{I} - \bar{\mathcal{Y}}]^{-1} \mathcal{V} \boldsymbol{\varepsilon}'. \tag{8.2.13b}$$

We should mention that the sum over k converges only if $|\lambda_i| < 1$, for all i^*.

8.2.3 Laplace Transforms

The formulas from the previous section allow us to find an expression for the Laplace transform of the convolution of two (correlated) variables. Let $T = X_n + X_{n+k}$, then, using (8.2.10a) the pdf, $f_T(t)$, is given by the convolution formula

$$f_T(t) = \int_{\mathrm{o}}^{t} f_{nk}(x, t-x)\, dx.$$

Even for renewal processes this is not very easy to do [see Equations (3.5.2)]. However, The Laplace transform can be evaluated in a fashion identical to that used to get (8.2.11c), giving:

$$F_T^*(s) := \int_{\mathrm{o}}^{\infty} e^{-st} f_T(t)\, dt$$

$$= \wp_{\mathrm{o}} \left[\mathcal{Y}^{n-1} [\mathcal{I} + s\mathcal{V}]^{-1} \mathcal{Y}^k [\mathcal{I} + s\mathcal{V}]^{-1} \right] \boldsymbol{\varepsilon}'. \tag{8.2.14}$$

Because of the term $\mathcal{Y}^k$, it is clear that the Laplace transform of the distribution of the sum of two random variables is not usually the product of their transforms if they are correlated. Only when k becomes large enough does $\mathcal{Y}^k \approx \boldsymbol{\varepsilon}' \wp$, yielding:

$$\lim_{k\to\infty} F_T^*(s) = \wp_{\mathrm{n}} \left[[\mathcal{I} + s\mathcal{V}]^{-1} \right] \boldsymbol{\varepsilon}' \, \wp \left[[\mathcal{I} + s\mathcal{V}]^{-1} \right] \boldsymbol{\varepsilon}' = F_{X_n}^*(s)\, F_X^*(s).$$

8.3 Some Examples

To clarify how the equations discussed in the previous sections can be applied to specific systems, we now present several examples of Markov renewal processes, each with a different matrix structure. We start with the simplest case, a renewal process.

8.3.1 Departures from Overloaded Server: Renewal Process

As in Chapter 3, consider a server S that can be represented by the ME pair $\langle\, \mathbf{p}\,, \mathbf{B}\,\rangle$. Furthermore, imagine that there is an infinite queue of customers waiting to use S. Then the state-space of the departure process is the same as the set of phases making up the matrix representation. (This is equivalent to Neuts' infinitesimal generator of PH-renewal processes and forms the substratum of his N-process [RAMASWAMI80]). It follows that

$$\boldsymbol{\mathcal{B}} = \mathbf{B}. \tag{8.3.1a}$$

The $\boldsymbol{\mathcal{L}}$ matrix can be derived as follows. $[\mathbf{B}\boldsymbol{\epsilon}']_i$ is the probability rate of leaving S from phase i, and $[\mathbf{p}]_j$ is the probability that the next customer will start in phase j. Therefore from its definition, we have

$$\boldsymbol{\mathcal{L}} = \mathbf{B}\boldsymbol{\epsilon}'\,\mathbf{p} = \mathbf{B}\mathbf{Q}, \tag{8.3.1b}$$

where $\mathbf{Q} = \boldsymbol{\epsilon}'\,\mathbf{p}$, with properties given by Lemma 3.5.1. Next,

$$\boldsymbol{\mathcal{Y}} = \mathbf{V}\mathbf{B}\mathbf{Q} = \mathbf{Q}. \tag{8.3.1c}$$

Clearly, this $\boldsymbol{\mathcal{Y}}$ has the appropriate property that $\boldsymbol{\mathcal{Y}}\boldsymbol{\epsilon}' = \boldsymbol{\epsilon}'$, and $\mathbf{p}$ is the steady-state start-up vector $\wp$, satisfying (8.2.7).

From (8.2.8a) we can find $\boldsymbol{\mathcal{Q}}$ for this example, namely

$$\boldsymbol{\mathcal{Q}} = \boldsymbol{\mathcal{B}} - \boldsymbol{\mathcal{L}} = \mathbf{B} - \mathbf{B}\mathbf{Q},$$

with left eigenvector

$$\boldsymbol{\pi} = \frac{1}{\Psi[\mathbf{V}]}\mathbf{p}\mathbf{V}.$$

This is the ***residual vector***, $\boldsymbol{\pi}_{\mathbf{r}}$, as given in (3.5.12a), and $\mathbf{B} - \mathbf{B}\mathbf{Q}$ is the matrix $\mathbf{B}_{\mathbf{r}}$ as given in the discussion following (3.5.11a). The reader is referred to Section 3.5.3.1 for a full discussion of their meaning.

Following Theorem 8.2.1, we insert the values for $\boldsymbol{\mathcal{V}}$, $\boldsymbol{\mathcal{B}}$, and $\boldsymbol{\mathcal{L}}$ from Equations (8.3.1) into (8.2.10a) and get (for $n > 1$)

$$\begin{aligned} f_{nk}(x,\, t) &= \mathbf{p}[\exp(-x\mathbf{B})\,\mathbf{B}]\,\mathbf{Q}\,[\exp(-t\mathbf{B})\,\mathbf{B}]\,\boldsymbol{\epsilon}' \\ &= \left[\mathbf{p}[\exp(-x\mathbf{B})\,\mathbf{B}]\boldsymbol{\epsilon}'\right]\left[\mathbf{p}[\exp(-t\mathbf{B})\,\mathbf{B}]\,\boldsymbol{\epsilon}'\right]. \end{aligned}$$

Using (3.1.7d), we get

$$f_{nk}(x,\, t) = f(x)\, f(t). \tag{8.3.2a}$$

This equation is true for all $n > 1$ and all $k > 0$, and is the condition that two random variables be ***independent variables***. For $n = 1$, the initial $\mathbf{p}$ is replaced by some initial vector $\wp_o$. Then (8.3.2a) becomes

$$f_{1k}(x,\, t) = f_{X_1}(x)\, f(t). \tag{8.3.2b}$$

As in Theorem 8.2.1, we see that all $\{X_i\}$ are mutually independent and (except perhaps for X_1), are taken from the same distribution. Therefore, as discussed in Section 3.5, this is a renewal process if $\wp_o = \mathbf{p}$. Otherwise it is called a ***delayed renewal process***, as defined by Feller [FELLER71]. It has also been called a ***generalized renewal process***. Needless to say, all autocovariances are equal to 0. Apparently, it is not generally realized (although well known in some circles) that the ***counting process*** (Definition 3.5.1) associated with any renewal process (with the Poisson process being the lone exception) does have a non-vanishing covariance. See Section 3.5.4.2 for an example that displays this correlation.

8.3.2 Markov Modulated (or Regulated) Processes

All the processes in the next few sections involve a ***token*** that in the course of its actions modulates, or regulates the customer departures. First we describe how the token behaves. Then we discuss several ways that the token can control traffic.

8.3.2.1 The Underlying Generator, $\mathcal{Q}$

Consider a closed system with M servers, $\{S_i \mid 1 \le i \le M\}$, each with service time T_i with distribution represented by $\langle\, \mathbf{p_i}\,,\, \mathbf{B_i}\,\rangle$ of dimension m_i. The representations are assumed to be mutually inequivalent. The token wanders from server to server, spending a time T_i at S_i and then with probability P_{ij} goes to S_j. The mean time the token spends at S_i is $\bar{t}_i := \mathbb{E}[T_i] = \mathbf{p_i}\,\mathbf{V_i}\,\boldsymbol{\epsilon}'_\mathbf{i}$. $\boldsymbol{P}$ is an M-dimensional Markov matrix with components $[\boldsymbol{P}]_{ij} = P_{ij}$. That is, $\boldsymbol{Pe}' = \boldsymbol{e}'$, where $\boldsymbol{e}'$ is an M-dimensional column vector, all of whose components are 1. As with all Markov matrices there is a vector $\boldsymbol{p}$ satisfying

$$\boldsymbol{pP} = \boldsymbol{p}, \quad \text{and} \quad \boldsymbol{pe}' = 1.$$

Only one server can be active at a time, therefore the set of states needed to describe this system is the union of the sets of states needed to describe each S_i. The vector space describing the process is the ***direct sum*** of the individual spaces. So if S_i is of dimension m_i, the full space is of dimension

$$M_m := \sum_{i=1}^{M} m_i.$$

We are dealing here with three levels of matrices. Each server S_i is described by a set of matrices (e.g., $\mathbf{B_i}$), the traffic between subsystems is governed by matrices (e.g., $\boldsymbol{P}_{ij}$), and the overall system has a matrix description (e.g., $\boldsymbol{\mathcal{P}}$). We hope to avoid confusion by standardizing our notation with the following definition.

Definition 8.3.1

Consider an overall system $\mathcal{S}$, which itself is made up of subsystems, S_i. Then matrices and vectors that refer to $\mathcal{S}$ as a whole are said to operate in ***Composite-space***, or simply ***C-space***, and are denoted by symbols of the form:

$$\boldsymbol{\wp},\ \boldsymbol{\pi},\ \boldsymbol{\mathcal{B}},\ \boldsymbol{\mathcal{I}},\ \boldsymbol{\mathcal{L}},\ \boldsymbol{\mathcal{P}},\ \boldsymbol{\mathcal{Q}},\ \boldsymbol{\mathcal{V}},\ \boldsymbol{\mathcal{Y}},\ \boldsymbol{\varepsilon}' \ (\textit{bold-faced } \boldsymbol{\mathcal{CALLIGRAPHIC}}).$$

Such matrices formally have dimension M, with components $[\boldsymbol{\mathcal{W}}]_{\mathbf{ij}}$, where $1 \le i,\ j \le M$. However, each $[\boldsymbol{\mathcal{W}}]_{\mathbf{ij}}$ is itself a matrix of dimension $m_i \times m_j$. Therefore, $\boldsymbol{\mathcal{W}}$ is really of dimension $M_m \times M_m$.

Matrices and vectors describing the individual subsystems S_i are denoted by symbols of the form:

$$\mathbf{p_i},\ \mathbf{B_i},\ \mathbf{I_i},\ \mathbf{L_i},\ \mathbf{P_i},\ \mathbf{Q_i},\ \mathbf{V_i},\ \mathbf{Y_i},\ \epsilon'_{\mathbf{i}}\ (\textbf{bold-faced Roman}).$$

These matrices have dimension m_i, with components $[\mathbf{W_i}]_{kl}$, where $1 \le i \le M$, and $1 \le k,\ l \le m_i$.

Matrices and vectors that refer to transitions between the $\{S_i\}$ are called ***interserver operators***, and operate in ***I*-*space***. They are denoted by symbols of the form:

$$\boldsymbol{a},\ \boldsymbol{p},\ \boldsymbol{B},\ \boldsymbol{I},\ \boldsymbol{P},\ \boldsymbol{V},\ \boldsymbol{Q},\ \boldsymbol{e'}\ (\textit{\textbf{bold-faced Italic}}).$$

These matrices are of dimension M, with components $[\boldsymbol{W}]_{ij} = W_{ij}$, where $1 \le i, j \le M$. In particular the transition matrix P_{ij}, referred to at the beginning of this section, is an element of $\boldsymbol{P}$; that is, $P_{ij} = [\boldsymbol{P}]_{ij}$.

If $m_i = 1$, for all i, then $\mathcal{S}$ reduces to an exponential network, and $\boldsymbol{\mathcal{C}}$-space collapses to $\boldsymbol{I}$-space ($M_m = M$). □

We find it useful in this section (as well as in Section 9.3) to use the following notation. Each S_i has its characteristic matrices, and often they appear as diagonal elements in the full space. We use the subscript "o" to denote such matrices. For instance:

$$\boldsymbol{\mathcal{B}}_{\mathrm{o}} := \begin{bmatrix} \mathbf{B}_1 & \mathbf{O} & \cdots & \mathbf{O} \\ \mathbf{O} & \mathbf{B}_2 & \cdots & \mathbf{O} \\ \cdots & \cdots & \cdots & \cdots \\ \mathbf{O} & \mathbf{O} & \cdots & \mathbf{B}_{\mathrm{M}} \end{bmatrix}, \tag{8.3.3a}$$

with inverse

$$\boldsymbol{\mathcal{V}}_{\mathrm{o}} = \boldsymbol{\mathcal{B}}_{\mathrm{o}}^{-1} = \begin{bmatrix} \mathbf{V}_1 & \mathbf{O} & \cdots & \mathbf{O} \\ \mathbf{O} & \mathbf{V}_2 & \cdots & \mathbf{O} \\ \cdots & \cdots & \cdots & \cdots \\ \mathbf{O} & \mathbf{O} & \cdots & \mathbf{V}_{\mathrm{M}} \end{bmatrix}. \tag{8.3.3b}$$

We also use the following notation

$$\boldsymbol{\mathcal{M}}_{\mathrm{o}} = \mathrm{Diag}[\mathbf{M_1},\ \mathbf{M_2},\ \ldots,\ \mathbf{M}_{\mathrm{M}}]$$

to denote matrices of diagonal form. The different objects satisfy the rules of Definition 8.3.1, namely, the (ij)th element of $\boldsymbol{\mathcal{B}}_{\mathrm{o}}$ is itself a matrix of dimension $m_i \times m_j$, where m_i is the dimension of the representation of S_i.

Given that the token wanders forever from server to server, it is governed by the same matrix described in Section 1.3.1, specifically, Equation (1.3.2c), except that there the every S_i was exponential. The token's position in time is governed by the rate matrix $\boldsymbol{\mathcal{Q}}$, satisfying $\boldsymbol{\mathcal{Q}} = \boldsymbol{\mathcal{M}}(\boldsymbol{\mathcal{I}} - \boldsymbol{\mathcal{P}})$. We should be able to construct it in a straightforward manner. Clearly, $\mathcal{M} = \mathcal{M}_o = \text{Diag}[\mathbf{M_1}, \mathbf{M_2} \ldots, \mathbf{M_M}]$. The identity matrix $\mathcal{I}$ is also of this form with identity matrices $\mathbf{I_i}$ of dimension m_i on the diagonal. The transition matrix can be seen to be

$$\mathcal{P} = \mathcal{P}_o + \begin{bmatrix} \mathbf{q_1'}P_{11}\mathbf{p_1} & \mathbf{q_1'}P_{12}\mathbf{p_2} & \cdots & \mathbf{q_1'}P_{1M}\mathbf{p_M} \\ \mathbf{q_2'}P_{21}\mathbf{p_1} & \mathbf{q_2'}P_{22}\mathbf{p_2} & \cdots & \mathbf{q_2'}P_{2M}\mathbf{p_M} \\ \cdots & \cdots & \cdots & \cdots \\ \mathbf{q_M'}P_{M1}\mathbf{p_1} & \mathbf{q_M'}P_{M2}\mathbf{p_2} & \cdots & \mathbf{q_M'}P_{MM}\mathbf{p_M} \end{bmatrix}. \tag{8.3.3c}$$

Consider a typical term $(\mathcal{P})_{\mathbf{ij}} = \mathbf{P_i}\delta_{ij} + \mathbf{q_i'}P_{ij}\mathbf{p_j}$. Say the token completes service in phase k of server S_i. He then either:

(1) Stays in S_i $[\delta_{ij}]$ and goes to phase l, $[(\mathbf{P_i})_{kl}]$, or

(2) Leaves S_i $[(\mathbf{q_i'})_k]$, goes to S_j $[P_{ij}]$, enters, and goes to phase l, $[(\mathbf{p_j})_l]$.

By thinking of $\boldsymbol{\varepsilon}'$ as the transpose of $\boldsymbol{\varepsilon} = [\boldsymbol{\epsilon_1}, \boldsymbol{\epsilon_2}, \ldots, \boldsymbol{\epsilon_M}]$, it is easy to show that $\mathcal{P}\boldsymbol{\varepsilon}' = \boldsymbol{\varepsilon}'$ when $\boldsymbol{P}\,\boldsymbol{e}' = \boldsymbol{e}'$ even though $\mathbf{P_i}\,\boldsymbol{\epsilon_i'} \neq \boldsymbol{\epsilon_i'}$.

Our next task is to find $\mathcal{Q} = \mathcal{M}(\mathcal{I} - \mathcal{P})$. The above equations, together with the properties $\mathbf{B_i} = \mathbf{M_i}(\mathbf{I_i} - \mathbf{P_i})$ and $\mathbf{M_i}\,\mathbf{q_i'} = \mathbf{B_i}\,\boldsymbol{\epsilon_i'}$ yield

$$\mathcal{Q} = \mathcal{M} - \mathcal{M}\mathcal{P}_o - \begin{bmatrix} \mathbf{M_1}\,\mathbf{q_1'}P_{11}\mathbf{p_1} & \mathbf{M_1}\,\mathbf{q_1'}P_{12}\mathbf{p_2} & \cdots & \mathbf{M_1}\,\mathbf{q_1'}P_{1M}\mathbf{p_M} \\ \mathbf{M_2}\,\mathbf{q_2'}P_{21}\mathbf{p_1} & \mathbf{M_2}\,\mathbf{q_2'}P_{22}\mathbf{p_2} & \cdots & \mathbf{M_2}\,\mathbf{q_2'}P_{2M}\mathbf{p_M} \\ \cdots & \cdots & \cdots & \cdots \\ \mathbf{M_M}\,\mathbf{q_M'}P_{M1}\mathbf{p_1} & \mathbf{M_M}\,\mathbf{q_M'}P_{M2}\mathbf{p_2} & \cdots & \mathbf{M_M}\,\mathbf{q_M'}P_{MM}\mathbf{p_M} \end{bmatrix}$$

$$= \mathcal{B}_o - \begin{bmatrix} \mathbf{B_1}\,\boldsymbol{\epsilon_1'}P_{11}\mathbf{p_1} & \mathbf{B_1}\,\boldsymbol{\epsilon_1'}P_{12}\mathbf{p_2} & \cdots & \mathbf{B_1}\,\boldsymbol{\epsilon_1'}P_{1M}\mathbf{p_M} \\ \mathbf{B_2}\,\boldsymbol{\epsilon_2'}P_{21}\mathbf{p_1} & \mathbf{B_2}\,\boldsymbol{\epsilon_2'}P_{22}\mathbf{p_2} & \cdots & \mathbf{B_2}\,\boldsymbol{\epsilon_2'}P_{2M}\mathbf{p_M} \\ \cdots & \cdots & \cdots & \cdots \\ \mathbf{B_M}\,\boldsymbol{\epsilon_M'}P_{M1}\mathbf{p_1} & \mathbf{B_M}\,\boldsymbol{\epsilon_m'}P_{M2}\mathbf{p_2} & \cdots & \mathbf{B_M}\,\boldsymbol{\epsilon_M'}P_{MM}\mathbf{p_M} \end{bmatrix},$$

or

$$\mathcal{Q} = \mathcal{B}_o - \mathcal{B}_o\langle \boldsymbol{P} \rangle = \mathcal{B}_o\left[\mathcal{I} - \langle \boldsymbol{P} \rangle\right], \tag{8.3.3d}$$

where we have introduced a new ***embedding operation***.

Definition 8.3.2

Let $\boldsymbol{W}$ be any $M \times M$ matrix with components $[\boldsymbol{W}]_{ij} = W_{ij}$. This can be embedded into the full $M_n \times M_n$ space of $\mathcal{S}$ in the following way.

$$\langle \boldsymbol{W} \rangle := \begin{bmatrix} W_{11}\,\boldsymbol{\epsilon_1'}\,\mathbf{p}_1 & W_{12}\,\boldsymbol{\epsilon_1'}\,\mathbf{p}_2 & \cdots & W_{1M}\,\boldsymbol{\epsilon_1'}\,\mathbf{p}_M \\ W_{21}\,\boldsymbol{\epsilon_2'}\,\mathbf{p}_1 & W_{22}\,\boldsymbol{\epsilon_2'}\,\mathbf{p}_2 & \cdots & W_{2M}\,\boldsymbol{\epsilon_2'}\,\mathbf{p}_M \\ \cdots & \cdots & \cdots & \cdots \\ W_{M1}\,\boldsymbol{\epsilon_M'}\,\mathbf{p}_1 & W_{M2}\,\boldsymbol{\epsilon_M'}\,\mathbf{p}_2 & \cdots & W_{MM}\,\boldsymbol{\epsilon_M'}\,\mathbf{p}_M \end{bmatrix}. \tag{8.3.4a}$$

Let $\boldsymbol{a}$ be any M-dimensional row vector with components $[\boldsymbol{a}]_i = a_i$; then the $\mathcal{C}$-space, M_n row vector is:

$$\langle\, \boldsymbol{a} \,| := [a_1\mathbf{p}_1,\; a_2\mathbf{p}_2,\; \ldots\; a_M\mathbf{p}_M]. \tag{8.3.4b}$$

Let $\boldsymbol{b}'$ be any M-dimensional column vector with components $[\boldsymbol{b}']_i = b_i$; then the $\boldsymbol{\mathcal{C}}$-space M_n column vector is:

$$\big|\, \boldsymbol{b}' \,\big\rangle := [b_1\boldsymbol{\epsilon}'_{\mathbf{1}},\; b_2\boldsymbol{\epsilon}'_{\mathbf{2}},\; \ldots\; b_M\boldsymbol{\epsilon}'_{\mathbf{M}}]. \tag{8.3.4c}$$

These operators can be very useful when dealing with networks of non-exponential servers. For instance,

$$\boldsymbol{\varepsilon}' = [\boldsymbol{\epsilon}'_{\mathbf{1}},\, \boldsymbol{\epsilon}'_{\mathbf{2}},\, \ldots,\, \boldsymbol{\epsilon}'_{\mathbf{M}}] = \big|\, \boldsymbol{e}' \,\big\rangle,$$

and suppose

$$\wp = \big\langle\, \boldsymbol{p} \,\big| := [p_1\, \mathbf{p}_1,\, p_2\, \mathbf{p}_2,\, \ldots,\, p_M\, \mathbf{p}_{\mathrm{M}}].$$

Let $\boldsymbol{\mathcal{W}}$ be any matrix in $\boldsymbol{\mathcal{C}}$-space, then

$$\wp \boldsymbol{\mathcal{W}} \boldsymbol{\varepsilon}' = \big\langle \boldsymbol{p} \,\big|\, \boldsymbol{\mathcal{W}} \,\big|\, \boldsymbol{e}' \big\rangle = \boldsymbol{p}\,\boldsymbol{W}\,\boldsymbol{e}'.$$

This algebra is discussed in full in Section 9.3. □

We now examine several ways in which the token can regulate customer traffic.

8.3.2.2 Markov Regulated Departure Process (MRDP)

We define a ***Markov Regulated Departure Process*** (MRDP) as one in which a customer departs every time the token leaves a server. It follows that the time for the ith epoch is determined by where the token is after customer $i-1$ leaves. We have already assumed that P_{ij} is a Markov matrix, but if all its rows are equal ($P_{ij} = P_{kj} = p_j$ for all i, j, k; i.e., $\boldsymbol{P} = \boldsymbol{e}'\boldsymbol{p}$) then the process reduces to the renewal process of Section 8.3.1.

An alternate but equivalent picture is of an infinite queue feeding into a network with M servers $\{S_i \,|\, 1 \le i \le M\}$, each with service time T_i from the distribution represented by $\langle\, \mathbf{p}_i\,,\, \mathbf{B}_i \,\rangle$ of dimension m_i. The customers enter, one at a time. When a customer departs from S_i he leaves the network and the next customer goes to S_j with probability P_{ij}.

For MRDPs $\boldsymbol{\mathcal{B}}$ is easy to express, because the time between customer departures is the same as the time the token spends at S_i. Therefore,

$$\boldsymbol{\mathcal{B}} = \boldsymbol{\mathcal{B}}_{\mathrm{o}} \quad \text{and} \quad \boldsymbol{\mathcal{V}} = \boldsymbol{\mathcal{V}}_{\mathrm{o}}. \tag{8.3.5a}$$

Now that we have shown from (8.3.3d) that $\boldsymbol{\mathcal{Q}} = \boldsymbol{\mathcal{B}}_{\mathrm{o}} - \boldsymbol{\mathcal{B}}_{\mathrm{o}}\big\langle \boldsymbol{P} \big\rangle$, $\boldsymbol{\mathcal{L}}$ and $\boldsymbol{\mathcal{Y}}$ follow directly:

$$\boldsymbol{\mathcal{L}} = \boldsymbol{\mathcal{B}} - \boldsymbol{\mathcal{Q}} = \boldsymbol{\mathcal{B}}_{\mathrm{o}}\big\langle \boldsymbol{P} \big\rangle \tag{8.3.5b}$$

and

$$\boldsymbol{\mathcal{Y}} = \boldsymbol{\mathcal{V}}\boldsymbol{\mathcal{L}} = \boldsymbol{\mathcal{V}}_{\mathrm{o}}\boldsymbol{\mathcal{B}}_{\mathrm{o}}\big\langle \boldsymbol{P} \big\rangle = \big\langle \boldsymbol{P} \big\rangle. \tag{8.3.5c}$$

Because $\sum_{j=1}^{M} P_{ij} = 1$ for all i ($\boldsymbol{P}\,\boldsymbol{e}' = \boldsymbol{e}'$), it follows that $\boldsymbol{\mathcal{Y}}\boldsymbol{\varepsilon}' = \boldsymbol{\varepsilon}'$. It is not hard to show that

$$\boldsymbol{\mathcal{Y}}^k = \big\langle \boldsymbol{P}^k \big\rangle,$$

which can be useful in calculating autocorrelation lag-k, or $\mathbb{E}[X_k]$. Note also that if $M = 1$ (only one server) then $\langle \boldsymbol{P} \rangle$ reduces to $\mathbf{Q} = \boldsymbol{\epsilon}'\,\mathbf{p}$.

The steady-state vector satisfying $\wp\,\mathcal{Y} = \wp$ is (see Definition 8.3.2):

$$\wp = \langle\, \boldsymbol{p} \,| \;:=\; [p_1\mathbf{p_1},\, p_2\mathbf{p_2},\, \ldots\, p_M\,\mathbf{p_M}], \tag{8.3.6a}$$

where p_i is the ith component of the left eigenvector of $\boldsymbol{P}$ with eigenvalue 1 (i.e., $\boldsymbol{p}\boldsymbol{P} = \boldsymbol{p}$). (Note that p_i is a component of the M-vector, $\boldsymbol{p}$ corresponding to the steady-state probability that the token will be found at S_i, and $\mathbf{p_i}$ is the m_i-vector whose kth component $[\mathbf{p_i}]_k$ is the probability that the token, upon entering S_i, will go to phase k.)

In anticipation of its usefulness later, we introduce the M-dimensional, I-space matrix,

$$\boldsymbol{V_o} := \text{Diag}\,[\bar{t}_1,\, \bar{t}_2,\, \ldots,\, \bar{t}_M\,],$$

where $\bar{t}_j = \mathbf{p}_\mathrm{j}\,\mathbf{V}_\mathrm{j}\,\boldsymbol{\epsilon}'_\mathbf{j}$ is the mean service time of S_j. It comes from

$$\wp\,\mathcal{V}_\mathrm{o}\,\mathcal{E}' = \langle \boldsymbol{p} \,|\, \mathcal{V}_\mathrm{o} \,|\, \boldsymbol{e}' \rangle = \boldsymbol{p}\,\boldsymbol{V_o}\,\boldsymbol{e}'.$$

We can now get $\boldsymbol{\pi}$ directly from (8.2.8b); that is,

$$\boldsymbol{\pi} = \frac{\wp\mathcal{V}}{\wp\mathcal{V}\mathcal{E}'} = \frac{1}{\wp\mathcal{V}_\mathrm{o}\,\mathcal{E}'}[p_1\mathbf{p_1}\,\mathbf{V_1},\, p_2\mathbf{p_2}\,\mathbf{V_2}, \ldots\, p_M\mathbf{p_M}\mathbf{V_M}]$$

$$=: \frac{1}{\boldsymbol{p}\,\boldsymbol{V_o}\boldsymbol{e}'}\langle\, \boldsymbol{p} \,|\, \mathcal{V}_\mathrm{o}. \tag{8.3.6b}$$

Given that $\boldsymbol{\pi}\mathcal{E}' = 1$, it follows that $\mathbb{E}[X] = \boldsymbol{p}\,\boldsymbol{V_o}\,\boldsymbol{e}' = \sum p_i\bar{t}_i$.

Let the initial vector be written in the form

$$\wp_\mathrm{o} = [a_1\,\mathbf{w}_1,\, a_2\,\mathbf{w}_2,\, \ldots,\, a_M\,\mathbf{w}_\mathrm{M}\,], \quad \text{with } \wp_\mathrm{o}\,\mathcal{E}' = 1, \tag{8.3.7}$$

where $\boldsymbol{a}$ is an M-vector such that $\boldsymbol{a}\,\boldsymbol{e}' = \sum_{i=1}^{M} a_i = 1$ and $\mathbf{w_i}\,\boldsymbol{\epsilon}'_\mathbf{i} = 1$. That is, the first customer is initially found at S_i with probability a_i, and in vector state $\mathbf{w}_\mathrm{i}$.

We defer actual derivation of these formulas to Section 9.3, but it follows from (8.2.10b) that

$$\mathbb{E}[X_n] = \boldsymbol{a}\,\boldsymbol{P}^{n-1}\boldsymbol{V_o}\,\boldsymbol{e}' = \sum_{i,j}^{M} a_i(\boldsymbol{P}^{n-1})_{ij}\,\bar{t}_j \quad \text{for } n > 1, \tag{8.3.8a}$$

but

$$\mathbb{E}[X_1] = \sum_{i,j}^{M} a_i\,[\mathbf{w_i}\,\mathbf{V_i}\,\boldsymbol{\epsilon}'_\mathbf{i}]. \tag{8.3.8b}$$

If n is very large, or the system started in its steady state ($a_j \to p_j$ and $\mathbf{w}_\mathrm{j} \to \mathbf{p}_\mathrm{j}$), then the mean interdeparture time becomes

$$\mathbb{E}[X] = \lim_{n\to\infty} \mathbb{E}[X_n] = \lim_{n\to\infty} \wp_\mathrm{o}\mathcal{Y}^n\mathcal{V}\mathcal{E}' = \wp\mathcal{V}\mathcal{E}' = \boldsymbol{p}\,\boldsymbol{V_o}\,\boldsymbol{e}' = \sum_{i=1}^{M} p_i\,\bar{t}_i. \tag{8.3.8c}$$

Recall that $\mathbb{E}[T_i^\ell] = \ell!\, \mathbf{p_i V_i^\ell \epsilon_i'} = \Psi_i[\mathbf{V_i}^\ell]$. Then

$$\mathbb{E}[X^2] = 2\wp\mathcal{V}^2\varepsilon' = 2\sum p_i\Psi_i[\mathbf{V_i}^2] = 2\boldsymbol{p}\,\boldsymbol{V_o^{(2)}}\boldsymbol{e}' = \sum p_i\mathbb{E}\left[T_i^2\right],$$

where

$$\begin{aligned}\boldsymbol{V_o^{(2)}} &:= \mathrm{Diag}[\Psi_1[\mathbf{V_1}^2],\, \Psi_2[\mathbf{V_2}^2],\, \cdots,\, \Psi_M[\mathbf{V_M}^2]] \\ &= \frac{1}{2}\mathrm{Diag}[\,\mathbb{E}[T_1^2],\, \mathbb{E}[T_2^2],\, \cdots,\, \mathbb{E}[T_M^2]\,].\end{aligned}$$

Note that $\boldsymbol{V_o^{(\ell)}} \neq \boldsymbol{V_o}^\ell$ unless all S_i are exponential.

The specific form for (8.2.12a) in this case is

$$\mathrm{Cov}(X,\, X_{+k}) = \boldsymbol{p}\,\boldsymbol{V_o}\,[\boldsymbol{P}^k - \boldsymbol{e}'\boldsymbol{p}]\,\boldsymbol{V_o}\,\boldsymbol{e}' = \sum_{i,j} p_i\,\bar{t}_i\,[\boldsymbol{P}^k - \boldsymbol{e}'\boldsymbol{p}]_{ij}\,\bar{t}_j \qquad (8.3.9a)$$

with interdeparture density

$$f(t) = \sum_{i=1}^{M} p_i\, f_i(t). \qquad (8.3.9b)$$

Some of the properties of these equations can best be seen by examining a particular subsystem. The steady-state interdeparture density for a subsystem with two servers ($M = 2$) follows.

Example 8.3.1: First, from $\boldsymbol{p}\boldsymbol{P} = \boldsymbol{p}$, it is seen that $p_1 = P_{21}/(P_{12} + P_{21})$ and $p_2 = 1 - p_1 = P_{12}/(P_{12} + P_{21})$, so (8.3.9b) becomes

$$f(t) = \frac{P_{21}\, f_1(t) + P_{12}\, f_2(t)}{P_{12} + P_{21}},$$

and from (8.3.8c), the mean interdeparture time is

$$\mathbb{E}[X] = \frac{P_{21}\,\bar{t}_1 + P_{12}\,\bar{t}_2}{P_{12} + P_{21}}.$$

Using $\mathbb{E}[X^\ell] = p_1\mathbb{E}[T_1^\ell] + p_2\mathbb{E}[T_2^\ell]$ and $\sigma^2 = \mathbb{E}[X^2] - (\mathbb{E}[X])^2$, it follows that

$$\sigma^2 = p_1\sigma_1^2 + p_2\sigma_2^2 + p_1 p_2(\bar{t}_1 - \bar{t}_2)^2.$$

From (8.3.9a), the steady-state covariance lag-k [$(1 - P_{12} - P_{21})$ is the other eigenvalue of P] becomes

$$\mathrm{Cov}(X,\, X_{+k}) = P_{12}\, P_{21}(1 - P_{12} - P_{21})^k \left(\frac{\bar{t}_1 - \bar{t}_2}{P_{12} + P_{21}}\right)^2,$$

and from (8.2.13b),

$$\sum_{k=1}^{\infty} \mathrm{Cov}(X,\, X_{+k}) = \frac{P_{12}\, P_{21}\,(1 - P_{12} - P_{21})}{P_{12} + P_{21}} \left(\frac{\bar{t}_1 - \bar{t}_2}{P_{12} + P_{21}}\right)^2.$$

It is clear that if the $\bar{t}_i$s are equal, then all covariances are 0. All covariances are also 0, if $P_{12} = P_{22}$. For then $P_{12} + P_{21} = 1$ and $\boldsymbol{P} = \boldsymbol{e}'\boldsymbol{p}$. That is, what happens in each epoch is independent of what happened in the previous epoch.

On the other hand, if $P_{12} = P_{21} = 1$ ($\boldsymbol{P}$ is cyclic), then

$$\text{Cov}(X, X_{+k}) = (-1)^k \left(\frac{\bar{t}_1 - \bar{t}_2}{2}\right)^2.$$

In this case, the limit as $k \to \infty$ does not exist, and the sum over k does not converge! [See Theorem 8.2.2.]

For a last word we look at the autocorrelations, $\hat{r}(k) = \text{Cov}(X, X_{+k})/\sigma^2$. They depend on S_1 and S_2 only through their variances. The bigger σ_1^2 and σ_2^2 are, the smaller is $\hat{r}(k)$. In the other direction, if the two distributions are deterministic, their variances equal 0 and

$$\hat{r}(k) = (1 - P_{12} - P_{21})^k.$$

The dependence on the distributions is completely gone; and all that remains is a "coin-flipping" game. The ***Bernoulli process*** corresponds to $P_{12} = P_{21}$ with $\hat{r}(k) = 0$. The probability of flipping a 1 is $P_{11} = P_{21}$. If P_{12} does not equal P_{21}, the game is biased in that the probability of a 1 depends on the result of the previous flip. ▲

What is most interesting about these processes is that their mean epoch times ($\mathbb{E}[X_n]$) and correlations depend only on the means ($\bar{t}_i$) of the different distributions, and not the distributions or even the higher moments. Thus, even two exponential servers regulated this way will produce a non-renewal process.

8.3.2.3 Markov Modulated Poisson Process (MMPP)

The most widely used SMPs are MMPPs. In particular, they have been used to model voice traffic, and recently, all telecommunications traffic (see, for instance, [Meier-Fischer92] and [Park-Will00]). In the previous section we defined the MRDP, where a "token" wanders from one server to another, spends a time T_j at S_j with distribution generated by $\langle \mathbf{p_j}, \mathbf{B_j} \rangle$, at which time one customer departs the system, and the token moves to another server according to the matrix $\boldsymbol{P}$ (8.3.5c). In this section the token still wanders from S_i to S_j, but now customers depart continuously at a Poisson rate of λ_j while the token is at S_j. That is, the time between departures is exponentially distributed, with mean $1/\lambda_j$, and on average, $\lambda_j \mathbb{E}[T_j]$ customers leave while the token is at j. Thus the token *modulates the rate* at which customers depart by moving from one station to another.

Most applications of MMPPs assume that each T_j is exponentially distributed. But here we assume that they are as described in Section 8.3.2.1 and have nonexponential distributions. Therefore, the token's behavior is governed by the $\boldsymbol{Q}$ of (8.3.3d). When viewed as an M-dimensional system, the time the token spends at S_i is indeed nonexponential. But if one looks at $\mathcal{Q}$ as an M_m-dimensional system, where each phase is thought of as a server, then the structure is again that of exponential servers. From a modeling point of view (that's what is important) we have a generalization of MMPPs. But from a purely mathematical view, this is still an MMPP (and a restricted one at that).

From its description, $\mathcal{L}$ is easy to write down, being:

$$\mathcal{L} = \mathcal{L}_o := \begin{bmatrix} \lambda_1\mathbf{I}_1 & \mathbf{O} & \cdots & \mathbf{O} \\ \mathbf{O} & \lambda_2\mathbf{I}_2 & \cdots & \mathbf{O} \\ \cdots & \cdots & \cdots & \cdots \\ \mathbf{O} & \mathbf{O} & \cdots & \lambda_M\mathbf{I}_M \end{bmatrix}. \tag{8.3.10a}$$

Note that adding a term of the form $\lambda_b\mathcal{I}$ to $\mathcal{L}$, doesn't change its structure and doesn't change $\mathcal{Q}$ either. But this can then be interpreted either as increasing the rate at each server, or as an MMPP with a background (or merged with a) Poisson process of rate λ_b. We also have occasion to use the M-dimensional matrix $\boldsymbol{L_o} := \text{Diag}[\lambda_1, \lambda_2, \ldots, \lambda_M]$.

We have another notational point to make. The matrices, $\mathcal{B}$, $\mathcal{V}$, $\mathcal{L}$, and $\mathcal{Q}$ have the same physical meaning from application to application, but they may have completely different structures. On the other hand, the matrices with subscript "o" (e.g., $\mathcal{L}_o$) are always block diagonal matrices, and may have no physical meaning in any particular application. For a summary of useful matrices, see Table 8.3.1 below.

In discussing overloaded servers in Section 8.3.1, we easily set up $\mathcal{B}$ and $\mathcal{L}$, and thereby were able to get $\mathcal{Q}$. In Section 8.3.2.2, for MRDPs we first set up $\mathcal{B}$ and $\mathcal{Q}$, from which $\mathcal{L}$ followed. Here we have set up $\mathcal{Q}$ and $\mathcal{L}$ for the MMPP and now have

$$\mathcal{B} = \mathcal{L} + \mathcal{Q} = \mathcal{L}_o + \mathcal{B}_o - \mathcal{B}_o\langle \boldsymbol{P} \rangle, \tag{8.3.10b}$$

where $\mathcal{Q}$ is from (8.3.3d) and $\mathcal{B}_o$ is from (8.3.3a).

The inverse of $\mathcal{B}$ can be found using a technique similar to that used in Lemma 4.2.1. We present the result here, and those who wish to know more about the algebra of $\mathcal{C}$ embeddings are referred to Section 9.3. First manipulate (8.3.10b), recalling that both $\mathcal{V}_o$ and $\mathcal{L}_o$ are block diagonal and commute with each other, but not with $\langle \boldsymbol{P} \rangle$. That is, $\mathcal{L}_o\mathcal{V}_o = \mathcal{V}_o\mathcal{L}_o$ but $\mathcal{L}_o\langle \boldsymbol{P} \rangle \neq \langle \boldsymbol{P} \rangle\mathcal{L}_o$. We get

$$\mathcal{V} = \mathcal{B}^{-1} = \left[\mathcal{I} - \mathcal{D}_o\langle \boldsymbol{P} \rangle\right]^{-1} \mathcal{V}_o\mathcal{D}_o, \tag{8.3.10c}$$

where

$$\mathcal{D}_o := [\mathcal{I} + \mathcal{L}_o\mathcal{V}_o]^{-1} = \text{Diag}[\mathbf{D_1}, \mathbf{D_2}, \ldots, \mathbf{D_M}]$$

with $\mathbf{D_i} = [\mathbf{I_i} + \lambda_i\mathbf{V_i}]^{-1}$. Furthermore,

$$\boldsymbol{D}_o := \text{Diag}[d_1, d_2, \ldots, d_M], \quad \text{where } d_i = \mathbf{p_i}\,\mathbf{D_i}\,\boldsymbol{\epsilon}'_\mathbf{i}.$$

We next make use of the special properties of $\langle\, P \,\rangle$ to take the inverse of an $M_m \times M_m$ matrix by embedding the inverse of an $M \times M$ matrix:

$$\left[\mathcal{I} - \mathcal{D}_{\rm o}\langle\, P \,\rangle\right]^{-1} = \mathcal{I} + \mathcal{D}_{\rm o}\langle\, (I - P\mathbf{D_o})^{-1}P \rangle$$

and put this into (8.3.10c) to get

$$\mathcal{V} = \left[\mathcal{I} + \mathcal{D}_{\rm o}\langle\, (I - P\mathbf{D_o})^{-1}P \rangle\right] \mathcal{V}_{\rm o}\mathcal{D}_{\rm o}. \qquad (8.3.10d)$$

As was shown in Theorem 3.1.1, $d_i = B^*(\lambda_i)$, the Laplace transform of the distribution generated by $\langle\, \mathbf{p_i},\ \mathbf{B_i} \rangle$ and can be interpreted as the probability that the token will leave S_i before any customers depart. We take a closer look at this in the next section.

The matrix $\mathcal{Y}$ comes easily:

$$\mathcal{Y} = \mathcal{V}\mathcal{L} = \left[\mathcal{I} + \mathcal{D}_{\rm o}\langle\, (I - P\mathbf{D_o})^{-1}P \rangle\right] \mathcal{V}_{\rm o}\mathcal{D}_{\rm o}\mathcal{L}_{\rm o}. \qquad (8.3.10e)$$

It is useful at times to use the identity $\mathcal{D}_{\rm o}\mathcal{V}_{\rm o}\mathcal{L}_{\rm o} = \mathcal{I} - \mathcal{D}_{\rm o}$, while noting that the three matrices commute with each other.

There are three advantages of using this notation. First, the internal structure of the matrices is more explicit (once one gets used to the notation). Second, the inverses of matrices are found by inverting matrices of smaller dimension. Third, one can go further by analytic manipulation rather than having to resort to numerical computation. The manipulations can occur without having to resort to a particular distribution representation; that is, the expressions are valid for all distributions.

We next find the steady-state mean interdeparture time. First we find $\wp$ and $\boldsymbol{\pi}$. We have actually done most of the work already. The $\mathcal{Q}$ of this section is the same as that in the previous section, therefore so is $\boldsymbol{\pi}$, as given in (8.3.6b). First multiply $\boldsymbol{\pi}$ by $\mathcal{L}$ [remembering that for MMPP, $\mathcal{L} = \mathcal{L}_{\rm o}$ from (8.3.10a)]

$$\boldsymbol{\pi}\mathcal{L} = \frac{1}{\sum p_i\bar{t}_i}[p_1\mathbf{p_1}\,\mathbf{V_1},\, p_2\mathbf{p_2}\,\mathbf{V_2}, \ldots,\, p_M\mathbf{p_M}\mathbf{V_M}]\mathcal{L}_{\rm o}$$

$$= \frac{1}{\sum p_i\bar{t}_i}[p_1\mathbf{p_1}\,\mathbf{V_1}\lambda_1,\, p_2\mathbf{p_2}\,\mathbf{V_2}\lambda_2, \ldots,\, p_M\mathbf{p_M}\mathbf{V_M}\lambda_M] = \frac{1}{\boldsymbol{p}\,\mathbf{V_o}\,\mathbf{e}'}\langle\, \boldsymbol{p} \,|\, \mathcal{V}_{\rm o}\mathcal{L}_{\rm o}.$$

Thus,

$$\boldsymbol{\pi}\mathcal{L}\boldsymbol{\varepsilon}' = \frac{\sum_{i=1}^{M} p_i\bar{t}_i\lambda_i}{\sum_{i=1}^{M} p_i\bar{t}_i} = \frac{\boldsymbol{p}\,\mathbf{V_o}\mathbf{L_o}\mathbf{e}'}{\boldsymbol{p}\,\mathbf{V_o}\mathbf{e}'}. \qquad (8.3.11a)$$

The steady-state vector comes directly from (8.2.8e) and satisfies $\wp\boldsymbol{\varepsilon}' = 1$.

$$\wp = \frac{\boldsymbol{\pi}\mathcal{L}}{\boldsymbol{\pi}\mathcal{L}\boldsymbol{\varepsilon}'} = \frac{1}{\boldsymbol{p}\,\mathbf{V_o}\mathbf{L_o}\mathbf{e}'}\langle\, \boldsymbol{p} \,|\, \mathcal{V}_{\rm o}\mathcal{L}_{\rm o}. \qquad (8.3.11b)$$

We can now find $\mathbb{E}[X] = \wp\mathcal{V}\boldsymbol{\varepsilon}'$. But wait; from (8.2.8c) and (8.3.11a) we already know what it is, namely:

$$\mathbb{E}[X] = \wp\mathcal{V}\boldsymbol{\varepsilon}' = \frac{1}{\boldsymbol{\pi}\mathcal{L}_{\rm o}\boldsymbol{\varepsilon}'} = \frac{\boldsymbol{p}\,\mathbf{V_o}\mathbf{e}'}{\boldsymbol{p}\,\mathbf{V_o}\mathbf{L_o}\mathbf{e}'}. \qquad (8.3.11c)$$

This has a straightforward physical interpretation. The numerator is the average time spent by the token per visit to some S_i, averaged over all servers. The term $\bar{t}_i\lambda_i = (\boldsymbol{V}_{\mathbf{o}}\boldsymbol{L}_{\mathbf{o}})_{ii}$ is the average number of departures while the token is at S_i. Thus the denominator is the average number of departures per token visit, averaged over all visits.

Keep in mind that (8.3.11c) is only valid for steady-state epochs. If the system is in some vector state, say $\wp_{\mathrm{o}}$, or $\wp_{\mathbf{n}} = \wp_{\mathrm{o}}\mathcal{Y}$ (the nth customer has just departed), then one must compute

$$\mathbb{E}[X_{n+1}] = \wp_{\mathbf{n}}\mathcal{V}\varepsilon'$$

using (8.3.10c). This takes some skill and practice to do analytically (see Section 9.3). However, all the moments, and even autocorrelation coefficients are easy to compute.

In the rest of this subsection we look at applying MMPP's to problems in telecommunications. We show how to use physical arguments to make mathematical changes to the model.

8.3.2.4 Augmented MMPP's (AMMPP)

There is one problem with this model, particularly for the ***ON-OFF processes*** we will be discussing later. As was mentioned in the discussion following (8.3.10c), d_i is the probability that the token will leave S_i without any packets departing (customers are now called ***packets***, or ***cells***). That is, sometimes a token's visit to S_i will result in no sent packets. If the mean number of packets per visit is large, then d_i will be small and nothing need be done. But if that is not the case, then some modifications must be made. After all, by definition each *ON* interval must have at least one packet. After all, it represents actual transmission, not merely permission to transmit.

Thus we introduce the ***Augmented MMPP*** (AMMPP). The token wanders through the system as usual. While it is at S_i, customers depart at rate λ_i. But when the token leaves S_i, another customer leaves. Thus, $\mathcal{Q}$ is the same as in the two previous sections, but $\mathcal{L}$ is the sum of the MRDP and MMPP $\mathcal{L}$s. (note that the resulting AMMPP is not an MMPP. That is [from (8.3.3d)]:

$$\mathcal{Q} = \mathcal{B}_{\mathrm{o}} - \mathcal{B}_{\mathrm{o}}\langle\, \mathbf{P}\,\rangle \tag{8.3.12a}$$

and [adding (8.3.5b) to (8.3.10a)]

$$\mathcal{L} = \mathcal{L}_{\mathrm{o}} + \mathcal{B}_{\mathrm{o}}\langle\, \mathbf{P}\,\rangle. \tag{8.3.12b}$$

Then

$$\mathcal{B} = \mathcal{Q} + \mathcal{L} = \mathcal{B}_{\mathrm{o}} - \mathcal{B}_{\mathrm{o}}\langle\, \mathbf{P}\,\rangle + \mathcal{B}_{\mathrm{o}}\langle\, \mathbf{P}\,\rangle + \mathcal{L}_{\mathrm{o}} = \mathcal{B}_{\mathrm{o}} + \mathcal{L}_{\mathrm{o}} \tag{8.3.12c}$$

and

$$\mathcal{V} = [\mathcal{B}_{\mathrm{o}} + \mathcal{L}_{\mathrm{o}}]^{-1} = \mathcal{V}_{\mathrm{o}}[\mathcal{I} + \mathcal{L}_{\mathrm{o}}\mathcal{V}_{\mathrm{o}}]^{-1} = \mathcal{V}_{\mathrm{o}}\mathcal{D}_{\mathrm{o}}. \tag{8.3.12d}$$

The various matrices for all three schemes are presented in Table 8.3.1 for comparison and reference.

Table 8.3.1. Comparison of Processes

	MRDP	MMPP	AMMPP
$\mathcal{Q}$	$\mathcal{B}_o - \mathcal{B}_o\langle \mathrm{P} \rangle$	$\mathcal{B}_o - \mathcal{B}_o\langle \mathrm{P} \rangle$	$\mathcal{B}_o - \mathcal{B}_o\langle \mathrm{P} \rangle$
$\mathcal{L}$	$\mathcal{B}_o\langle \mathrm{P} \rangle$	$\mathcal{L}_o$	$\mathcal{L}_o + \mathcal{B}_o\langle \mathrm{P} \rangle$
$\mathcal{B}$	$\mathcal{B}_o$	$\mathcal{L}_o + \mathcal{B}_o - \mathcal{B}_o\langle \mathrm{P} \rangle$	$\mathcal{B}_o + \mathcal{L}_o$
$\mathcal{V}$	$\mathcal{V}_o$	$\mathcal{X}_o\mathcal{V}_o\mathcal{D}_o$	$\mathcal{V}_o\mathcal{D}_o$
$\mathcal{Y}$	$\langle \mathrm{P} \rangle$	$\mathcal{X}_o\mathcal{V}_o\mathcal{D}_o\mathcal{L}_o$	$\mathcal{I} - \mathcal{D}_o + \mathcal{D}_o\langle \mathrm{P} \rangle$
$\boldsymbol{\pi}$	$\kappa_o\langle \mathbf{p} \| \mathcal{V}_o$	$\kappa_o\langle \mathbf{p} \| \mathcal{V}_o$	$\kappa_o\langle \mathbf{p} \| \mathcal{V}_o$
$\wp$	$\langle \mathbf{p} \|$	$\kappa_1\langle \mathbf{p} \| \mathcal{V}_o\mathcal{L}_o$	$\kappa_2\langle \mathbf{p} \| (\mathcal{I} + \mathcal{V}_o\mathcal{L}_o)$
$\wp\mathcal{V}$	$\langle \mathbf{p} \| \mathcal{V}_o$	$\kappa_1\langle \mathbf{p} \| \mathcal{V}_o$	$\kappa_2\langle \mathbf{p} \| \mathcal{V}_o$
$\mathbb{E}[X]$	$\mathbf{p}\,\mathbf{V_o}\mathbf{e}'$	κ_1/κ_o	κ_2/κ_o

Notes:
1. All three have the same $\mathcal{Q}$, and therefore the same $\boldsymbol{\pi}$;
2. Given $\wp = c\boldsymbol{\pi}\mathcal{B}$ [from (8.2.8e)], the vectors, $\wp\mathcal{V}$, must be proportional to $\boldsymbol{\pi}$ and to each other;
3. The number of departures per visit for the augmented process is one more than that for the MMPP, and of course, the number of departures per visit for the MRDP is 1 (see the denominators of $\mathbb{E}[X]$);
4. $\mathcal{X}_o := [\mathcal{I} - \mathcal{D}_o\langle P \rangle]^{-1} = \mathcal{I} + \mathcal{D}_o\langle P(I - D_oP)^{-1} \rangle$;
5. $\kappa_o := (\mathbf{p}\,\mathbf{V_o}\mathbf{e}')^{-1}$;
6. $\kappa_1 := (\mathbf{p}\,\mathbf{V_o}\mathbf{L_o}\mathbf{e}')^{-1}$;
7. $\kappa_2 := (\mathbf{p}\,\mathbf{V_o}\mathbf{L_o}\mathbf{e}' + 1)^{-1}$

8.3.2.5 ON-OFF Models (Bursty Traffic)

Researchers in telecommunications have long been aware that information traffic (e.g., voice communication or transmission of data packets) is very non-uniform. (see, e.g., Leland et al. [LELANDETAL94].) That is, the amount of traffic from time interval to time interval fluctuates enormously. This kind of behavior is called ***bursty***. It is explained, at least for voice, as follows. While someone is speaking, data flows at a ***peak rate***, but when that person stops speaking, no data are transmitted until someone speaks again. This can satisfactorily be modeled by a 2-state MMPP model, where, say, $\lambda_1 = \lambda_p$ is the peak rate at which information flows when someone is talking (S_1 represents the ***ON time***), and $\lambda_2 = 0$ when there is silence (S_2 represents the

OFF time). This has been called a ***one-burst process***. If the times between packets during an *ON* time are exponentially distributed (the usual assumption) the system is also called an ***Interrupted Poisson Process*** (IPP) (see, e.g., [LEE-LIEF-WALLACE00]). When one analyzes the superposition of several voice streams, it is difficult to tell where the *ON* and *OFF* periods are, but the burstiness remains. Still, satisfactory MMPP models were constructed where several servers, corresponding to 1, 2, ..., n simultaneous voice streams were included. In this case, $\lambda_n = n\lambda_1$. Reasonable $\boldsymbol{P}$ matrices were constructed to reflect the probability that a new voice stream will join in, or a present one will stop. We might call these ***ON-OFF MMPP***'s (OOMMPP).

As data transmission became more common the MMPP models were found to be less and less useful. Further examination of data streams showed that there was ***long-range autocorrelation*** [CROVELLABESTAVROS96]. That is, $\hat{r}(k)$ [see (8.2.12c)] remains measurable for very large k. This could not be modeled by the then-existing models. But further measurements of data revealed that the size of transmitted files is power-tailed for many orders of magnitude; see Hatem [HATEM97], Lipsky [LIPGARGROBBERT92], and Crovella [CROVELLABESTAVROS96]. See Section 3.3 for a full discussion, including the TPTs. When files are to be transmitted they are first broken up into packets. The packets are then sent in a smooth (Poisson?) manner, for a period of time which is PT. That is, the *ON* times must be power-tail distributed. The model presented in Section 8.3.2.3 is adequate, even reproducing the long-range autocorrelation, if a good representation of PT distributions is used. Strictly speaking, PT functions require infinite representations, but in Section 3.3.6.2 we present a truncated variety that has been shown to be more than adequate (see Schwefel [SCHWEFEL00]).

Perhaps the best way to become familiar with all the above matrices is by an example. Let us consider a simple *ON-OFF* model. It shows that previously unknown properties can be discovered without actually having to specify the PDFs of the S_is. In fact, we come up with some interesting results.

Example 8.3.2: Consider a system with two servers S_1 and S_2, with distributions represented by $\langle\, \mathbf{p}_1,\, \mathbf{B_1} \,\rangle$ and $\langle\, \mathbf{p}_2,\, \mathbf{B_2} \,\rangle$, respectively. While the token is at S_1 a data source sends a ***burst of packets*** at a peak rate of λ_p for a time T_1. When the burst is over, the token goes to S_2 for a time T_2, during which time no packets are sent ($\lambda_2 = 0$). The token then returns to S_1, repeating the process indefinitely. The matrices describing the system are:

$$\boldsymbol{P} = \begin{bmatrix} 0 & 1 \\ 1 & 0 \end{bmatrix}, \qquad \langle\, \boldsymbol{P} \,\rangle = \begin{bmatrix} \mathbf{0}_1 & \boldsymbol{\epsilon}_1' \,\mathbf{p}_2 \\ \boldsymbol{\epsilon}_2' \,\mathbf{p}_1 & \mathbf{0}_2 \end{bmatrix},$$

$$\boldsymbol{p} = \begin{bmatrix} \frac{1}{2}, \frac{1}{2} \end{bmatrix}, \qquad \boldsymbol{\varepsilon}' = \begin{bmatrix} \boldsymbol{\epsilon}_1' \\ \boldsymbol{\epsilon}_2' \end{bmatrix} = |\, \boldsymbol{e}' \,\rangle,$$

and (using $\boldsymbol{\mathcal{D}}_{\rm o} = [\boldsymbol{\mathcal{I}} + \boldsymbol{\mathcal{L}}_{\rm o}\boldsymbol{\mathcal{V}}_{\rm o}]^{-1}$ with $\mathbf{D_1} = [\mathbf{I} + \lambda_p \mathbf{V_1}]^{-1}$)

$$\boldsymbol{\mathcal{L}}_{\rm o} = \begin{bmatrix} \lambda_p \mathbf{I}_1 & \mathbf{0} \\ \mathbf{0} & \mathbf{0} \end{bmatrix}, \qquad \boldsymbol{\mathcal{B}}_{\rm o} = \begin{bmatrix} \mathbf{B}_1 & \mathbf{0} \\ \mathbf{0} & \mathbf{B_2} \end{bmatrix},$$

$$\mathcal{V}_{\mathrm{o}} = \begin{bmatrix} \mathbf{V}_1 & \mathbf{0} \\ \mathbf{0} & \mathbf{V}_2 \end{bmatrix}, \qquad \mathcal{D}_{\mathrm{o}} = \begin{bmatrix} \mathbf{D}_1 & \mathbf{0} \\ \mathbf{0} & \mathbf{I}_2 \end{bmatrix}.$$

The matrices governing the 2-server MMPP ***ON-OFF process*** follow.

$$\mathcal{L} = \mathcal{L}_{\mathrm{o}}, \qquad \mathcal{Q} = \begin{bmatrix} \mathbf{B}_1 & -\mathbf{B}_1\boldsymbol{\epsilon}_1'\mathbf{p}_2 \\ -\mathbf{B}_2\boldsymbol{\epsilon}_2'\mathbf{p}_1 & \mathbf{B}_2 \end{bmatrix},$$

$$\mathcal{B} = \begin{bmatrix} \mathbf{B}_1 + \lambda_p\mathbf{I}_1 & -\mathbf{B}_1\boldsymbol{\epsilon}_1'\mathbf{p}_2 \\ -\mathbf{B}_2\boldsymbol{\epsilon}_2'\mathbf{p}_1 & \mathbf{B}_2 \end{bmatrix},$$

(using $d := \mathbf{p}_1\mathbf{D}_1\boldsymbol{\epsilon}_1'$)

$$\mathcal{V} = \begin{bmatrix} \mathbf{V}_1\mathbf{D}_1 + \frac{1}{1-d}\mathbf{D}_1\boldsymbol{\epsilon}_1'\mathbf{p}_1\mathbf{V}_1\mathbf{D}_1 & \frac{1}{1-d}\mathbf{D}_1\boldsymbol{\epsilon}_1'\mathbf{p}_2\mathbf{V}_2 \\ \frac{1}{1-d}\boldsymbol{\epsilon}_2'\mathbf{p}_1\mathbf{V}_1\mathbf{D}_1 & \mathbf{V}_2 + \frac{d}{1-d}\boldsymbol{\epsilon}_2'\mathbf{p}_2\mathbf{V}_2 \end{bmatrix},$$

$$\wp = \frac{1}{\bar{t}_1}[\mathbf{p}_1\mathbf{V}_1,\ \mathbf{o}], \qquad \mathcal{Y} = \lambda_p \begin{bmatrix} \mathbf{V}_1\mathbf{D}_1 + \frac{1}{1-d}\mathbf{D}_1\boldsymbol{\epsilon}_1'\mathbf{p}_1\mathbf{V}_1\mathbf{D}_1 & \mathbf{0} \\ \frac{1}{1-d}\boldsymbol{\epsilon}_2'\mathbf{p}_1\mathbf{V}_1\mathbf{D}_1 & \mathbf{0} \end{bmatrix}.$$

$$\boldsymbol{\pi} = \frac{1}{\boldsymbol{p}\mathcal{V}_{\mathbf{o}}\boldsymbol{e}'}\langle \boldsymbol{p} \,|\, \mathcal{V}_{\mathrm{o}} = \frac{1}{\bar{t}_1 + \bar{t}_2}[\mathbf{p}_1\mathbf{V}_1,\ \mathbf{p}_2\mathbf{V}_2],$$

$$\wp\mathcal{V} = \frac{1}{\boldsymbol{p}\mathcal{V}_{\mathbf{o}}\boldsymbol{e}'}\langle \boldsymbol{p} \,|\, \mathcal{V}_{\mathbf{o}} = \frac{1}{\lambda_p\bar{t}_1}[\mathbf{p}_1\mathbf{V}_1,\ \mathbf{p}_2\mathbf{V}_2].$$

We now find the mean and variance of the interdeparture times. The mean is simple enough to evaluate. It is

$$\mathbb{E}[X] = \wp\mathcal{V}\boldsymbol{\varepsilon}' = \frac{\bar{t}_1 + \bar{t}_2}{\bar{n}_p}, \tag{8.3.13a}$$

where $\bar{n}_p := \lambda_p\bar{t}_1$ is the mean number of packets per cycle and the numerator is the total time for one cycle. Considered as a flow of packets, the mean flow rate κ [see 8.2.8d] is [the same as $1/(\wp\mathcal{V}\boldsymbol{\varepsilon}')$]:

$$\kappa := \boldsymbol{\pi}\mathcal{L}\boldsymbol{\varepsilon}' = \left[\frac{\bar{t}_1}{\bar{t}_1 + \bar{t}_2}\right]\lambda_p.$$

In many applications it is possible to change λ_p, by for instance, increasing the transmission speed of data. At that moment, the amount of data to be sent is fixed, therefore $\bar{t}_1$ decreases in such a way that $\bar{n}_p$ remains constant. Therefore, at least for *ON-OFF* models, it is appropriate to replace $\lambda_p\bar{t}_1$ by $\bar{n}_p$. The typical picture is of data being prepared for transmission and then sent to the transmitter. In this scenario, even if the data are transmitted more rapidly, the next batch of data won't be ready for transmission until one full cycle later. In other words $\bar{t}_1 + \bar{t}_2$, like $\bar{n}_p$, is constant. In such cases the ***burst parameter, b***, can be a useful variable for describing the performance of the application.

$$b := \frac{\bar{t}_2}{\bar{t}_1 + \bar{t}_2} = 1 - \frac{\kappa}{\lambda_p}. \tag{8.3.13b}$$

When $b = 0$, $\lambda_p = \kappa$, and the *OFF* time is 0; that is, there is no burstiness and the traffic is pure Poisson. As λ_p increases unboundedly, $b \to 1$, and in the limit, all the packets are sent at the same time, that is, in ***bulk***. When packets arrive at a server in this manner, it is called a ***bulk arrival process***, or ***batch arrival process***. (See, e.g., [GROSS-HARRIS98].)

Perhaps the easiest way to find the variance is to first evaluate $\mathcal{V}\varepsilon'$. We do that now, finding

$$\mathcal{V}\varepsilon' = \begin{bmatrix} \frac{1}{\lambda_p}\boldsymbol{\epsilon}_1' + \frac{\bar{t}_2}{1-d}\mathbf{D}_1\boldsymbol{\epsilon}_1' \\ \\ \frac{1}{\lambda_p}\boldsymbol{\epsilon}_2' + \frac{\bar{t}_2 d}{1-d}\boldsymbol{\epsilon}_2' + \mathbf{V}_2\boldsymbol{\epsilon}_2' \end{bmatrix}.$$

We know that $\mathbb{E}[X^2] = 2\wp\mathcal{V}^2\varepsilon'$, so

$$\sigma_X^2 = 2(\wp\mathcal{V})(\mathcal{V}\varepsilon') - [\mathbb{E}[X]]^2$$

$$= \frac{1}{\lambda_p \bar{t}_1}\sigma_2^2 + \frac{1}{(\lambda_p \bar{t}_1)^2}\left[\bar{t}_1^2 + 2\bar{t}_1\bar{t}_2 + (\lambda_p\bar{t}_1 - 1)\bar{t}_2^2 + \frac{2\lambda_p d}{1-d}\bar{t}_1\bar{t}_2^2\right]$$

$$= \frac{1}{\bar{n}_p}\sigma_2^2 + \left(\frac{1}{\bar{n}_p}\right)^2\left[(\bar{t}_1 + \bar{t}_2)^2 + \frac{2\bar{n}_p\bar{t}_2^2}{1-d} - (\bar{n}_p + 2)\bar{t}_2^2\right]. \qquad (8.3.13c)$$

This somewhat unwieldy expression can be brought into simpler form by looking at the squared coefficient of variation:

$$C_X^2 := \frac{\sigma_X^2}{\mathbb{E}[X]^2} = 1 + b^2\left[\bar{n}_p C_2^2 + \frac{2\bar{n}_p}{1-d} - (\bar{n}_p + 2)\right]. \qquad (8.3.13d)$$

If $b = 0$ ($\bar{t}_2 = 0$), then $C_X^2 = 1$ corresponding to a Poisson process.

The dependence of C_X^2 on the *OFF* time distribution is explicit in C_2^2, but the dependence on the *ON* time is implicitly contained in the behavior of d. In fact, all properties of this *ON-OFF* model depend on the *ON* time distribution through powers of $\mathbf{D_1} = (\mathbf{I_1} + \lambda_\mathbf{p}\mathbf{V_1})^{-1}$. This, in turn, seems to depend on the peak rate λ_p as well. But in our model the two are intimately connected, not merely through $\bar{n}_p = \lambda_p\bar{t}_1$. After all, during an *ON* time a certain number of packets are transmitted, and that should be independent of how fast they are sent. That is, the distribution of T_1 depends on the distribution of the number of packets in a burst.

In Definition 3.2.1 we introduced the equivalence relation that groups together functions that have the same shape. Let $\hat{\mathbf{V}}_\mathbf{1}$ generate a function with the same shape as $\mathbf{V_1}$, but with mean $\mathbf{p_1}\hat{\mathbf{V}}_\mathbf{1}\boldsymbol{\epsilon}_\mathbf{1}' = 1$. Then T_1 has a distribution generated by $\langle\, \mathbf{p}_1,\, \bar{t}_1\hat{\mathbf{V}}_1 \,\rangle$, with mean $\mathbb{E}[T_1] = \bar{t}_1$. We see, then, that

$$\mathbf{D_1} = (\mathbf{I_1} + \lambda_p\bar{t}_1\hat{\mathbf{V}}_1)^{-1} = (\mathbf{I_1} + \bar{n}_p\hat{\mathbf{V}}_1)^{-1}.$$

$\bar{n}_p$ is assumed to be the same irrespective of the peak rate; consequently we see that $\mathbf{D_1}$ is also independent of λ_p.

We now go one step further. In Section 4.4.1 we found a relationship between the ***exponential moments*** $\alpha_k(s)$ and the matrices, $\mathbf{D}^k$. From (4.4.1a) we have

$$\alpha_k(s) = \int_0^\infty \frac{(sx)^k}{k!} e^{-sx}\, b(x)\, dx = \Psi[(\mathbf{I} - \mathbf{D})^k \mathbf{D}] = \Psi[(s\mathbf{V}\mathbf{D})^k \mathbf{D}].$$

If we identify s with λ_p and $\mathbf{D}(s)$ with $\mathbf{D_1}(\lambda_p)$, we can interpret α_k to be the probability that exactly k packets are sent during an *ON* period. Given that $\mathbf{D_1}$ is independent of λ_p, so is α_k. This can also be seen directly from the integral term. From Definition 3.2.1 we have $b(x) = \hat{b}(x/\bar{t}_1)/\bar{t}_1$. We put this into the equation above, let $x = \bar{t}_1 u$, recognize that $\lambda_p \bar{t}_1 = \bar{n}_p$, and get:

$$\alpha_k(\bar{n}_p) = \int_0^\infty \frac{(\bar{n}_p u)^k}{k!} e^{-\bar{n}_p u}\, b(u)\, du.$$

Thus, the number of packets per *ON* time does not depend on λ_p or $\bar{t}_1$ independently.

As a specific example, if T_1 is exponentially distributed, we get

$$d_e = \Psi[(\mathbf{I} + \lambda_\mathbf{p} \mathbf{V_1})^{-1}] = \frac{1}{1 + \bar{n}_p}$$

and C_X^2 simplifies to $C_{X_e}^2 = 1 + \bar{n}_p\, b^2 (C_2^2 + 1)$.

If all *ON* times are the same ($T_1 = \bar{t}_1$; i.e., the **d**eterministic distribution), then $d_d = e^{-\bar{n}_p}$ and

$$C_{X_d}^2 = 1 + b^2 \left[\bar{n}_p C_2^2 + \frac{2\bar{n}_p}{1 - e^{-\bar{n}_p}} - (\bar{n}_p + 2) \right] \cdot$$

For fixed b, $\bar{n}_p$, and C_2^2 this expression provides a lower bound on C_X^2, but there is no upper bound. Recall that d is the probability that an *ON* time will end without any packets. Also, distributions where the vast majority of *ON* times are very small are possible, leading to a value for d that can be very close to 1, making $1/(1 - d)$ arbitrarily large in (8.3.13d). ▲

The formula for the autocovariance leads to two interesting results, which we state as theorems. The following is really a corollary to Theorem 8.2.1.

Theorem 8.3.1: For any pure MMPP ***ON-OFF arrival process***, if the *ON*-time distribution is exponentially distributed, then the process is a renewal process (the interarrival times are iid). This is true irrespective of the *OFF*-time distribution. The interarrival times are represented by $\langle \boldsymbol{\wp}, \boldsymbol{\mathcal{B}} \rangle$, where

$$\boldsymbol{\mathcal{B}} = \begin{bmatrix} \mu_1 + \lambda_p & -\mu_1 \mathbf{p}_2 \\ -\mathbf{B_2} \boldsymbol{\epsilon}_2' & \mathbf{B_2} \end{bmatrix}$$

and $\wp = [1, 0, \ldots, 0]$. ■

Proof: The formulas of Example 8.3.2 apply here with the following substitutions: $\mathbf{I_1} \to 1$, $\mathbf{B_1} \to \mu_1 := 1/\bar{t}_1$, $\mathbf{V_1} \to \bar{t}_1$, $\mathbf{p}_1 \to 1$ $\mathbf{D_1} \to 1/(1+\bar{n}_p)$, and $\boldsymbol{\epsilon}'_1 \to 1$. Then

$$\boldsymbol{\mathcal{L}} \Longrightarrow \lambda_p \begin{bmatrix} 1 & \mathbf{o} \\ \mathbf{o}' & \mathbf{0} \end{bmatrix} = \lambda_p \begin{bmatrix} 1 \\ \mathbf{o}' \end{bmatrix} \wp;$$

that is, $[\boldsymbol{\mathcal{L}}]_{11} = 1$ and all other elements are 0. Also,

$$\boldsymbol{\mathcal{Y}} \Longrightarrow \begin{bmatrix} 1 & \mathbf{o} \\ \boldsymbol{\epsilon}'_2 & \mathbf{0} \end{bmatrix} = \boldsymbol{\varepsilon}' \wp.$$

This makes $\boldsymbol{\mathcal{L}}$ and $\boldsymbol{\mathcal{Y}}$ rank-1 matrices. Therefore by Theorem 8.2.1 the process is a renewal process. Each departure epoch (time between departures) can be described in the following way. The customer starts in S_1. Because it is exponential no $\mathbf{p}_1$ vector is necessary. Then, after mean time $\bar{t}_1$ he either departs [with probability $\bar{n}_p/(1+\bar{n}_p)$] or goes to S_2. After a mean time of $\bar{t}_2 = \mathbf{p}_2\mathbf{V_2}\boldsymbol{\epsilon}'_2$, he returns to S_1. The cycle continues until he finally departs. Each new customer begins at the exponential server, so the interdeparture times are iid. **QED**

The second interesting result concerns autocovariance and autocorrelation, and is given in the following.

Theorem 8.3.2: The $\mathrm{Cov}(X, X_{+k})$s are independent of the *OFF-time* distribution. Also, $\hat{r}(k)$ varies inversely with σ^2_{OFF} but no other moments. ■

Proof: The autocovariance lag-k is given by (8.2.12b), but first we look at (8.2.12a). From the previous example we see that $\boldsymbol{\mathcal{Y}}$ is of the form

$$\boldsymbol{\mathcal{Y}} = \begin{bmatrix} \mathbf{A} & \mathbf{0} \\ \mathbf{B} & \mathbf{0} \end{bmatrix}.$$

Direct multiplication shows that

$$\boldsymbol{\mathcal{Y}}^k = \begin{bmatrix} \mathbf{A}^k & \mathbf{0} \\ \mathbf{B}\,\mathbf{A}^{k-1} & \mathbf{0} \end{bmatrix} = \begin{bmatrix} \mathbf{A} & \mathbf{0} \\ \mathbf{B} & \mathbf{0} \end{bmatrix} \begin{bmatrix} \mathbf{A}^{k-1} & \mathbf{0} \\ \mathbf{0} & \mathbf{0} \end{bmatrix}$$

and $\wp\boldsymbol{\mathcal{V}}\boldsymbol{\mathcal{Y}}$ is of the form $[\mathbf{a}_1, \mathbf{o}]$. Thus, from (8.2.12a), $\mathbb{E}[X, X_{+k}]$ is of the form

$$[\wp\boldsymbol{\mathcal{V}}\boldsymbol{\mathcal{Y}}]\,\boldsymbol{\mathcal{Y}}^{k-1}\,[\boldsymbol{\mathcal{V}}\boldsymbol{\varepsilon}'] = [\mathbf{a}_1, \mathbf{o}] \begin{bmatrix} \mathbf{A}^{k-1} & \mathbf{0} \\ \mathbf{0} & \mathbf{0} \end{bmatrix} \begin{bmatrix} \mathbf{c}'_1 \\ \mathbf{d}'_2 \end{bmatrix} = \mathbf{a}_1\,\mathbf{A}^{k-1}\mathbf{c}'_1,$$

where

$$\mathbf{a}_1 = \frac{1}{\lambda_p \bar{t}_1}\left[\mathbf{p}_1\mathbf{V}_1 + \frac{\bar{t}_2}{1-d}\mathbf{p}_1(\mathbf{I}_1 - \mathbf{D}_1)\right],$$

$$\mathbf{A} = \lambda_p\left[\mathbf{V}_1\mathbf{D}_1 + \frac{1}{1-d}\mathbf{D}_1\boldsymbol{\epsilon}'_1\mathbf{p}_1\mathbf{V}_1\mathbf{D}_1\right],$$

and

$$\mathbf{c}_1' = \left[\frac{1}{\lambda_p}\boldsymbol{\epsilon}_1' + \frac{\bar{t}_2}{1-d}\mathbf{D}_1\boldsymbol{\epsilon}_1'\right].$$

The calculations can be done entirely in S_1 space. Next, from (8.2.12b) and (8.3.13a),

$$\mathrm{Cov}(X, X_{+k}) = \mathbf{a}_1\,\mathbf{A}^{k-1}\mathbf{c}_1' - \left[\frac{\bar{t}_1 + \bar{t}_2}{\lambda_p \bar{t}_1}\right]^2. \tag{8.3.14a}$$

By looking at $\mathbf{A}$, $\mathbf{a}_1$, $\mathbf{c}_1'$, and $\mathbb{E}[X]$ it is clear that $\mathrm{Cov}(X, X_{+k})$ does not depend on the *OFF*-time distribution, except for $\bar{t}_2$. In other words, it is the same for every *OFF*-time distribution with the same mean. However, it depends very heavily on the *ON*-time distribution through the operators $\mathbf{V}_1$ and $\mathbf{D}_1$, and is different for each value of k because they will appear in ever-increasing powers with increasing k.

The autocorrelation coefficient lag-k is found from (8.2.12c) and (8.3.13c) by evaluating:

$$\hat{r}(k) = \frac{\mathrm{Cov}(X, X_{+k})}{\sigma_X^2}. \tag{8.3.14b}$$

$\hat{r}(k)$ behaves in a manner similar to $\mathrm{Cov}(X, X_{+k})$ in that systems with different *OFF*-time distributions will show proportional behavior for all k. Interestingly, if the *OFF*-time is PT, with $\sigma_2^2 = \infty$, then $\sigma_X^2 = \infty$ and $\hat{r}(k) = 0$ even though the autocovariance is finite and measurable. Even if the PT is truncated, σ_2^2 may be extremely large, and $\hat{r}(k)$ may be too small to measure. **QED**

But if there is some background Poisson traffic, then all bets are off. Customers depart during the *OFF*-times, and all those components that were identically 0 are now finite. Several researchers have observed behavior such as that described here [AntoniosSchwefelLip07]. Perhaps this analysis will explain those results. We go into this further after the following example.

Example 8.3.3: Here we find an explicit algebraic expression for $\hat{r}(1)$. From (8.3.14a),

$$\mathrm{Cov}(X, X_{+1})$$
$$= \frac{1}{\bar{n}_p}\left[\mathbf{p}_1\mathbf{V}_1 + \frac{\bar{t}_2}{1-d}\mathbf{p}_1(\mathbf{I}_1 - \mathbf{D}_1)\right]\left[\frac{1}{\lambda_p}\boldsymbol{\epsilon}_1' + \frac{\bar{t}_2}{1-d}\mathbf{D}_1\boldsymbol{\epsilon}_1'\right] - \left[\frac{\bar{t}_1 + \bar{t}_2}{\bar{n}_p}\right]^2.$$

From Example 8.3.2, $d = \alpha_o(\bar{n}_p)$ and the covariance can be written as

$$\mathrm{Cov}(X, X_{+1}) = \left[\frac{\bar{t}_2}{\bar{n}_p}\right]^2\left[\frac{\bar{n}_p\alpha_1(\bar{n}_p)}{[1-\alpha_o(\bar{n}_p)]^2} - 1\right].$$

Combining this with (8.3.13c), we get

$$\hat{r}(1) = \frac{b^2\left[\frac{\bar{n}_p\alpha_1}{(1-\alpha_o)^2} - 1\right]}{1 + b^2\left[\bar{n}_p C_2^2 + \frac{2\bar{n}_p}{1-\alpha_o} - (\bar{n}_p + 2)\right]}.$$

Well, it could have turned out messier. It does display the properties we established previously. For instance, if $b \to 0$ then $\hat{r}(1) = 0$, as should be the case for all $\hat{r}(k)$, because in that limit the process becomes a Poisson process. Furthermore, it depends on S_2 only through C_2^2 and decreases with increasing variance. In addition, it only depends on the probabilities of having 0 or 1 packet in the *ON* period.

Last, for exponential *ON* times,

$$\alpha_k(\bar{n}_p) = \left[\frac{\bar{n}_p}{\bar{n}_p + 1}\right]^k \frac{1}{\bar{n}_p + 1}.$$

As would be expected, geometric distribution of packets per burst yields exponential *ON* times, and it is independent of λ_p and $\bar{t}_1$. It also follows that $\hat{r}(1) = 0$, consistent with Theorem 8.3.1. ▲

MRP's with Background Poisson Traffic Added

We now return to the question of what happens when there is background Poisson traffic. Here, for any MRP, whatever phase the token is in, the background source produces at the rate λ_b. The $\boldsymbol{\mathcal{Q}}$ matrix doesn't change, and $\boldsymbol{\mathcal{L}}$ is modified to:

$$\boldsymbol{\mathcal{L}}_{\mathbf{b}} = \boldsymbol{\mathcal{L}} + \lambda_b \boldsymbol{\mathcal{I}}$$

and $\boldsymbol{\mathcal{B}}$ is modified to

$$\boldsymbol{\mathcal{B}}_{\mathbf{b}} = \boldsymbol{\mathcal{Q}} + \boldsymbol{\mathcal{L}}_{\mathbf{b}} = \boldsymbol{\mathcal{B}} + \lambda_b \boldsymbol{\mathcal{I}}.$$

We look at the special case of merging renewal processes in Section 8.3.3. If one of them is Poisson, then that is equivalent to what we have here. But right now we are interested in what happens to an *ON-OFF* process. If the term $\lambda_b \boldsymbol{\mathcal{I}}$ is added to $\boldsymbol{\mathcal{L}}$ in Example 8.3.2, then the result is a process that looks exactly like any 2-server MMPP. This leads us to the following theorem.

Theorem 8.3.3: Every MMPP is equivalent to some *ON-OFF* MMPP with background Poisson traffic. ■

Proof: Consider any MMPP with $\boldsymbol{\mathcal{Q}}$, $\boldsymbol{\mathcal{L}}$, and $\boldsymbol{\mathcal{B}}$ given. Because the process is MMPP,

$$\boldsymbol{\mathcal{L}} = \text{Diag}[\lambda_1 \mathbf{I_1}, \lambda_2 \mathbf{I_2}, \cdots, \lambda_M \mathbf{I_M}].$$

Define λ_b as the smallest λs. That is

$$\lambda_b := \text{Min}\{\lambda_i | 1 \le i \le M\}.$$

We now construct an *ON-OFF* process (using subscript "**oo**") as follows. Let

$$\boldsymbol{\mathcal{L}}_{\mathbf{oo}} = \boldsymbol{\mathcal{L}} - \lambda_b \boldsymbol{\mathcal{I}}, \qquad \boldsymbol{\mathcal{Q}}_{\mathbf{oo}} = \boldsymbol{\mathcal{Q}}, \quad \text{and} \quad \boldsymbol{\mathcal{B}}_{\mathbf{oo}} = \boldsymbol{\mathcal{B}} - \lambda_b \boldsymbol{\mathcal{I}}.$$

Then $\{\boldsymbol{\mathcal{L}}_{\mathbf{oo}}, \boldsymbol{\mathcal{B}}_{\mathbf{oo}}, \boldsymbol{\mathcal{Q}}_{\mathbf{oo}}\}$ is an *ON-OFF* process. After all, while the token is visiting the server corresponding to λ_b no packets are leaving; that is, it's *OFF*. We can now reverse the process by adding $\lambda_b \boldsymbol{\mathcal{I}}$ to the *ON-OFF* process and end up with the original MMPP. **QED**

One might ask if this is true in general. The answer is "No." It is true for MMPP's because of the particular structure of $\mathcal{L}$, but each process must be examined individually. We show this in what follows.

Modified Augmented ON-OFF MMPP Model (MAOOMMPP)

We next examine the augmented MMPP that is also an *ON-OFF* process (MAOOMMPP). This process forces the *ON* server to yield at least one packet per token visit. But it cannot be a special case of the AMMPP model presented in Section 8.3.2.4. There, every token visit to every server produced at least one packet. This must not be allowed to happen at the *OFF* server. The way we augmented the MMPP model was to add $\mathcal{B}_o\langle \boldsymbol{P}\rangle$ to $\mathcal{L}$. A particular term in that matrix is $\mathbf{B_i}\boldsymbol{\epsilon}'_\mathbf{i}P_{ij}\mathbf{p_j}$, or $\mathbf{M_i}\,\mathbf{q}'_\mathbf{i}P_{ij}\mathbf{p_j}$. Its interpretation is as follows. Start with the token finishing in phase k of server S_i $[(\mathbf{M_i})_{kk}]$, leaving S_i $[(\mathbf{q_i})_k]$, going to S_j $[(\boldsymbol{P})_{ij}]$, and finally going to phase ℓ in S_j $[(\mathbf{p}_j)_\ell]$. Because this is a term in the $\mathcal{L}$ matrix, it causes a customer to depart. If S_i is the *OFF* server, then this shouldn't happen. Therefore we *modify* the augmented model by setting that corresponding row (now call it ℓ) to $\mathbf{0}$. That is, the matrix block $\mathcal{B}_{\ell \mathbf{j}} = \mathcal{O}$. This can be done formally by defining $\mathcal{I}_{oo}$ as

$$\mathcal{I}_{oo} := \text{Diag}[\mathbf{I}_1, \ldots, \mathbf{I}_{\ell-1}, \mathbf{0}, \mathbf{I}_{\ell+1}, \cdots, \mathbf{I}_\mathbf{M}].$$

Then the *Modified Augmented ON-OFF MMPP* (MAOOMMPP) model is:

$$\begin{aligned} \mathcal{Q} &= \mathcal{B}_o - \mathcal{B}_o\langle \boldsymbol{P}\rangle; \\ \mathcal{L} &= \mathcal{L}_o + \mathcal{B}_o\mathcal{I}_{oo}\langle \boldsymbol{P}\rangle; \qquad (8.3.15) \\ \mathcal{B} &= \mathcal{B}_o + \mathcal{L}_o - \mathcal{B}_o(\mathcal{I}_o - \mathcal{I}_{oo})\langle \boldsymbol{P}\rangle. \end{aligned}$$

Compare with the comparable entries in Table 8.3.1. We now explore the two-server system in the following example.

Example 8.3.4: Consider a system as in Example 8.3.2, but now the *ON* time must have at least one packet, and the *OFF* time must have none. Assume that when the token leaves the *ON* server he emits a packet, giving the MAOOMMPP. Let $M = 2$, then (8.3.15) becomes

$$\mathcal{L} = \begin{bmatrix} \lambda_p\mathbf{I}_1 & \mathbf{B}_1\boldsymbol{\epsilon}'_1\mathbf{p}_2 \\ 0 & 0 \end{bmatrix}, \qquad \mathcal{B} = \begin{bmatrix} \mathbf{B}_1 + \lambda_p\mathbf{I}_1 & 0 \\ -\mathbf{B}_2\boldsymbol{\epsilon}'_2\mathbf{p}_1 & \mathbf{B}_2 \end{bmatrix},$$

$$\mathcal{Q} = \begin{bmatrix} \mathbf{B}_1 & -\mathbf{B}_1\boldsymbol{\epsilon}'_1\mathbf{p}_2 \\ -\mathbf{B}_2\boldsymbol{\epsilon}'_2\mathbf{p}_1 & \mathbf{B}_2 \end{bmatrix}.$$

It is straightforward to set up $\mathcal{V}$ and $\mathcal{Y}$.

$$\mathcal{V} = \begin{bmatrix} \mathbf{V}_1\mathbf{D}_1 & 0 \\ \boldsymbol{\epsilon}'_2\mathbf{p}_1\mathbf{V}_1\mathbf{D}_1 & \mathbf{V}_2 \end{bmatrix} \quad \text{and} \quad \mathcal{Y} = \begin{bmatrix} \mathbf{I}_1 - \mathbf{D}_1 & \mathbf{D}_1\boldsymbol{\epsilon}'_1\mathbf{p}_2 \\ \boldsymbol{\epsilon}'_2\mathbf{p}_1(\mathbf{I}_1 - \mathbf{D}_1) & d\boldsymbol{\epsilon}'_2\mathbf{p}_2 \end{bmatrix}.$$

$\mathcal{Q}$ is the same as before. Therefore we already know what $\boldsymbol{\pi}$ is, and get $\boldsymbol{\wp}$ from that.

$$\boldsymbol{\pi} = \frac{1}{\bar{t}_1 + \bar{t}_2}[\mathbf{p}_1\mathbf{V}_1, \mathbf{p}_2\mathbf{V}_2] \quad \text{and} \quad \boldsymbol{\wp} = \frac{1}{1 + \lambda_p\bar{t}_1}[\lambda_p\mathbf{p}_1\mathbf{V}_1, \mathbf{p}_2].$$

The flow rate is

$$\kappa = \boldsymbol{\pi}\boldsymbol{\mathcal{L}}\boldsymbol{\varepsilon}' = \frac{1}{\boldsymbol{\wp}\boldsymbol{\mathcal{V}}\boldsymbol{\varepsilon}'} = \frac{1+\lambda_p\bar{t}_1}{\bar{t}_1+\bar{t}_2}.$$

The denominator is the mean cycle time, so the mean number of packets per burst is one more than in the pure *ON-OFF* MMPP model, as we would have hoped.

Before going on, we examine $\boldsymbol{\mathcal{Y}}$. Although it is more complex than the $\boldsymbol{\mathcal{Y}}$ for the pure MMPP *ON-OFF* process in Example 8.3.2, it has the same rank. The other $\boldsymbol{\mathcal{Y}}$ has m_2 columns of all zeroes. Also its $\boldsymbol{\mathcal{Y}}_{11}$ block matrix has an inverse. Therefore it must be of rank m_1. This $\boldsymbol{\mathcal{Y}} = \boldsymbol{\mathcal{V}}\boldsymbol{\mathcal{L}}$, as it must. $\boldsymbol{\mathcal{L}}$ has m_2 rows of 0, and so must be of rank m_1. Therefore, $\boldsymbol{\mathcal{Y}}$ must also have rank m_1.

If in particular, the *ON* time is exponentially distributed then $m_1 = 1$ and $\boldsymbol{\mathcal{Y}}$ is of rank 1, just as in Theorem 8.3.1. Therefore, here too, if the *ON*-time distribution is exponential, the process is a renewal process. Direct substitution shows that $\boldsymbol{\mathcal{L}}$ and $\boldsymbol{\mathcal{Y}}$ reduce to

$$\boldsymbol{\mathcal{L}} = \begin{bmatrix} \lambda_p & (1/\bar{t}_1)\mathbf{p}_2 \\ \mathbf{o}' & \mathbf{0} \end{bmatrix}$$

and

$$\boldsymbol{\mathcal{Y}} = \begin{bmatrix} 1-d & d\,\mathbf{p}_2 \\ (1-d)\boldsymbol{\epsilon}_2' & d\boldsymbol{\epsilon}_2' \end{bmatrix} = \begin{bmatrix} 1 \\ \boldsymbol{\epsilon}_2' \end{bmatrix} [1-d,\, d\,\mathbf{p}_2] = \boldsymbol{\varepsilon}'\boldsymbol{\wp},$$

whereas $\boldsymbol{\mathcal{B}}$ and $\boldsymbol{\mathcal{V}}$ reduce to

$$\boldsymbol{\mathcal{B}} = \begin{bmatrix} 1/\bar{t}_1\, d & \mathbf{o} \\ -\mathbf{B}_2\boldsymbol{\epsilon}_2' & \mathbf{B}_2 \end{bmatrix} \quad \text{and} \quad \boldsymbol{\mathcal{V}} = \begin{bmatrix} \bar{t}_1 d & \mathbf{o} \\ \bar{t}_1\, d\boldsymbol{\epsilon}_2' & \mathbf{V}_2 \end{bmatrix},$$

where $d = 1/(1+\lambda_p\bar{t}_1)$. As already stated, this is a renewal process with interdeparture times generated by $\langle\, \boldsymbol{\wp}, \boldsymbol{\mathcal{B}}\rangle$. The reader should show directly that

$$\mathbb{E}[X] = \boldsymbol{\wp}\boldsymbol{\mathcal{V}}\boldsymbol{\varepsilon}' = d(\bar{t}_1+\bar{t}_2) \quad \text{and}$$
$$\sigma_X^2 = d\,\sigma_2^2 + d^2\,\bar{t}_1^2 + d(1-d)\bar{t}_2^2.$$

We return now to nonexponential *ON* times, The formulas get quite messy as we attempt to find σ_X^2 and other properties. We find that

$$\boldsymbol{\wp}\boldsymbol{\mathcal{V}} = \frac{1}{1+\lambda_p\bar{t}_1}[\mathbf{p}_1\mathbf{V}_1,\ \mathbf{p}_2\mathbf{V}_2]$$

and

$$\boldsymbol{\mathcal{V}}\boldsymbol{\varepsilon}' = \begin{bmatrix} \mathbf{V}_1\mathbf{D}_1\boldsymbol{\epsilon}_1' \\ \Psi[\mathbf{V}_1\mathbf{D}_1]\boldsymbol{\epsilon}_2' + \mathbf{V}_2\boldsymbol{\epsilon}_2' \end{bmatrix}.$$

It is easy enough to evaluate $\boldsymbol{\wp}\boldsymbol{\mathcal{V}}\boldsymbol{\mathcal{V}}\boldsymbol{\varepsilon}'$ numerically for any specific values of the various parameters, but the analytic expression is somewhat long and not too informative. However, it can be seen that it, and therefore σ_X^2, depends on the *OFF* time explicitly through $\mathbf{p_2 V_2^2 \epsilon_2'}$ and $\bar{t}_2$ only, similar to (8.3.13c). For autocorrelation $\mathcal{Y}$ is not as simple as that in Example 8.3.2, but it does not contain any information about the *OFF*-time. It pays for us to look at

$$\wp\mathcal{V}\mathcal{Y} = \frac{1}{1+\lambda_p \bar{t}_1}[\mathbf{p}_1[(\mathbf{V_1} + \bar{t}_2\mathbf{I_1}(\mathbf{I_1} - \mathbf{D_1})],\ (\Psi[\mathbf{V_1 D_1}] + d\bar{t}_2)\mathbf{p}_2].$$

This also has no dependence on the *OFF*-time distribution except for its mean. $\mathcal{V}\varepsilon'$ does contain $\mathbf{V_2}$, but $\mathcal{Y}\mathcal{V}\varepsilon'$ does not, as displayed below.

$$\mathcal{Y}\mathcal{V}\varepsilon' = \begin{bmatrix} [(\mathbf{I_1} - \mathbf{D_1})\mathbf{V_1 D_1} + \Psi[\mathbf{V_1 D_1}] + \bar{t}_2\mathbf{D_1}]\,\boldsymbol{\epsilon}_1' \\ \\ [\Psi[(\mathbf{I_1} - \mathbf{D_1})\mathbf{V_1 D_1}] + d\Psi[\mathbf{V_1 D_1}] + \bar{t}_2 d]\,\boldsymbol{\epsilon}_2' \end{bmatrix}.$$

the autocorrelation lag-k depends on $(\wp\mathcal{V}\mathcal{Y})\mathcal{Y}^{k-2}(\mathcal{Y}\mathcal{V}\varepsilon')$, and given that none of the bracketed terms depends on $\mathbf{V_2}$, it therefore follows that the MAOOMMPP does not depend on the *OFF*-time distribution, similar to the unmodified process in Theorem 8.3.2.

We have seen that although the OOMMPP and MAOOMMPP processes have similar behavior, they are not equivalent. After all, they do have different mean interdeparture times. Furthermore, the OOMMPP is an MMPP, but the MAOOMMPP is not. In the next subsection we quickly look at another variation.

Alternative Modified Augmented *ON-OFF* Model

This process abbreviates to AMAOOMMPP. (YES, we have been carried away with acronyms, but they do carry some meaning.) We finally present our last variation of Markov modulated processes. Our purpose (besides generating long strings) is to show how physical ideas can be implemented into mathematical models, and also to see that systems that are differently described can still produce physically identical results even though they appear to be different mathematically. In Section 3.4 we showed, through ***isometric transformations***, that a single ME distribution can have an infinite number of distinct representations. The same could be true for more general systems.

In the MAOOMMPP model each *ON*-time ends with a packet transmission. An outside observer cannot tell for sure when that *ON*-time began, because the motion of the token is not observable, but the final packet could tell her when it ended if marking of packets were allowed. In this section we look at a different scenario, namely, each *ON*-time begins with a packet transmission. We do this by allowing the token to send a packet whenever it leaves the *OFF* server. Then that packet can be considered to be the first of the next *ON* period for whichever server the token moves to next.

Let S_ℓ be the *OFF* server. In the previous section by setting the matrix block $\mathcal{B}_{\ell \mathrm{j}}$ to 0, we were able to have the token not emit a packet as he left S_ℓ. Now, instead, we want the token not to emit a packet as he enters S_ℓ.

Then $\boldsymbol{\mathcal{B}}_{\mathbf{j}\boldsymbol{\ell}} = \mathbf{0}$ for all j. This can be done in the following way. In analogy with Equations (8.3.15) we have

$$\begin{aligned} \boldsymbol{\mathcal{Q}} &= \boldsymbol{\mathcal{B}}_{\text{o}} - \boldsymbol{\mathcal{B}}_{\text{o}}\langle P \rangle \\ \boldsymbol{\mathcal{L}} &= \boldsymbol{\mathcal{L}}_{\text{o}} + \boldsymbol{\mathcal{B}}_{\text{o}}\langle P \rangle \boldsymbol{\mathcal{I}}_{\text{oo}} \qquad (8.3.16) \\ \boldsymbol{\mathcal{B}} &= \boldsymbol{\mathcal{B}}_{\text{o}} + \boldsymbol{\mathcal{L}}_{\text{o}} - \boldsymbol{\mathcal{B}}_{\text{o}}\langle P \rangle (\boldsymbol{\mathcal{I}}_{\text{o}} - \boldsymbol{\mathcal{I}}_{\text{oo}}). \end{aligned}$$

We now consider the two-server system where the token emits a packet upon entering the *ON* server (or leaving the *OFF* server).

Example 8.3.5: Consider a system as in Example 8.3.4, but now a packet is emitted as the token enters the *ON* state. Then

$$\boldsymbol{\mathcal{L}} = \begin{bmatrix} \lambda_p \mathbf{I_1} & \mathbf{0} \\ \mathbf{B_2}\boldsymbol{\epsilon}_2'\mathbf{p}_1 & \mathbf{0} \end{bmatrix}, \qquad \boldsymbol{\mathcal{Q}} = \begin{bmatrix} \mathbf{B_1} & -\mathbf{B_1}\boldsymbol{\epsilon}_1'\mathbf{p}_2 \\ -\mathbf{B_2}\boldsymbol{\epsilon}_2'\mathbf{p}_1 & \mathbf{B_2} \end{bmatrix},$$

$$\boldsymbol{\mathcal{B}} = \begin{bmatrix} \mathbf{B_1} + \lambda_p \mathbf{I_1} & -\mathbf{B_1}\boldsymbol{\epsilon}_1'\mathbf{p}_2 \\ \mathbf{0} & \mathbf{B_2} \end{bmatrix}.$$

It is straightforward to set up $\boldsymbol{\mathcal{V}}$ and $\boldsymbol{\mathcal{Y}}$:

$$\boldsymbol{\mathcal{V}} = \begin{bmatrix} \mathbf{V_1 D_1} & \mathbf{D_1}\boldsymbol{\epsilon}_1'\mathbf{p_2 V_2} \\ \mathbf{0} & \mathbf{V_2} \end{bmatrix} \quad \text{and} \quad \boldsymbol{\mathcal{Y}} = \begin{bmatrix} \mathbf{I_1} - \mathbf{D_1} + \mathbf{D_1}\boldsymbol{\epsilon}_1'\mathbf{p}_1 & \mathbf{0} \\ \boldsymbol{\epsilon}_2'\mathbf{p}_1 & \mathbf{0} \end{bmatrix}.$$

Once again $\boldsymbol{\mathcal{Q}}$ is the same as before, so we get

$$\boldsymbol{\pi} = \frac{1}{\bar{t}_1 + \bar{t}_2}[\mathbf{p_1 V_1},\, \mathbf{p_2 V_2}] \quad \text{and} \quad \wp = \frac{1}{1 + \lambda_p \bar{t}_1}[p_1(\mathbf{I_1} + \lambda_p \mathbf{V_1}),\, \mathbf{o}].$$

The flow rate is the same as that for the MAOOMMPP, namely

$$\kappa = \boldsymbol{\pi}\boldsymbol{\mathcal{L}}\boldsymbol{\mathcal{E}}' = \frac{1}{\wp \boldsymbol{\mathcal{V}}\boldsymbol{\mathcal{E}}'} = \frac{1 + \lambda_p \bar{t}_1}{\bar{t}_1 + \bar{t}_2}.$$

We can also show that the two processes have the same variance.

So, what have we here? Observe that $\boldsymbol{\mathcal{Y}}$ and $\boldsymbol{\mathcal{L}}$ have zeroes in their second columns. It is that property we used to prove Theorems 8.3.1 and 8.3.2 for the pure *ON-OFF* process. Therefore, those theorems must apply here as well. ▲

We summarize this section with a theorem and a conjecture which is very likely true.

Theorem 8.3.4: Markov modulated *ON-OFF* processes, with and without the modifications discussed above, share the following properties.

1. The autocovariance lag-k is independent of the *OFF*-time distribution;

2. The variance for the interdeparture times σ_X^2 depends on the *OFF*-time distribution only through its variance σ_{0FF}^2. Therefore, the $\hat{r}(k)$s are proportional for all *OFF-time* distributions with the same mean;
3. If the *ON*-time is exponentially distributed, then the process is a renewal process.

Conjecture: Although the MAOOMMPP and AMOOAMMPP processes have different representations (Examples 8.3.4 and 8.3.5), they are equivalent.
Evidence: They have the same mean and variance; They both satisfy 1. to 3. above, their $\boldsymbol{\mathcal{B}}$ matrices have the same set of eigenvalues, and therefore there exists an isometric transformation that connects them, their $\boldsymbol{\mathcal{Y}}$s have the same rank (m_1), they have the same $\hat{r}(1)$, previous calculations ([SCHWEFEL00]) of specific models have yielded results that are the same to within calculation error. ■

8.3.3 Merging Renewal Processes

It would seem at first thought that the merging of two independent renewal streams would produce a composite stream with zero covariance. Except for Poisson processes, this is not the case. In fact, this is more complicated to describe than the processes of the previous sections. In what follows, we restrict ourselves to two processes, although a generalization to more streams is straightforward.

Visualize an infinite queue feeding into two general servers S_1 and S_2 represented, respectively, by $\langle\, \mathbf{p}_j\,,\, \mathbf{B}_j\,\rangle$, $j = 1, 2$. Then two customers are being served simultaneously and independently. Thus the state space needed must be a ***direct product*** of the spaces needed to describe each. We use the standard ***Kronecker product*** representation here (see Chapter 7 and, e.g., [GRAHAM81]). The following are square matrices of dimension $m_1\, m_2$.

$$\begin{aligned} \hat{\mathbf{B}}_1 &:= \mathbf{B}_1 \otimes \mathbf{I}_2 \\ \hat{\mathbf{B}}_2 &:= \mathbf{I}_1 \otimes \mathbf{B}_2. \end{aligned} \tag{8.3.17}$$

Then the generator matrix for the interdeparture times is

$$\boldsymbol{\mathcal{B}} = \hat{\mathbf{B}}_1 + \hat{\mathbf{B}}_2, \quad \text{and} \tag{8.3.18a}$$

$$\boldsymbol{\mathcal{V}} = [\hat{\mathbf{B}}_1 + \hat{\mathbf{B}}_2]^{-1} = \hat{\mathbf{V}}_1\hat{\mathbf{V}}_2[\hat{\mathbf{V}}_1 + \hat{\mathbf{V}}_2]^{-1}. \tag{8.3.18b}$$

From its definition, the $\boldsymbol{\mathcal{L}}$ matrix is (where $\mathbf{Q_j} = \boldsymbol{\epsilon}'_{\mathbf{j}}\, \mathbf{p_j}$)

$$\boldsymbol{\mathcal{L}} = \hat{\mathbf{B}}_1\, \hat{\mathbf{Q}}_1 + \hat{\mathbf{B}}_2\, \hat{\mathbf{Q}}_2 \tag{8.3.18c}$$

which certainly satisfies (8.2.1). Then from (8.2.2),

$$\boldsymbol{\mathcal{Y}} = [\hat{\mathbf{B}}_1 + \hat{\mathbf{B}}_2]^{-1}\, [\hat{\mathbf{B}}_1\, \hat{\mathbf{Q}}_1 + \hat{\mathbf{B}}_2\, \hat{\mathbf{Q}}_2] = [\hat{\mathbf{V}}_1 + \hat{\mathbf{V}}_2]^{-1}\, [\hat{\mathbf{V}}_2\, \hat{\mathbf{Q}}_1 + \hat{\mathbf{V}}_1\, \hat{\mathbf{Q}}_2], \tag{8.3.19a}$$

and by (8.2.8a)

$$\mathcal{Q} = \mathcal{B} - \mathcal{L} = \hat{\mathbf{B}}_1(\mathbf{I} - \hat{\mathbf{Q}}_1) + \hat{\mathbf{B}}_2(\mathbf{I} - \hat{\mathbf{Q}}_2). \tag{8.3.19b}$$

By direct substitution, it can be shown that

$$\wp = \frac{1}{\bar{x}_1 + \bar{x}_2}(\mathbf{p}_1 \otimes \mathbf{p}_2)(\hat{\mathbf{V}}_1 + \hat{\mathbf{V}}_2) \tag{8.3.20a}$$

and satisfies $\wp \mathcal{Y} = \wp$. Also, from (8.2.8b)

$$\boldsymbol{\pi} = c\,\wp \mathcal{V} = \frac{1}{\bar{x}_1\,\bar{x}_2}(\mathbf{p}_1 \otimes \mathbf{p}_2)(\hat{\mathbf{V}}_1\,\hat{\mathbf{V}}_2), \tag{8.3.20b}$$

$$\begin{aligned} \mathbb{E}[X] &= \wp[\hat{\mathbf{B}}_1 + \hat{\mathbf{B}}_2]^{-1}\boldsymbol{\varepsilon}' = \wp[\hat{\mathbf{V}}_1 + \hat{\mathbf{V}}_2]^{-1}\,\hat{\mathbf{V}}_1\,\hat{\mathbf{V}}_2\,\boldsymbol{\varepsilon}' \\ &= \frac{\bar{x}_1\,\bar{x}_2}{\bar{x}_1 + \bar{x}_2} = \frac{1}{(1/\bar{x}_1 + 1/\bar{x}_2)}. \end{aligned} \tag{8.3.20c}$$

Clearly, the mean arrival rate $(1/\bar{x})$ is equal to the sum of the arrival rates $[(1/\bar{x_1} + 1/\bar{x_2})]$ of the two streams. This is only true for the steady state, or when many customers have already departed.

These equations are perfectly amenable to numerical computation, but we can get analytical results if S_1 or S_2 is an exponential server (or equivalently, if one of the processes is Poisson). Let $m_2 = 1$. Then $\mathbf{B}_2$ is a scalar, say λ, and we can drop the subscript for S_1. The product space is now the same as the state-space for S_1. The above equations become

$$\mathcal{B} = \mathbf{B} + \lambda \mathbf{I}, \tag{8.3.21a}$$

$$\mathcal{L} = \mathbf{B}\,\mathbf{Q} + \lambda \mathbf{I}, \qquad \mathcal{Q} = \mathbf{B} - \mathbf{B}\,\mathbf{Q}, \tag{8.3.21b}$$

and

$$\mathcal{Y} = [\lambda \mathbf{I} + \mathbf{B}]^{-1}\,[\lambda \mathbf{I} + \mathbf{B}\,\mathbf{Q}] = [\mathbf{I} + \lambda \mathbf{V}]^{-1}\,[\lambda \mathbf{V} + \mathbf{Q}]. \tag{8.3.21c}$$

Then (8.3.20a) becomes

$$\wp = \frac{1}{1 + \lambda \bar{x}}\mathbf{p}(\mathbf{I} + \lambda \mathbf{V}), \tag{8.3.21d}$$

satisfying $\wp \mathcal{Y} = \wp$ and $\wp \epsilon' = 1$. Also, from (8.3.20c), it follows that

$$\mathbb{E}[X] = \frac{\bar{x}}{1 + \lambda \bar{x}}. \tag{8.3.22a}$$

This process can be considered to be an AMMPP with one server where an additonal customer departs when the token leaves the server and then returns. (See Section 8.3.2.4 and let $M = 1$. See also Theorem 8.3.3.) Define $\mathbf{D} := [\mathbf{I} + \lambda \mathbf{V}]^{-1}$. Then the autocovariance lag-1 turns out to be

$$\lambda^2\,\mathrm{Cov}(X,\, X_{+1})$$

$$= \frac{1}{1+\lambda\bar{x}}\left[(\Psi[\lambda\mathbf{V}\mathbf{D}])^2 + \Psi[\lambda^3\,\mathbf{V}^3\,\mathbf{D}^2]\right] - \left[\frac{\lambda\bar{x}}{1+\lambda\bar{x}}\right]^2. \tag{8.3.22b}$$

Recall that $\lambda\mathbf{V}\mathbf{D} = \mathbf{I} - \mathbf{D}$, so from (4.4.1c)

$$\alpha_k(\lambda) := \Psi[(\lambda\mathbf{V}\mathbf{D})^k\,\mathbf{D}] = \int_{\mathrm{o}}^{\infty} \frac{(\lambda x)^k}{k!}\, e^{-\lambda x}\, f(x)\, dx. \tag{8.3.22c}$$

The integral clearly shows that $\alpha_k(\lambda)$ is the probability that there will be k departures from S_2 between departures from S_1. For future reference, it is not hard to see (in at least two different ways) that $\sum_{k=\mathrm{o}}^{\infty} \alpha_k(\lambda) = 1$.

Finally it can be shown that

$$\lambda^2\,\mathrm{Cov}(X,\, X_{+1}) = \frac{\alpha_{\mathrm{o}}^2 + \alpha_1}{1+\lambda\bar{x}} - \frac{1}{[1+\lambda\bar{x}]^2}. \tag{8.3.22d}$$

If $f(x)$ is exponential (two Poisson processes), then $\alpha_{\mathrm{o}} = 1/(1+\lambda\bar{x})$, $\alpha_1 = \lambda\bar{x}/(1+\lambda\bar{x})^2$, and the covariance is 0. Of course in this case, (8.3.21c) clearly shows that $\mathcal{Y}$ reduces to 1, and all correlations are 0. Thus we reprove the well-known theorem that the merging of Poisson processes is a Poisson process with mean arrival rate equal to the sum of the arrival rates of the individual processes.

Similar expressions can be derived for lag-2 or more, but with increasing difficulty. Note, however, that the last equation does not depend on any ME representation, so it is true for all distributions.

8.3.4 Departures from Overloaded Multiprocessor Systems

In Chapter 6 we discussed "generalized X/G/C-type systems". Such systems can be C identical servers, or even an arbitrary ***Jackson networklike*** collection of load-dependent exponential servers, for which only C customers can be active at once. The other customers must queue up. The matrices needed here are already defined in that chapter. The correspondence is as follows, where all matrices with subscript c are the ***reduced-product space*** operators explicitly defined in Chapter 6.

$$\begin{aligned} \mathcal{B} &= \mathbf{B}_c \\ \mathcal{L} &= \mathbf{M}_c\,\mathbf{Q}_c\,\mathbf{R}_c \\ \mathcal{Y} &= \mathbf{V}_c\,\mathbf{M}_c\,\mathbf{Q}_c\,\mathbf{R}_c \\ \wp_{\mathrm{o}} &= \mathbf{p}\,\mathbf{R}_2\,\mathbf{R}_3\,\cdots\,\mathbf{R}_c \\ \wp &= \pi_c. \end{aligned} \tag{8.3.23}$$

Imagine a large number of customers waiting to be served with C of them entering service simultaneously at the start. Then $\wp_{\mathrm{o}}$ is the initial vector, and many properties, including the mean time to drain the queue, as well as the interdeparture distributions and correlations can be calculated according to the formulas in this chapter.

8.3.5 Departures from ME/ME/1 Queues

Consider two servers S_1 and S_2 represented by vector-matrix pairs, $\langle\, \mathbf{p}_i\,,\, \mathbf{B}_i\,\rangle$, with dimension m_i. Further suppose that there is an infinite queue of customers waiting to be served one at a time by S_2. As was shown in Section 8.3.1, departures from S_2 constitute a renewal process. After being served, a customer moves "downstream" to S_1. The behavior of the queue at S_1 constitutes a G/G/1 queue. Assuming that $\mathbb{E}[T_2] > \mathbb{E}[T_1]$, S_1 will sometimes be empty, so the departure process from S_1 (almost always) is not a renewal process. It is this process that we analyze here. The subsystem includes everything upstream from the departure point of S_1. We must now deal with an infinite state-space, because not only must the states of the customers in service be tracked, but also the length of the queue at S_1.

8.3.5.1 If S_2 Is Exponential (M/ME/1 Queues)

Let S_2 be an exponential server with service rate λ. Then it generates a Poisson arrival process to S_1, now represented without subscripts by an m-dimensional vector-matrix pair, $\langle\, \mathbf{p}\,,\, \mathbf{B}\,\rangle$. The full-system matrices in this section (e.g., $\boldsymbol{\mathcal{L}}$, $\boldsymbol{\mathcal{Y}}$, $\boldsymbol{\mathcal{V}}$, $\boldsymbol{\mathcal{B}}$, and $\wp$) have elements that are of different size, because an empty queue is represented by a single state. Thus the $\{1,\ 1\}$ element of the $\boldsymbol{\mathcal{B}}$ matrix below is a scalar, whereas the other elements in row 1 are m-dimensional row vectors. Similarly, the other elements in the first column are column m-vectors. All other elements are $m \times m$ matrices. Analogous conditions hold for row- and column-vectors (e.g., $\wp$ and $\boldsymbol{\varepsilon}'$).

$$\boldsymbol{\mathcal{B}} = \begin{bmatrix} \lambda & -\lambda\mathbf{p} & \mathbf{o} & \mathbf{o} & \cdots \\ \mathbf{o}' & \mathbf{B}+\lambda\mathbf{I} & -\lambda\mathbf{I} & \mathbf{O} & \cdots \\ \mathbf{o}' & \mathbf{O} & \mathbf{B}+\lambda\mathbf{I} & -\lambda\mathbf{I} & \cdots \\ \mathbf{o}' & \mathbf{O} & \mathbf{O} & \mathbf{B}+\lambda\mathbf{I} & \cdots \\ \cdots & \cdots & \cdots & \cdots & \cdots \end{bmatrix} \tag{8.3.24a}$$

and thus

$$\boldsymbol{\mathcal{B}}\,\boldsymbol{\varepsilon}' = \begin{bmatrix} 0 \\ \mathbf{B}\boldsymbol{\epsilon}' \\ \mathbf{B}\boldsymbol{\epsilon}' \\ \mathbf{B}\boldsymbol{\epsilon}' \\ \cdots \end{bmatrix}.$$

As in the previous subsections, let $\mathbf{D} = [\mathbf{I} + \lambda\mathbf{V}]^{-1}$, then it can be shown that $\boldsymbol{\mathcal{B}}^{-1}$ is

$$\boldsymbol{\mathcal{V}} = \frac{1}{\lambda}\begin{bmatrix} 1 & \mathbf{p}\lambda\mathbf{V}\mathbf{D} & \mathbf{p}(\lambda\mathbf{V}\mathbf{D})^2 & \mathbf{p}(\lambda\mathbf{V}\mathbf{D})^3 & \cdots \\ \mathbf{o}' & \lambda\mathbf{V}\mathbf{D} & (\lambda\mathbf{V}\mathbf{D})^2 & (\lambda\mathbf{V}\mathbf{D})^3 & \cdots \\ \mathbf{o}' & \mathbf{O} & \lambda\mathbf{V}\mathbf{D} & (\lambda\mathbf{V}\mathbf{D})^2 & \cdots \\ \mathbf{o}' & \mathbf{O} & \mathbf{O} & \lambda\mathbf{V}\mathbf{D} & \cdots \\ \cdots & \cdots & \cdots & \cdots & \cdots \end{bmatrix}. \tag{8.3.24b}$$

It is not hard to see that the departure matrix is

$$\mathcal{L} = \begin{bmatrix} 0 & \mathrm{o} & \mathrm{o} & \mathrm{o} & \cdots \\ \mathbf{B}\epsilon' & \mathbf{O} & \mathbf{O} & \mathbf{O} & \cdots \\ \mathrm{o}' & \mathbf{BQ} & \mathbf{O} & \mathbf{O} & \cdots \\ \mathrm{o}' & \mathbf{O} & \mathbf{BQ} & \mathbf{O} & \cdots \\ \cdots & \cdots & \cdots & \cdots & \cdots \end{bmatrix} \quad \text{and} \quad \mathcal{L}\varepsilon' = \begin{bmatrix} 0 \\ \mathbf{B}\epsilon' \\ \mathbf{B}\epsilon' \\ \mathbf{B}\epsilon' \\ \cdots \end{bmatrix} = \mathcal{B}\varepsilon'. \quad (8.3.25a)$$

The matrix $\mathcal{Y}$ can now be written down:

$$\mathcal{Y} = \mathcal{V}\mathcal{L} =$$

$$\begin{bmatrix} \Psi[\mathbf{D}] & \Psi[\lambda\mathbf{V}\mathbf{D}^2]\,\mathbf{p} & \Psi[(\lambda\mathbf{V}\mathbf{D})^2\,\mathbf{D}]\,\mathbf{p} & \Psi[(\lambda\mathbf{V}\mathbf{D})^3\,\mathbf{D}]\,\mathbf{p} & \cdots \\ \mathbf{D}\epsilon' & (\lambda\mathbf{V}\mathbf{D})\mathbf{D}\mathbf{Q} & (\lambda\mathbf{V}\mathbf{D})^2\mathbf{D}\mathbf{Q} & (\lambda\mathbf{V}\mathbf{D})^3\mathbf{D}\mathbf{Q} & \cdots \\ \mathrm{o}' & \mathbf{D}\mathbf{Q} & (\lambda\mathbf{V}\mathbf{D})\mathbf{D}\mathbf{Q} & (\lambda\mathbf{V}\mathbf{D}^2)\mathbf{D}\mathbf{Q} & \cdots \\ \mathrm{o}' & \mathbf{O} & \mathbf{D}\mathbf{Q} & (\lambda\mathbf{V}\mathbf{D})\mathbf{D}\mathbf{Q} & \cdots \\ \cdots & \cdots & \cdots & \cdots & \cdots \end{bmatrix}. \quad (8.3.25b)$$

Using $\lambda\mathbf{V}\mathbf{D} = \mathbf{I} - \mathbf{D}$, one can show that $\mathcal{Y}\varepsilon' = \varepsilon'$ by recognizing that the matrix geometric series sum over n of $(\lambda\,\mathbf{V}\mathbf{D})^n$ converges to

$$\begin{aligned} \mathbf{I} + \lambda\mathbf{V}\mathbf{D} + (\lambda\mathbf{V}\mathbf{D})^2 + \cdots &= [\mathbf{I} - \lambda\mathbf{V}\mathbf{D}]^{-1} \\ &= [\mathbf{I} - (\mathbf{I} - \mathbf{D})]^{-1} = \mathbf{D}^{-1} = \mathbf{I} + \lambda\mathbf{V}. \end{aligned}$$

The vector $\mathcal{V}\varepsilon'$ can also be evaluated from the above. We use the utilization parameter $\rho = \lambda\bar{x}$ and get

$$\lambda\mathcal{V}\varepsilon' = \begin{bmatrix} 1 \\ \mathrm{o}' \\ \mathrm{o}' \\ \mathrm{o}' \\ \cdots \end{bmatrix} + \begin{bmatrix} \rho \\ \lambda\mathbf{V}\epsilon' \\ \lambda\mathbf{V}\epsilon' \\ \lambda\mathbf{V}\epsilon' \\ \cdots \end{bmatrix}. \quad (8.3.26)$$

From Theorems 4.2.3 and 4.2.4, the steady-state departure vectors for the M/ME/1 queue are given by

$$\mathbf{d}(n) = (1-\rho)\Psi[\mathbf{U}^n]\,\mathbf{p},$$

where from Equations (4.1.4)

$$\mathbf{U}^{-1} := \mathbf{A} := \mathbf{I} + \frac{1}{\lambda}\mathbf{B} - \mathbf{Q}. \quad (8.3.27)$$

Given that $\sum_{n=\mathrm{o}}^{\infty} \mathbf{d}(n) = \mathbf{p}$, it must be true that $\sum_{n=\mathrm{o}}^{\infty} \Psi[\mathbf{U}^n] = \Psi[(\mathbf{I} - \mathbf{U})^{-1}] = (1-\rho)^{-1}$, which it is [see (4.2.3)]. We also mention that $\Psi[\mathbf{U}] = (1-\alpha_{\mathrm{o}})/\alpha_{\mathrm{o}}$.

The steady-state vector over all states is given by

$$\wp = (1-\rho)\,\left[1,\, \Psi[\mathbf{U}]\,\mathbf{p},\, \Psi[\mathbf{U}^2]\,\mathbf{p},\, \Psi[\mathbf{U}^3]\,\mathbf{p},\, \ldots\right]. \quad (8.3.28)$$

where $\wp\mathcal{E}' = 1$. With some algebraic manipulation it can be shown that $\wp\mathcal{Y} = \wp$.

Note, it is the departure vectors of the M/G/1 queue, $\mathbf{d}(n)$ (see theorem 4.2.4), not the steady-state vectors $\pi(n)$, that make up $\wp$, the left eigenvector of $\mathcal{Y}$. Also note that if the elements of $\mathcal{Y}$ are reduced to scalars by pre- and postmultiplying them by appropriately dimensioned $\mathbf{p}$ (or 1) and $\boldsymbol{\epsilon}'$ (or 1), the following matrix results [see (8.3.22c)].

$$\bar{\mathcal{Y}} := \begin{bmatrix} \alpha_o & \alpha_1 & \alpha_2 & \alpha_3 & \alpha_4 & \cdots \\ \alpha_o & \alpha_1 & \alpha_2 & \alpha_3 & \alpha_4 & \cdots \\ 0 & \alpha_o & \alpha_1 & \alpha_2 & \alpha_3 & \cdots \\ 0 & 0 & \alpha_o & \alpha_1 & \alpha_2 & \cdots \\ \cdots & \cdots & \cdots & \cdots & \cdots & \cdots \end{bmatrix}. \tag{8.3.29}$$

Finding the left-eigenvector of this matrix is the standard way one finds the scalar steady-state probabilities, as given in [KLEINROCK75] (see also Section 4.4.3). But its derivation depends on the knowledge that a random observer sees the same probabilities as a departing customer for the M/G/1 queue. This, in turn, is only true because the arrival process to S_1 is Poisson.

Returning to evaluation of the various covariances, we need expressions for $\mathcal{Y}\mathcal{V}\mathcal{E}'$ and $\mathcal{V}\mathcal{Y}\mathcal{V}\mathcal{E}'$. It does not take too much effort to get them. They are:

$$\lambda\mathcal{Y}\mathcal{V}\mathcal{E}' = \begin{bmatrix} \alpha_o \\ \mathbf{D}\boldsymbol{\epsilon}' \\ \mathbf{o}' \\ \mathbf{o}' \\ \cdots \end{bmatrix} + \rho\mathcal{E}' \tag{8.3.30a}$$

and

$$\lambda\mathcal{V}\mathcal{Y}\mathcal{V}\mathcal{E}' = \begin{bmatrix} \alpha_o + \alpha_1 \\ (\lambda\mathbf{V}\mathbf{D})\mathbf{D}\boldsymbol{\epsilon}' \\ \mathbf{o}' \\ \mathbf{o}' \\ \cdots \end{bmatrix} + \rho \begin{bmatrix} 1 \\ \mathbf{o}' \\ \mathbf{o}' \\ \mathbf{o}' \\ \cdots \end{bmatrix} + \rho \begin{bmatrix} \rho \\ \lambda\mathbf{V}\boldsymbol{\epsilon}' \\ \lambda\mathbf{V}\boldsymbol{\epsilon}' \\ \lambda\mathbf{V}\boldsymbol{\epsilon}' \\ \cdots \end{bmatrix}. \tag{8.3.30b}$$

Three different initial conditions are presented here for $\wp_o$. They are:

1. The process starts with an empty queue (designated by subscript "a"),

2. The process starts with the arrival of a customer to an empty queue (subscript "b"),

3. The process starts in its steady state (8.3.28) (no subscript).

The first two are:

$$\wp_{\mathbf{a}} = [1, \mathbf{o}, \mathbf{o}, \mathbf{o}, \ldots] \tag{8.3.31a}$$

and

$$\wp_{\mathbf{b}} = [0, \mathbf{p}, \mathbf{o}, \mathbf{o}, \ldots]. \tag{8.3.31b}$$

The formulas for the various mean values and covariances are shown in Table 8.3.2, together with the equivalent covariances for the M/M/1 queue.

Table 8.3.2. Comparison of Means and Covariances

$\wp_x \mathbf{X}\varepsilon'$	System a	System b	Steady − State
$\lambda \wp_x \mathcal{V}\varepsilon'$	$1+\rho$	ρ	1
$\lambda \wp_x \mathcal{Y}\mathcal{V}\varepsilon'$	$\alpha_o+\rho$	$\alpha_o+\rho$	1
$\lambda^2 \wp_x \mathcal{V}\mathcal{Y}\mathcal{V}\varepsilon'$	$\alpha_o+\alpha_1+\rho+\rho^2$	$\alpha_1+\rho^2$	$\frac{(1-\rho)}{\alpha_o}\left[\alpha_o^2+\alpha_1\right]+\rho$
$\lambda^2\,\mathrm{Cov}_x(X_1,\,X_2)$	$\alpha_1-\rho\alpha_o$	$\alpha_1-\rho\,\alpha_o$	$\frac{1-\rho}{\alpha_o}[\alpha_o(\alpha_o-1)+\alpha_1]$
$\lambda^2\,\mathrm{Cov}_x(\exp)$	$-\left[\frac{\rho}{1+\rho}\right]^2$	$-\left[\frac{\rho}{1+\rho}\right]^2$	0

Note that the covariances for systems a and b are identical. Some of these results are already known, and can be found in, for example, [DisneyKiessler87] and [Saito90].

8.3.5.2 If S_1 Is Exponential (ME/M/1 Queues)

The open G/M/1 queue is actually somewhat easier to set up than the M/G/1 queue, because all the blocks in the various matrices are the same size. The complications come in when one must select the initial vector. Let S_1 be an exponential server with service rate λ, and S_2 (again dropping subscripts) is represented by the vector matrix pair $\langle\, \mathbf{p}\,,\, \mathbf{B}\,\rangle$.

First we establish the $\mathcal{B}$ matrix. Here,

$$\mathcal{B} = \begin{bmatrix} \mathbf{B} & -\mathbf{BQ} & \mathbf{O} & \mathbf{O} & \cdots \\ \mathbf{O} & \mathbf{B}+\lambda\mathbf{I} & -\mathbf{BQ} & \mathbf{O} & \cdots \\ \mathbf{O} & \mathbf{O} & \mathbf{B}+\lambda\mathbf{I} & -\mathbf{BQ} & \cdots \\ \mathbf{O} & \mathbf{O} & \mathbf{O} & \mathbf{B}+\lambda\mathbf{I} & \cdots \\ \cdots & \cdots & \cdots & \cdots & \cdots \end{bmatrix} \tag{8.3.32a}$$

and thus

$$\mathcal{B}\varepsilon' = \lambda \begin{bmatrix} \mathbf{o}' \\ \epsilon' \\ \epsilon' \\ \epsilon' \\ \cdots \end{bmatrix}. \tag{8.3.32b}$$

It can be shown that $\mathcal{B}^{-1}$ is

$$\mathcal{V} = \begin{bmatrix} \mathbf{V} & \mathbf{QVD} & d\mathbf{QVD} & d^2\mathbf{QVD} & d^3\mathbf{QVD} & \cdots \\ \mathbf{O} & \mathbf{VD} & \mathbf{DQVD} & d\mathbf{DQVD} & d^2\mathbf{DQVD} & \cdots \\ \mathbf{O} & \mathbf{O} & \mathbf{VD} & \mathbf{DQVD} & d\mathbf{DQVD} & \cdots \\ \mathbf{O} & \mathbf{O} & \mathbf{O} & \mathbf{VD} & \mathbf{DQVD} & \cdots \\ \cdots & \cdots & \cdots & \cdots & \cdots & \cdots \end{bmatrix} \tag{8.3.32c}$$

and

$$\mathcal{V}\varepsilon' = \frac{1}{\lambda}\varepsilon' + \begin{bmatrix} \mathbf{V}\epsilon' \\ \mathbf{o}' \\ \mathbf{o}' \\ \mathbf{o}' \\ \cdots \end{bmatrix}, \tag{8.3.32d}$$

where $\mathbf{D} := [\mathbf{I} + \lambda\mathbf{V}]^{-1}$ and $d := \alpha_o = \Psi[\mathbf{D}]$ [see (8.3.22c)]. We also have occasion once again to use $\lambda\mathbf{VD} = \mathbf{I} - \mathbf{D}$. It is not hard to see that the departure matrix is

$$\mathcal{L} = \begin{bmatrix} \mathbf{O} & \mathbf{O} & \mathbf{O} & \mathbf{O} & \cdots \\ \lambda\mathbf{I} & \mathbf{O} & \mathbf{O} & \mathbf{O} & \cdots \\ \mathbf{O} & \lambda\mathbf{I} & \mathbf{O} & \mathbf{O} & \cdots \\ \mathbf{O} & \mathbf{O} & \lambda\mathbf{I} & \mathbf{O} & \cdots \\ \cdots & \cdots & \cdots & \cdots & \cdots \end{bmatrix} \quad \text{and} \quad \mathcal{L}\varepsilon' = \lambda \begin{bmatrix} \mathbf{o}' \\ \epsilon' \\ \epsilon' \\ \epsilon' \\ \cdots \end{bmatrix} = \mathcal{B}\varepsilon'. \tag{8.3.33a}$$

We see, then, that (8.2.1) is satisfied. We can calculate $\mathcal{Y}$ and, with some effort, we can also show that it is isometric,

$$\mathcal{Y} = \mathcal{V}\mathcal{L} = \lambda \begin{bmatrix} \mathbf{QVD} & d\mathbf{QVD} & d^2\mathbf{QVD} & d^3\mathbf{QVD} & \cdots \\ \mathbf{VD} & \mathbf{DQVD} & d\mathbf{DQVD} & d^2\mathbf{DQVD} & \cdots \\ \mathbf{O} & \mathbf{VD} & \mathbf{DQVD} & d\mathbf{DQVD} & \cdots \\ \mathbf{O} & \mathbf{O} & \mathbf{VD} & \mathbf{DQVD} & \cdots \\ \cdots & \cdots & \cdots & \cdots & \cdots \end{bmatrix} \tag{8.3.33b}$$

and $\mathcal{Y}\varepsilon' = \varepsilon'$. To fully define the process, the initial vector $\wp_o$ must be specified. We present three interesting options here. First, we can imagine the process beginning immediately after an arrival to an empty queue (the beginning of a busy period). Then

$$\wp_a := [\mathbf{o}, \mathbf{p}, \mathbf{o}, \mathbf{o}, \ldots]. \tag{8.3.34}$$

Each element is itself a vector of dimension m.

A second interesting case occurs at the end of a busy period, that is, when a customer leaves an empty queue behind. Consider the matrix $\mathbf{A}$, defined in (8.3.27), and let s be its smallest eigenvalue between 0 and 1, with left eigenvector $\hat{\mathbf{u}}$ (i.e., $\hat{\mathbf{u}}\,\mathbf{A} = s\,\hat{\mathbf{u}}$). From Corollary 5.1.2 we know that the arrival process (at S_1) is in vector state

$$\hat{\mathbf{u}} := \lambda\mathbf{pV}[\mathbf{I} + \lambda(1-s)\mathbf{V}]^{-1} \tag{8.3.35}$$

at that moment, so

$$\wp_b := [\hat{\mathbf{u}}, \mathbf{o}, \mathbf{o}, \mathbf{o}, \ldots]. \tag{8.3.36}$$

Pictorially, S_2 is in state i with probability $[\hat{\mathbf{u}}]_i$ at the moment a customer leaves an empty queue behind at S_1. The requirement that $\hat{\mathbf{u}}\epsilon' = 1$ is equivalent to requiring that s satisfy the equation

$$s = F^*(\lambda(1-s)).$$

The geometric parameter for the steady-state G/M/1 queue s is the smallest root between 0 and 1 that satisfies the above.

The most important example is the steady-state vector. Again from Theorem 5.1.3 we know that the steady-state vector probability of having k customers at S_1 at the time of a departure is

$$\mathbf{d}(k) = (1-s)s^k\,\hat{\mathbf{u}}.$$

Therefore, the infinite steady-state vector over all queue lengths is

$$\wp = (1-s)[\hat{\mathbf{u}},\, s\hat{\mathbf{u}},\, s^2\hat{\mathbf{u}},\, s^3\hat{\mathbf{u}},\, \ldots]. \tag{8.3.37}$$

One can show by direct calculation that this $\wp$ satisfies (8.2.7) ($\wp\mathcal{Y} = \wp$), as it must. Of course, all three vectors have "length" 1; that is,

$$\wp_{\rm a}\,\varepsilon' = \wp_{\rm b}\,\varepsilon' = \wp\varepsilon' = 1.$$

In order to calculate the covariance for each of the three cases, we need:

$$\wp_{\rm x}\,[\mathcal{V}]\,\varepsilon', \qquad \wp_{\rm x}\,[\mathcal{Y}\mathcal{V}]\,\varepsilon', \quad \text{and} \quad \wp_{\rm x}\,[\mathcal{V}\mathcal{Y}\mathcal{V}]\,\varepsilon',$$

where $\mathbf{x} = \mathbf{a}$, $\mathbf{b}$, and *blank*. This is easiest done by first setting up $[\mathcal{V}\varepsilon']$, $[\mathcal{Y}\mathcal{V}\varepsilon']$, and $[\mathcal{V}\mathcal{Y}\mathcal{V}\varepsilon']$. We already know $[\mathcal{V}\varepsilon']$ from (8.3.32d). The second term is

$$\mathcal{Y}\mathcal{V}\varepsilon' = \mathcal{Y}\,[\mathcal{V}\varepsilon'] = \frac{1}{\lambda}\mathcal{Y}\varepsilon' + \mathcal{Y}\begin{bmatrix} \mathbf{V}\boldsymbol{\epsilon}' \\ \mathbf{o}' \\ \mathbf{o}' \\ \mathbf{o}' \\ \cdots \end{bmatrix} = \frac{1}{\lambda}\varepsilon' + \lambda\begin{bmatrix} \Psi[\mathbf{V}^2\,\mathbf{D}]\,\boldsymbol{\epsilon}' \\ \mathbf{V}^2\,\mathbf{D}\boldsymbol{\epsilon}' \\ \mathbf{o}' \\ \mathbf{o}' \\ \cdots \end{bmatrix}. \tag{8.3.38a}$$

The third term can be evaluated in a similar fashion

$$\mathcal{V}\mathcal{Y}\mathcal{V}\varepsilon' = \mathcal{V}\,[\mathcal{Y}\mathcal{V}\varepsilon'] = \frac{1}{\lambda}\mathcal{V}\varepsilon' + \lambda\mathcal{V}\begin{bmatrix} \Psi[\mathbf{V}^2\,\mathbf{D}]\,\boldsymbol{\epsilon}' \\ \mathbf{V}^2\,\mathbf{D}\boldsymbol{\epsilon}' \\ \mathbf{o}' \\ \mathbf{o}' \\ \cdots \end{bmatrix}$$

$$= \frac{1}{\lambda^2}\varepsilon' + \frac{1}{\lambda}\begin{bmatrix} \mathbf{V}\boldsymbol{\epsilon}' \\ \mathbf{o}' \\ \mathbf{o}' \\ \mathbf{o}' \\ \cdots \end{bmatrix} + \lambda\begin{bmatrix} \Psi[\mathbf{V}^2\,\mathbf{D}]\,\mathbf{V}\boldsymbol{\epsilon}' + \Psi[\mathbf{V}^3\,\mathbf{D}^2]\boldsymbol{\epsilon}' \\ \mathbf{V}^3\,\mathbf{D}^2\,\boldsymbol{\epsilon}' \\ \mathbf{o}' \\ \mathbf{o}' \\ \cdots \end{bmatrix}. \tag{8.3.38b}$$

Next, define the random variables X_{an}, X_{bn}, and X_n, where $n = 1, 2 \ldots$. Then combining (8.3.34), (8.3.36), and (8.3.37) with (8.3.32d), we get for the departure time of the first customer:

$$\begin{aligned} \lambda\mathbb{E}[X_{a1}] &= 1 \\ \lambda\mathbb{E}[X_{b1}] &= 1 + \lambda\,(\hat{\mathbf{u}}\,\mathbf{V}\boldsymbol{\epsilon}') \\ \lambda\mathbb{E}[X_1] &= 1 + \lambda\,(1-s)(\hat{\mathbf{u}}\,\mathbf{V}\boldsymbol{\epsilon}'). \end{aligned} \qquad (8.3.39a)$$

Next, combining (8.3.34) and (8.3.36) with (8.3.38a), and recalling that $\wp\mathcal{Y} = \wp$ [from (8.2.7)], the mean interdeparture time for the second customer is

$$\begin{aligned} \lambda\mathbb{E}[X_{a2}] &= 1 + \lambda^2\,\Psi[\mathbf{V}^2\,\mathbf{D}] \\ \lambda\mathbb{E}[X_{b2}] &= \lambda\mathbb{E}[X_{a2}] \\ \lambda\mathbb{E}[X_2] &= \lambda\mathbb{E}[X_1]. \end{aligned} \qquad (8.3.39b)$$

Finally, the same three equations are combined with (8.3.38b) to get the double expectations

$$\begin{aligned} \lambda^2\,\mathbb{E}[X_{a1}\,X_{a2}] &= 1 + \lambda^3\,\Psi[\mathbf{V}^3\,\mathbf{D}^2] \\ \lambda^2\,\mathbb{E}[X_{b1}\,X_{b2}] &= \lambda^2\,\mathbb{E}[X_{a1}\,X_{a2}] + \lambda^2\,(\hat{\mathbf{u}}\,\mathbf{V}\boldsymbol{\epsilon}')\,\mathbb{E}[X_{a2}] \\ \lambda^2\,\mathbb{E}[X_1\,X_2] &= s + (1-s)\lambda^2\,\mathbb{E}[X_{b1}\,X_{b2}] + \lambda^3\,s(1-s)\,(\hat{\mathbf{u}}\,\mathbf{V}^3\,\mathbf{D}^2\,\boldsymbol{\epsilon}'). \end{aligned} \qquad (8.3.39c)$$

(See also Section 4.4.1). The matrix terms $\Psi[\mathbf{V}^2\,\mathbf{D}]$, $\Psi[\mathbf{V}^3\,\mathbf{D}^2]$, $(\hat{\mathbf{u}}\,\mathbf{V}\boldsymbol{\epsilon}')$ and $(\hat{\mathbf{u}}\,\mathbf{V}^3\,\mathbf{D}^2\,\boldsymbol{\epsilon}')$ can be written as nonmatrix expressions by algebraic manipulation of $\lambda\mathbf{V}\mathbf{D} = \mathbf{I} - \mathbf{D}$,

$$\lambda\,\Psi[\mathbf{V}^2\,\mathbf{D}] = \lambda\,\Psi[\mathbf{V}(\mathbf{I}-\mathbf{D})] = \lambda\bar{x} - \Psi[\mathbf{I}-\mathbf{D}] = \lambda\bar{x} + \alpha_o - 1.$$

Similarly,

$$\lambda^3\,\Psi[\mathbf{V}^3\,\mathbf{D}^2] = \lambda\bar{x} + 2\alpha_o + \alpha_1 - 2.$$

The $\hat{\mathbf{u}}$ terms are more difficult, but straightforward when using $\hat{\mathbf{u}}[\mathbf{I} + \lambda(1-s)\mathbf{V}] = \lambda\,\mathbf{p}\mathbf{V}$, from (8.3.35). Algebraic manipulation yields

$$\begin{aligned} s\,\hat{\mathbf{u}}\,\mathbf{D} &= \lambda\,\mathbf{p}\mathbf{V}\mathbf{D} - (1-s)\hat{\mathbf{u}} \\ \lambda\,(1-s)\hat{\mathbf{u}}\,\mathbf{V} &= \lambda\,\mathbf{p}\mathbf{V} - \hat{\mathbf{u}} \\ \lambda\,s\hat{\mathbf{u}}\mathbf{V}\mathbf{D} &= \hat{\mathbf{u}} - \lambda\,\mathbf{p}\mathbf{V}\mathbf{D}. \end{aligned}$$

From these, on multiplying from the right with any powers of $\mathbf{V}$ and $\mathbf{D}$, and then with $\boldsymbol{\epsilon}'$, all terms of the form $[\hat{\mathbf{u}}\,\mathbf{V}^k\,\mathbf{D}^j\,\boldsymbol{\epsilon}']$ can be expressed. In particular,

$$\lambda\,(1-s)\,[\hat{\mathbf{u}}\,\mathbf{V}\boldsymbol{\epsilon}'] = \lambda\,\bar{x} - 1$$

and

$$\lambda^3\,s^2(1-s)\,[\hat{\mathbf{u}}\,\mathbf{V}^3\,\mathbf{D}^2\,\boldsymbol{\epsilon}'] = \lambda\,\bar{x}\,s^2 - 1 + (1-\alpha_o)(1-s)(1+2s) - s(1-s)\alpha_1.$$

After all of the above are put into (8.2.11a) with $n = k = 1$, we get for the covariance lag-1

$$\begin{aligned} \lambda^2 \operatorname{Cov}(X_{a1}, X_{a2}) &= \alpha_o + \alpha_1 - 1 \\ \lambda^2 \operatorname{Cov}(X_{b1}, X_{b2}) &= \lambda^2 \operatorname{Cov}(X_{a1}, X_{a2}) \\ s\lambda^2 \operatorname{Cov}(X_1, X_2) &= \alpha_o (\lambda s\bar{x} - 1). \end{aligned} \tag{8.3.39d}$$

The steady-state covariance formula is particularly interesting. Only if $\lambda s\bar{x} = 1$ is the covariance equal to 0. For G/M/1 queues, the utilization factor, ρ is equal to $1/(\lambda\bar{x})$. The only interarrival process for which $s = \rho$ for all ρ is the Poisson process, but it is possible for the covariance lag-1 to vanish for some values of ρ.

8.3.5.3 Both S_1 and S_2 Are Nonexponential

It is possible to generalize from the two previous sections what $\boldsymbol{\mathcal{B}}$, $\boldsymbol{\mathcal{V}}$, $\boldsymbol{\mathcal{L}}$, and $\boldsymbol{\mathcal{Y}}$ are for the G/G/1 queue. Furthermore, given that $\boldsymbol{\mathcal{Y}}$ is subtriangular, the steady-state departure vector $\wp$ can be computed recursively. The notation is the same as that for Section 8.3.3, where subscript 2 refers to the arrival process, and subscript 1 refers to the service process. The relevant matrices are again ordered according to the number of customers at S_1, and the entries themselves are matrices. The 00 element is an $m_2 \times m_2$ matrix, the other $0n$ elements are $m_2 \times m_1 m_2$ matrices, the other $n0$ matrices are $m_1 m_2 \times m_2$-dimensional, and all other elements are $m_1 m_2 \times m_1 m_2$ matrices. Generalizing from (8.3.24a) and (8.3.32a), we write

$$\boldsymbol{\mathcal{B}} = \begin{bmatrix} \mathbf{B}_2 & -\hat{\mathbf{p}}_1 \hat{\mathbf{B}}_2\hat{\mathbf{Q}}_2 & \mathbf{O} & \mathbf{O} & \cdots \\ \mathbf{O} & \hat{\mathbf{B}}_1 + \hat{\mathbf{B}}_2 & -\hat{\mathbf{B}}_2\hat{\mathbf{Q}}_2 & \mathbf{O} & \cdots \\ \mathbf{O} & \mathbf{O} & \hat{\mathbf{B}}_1 + \hat{\mathbf{B}}_2 & -\hat{\mathbf{B}}_2\hat{\mathbf{Q}}_2 & \cdots \\ \mathbf{O} & \mathbf{O} & \mathbf{O} & \hat{\mathbf{B}}_1 + \hat{\mathbf{B}}_2 & \cdots \\ \cdots & \cdots & \cdots & \cdots & \cdots \end{bmatrix}. \tag{8.3.40a}$$

It can be verified by direct multiplication that (now let $\mathbf{D} := [\hat{\mathbf{B}}_1 + \hat{\mathbf{B}}_2]^{-1}$)

$$\boldsymbol{\mathcal{V}} = \begin{bmatrix} \mathbf{V}_2 & \hat{\mathbf{p}}_1\hat{\mathbf{Q}}_2\mathbf{D} & \hat{\mathbf{p}}_1\hat{\mathbf{Q}}_2\mathbf{D}\mathbf{X} & \hat{\mathbf{p}}_1\hat{\mathbf{Q}}_2\mathbf{D}\mathbf{X}^2 & \hat{\mathbf{p}}_1\hat{\mathbf{Q}}_2\mathbf{D}\mathbf{X}^3 & \cdots \\ \mathbf{o}' & \mathbf{D} & \mathbf{D}\mathbf{X} & \mathbf{D}\mathbf{X}^2 & \mathbf{D}\mathbf{X}^3 & \cdots \\ \mathbf{o}' & \mathbf{O} & \mathbf{D} & \mathbf{D}\mathbf{X} & \mathbf{D}\mathbf{X}^2 & \cdots \\ \mathbf{o}' & \mathbf{O} & \mathbf{O} & \mathbf{D} & \mathbf{D}\mathbf{X} & \cdots \\ \cdots & \cdots & \cdots & \cdots & \cdots & \cdots \end{bmatrix}, \tag{8.3.40b}$$

where for ease of notation we have set $\mathbf{X} := \hat{\mathbf{B}}_2\hat{\mathbf{Q}}_2\mathbf{D}$.

In a similar fashion the departure matrix $\boldsymbol{\mathcal{L}}$ can be generalized from (8.3.25a) and (8.3.33a) to give

$$\boldsymbol{\mathcal{L}} = \begin{bmatrix} \mathbf{O} & \mathbf{O} & \mathbf{O} & \mathbf{O} & \mathbf{O} & \cdots \\ \hat{\mathbf{B}}_1\hat{\epsilon}_1' & \mathbf{O} & \mathbf{O} & \mathbf{O} & \mathbf{O} & \cdots \\ \mathbf{O} & \hat{\mathbf{B}}_1\hat{\mathbf{Q}}_1 & \mathbf{O} & \mathbf{O} & \mathbf{O} & \cdots \\ \mathbf{O} & \mathbf{O} & \hat{\mathbf{B}}_1\hat{\mathbf{Q}}_1 & \mathbf{O} & \mathbf{O} & \cdots \\ \cdots & \cdots & \cdots & \cdots & \cdots & \cdots \end{bmatrix}. \tag{8.3.40c}$$

Finally, we have

$$\mathcal{Y} = \mathcal{V}\mathcal{L}$$

$$= \begin{bmatrix} \hat{\mathbf{p}}_1\hat{\mathbf{B}}_1\hat{\mathbf{Q}}_2\mathbf{D}\hat{\epsilon}_1' & \hat{\mathbf{p}}_1\hat{\mathbf{B}}_1\hat{\mathbf{Q}}_2\mathbf{D}\mathbf{X}\hat{\mathbf{Q}}_1 & \hat{\mathbf{p}}_1\hat{\mathbf{B}}_1\hat{\mathbf{Q}}_2\mathbf{D}\mathbf{X}^2\hat{\mathbf{Q}}_1 & \cdots \\ \hat{\mathbf{B}}_1\mathbf{D}\hat{\epsilon}_1' & \hat{\mathbf{B}}_1\mathbf{D}\mathbf{X}\hat{\mathbf{Q}}_1 & \hat{\mathbf{B}}_1\mathbf{D}\mathbf{X}^2\hat{\mathbf{Q}}_1 & \cdots \\ \mathbf{O} & \hat{\mathbf{B}}_1\mathbf{D}\hat{\mathbf{Q}}_1 & \hat{\mathbf{B}}_1\mathbf{D}\mathbf{X}\hat{\mathbf{Q}}_1 & \cdots \\ \mathbf{O} & \mathbf{O} & \hat{\mathbf{B}}_1\mathbf{D}\hat{\mathbf{Q}}_1 & \cdots \\ \cdots & \cdots & \cdots & \cdots \end{bmatrix} \quad (8.3.40d)$$

and $\mathcal{Y}\varepsilon' = \varepsilon'$. We have made use of the fact that all subscripted matrices commute with matrices with different subscripts (i.e., $\hat{\mathbf{B}}_1\hat{\mathbf{Q}}_2 = \hat{\mathbf{Q}}_2\hat{\mathbf{B}}_1$ but $\hat{\mathbf{B}}_1\hat{\mathbf{Q}}_1 \neq \hat{\mathbf{Q}}_1\hat{\mathbf{B}}_1$). Also, $\hat{\mathbf{B}}_1$ and $\hat{\mathbf{B}}_2$ commute with $\mathbf{D}$, but $\hat{\mathbf{Q}}_1$ and $\hat{\mathbf{Q}}_2$ do not.

Note that $\mathcal{Y}$ in (8.3.40d) is a stochastic matrix (if its elements are all nonnegative) which satisfies the canonical form described as "M/G/1-type" by M. Neuts [NEUTS81]. Thus there exist standard numerical procedures for solving the equation $\wp\mathcal{Y} = \wp$. The nth component of $\wp$ is itself a vector, the sum of whose elements is the probability $d(n)$ that a departing customer will leave n other customers behind at S_1. Each component must be of the form $d(n)\mathbf{p}_1 \times \mathbf{v}_2(n)$, where $\mathbf{v}_2(n)$ is the vector state of S_2 at the moment of the departure.

8.3.5.4 M/M/1//N Queues

It has long been well known that the departure process from a steady-state open M/M/1 queue is itself a Poisson process. We give here a simple demonstration of why this is so. The expressions also show that this is an exceptional property, and that in general, except for the steady-state M/M/1 queue (see [DISNEYKIESSLER87] for minor exceptions), there *is* correlation. This includes departures from servers in closed systems and also finite buffered queues (i.e., departures from queued servers are not generally renewal processes).

Let λ be the arrival rate of the Poisson process to an exponential server whose rate is $\mu = 1/\bar{x}$. The formulas of the previous sections simplify when the following substitutions are made. $\mathbf{Q} \to 1$, $\mathbf{V} \to 1/\mu$, $\mathbf{B} \to \mu$, and $\mathbf{D} \to 1/(1+\lambda/\mu)$. If the formulas from the M/G/1 section are used, then the utilization factor is $\rho = \lambda/\mu$. But if the formulas from the G/M/1 section are used, the roles of λ and μ must be interchanged; then $\rho = \mu/\lambda$. In either case, the subsystem $\mathcal{V}$ and $\mathcal{Y}$ matrices become:

$$\mathcal{V} = \frac{\bar{x}}{1+\rho} \begin{bmatrix} 1/\alpha & 1 & \alpha & \alpha^2 & \alpha^3 & \cdots \\ 0 & 1 & \alpha & \alpha^2 & \alpha^3 & \cdots \\ 0 & 0 & 1 & \alpha & \alpha^2 & \cdots \\ 0 & 0 & 0 & 1 & \alpha & \cdots \\ 0 & 0 & 0 & 0 & 1 & \cdots \\ \cdots & \cdots & \cdots & \cdots & \cdots & \cdots \end{bmatrix} \quad (8.3.41a)$$

and

$$\mathcal{Y} = \frac{1}{1+\rho}\begin{bmatrix} 1 & \alpha & \alpha^2 & \alpha^3 & \alpha^4 & \cdots \\ 1 & \alpha & \alpha^2 & \alpha^3 & \alpha^4 & \cdots \\ 0 & 1 & \alpha & \alpha^2 & \alpha^3 & \cdots \\ 0 & 0 & 1 & \alpha & \alpha^2 & \cdots \\ 0 & 0 & 0 & 1 & \alpha & \cdots \\ \cdots & \cdots & \cdots & \cdots & \cdots & \cdots \end{bmatrix}, \tag{8.3.41b}$$

where $\alpha := \rho/(1+\rho)$. Equations (8.3.25b), (8.3.29) and (8.3.33b) all reduce to this one for the M/M/1 queue. The steady-state probabilities are $p(n) = (1-\rho)\rho^n$, so

$$\wp = (1-\rho)[1, \rho, \rho^2, \rho^3, \rho^4, \ldots]. \tag{8.3.42a}$$

The extraordinary property is that $\wp$ is a left eigenvector of both $\mathcal{V}$ and $\mathcal{Y}$. That is,

$$\wp\mathcal{Y} = \wp, \tag{8.3.42b}$$

as it should. But it is also true that

$$\wp\mathcal{V} = \frac{1}{\lambda}\wp. \tag{8.3.42c}$$

Clearly, then, $\wp\mathcal{V}\boldsymbol{\varepsilon}' = 1/\lambda$. Equation (8.2.11c), with $\wp$ replacing $\wp_o$, simplifies to

$$\mathbb{E}[X_n\, X_{n+k}] = \wp\,[\mathcal{V}\, Y^k\, \mathcal{V}]\,\boldsymbol{\varepsilon}' = \frac{1}{\lambda}\wp\,[\mathcal{Y}^k\, \mathcal{V}]\,\boldsymbol{\varepsilon}' = \frac{1}{\lambda}\wp\,[\mathcal{V}]\,\boldsymbol{\varepsilon}' = \frac{1}{\lambda^2} \tag{8.3.43}$$

for all n and all k. This, together with (8.2.10d) and (8.2.11a) shows that the autocovariance is 0 for all n and all k. Be reminded, though, that this assumes the subsystem to be in its steady state initially. If the initial vector is not $\wp$, then all bets are off. For the finite customer (M/M/1//N) and finite buffer (M/M/1/N) queues,. the last column of $\mathcal{V}$ does not fit the pattern for the other elements, so (8.3.42c) is not satisfied. Thus only the steady-state, open M/M/1 queue yields a Poisson departure process.

8.4 MRP/M/1 Queues

All the examples given can be used as arrival processes to a queueing system. We discuss how to do this here, where the queue feeds to an exponential server. The general method is also applicable to M/G/1 (Chapter 4), G/M/1 queues (Chapter 5), and with some extension, generalized M/G/C and G/G/1 queues (Chapters 6 and 7). Whereas previously we were able to find explicit solutions, now we must find the correct solution by iteration. The method depends on a very powerful theorem by Wallace [WALLACE69] on ***QBD processes*** of which all of these are special cases. Recall that ***Birth-Death*** Processes are those for which the population grows and contracts by single steps (arrivals and departures). For QBD processes the steps are multistate sets, exactly as we have been dealing with here.

Let $\boldsymbol{\pi}(n)$ be the steady-state vector probability that the system is in vector state $\{i, n\}$ and $r(n) = \boldsymbol{\pi}(n)\boldsymbol{\varepsilon}'$ is the associated scalar probability. The theorem states that if the matrices that govern the transitions are independent of the population n, then

$$\boldsymbol{\pi}(n) = c\boldsymbol{u}\boldsymbol{\mathcal{R}}^n \quad \text{and} \quad r(n) = \boldsymbol{\pi}(n)\boldsymbol{\varepsilon}',$$

where $\boldsymbol{\mathcal{R}}$ is a matrix satisfying some ***matrix quadratic equation***, $\boldsymbol{u}$ is a special vector with $\boldsymbol{u}\boldsymbol{\varepsilon}' = 1$, and c is determined by the normalization condition, $\sum_{n=o}^{\infty} r(n) = 1$.

We next consider queueing systems where the arrivals to an exponential server are generated by some MRP satisfying the rules defined in this chapter. By "system" we mean the combination of the arrival process, the exponential server, and the customers in the queue.

8.4.1 Balance Equations

Let n be the number of customers at an exponential server (called S_ν) with service rate ν. The arrival process is described by the matrices $\boldsymbol{\mathcal{B}}$, $\boldsymbol{\mathcal{Q}}$, and $\boldsymbol{\mathcal{L}}$, as defined previously. The ith component of the ss vector, $\boldsymbol{\pi}_i(n)$, refers to the state the MRP is in when there are n customers at S_ν. This is a straightfoward generalization of the description we gave in Chapter 5 from the G/M/1 queue. The system can leave state $\{i\,;n\}$ by either a change at the MRP $[\boldsymbol{\pi}_i(n)(\boldsymbol{\mathcal{M}})_{ii}]$ or a customer completion at S_ν $[\boldsymbol{\pi}_i(n)\nu]$. The system can enter this state by one of three ways:

1. A change of state from some j to i in the arrival process $[\boldsymbol{\pi}_j(n)(\boldsymbol{\mathcal{M}})_{jj}(\boldsymbol{\mathcal{P}})_{ji}]$,
2. A customer completion at S_ν when there are $n+1$ customers there $[\boldsymbol{\pi}_i(n+1)\nu]$,
3. The MRP has a departure when there are $n-1$ customers at S_ν $[\boldsymbol{\pi}_j(n-1)(\boldsymbol{\mathcal{L}})_{ji}]$.

By summing over all intermediate subscripts we get the vector balance equations:

$$\boldsymbol{\pi}(n)(\boldsymbol{\mathcal{M}} + \mu\boldsymbol{\mathcal{I}}) = \boldsymbol{\pi}(n)\boldsymbol{\mathcal{M}}\boldsymbol{\mathcal{P}} + \boldsymbol{\pi}(n+1)\nu + \boldsymbol{\pi}(n-1)\boldsymbol{\mathcal{L}}.$$

Making use of the relation, $\boldsymbol{\mathcal{B}} = \boldsymbol{\mathcal{M}} - \boldsymbol{\mathcal{M}}\boldsymbol{\mathcal{P}}$ we get for $n \geq 1$,

$$\boldsymbol{\pi}(n+1)\nu - \boldsymbol{\pi}(n)(\boldsymbol{\mathcal{B}} + \nu\boldsymbol{\mathcal{I}}) + \boldsymbol{\pi}(n-1)\boldsymbol{\mathcal{L}} = 0. \tag{8.4.1a}$$

[Compare with (4.1.3d).] For $n = 0$ there is no possibility for a customer to complete service, so instead we have

$$\boldsymbol{\pi}(1)\nu = \boldsymbol{\pi}(0)\boldsymbol{\mathcal{B}}. \tag{8.4.1b}$$

We now substitute $\boldsymbol{\pi}(n) = \boldsymbol{\pi}\boldsymbol{\mathcal{R}}^n$ into (8.4.1a), but $\boldsymbol{\pi}$ and $\boldsymbol{\mathcal{R}}$ are yet to be determined. For $n > 1$,

$$\boldsymbol{\pi}(1)\left[\nu\boldsymbol{\mathcal{R}}^{n+1} - \boldsymbol{\mathcal{R}}^n(\boldsymbol{\mathcal{B}} + \nu\boldsymbol{\mathcal{I}}) + \boldsymbol{\mathcal{R}}^{n-1}\boldsymbol{\mathcal{L}}\right] = 0.$$

Because this must be true for all $n > 1$ and $\boldsymbol{\pi}(1)$ cannot be 0, the expression in square brackets must be 0. Therefore

$$\mathcal{R}^{n-1}\left[\nu\mathcal{R}^2 - \mathcal{R}(\mathcal{B} + \nu\mathcal{I}) + \mathcal{L}\right] = 0.$$

Again, if $\mathcal{R}$ has an inverse (something that is not always true, as we show below) then the expression in square brackets must be 0. Thus

$$\nu\mathcal{R}^2 - \mathcal{R}(\mathcal{B} + \nu\mathcal{I}) + \mathcal{L} = 0. \tag{8.4.2a}$$

This equation doesn't hold for $n = 1$, so we must go back to (8.4.1a), using $\boldsymbol{\pi}(2) = \boldsymbol{\pi}(1)\mathcal{R}$, $\mathcal{Y} = \mathcal{V}\mathcal{L}$, and (8.4.1b) to get

$$\boldsymbol{\pi}(1)\left[\nu\mathcal{R} - \mathcal{B} - \nu\mathcal{I} + \nu\mathcal{Y}\right] = 0. \tag{8.4.2b}$$

Ah, if only we could argue that the expression in square brackets is zero, we would have an explicit expression for $\mathcal{R}$. But it is, instead, an eigenvector equation for $\boldsymbol{\pi}(1)$ (once we know what $\mathcal{R}$ is). A necessary and sufficient condition that $\mathcal{R} = \mathcal{I} + \mathcal{B}/\nu - \mathcal{Y}$ satisfy (8.4.2a) is that $\mathcal{Y}^2 = \mathcal{Y}$. From (8.2.12c) this condition leads to $\text{Cov}(X, X_{+k})$ = constant, independent of k. Furthermore, all the eigenvalues of $\mathcal{Y}$ must be either 0 or 1, the number of unit eigenvalues being equal to the rank of $\mathcal{Y}$. The only processes of interest to us that have these properties are the renewal processes, where the covariance equals 0 for all k and $\mathcal{Y} = \boldsymbol{\varepsilon}'\boldsymbol{\wp}$ has one unit eigenvalue. In fact this is exactly what we used in Chapters 4 and 5. But that does not work here, for we are now interested in the more general MRPs. We discuss this in Section 8.4.3.

Equation (8.4.2a) is the defining equation for $\mathcal{R}$, but it is not that easy to solve. First we search for some other properties. We multiply this equation from the right by $\boldsymbol{\varepsilon}'$ and note that $\mathcal{L}\boldsymbol{\varepsilon}' = \mathcal{B}\boldsymbol{\varepsilon}'$ to get:

$$\nu(\mathcal{R} - \mathcal{I})\mathcal{R}\boldsymbol{\varepsilon}' = (\mathcal{R} - \mathcal{I})\mathcal{B}\boldsymbol{\varepsilon}'.$$

But $(\mathcal{R} - \mathcal{I})$ must have an inverse unless at least one of the eigenvalues of $\mathcal{R}$ equals 1. This happens when the arrival rate ($\kappa = \boldsymbol{\pi}\mathcal{L}\boldsymbol{\varepsilon}'$) equals ν, in which case the system is unstable and there is no steady-state solution. Otherwise, a unit eigenvalue implies decomposability, a property which we assume has been removed *a priori*. So, assuming that $(\mathcal{I} - \mathcal{R})^{-1}$ exists, we get

$$\nu\mathcal{R}\boldsymbol{\varepsilon}' = \mathcal{B}\boldsymbol{\varepsilon}'. \tag{8.4.3}$$

This relation also satisfies (8.4.2b).

The $\boldsymbol{\pi}$ vectors must still satisfy the normalization property $\sum r(n) = 1$. But more than that, we can assume that if the MRP is observed without reference to queue length it must be found in state i with the same probability as the residual vector. That is,

$$\sum_{n=o}^{\infty} \boldsymbol{\pi}(n) = \boldsymbol{\pi},$$

where $\boldsymbol{\pi}$ (no argument) is defined by (8.2.8b), namely, $\boldsymbol{\pi}\boldsymbol{\mathcal{Q}} = \mathbf{o}$, and $\boldsymbol{\pi}\boldsymbol{\varepsilon}' = 1$. Thus [note that $\boldsymbol{\pi}(0)$ may not be of the same form as the other vector probabilities]

$$\boldsymbol{\pi} = \sum_{n=1}^{\infty} \boldsymbol{\pi}(1)\boldsymbol{\mathcal{R}}^{n-1} + \boldsymbol{\pi}(0) = \boldsymbol{\pi}(1)\left[(\boldsymbol{\mathcal{I}} - \boldsymbol{\mathcal{R}})^{-1} + \nu\boldsymbol{\mathcal{V}}\right]$$

or

$$\boldsymbol{\pi}(1)[\boldsymbol{\mathcal{I}} + \nu\boldsymbol{\mathcal{V}}(\boldsymbol{\mathcal{I}} - \boldsymbol{\mathcal{R}})] = \boldsymbol{\pi}(\boldsymbol{\mathcal{I}} - \boldsymbol{\mathcal{R}}). \tag{8.4.4}$$

But equations (8.4.2a), (8.4.2b), (8.4.3), and (8.4.4) together are not sufficient to uniquely determine the vector-matrix pair $\langle \boldsymbol{u}, \boldsymbol{\mathcal{R}} \rangle$. In fact, there may be multiple distinct solutions, all of which produce the same queue-length probabilities $\boldsymbol{\pi}(n)$.

At this point, following [MEIER-FISCHER92], we assume that

$$c\boldsymbol{u} = \boldsymbol{\pi}(\boldsymbol{\mathcal{I}} - \boldsymbol{\mathcal{R}}).$$

From this we have

$$\boldsymbol{\pi}(n) = \boldsymbol{\pi}(\boldsymbol{\mathcal{I}} - \boldsymbol{\mathcal{R}})\boldsymbol{\mathcal{R}}^n \quad \text{and} \quad r(n) = \boldsymbol{\pi}(\boldsymbol{\mathcal{I}} - \boldsymbol{\mathcal{R}})\boldsymbol{\mathcal{R}}^n\boldsymbol{\varepsilon}'. \tag{8.4.5}$$

This equation clearly satisfies $\sum \boldsymbol{\pi}(n) = \boldsymbol{\pi}$, which then implies that $\sum r(n) = 1$. But, we still don't know how to solve for $\boldsymbol{\mathcal{R}}$.

A standard procedure for finding $\boldsymbol{\mathcal{R}}$ follows.

Algorithm 8.4.1: First rewrite (8.4.2a) as

$$\boldsymbol{\mathcal{R}} = \nu\boldsymbol{\mathcal{R}}^2\boldsymbol{\mathcal{D}} + \boldsymbol{\mathcal{L}}\boldsymbol{\mathcal{D}},$$

where $\boldsymbol{\mathcal{D}} := (\nu\boldsymbol{\mathcal{I}} + \boldsymbol{\mathcal{B}})^{-1}$. Consider this to be a formula for ***fixed point iteration***. That is, let $\boldsymbol{\mathcal{R}}_{\text{o}} = \mathbf{0}$ and

$$\boldsymbol{\mathcal{R}}_{\ell+1} = \nu(\boldsymbol{\mathcal{R}}_\ell)^2\boldsymbol{\mathcal{D}} + \boldsymbol{\mathcal{L}}\boldsymbol{\mathcal{D}}, \quad \text{for } \ell \geq 0.$$

Iterate on ℓ until $(\boldsymbol{\mathcal{R}}_{\ell+1} - \boldsymbol{\mathcal{R}}_\ell)$ is "sufficiently small" by some pre-established criterion.

This procedure is guaranteed to converge if the MRP was constructed from PH representations, but may not converge otherwise. Nonconvergence does not mean there is no solution, just that another method, or a different $\boldsymbol{\mathcal{R}}_{\text{o}}$, must be chosen. Furthermore, this is not the unique solution to (8.4.2a). Given that this is a quadratic equation, one might expect to find two independent solutions. But this is a ***matrix quadratic*** equation, for which the number of independent solutions is given by

$$\begin{pmatrix} 2M \\ M \end{pmatrix}, \quad \text{where } M = \text{Dim}(\boldsymbol{\mathcal{R}}).$$

We can say that the algorithm produces an $\boldsymbol{\mathcal{R}}$ whose eigenvalues are all less than 1 in magnitude, otherwise the algorithm would not converge. For more information, see [LATOUCHE-RAM99] or [NEUTS89]. We give an example of this ambiguity when we look at the G/M/1 queue from the point-of-view of this chapter.

Before showing how to calculate various performance measures we prove the following.

Theorem 8.4.1: The matrix $\boldsymbol{\mathcal{R}}$, as found by the iterative method described above, must be of the form

$$\boldsymbol{\mathcal{R}} = \boldsymbol{\mathcal{L}}\boldsymbol{\mathcal{X}}, \tag{8.4.6}$$

and has at most the same rank as $\boldsymbol{\mathcal{L}}$. Therefore if $\boldsymbol{\mathcal{L}}$ has no inverse, then $\boldsymbol{\mathcal{R}}$ has no inverse. But there may be another solution of (8.4.2a) that is invertible. ■

Proof: Observe that $\boldsymbol{\mathcal{R}}_1 = \boldsymbol{\mathcal{L}}\boldsymbol{\mathcal{D}}$. Next assume that $\boldsymbol{\mathcal{R}}_k = \boldsymbol{\mathcal{L}}\boldsymbol{\mathcal{X}}_k$ for $k \le \ell$ where $\boldsymbol{\mathcal{X}}_\ell$ follows from the recursive formula. Then

$$\boldsymbol{\mathcal{R}}_{\ell+1} = \nu\boldsymbol{\mathcal{L}}\boldsymbol{\mathcal{X}}_\ell\boldsymbol{\mathcal{L}}\boldsymbol{\mathcal{X}}_\ell\boldsymbol{\mathcal{D}} + \boldsymbol{\mathcal{L}}\boldsymbol{\mathcal{D}} = \boldsymbol{\mathcal{L}}[\nu\boldsymbol{\mathcal{X}}_\ell\boldsymbol{\mathcal{L}}\boldsymbol{\mathcal{X}}_\ell\boldsymbol{\mathcal{D}} + \boldsymbol{\mathcal{D}}] = \boldsymbol{\mathcal{L}}\boldsymbol{\mathcal{X}}_{\ell+1}.$$

Therefore, $\boldsymbol{\mathcal{R}}_\ell = \boldsymbol{\mathcal{L}}\boldsymbol{\mathcal{X}}_\ell$ for all ℓ. Furthermore, the limit (if it exists) is

$$\boldsymbol{\mathcal{R}} = \lim_{\ell\to\infty} \boldsymbol{\mathcal{L}}\boldsymbol{\mathcal{X}}_\ell = \boldsymbol{\mathcal{L}}\boldsymbol{\mathcal{X}},$$

where

$$\boldsymbol{\mathcal{X}} := \lim_{\ell\to\infty} \boldsymbol{\mathcal{X}}_\ell.$$

Therefore, $\text{Rank}(\boldsymbol{\mathcal{R}}) \le \text{Rank}(\boldsymbol{\mathcal{L}})$.

The method described here may not apply to some more general systems, but it does apply to all MRP/M/1 queues.

8.4.2 Some Performance Measures

As in previous chapters, given $\boldsymbol{\pi}(n)$ one can compute the mean queue length, the mean system time, and probability of overflow. We do that now.

Let N be the r.v. denoting the number of customers queued at S_ν; then

$$\bar{q} := \mathbf{E}[N] = \sum_{n=1}^{\infty} n\, r(n) = \boldsymbol{\pi}(\boldsymbol{\mathcal{I}}-\boldsymbol{\mathcal{R}}) \left[\sum_{n=1}^{\infty} n\boldsymbol{\mathcal{R}}^n\right] \boldsymbol{\varepsilon}' = \boldsymbol{\pi}\boldsymbol{\mathcal{R}}[\boldsymbol{\mathcal{I}}-\boldsymbol{\mathcal{R}}]^{-1}\boldsymbol{\varepsilon}'. \tag{8.4.7a}$$

The *mean system time* is given by Little's formula (1.1.2). This is also called ***Mean Cell Delay*** (MCD) or ***Mean Packet Delay*** (MPD) when studying telecommunications traffic. We need κ, the arrival rate of cells to S_ν, to use Little's formula. This is given by (8.2.8d).

$$MCD = \frac{\mathbf{E}[N]}{\kappa} = (\boldsymbol{\wp}\boldsymbol{\mathcal{V}}\boldsymbol{\varepsilon}')\,\boldsymbol{\pi}\boldsymbol{\mathcal{R}}[\boldsymbol{\mathcal{I}}-\boldsymbol{\mathcal{R}}]^{-1}\boldsymbol{\varepsilon}'. \tag{8.4.7b}$$

Recall from Section 4.2.4 what is meant by ***buffer overflow probability*** (BOP), namely $\mathbf{Pr}(N \ge B_s)$, where B_s is the size of the primary buffer. The probability that an arriving customer will see n customers at S_ν is needed to find this. $[\boldsymbol{\pi}(n)]_i$ is the steady-state probability that there are n cells already at S_ν and the MRP is in state i. Multiplying by $\mathcal{L}\varepsilon'$ gives the probability rate that a new cell will arrive under these conditions. Upon dividing by the overall arrival rate, we get the arrival probability.

$$a(n) = (\wp\mathcal{V}\varepsilon')\,\boldsymbol{\pi}[(\mathcal{I} - \mathcal{R})\mathcal{R}^n\,\mathcal{L}]\varepsilon'. \tag{8.4.8a}$$

Then the BOP is

$$\begin{aligned}\mathbb{P}\mathbf{r}(N \geq B_s) &= \sum_{n=B_s}^{\infty} a(n) = (\wp\mathcal{V}\varepsilon')\,\boldsymbol{\pi}\,(\mathcal{I} - \mathcal{R})\left[\sum_{n=B_s}^{\infty} \mathcal{R}^n\right]\mathcal{L}\varepsilon' \\ &= (\wp\mathcal{V}\varepsilon')\boldsymbol{\pi}[\mathcal{R}^{B_s}\mathcal{L}]\varepsilon'.\end{aligned} \tag{8.4.8b}$$

For further information of the utility of these formulas see, for instance, [SCHWEFEL00], [SCHWEFEL-LIP01], and [PARK-WILL00].

8.4.3 The G/M/1 Queue as an Example

Recall that in Chapters 4 and 5 we solved the M/G/1 and G/M/1 queues by finding the special matrices (replacing λ with ν) $\mathbf{A} = \mathbf{I} + \mathbf{B}/\nu - \mathbf{Q}$ and $\mathbf{U} = \mathbf{A}^{-1}$ in (4.1.4a), yielding $r(n) = (1-\rho)\mathbf{p}\mathbf{U}^n\boldsymbol{\epsilon}'$ for the M/G/1 queue. The G/M/1 queue was more difficult, and the limit in going from the G/M/1//N to the open G/M/1 queue for $N \to \infty$ has to be taken very carefully. But we found the solution in Theorem 5.1.3 to be

$$\boldsymbol{\pi}(0) = (1 - \varrho)\frac{\hat{\mathbf{u}}\mathbf{V}}{\hat{\mathbf{u}}\mathbf{V}\boldsymbol{\epsilon}'} \quad \text{and}$$
$$\boldsymbol{\pi}(k) = (1 - s)\varrho\, s^{k-1}\hat{\mathbf{u}},$$

where $\varrho = 1/(\nu\Psi[\mathbf{V}])$ is the utilization parameter of Chapter 5, and

$$\hat{\mathbf{u}} = \nu\mathbf{p}\,[\nu(1 - s)\mathbf{I} + \mathbf{B}]^{-1}$$

with normalization, $\hat{\mathbf{u}}\boldsymbol{\epsilon}' = 1$. s is the smallest positive root of the equation

$$s = B^*[\nu(1 - s)] = \mathbf{p}\mathbf{B}(\mathbf{B} + \nu(1 - s)\mathbf{I})^{-1}\boldsymbol{\epsilon}'.$$

Of more relevance to us here, we also showed that $\hat{\mathbf{u}}\mathbf{A} = s\,\hat{\mathbf{u}}$, that is, s is the smallest positive eigenvalue of $\mathbf{A}$, with left eigenvector $\hat{\mathbf{u}}$. Because of this, the solution could be written in matrix geometric form as

$$\boldsymbol{\pi}(k) = (1 - s)\varrho\,\hat{\mathbf{u}}\mathbf{A}^{k-1}.$$

Interestingly enough, $\mathbf{A}$ has eigenvalues that are greater than 1 in magnitude, so $\mathbf{A}^k$ grows unboundedly large with k. But $\hat{\mathbf{u}}$ is orthogonal to all the corresponding eigenvectors, so $\hat{\mathbf{u}}\mathbf{A}^k = \hat{\mathbf{u}}\,s^k \to 0$. Its relevance here is that $\mathbf{A}$ satisfies (8.4.2a) with $\mathcal{L} = \mathbf{BQ}$, yet it does not satisfy Theorem 8.4.1. That is,

$$\nu\mathbf{A}^2 - \mathbf{A}(\mathbf{B} + \nu\mathbf{I}) + \mathbf{BQ} = 0.$$

(Recall that here, $\mathbf{Q} = \boldsymbol{\epsilon}'\mathbf{p}$.) But although $\mathbf{BQ}$ is of rank 1, Rank($\mathbf{A}$) = Dim($\mathbf{A}$) > 1 if the renewal process is not Poisson.

We now use Algorithm 8.4.1 (well, not quite) to find a solution of (8.4.2a). We know from Theorem 8.4.1 that $\mathbf{R}$ must be of rank 1, because $\mathbf{BQ}$ is of rank 1. Therefore, $\mathbf{R}$ must be of the form $s\mathbf{v}'\mathbf{u}$ where $\mathbf{u}\,\mathbf{v}' = 1$. Its one non-zero eigenvalue is s. Given that we know its form so precisely, we can substitute it into (8.4.2a) and find what s, $\mathbf{u}$, and $\mathbf{v}'$ are. Note that$(s\mathbf{v}'\mathbf{u})^2 = s^2\mathbf{v}'\mathbf{u}$, therefore $\mathbf{R}^2 = s\mathbf{R}$. (In fact, for any $n > 0$, $\mathbf{R}^n = s^{n-1}\mathbf{R}$.) Then

$$\nu\mathbf{R}^2 - \mathbf{R}(\mathbf{B} + \nu\mathbf{I}) + \mathbf{BQ} = \nu s\mathbf{R} - \mathbf{R}(\mathbf{B} + \nu\mathbf{I}) + \mathbf{BQ} = \mathbf{BQ} - \mathbf{R}(\mathbf{B} + \nu(1-s)\mathbf{I}) = 0.$$

Rearranging the terms and multiplying from the right by $(\mathbf{B} + \nu(1 - s)\mathbf{I})^{-1}$ yields

$$\mathbf{R} = \mathbf{B}\boldsymbol{\epsilon}'[\mathbf{p}(\mathbf{B} + \nu(1 - s)\mathbf{I})].$$

But if s is right, the expression in square brackets is precisely what was defined above as $\hat{\mathbf{u}}/\nu$. In order to have $\mathbf{R} = s\mathbf{v}'\hat{\mathbf{u}}$ it must follow that $\hat{\mathbf{u}}\mathbf{B}\boldsymbol{\epsilon}' = s\nu$. But this reduces to the expression $s = \mathbf{pB}(\mathbf{B} + \nu(1 - s)\mathbf{I})^{-1}\boldsymbol{\epsilon}'$, the equation that defined s. Therefore $s\nu\mathbf{v}' = \mathbf{B}\boldsymbol{\epsilon}'$, and because $\mathbf{B}\boldsymbol{\epsilon}' = \boldsymbol{\mathcal{L}}\boldsymbol{\epsilon}'$,

$$\mathbf{R} = \frac{1}{\nu}\mathbf{B}\boldsymbol{\epsilon}'\hat{\mathbf{u}} = \frac{1}{\nu}\boldsymbol{\mathcal{L}}\boldsymbol{\epsilon}'\hat{\mathbf{u}} = \mathbf{A}\boldsymbol{\epsilon}'\hat{\mathbf{u}},$$

thereby explicitly satisfying Theorem 8.4.1. The rightmost expression for $\mathbf{R}$ explicitly yields the idempotent property for $\mathbf{R}$. That is,

$$\mathbf{R}^2 = (\mathbf{A}\boldsymbol{\epsilon}'\hat{\mathbf{u}})(\mathbf{A}\boldsymbol{\epsilon}'\hat{\mathbf{u}}) = \mathbf{A}\boldsymbol{\epsilon}'(\hat{\mathbf{u}}\mathbf{A}\boldsymbol{\epsilon}')\hat{\mathbf{u}} = s\mathbf{A}\boldsymbol{\epsilon}'\hat{\mathbf{u}} = s\mathbf{R},$$

and thus,

$$\mathbf{R}^n = s^{n-1}\mathbf{R}.$$

Using what we have found so far we can say that, for $n > 0$,

$$\boldsymbol{\pi}(n) = \boldsymbol{\pi}(\mathbf{I} - \mathbf{R})\mathbf{R}^n = s^{n-1}\boldsymbol{\pi}(\mathbf{R} - \mathbf{R}^2) = s^{n-1}(1 - s)\boldsymbol{\pi}\mathbf{R}.$$

Next we look at $\boldsymbol{\pi}\mathbf{R}$,

$$\boldsymbol{\pi}\mathbf{R} = \left(\frac{1}{\mathbf{pV}\boldsymbol{\epsilon}'}\mathbf{pV}\right)\left(\frac{1}{\nu}\mathbf{B}\boldsymbol{\epsilon}'\hat{\mathbf{u}}\right) = \varrho\,\hat{\mathbf{u}}.$$

This yields

$$\boldsymbol{\pi}(n) = (1 - s)s^{n-1}\varrho\,\hat{\mathbf{u}} \quad \text{for } n \geq 1,$$

exactly the same as Chapter 5. With some contortions (identical with those we did in Chapter 5) we can reproduce the expression for $\boldsymbol{\pi}(0)$ given above.

In conclusion, we have found two completely distinct solutions for the simplest nontrivial MRP/M/1 queue, and have shown that they produce identical results. For more complicated systems it may be impossible to show that two different solutions yield the same results except by direct computation, but then we can only be sure to within numerical accuracy, and even then only for the particular parameters chosen.

Chapter 9

LAQT

A theory should be as simple as possible, but no simpler
Albert Einstein

In the previous chapters we saw that matrix relations continually occur, independently of probabilistic interpretations. Surely this is not an accident. We now attempt to create a linear algebraic formulation that is not merely an algorithmic or computational aid but could lead to a complete formal procedure for dealing with nonexponential queues. The idea is to avoid resorting to any particular basis set, a common technique in linear algebra. We have not been entirely successful, but some interesting results, particularly in Section 9.3, are presented. The rest is open to discussion and review.

We first show that most, if not all, the equations in this book are invariant to the isometric transformations we introduced in Section 3.4.2. This invariance property implies that a basis-free formulation is possible. In some sense this chapter serves as a review of the book, but now all the properties of the servers and queues are in terms of linear operators that modify the state vector of the system when things happen. This change in viewpoint may appear self-evident to some readers, and if so, fine, but it is important to mention, nonetheless. We do not claim that we are doing this in the best or most efficient way to set up the algebraic structure. Surely some readers can do better. We merely wish to show that it can be done. Therefore, questions that may arise should not be considered to be weaknesses of the theory but issues to be cleared up or clarified, which may actually lead to new insights.

One problem we have is that density functions have the constraint that $f(x) \geq 0$ for all pdfs. Thus the difference of pdfs does not always lead to a function that is greater than or equal to 0 for all x. Therefore the set of all pdfs is not truly a ***vector space*** even though the set of all integrable functions is. In various areas of applied mathematics, functions are expanded in terms of orthogonal functions which serve as the ***basis vectors***. See Section 4.4.2 for the example of Laguerre polynomials and the discussion therein. Usually the accepted metric is defined in L_2 space, that is, the "length" of a vector (function) is

$$\left[\int_0^\infty |f(x)|^2 dx\right]^{1/2}$$

L. Lipsky, *Queueing Theory*, DOI 10.1007/978-0-387-49706-8_9,

and ***orthogonal basis functions***, $\{\phi_j(x)\}$ satisfy the property:

$$\int_0^\infty \phi_j(x)\phi_i'(x)dx = \delta_{ij}.$$

For this orthogonality condition to occur, all but one of the ϕ_is must be negative for some values of x. Therefore they cannot be interpreted as pdfs.

In quantum mechanics the ψ functions are interpreted as ***probability amplitudes*** (i.e., $|\psi(x)|^2$ is a probability density), and $\psi(x)$ can even be complex. How fortunate for physics that nature works this way for subatomic particles. But we are stuck with classical probability and as a substitute must use phases as basis functions, and isometric transformations as a substitute for preserving lengths. So don't try too hard to give physical meaning to individual phases.

9.1 Isometric Transformations

In Section 3.4.2 (Theorem 3.4.1), we showed that if $\langle \mathbf{p}, \mathbf{B} \rangle$ is a faithful representation of a given distribution function, so is $\langle \mathbf{pS}^{-1}, \mathbf{SBS}^{-1} \rangle$, where $\mathbf{S}$ is any isometric invertible matrix. That is, $B(t)$, $R(t)$, $b(t)$, and $B^*(s)$ remain unchanged by such transformations. These isometric transformations go beyond the description of a single server. We now extend this idea to any row vector $\mathbf{u}$, column vector $\mathbf{v}'$, and square matrix $\mathbf{X}$, and define the following mapping.

Definition 9.1.1

Let $\mathbf{S}$ be any nonsingular ***isometric matrix***, then the following mapping (or similarity transformation) is called an *isometric transformation*:

$$\tilde{\mathbf{u}} := \mathbf{uS}^{-1}, \qquad \tilde{\mathbf{v}}' = \mathbf{Sv}',$$

and

$$\tilde{\mathbf{X}} := \mathbf{SXS}^{-1},$$

for every row vector, column vector, and matrix of interest. Because $\mathbf{S}$ is isometric, $\boldsymbol{\epsilon}'$ does not change under any transformation. Note that

$$\tilde{\mathbf{u}}\tilde{\mathbf{v}}' = \mathbf{uS}^{-1}\mathbf{Sv}' = \mathbf{uv}' \quad \text{and} \quad \tilde{\Psi}\left[\tilde{\mathbf{X}}\right] := \tilde{\mathbf{p}}\tilde{\mathbf{X}}\boldsymbol{\epsilon}' = \Psi\left[\mathbf{X}\right].$$

These equations show us that inner products and $\Psi[\cdot]$ operations remain unchanged (are invariant) under isometric transformations. In general, we say that an "equation is invariant" if it is identical in form for the transformed objects as it is for the original objects. □

We showed in Section 4.1.2 that the steady-state solutions of M/G/1 queues (both open and closed) depend on the matrix $\mathbf{A}$ and its inverse $\mathbf{U}$, defined by

$$\mathbf{A} := \mathbf{U}^{-1} := \mathbf{I} + \frac{1}{\lambda}\mathbf{B} - \mathbf{Q}, \tag{9.1.1}$$

where λ is the service rate of S_2 (or the Poisson arrival rate to S_1), and $\mathbf{Q} := \boldsymbol{\epsilon}'\,\mathbf{p}$. Given that $\mathbf{S}\boldsymbol{\epsilon}' = \boldsymbol{\epsilon}'$, it follows from their definitions that

$$\tilde{\mathbf{Q}} = \mathbf{S}\mathbf{Q}\mathbf{S}^{-1} = \mathbf{S}\boldsymbol{\epsilon}'\,\mathbf{p}\,\mathbf{S}^{-1} = \boldsymbol{\epsilon}'\,\tilde{\mathbf{p}}$$

and

$$\tilde{\mathbf{A}} = \mathbf{S}\mathbf{A}\mathbf{S}^{-1} = \mathbf{I} + \frac{1}{\lambda}\tilde{\mathbf{B}} - \tilde{\mathbf{Q}}.$$

Thus the equations defining $\mathbf{Q}$ and $\mathbf{A}$ are invariant to isometric transformations. From Theorem 4.1.2, the steady-state vector and scalar probabilities for the open queue are

$$\boldsymbol{\pi}(n) = (1-\rho)\mathbf{p}\,\mathbf{U}^n \tag{9.1.2a}$$

and

$$r(n) = \boldsymbol{\pi}(n)\boldsymbol{\epsilon}' = (1-\rho)\Psi\left[\mathbf{U}^n\right]. \tag{9.1.2b}$$

Any isometric transformation $\mathbf{S}$ will produce the following.

$$\tilde{\boldsymbol{\pi}}(n) := \boldsymbol{\pi}(n)\mathbf{S}^{-1} = (1-\rho)\mathbf{p}\mathbf{S}^{-1}\mathbf{S}\,\mathbf{U}^n\,\mathbf{S}^{-1} = (1-\rho)\tilde{\mathbf{p}}\,\tilde{\mathbf{U}}^n$$

and (note that $\mathbf{S}\mathbf{U}^2\mathbf{S}^{-1} = \mathbf{S}\mathbf{U}\mathbf{S}^{-1}\mathbf{S}\mathbf{U}\mathbf{S}^{-1} = \tilde{\mathbf{U}}^{-2}$, etc. for all n)

$$\tilde{r}(n) := \tilde{\boldsymbol{\pi}}(n)\boldsymbol{\epsilon}' = (1-\rho)\tilde{\Psi}\left[\tilde{\mathbf{U}}^n\right] = (1-\rho)\Psi\left[\mathbf{U}^n\right] = r(n).$$

Clearly, the vector and scalar probabilities, $\boldsymbol{\pi}(n)$ and $r(n)$, are also invariant to isometric transformations. In particular, we see that for scalars [e.g., $r(n)$], "invariance" means "no change."

We mentioned in Section 4.4 that the standard algorithm for evaluating the steady-state probabilities for the M/G/1 queue requires the ***exponential moments*** defined by

$$\alpha_n(s) := \int_0^\infty \frac{(sx)^n}{n!} e^{-sx} b(x)dx.$$

We then showed that [Equations (4.4.1)]

$$\alpha_n(s) = \Psi\left[(s\mathbf{V}\mathbf{D})^n\mathbf{D}\right],$$

where $\mathbf{D} := (\mathbf{I} + \mathbf{s}V)^{-1}$. Clearly, these expressions are invariant to isometric transformations, so the results one gets with one representation will be identical to the results one gets with any similar representation. For instance [using $(\mathbf{S}\mathbf{X}\mathbf{S}^{-1})^{-1} = (\mathbf{S}^{-1})^{-1}\mathbf{X}^{-1}\mathbf{S}^{-1} = \mathbf{S}\mathbf{X}^{-1}\mathbf{S}^{-1}$],

$$\begin{aligned}\tilde{\mathbf{D}} := \mathbf{S}\mathbf{D}\mathbf{S}^{-1} &= \mathbf{S}[\mathbf{I} + \mathbf{s}\mathbf{V}]^{-1}\mathbf{S}^{-1} = [\mathbf{S}(\mathbf{I} + \mathbf{s}\mathbf{V})\mathbf{S}^{-1}]^{-1}\\ &= [\mathbf{I} + \mathbf{s}\mathbf{S}\mathbf{V}\mathbf{S}^{-1}]^{-1} = [\mathbf{I} + \mathbf{s}\tilde{\mathbf{V}}]^{-1}.\end{aligned}$$

We mention that the various formulas describing the M/ME/1 queue are very similar to those for the M/M/1 queue and would generalize trivially were it not for the fact that $\mathbf{Q}$ and $\mathbf{B}$ do not commute! On the other hand, things would have been a lot worse if $\mathbf{Q}$ did not have rank one, which is the case for M/G/C//N systems.

9.2 Linear Algebraic Formulation

We now attempt to formulate queueing processes without resorting to individual components or phases. First we look at a single isolated (general) server S. To do this we change the meaning of our notation somewhat. In general, one can start with a set of independent basis vectors (the equivalent of our phases) and then generate the entire vector space by taking all possible linear combinations of the basis vectors. Alternatively, we can start with an abstract vector space, and then, if we need one, select a basis set. We did the former in previous chapters. We do the latter here. We assume, as we did throughout this book, that all systems of interest are ***stationary*** in that all the primitive operators are independent of time [FELLER71].

9.2.1 Description of a Single Server

Let $\mathbf{r}$ be a vector in some discrete (in our case, finite-dimensional) vector space Ξ that contains all we know about S. Previously, we considered Ξ to be the set of phases of S and then constructed the vectors from them. Now, we let Ξ be the set of all vectors. In doing this we are actually tightening up our mathematics. Keep in mind, though, that not every vector in Ξ has physical meaning.

Let the "length" of any vector in Ξ be its "dot product" with a special unique vector from the ***adjoint space*** Ξ', denoted by $\boldsymbol{\epsilon}'$.*

Then, for one thing,

$$R := \mathbf{r}\,\boldsymbol{\epsilon}' = \text{probability that S is busy.}$$

R is a measurable quantity, but the components of $\mathbf{r}$ need not be. From an outside observer's point of view, S can only be in one of two *external states*: either it is busy or it is not. What goes on inside is hidden from view until S stops, in which case $\mathbf{r}$ becomes the null vector, $\mathbf{o}$. (Of course, if an observer really can look inside, S must truly be a phase distribution.)

From the basic Markov property, only one thing can happen at a time, and it can only depend on the state the system is in when it happens. Also, a transition that does not change the length of $\mathbf{r}$ is not directly observable. Let $\mathbf{P}$ be a linear operator on Ξ which moderates internal transitions, while $\mathbf{q}'$ moderates completion of service. That is, given that something has occurred, $\mathbf{r}\mathbf{q}'$ is the probability that service ended, $\mathbf{r}\mathbf{P}$ is the new state S is in if service has not ended, and $\mathbf{r}\mathbf{P}\,\boldsymbol{\epsilon}'$ is the probability that service did not end. Nothing else can occur, so we must have

$$\mathbf{r}\mathbf{q}' + \mathbf{r}\,\mathbf{P}\,\boldsymbol{\epsilon}' = \mathbf{r}\,\boldsymbol{\epsilon}'.$$

*Technically, objects in Ξ' are ***linear functionals*** that map vectors in Ξ into the complex numbers. It is well known that this is also a vector space (see, e.g., [HALMOS55]) and is isomorphic to (i.e., has the same dimension as) Ξ. When one is working with an explicit basis, one thinks of row and column vectors, and the scalar mapping is the dot product.

This equation must be true for all $\mathbf{r} \in \Xi$ which have physical meaning, so it follows that $\mathbf{q}' + \mathbf{P}\boldsymbol{\epsilon}' = \boldsymbol{\epsilon}'$. Put differently, this equation can be rewritten as

$$\mathbf{r}[\mathbf{q}' + \mathbf{P}\boldsymbol{\epsilon}' - \boldsymbol{\epsilon}'] = 0.$$

Then if it is true for m linearly independent $\mathbf{r}$ vextors, the term in brackets must be identically equal to $\mathbf{o}'$. (m is the dimension of vector space Ξ.) Thus $\mathbf{q}'$ and $\mathbf{P}$ are related by the relation

$$\mathbf{q}' = (\mathbf{I} - \mathbf{P})\boldsymbol{\epsilon}'. \tag{9.2.1}$$

The time scale for the behavior of S comes in through the operator $\mathbf{T}$, where $\mathbf{rT}\boldsymbol{\epsilon}'$ is the mean time to the next event. Also, let $\boldsymbol{\tau}' \in \Xi'$ be a linear functional such that $\mathbf{r}\boldsymbol{\tau}'$ is the mean time until service terminates, given that S is initially busy, and described by state vector $\mathbf{r}$, where $\mathbf{r}\boldsymbol{\epsilon}' = 1$. Then we can write

$$\mathbf{r}\boldsymbol{\tau}' = \mathbf{rT}\boldsymbol{\epsilon}' + \mathbf{rP}\boldsymbol{\tau}'.$$

In words, the time for service to complete is made up of two parts. First there is the time until the next event [$\mathbf{rT}\boldsymbol{\epsilon}'$], and if that event was not a termination [$\mathbf{rP}\boldsymbol{\epsilon}'$], then S changes its internal state [$\mathbf{rP}$], and completes service from there [$\boldsymbol{\tau}'$]. Given that this equation is valid for all $\mathbf{r} \in \Xi$, we can once again discard $\mathbf{r}$ and solve for $\boldsymbol{\tau}'$ to get

$$\boldsymbol{\tau}' = (\mathbf{I} - \mathbf{P})^{-1}\mathbf{T}\boldsymbol{\epsilon}' = \mathbf{V}\boldsymbol{\epsilon}', \tag{9.2.2}$$

where $\mathbf{V} := (\mathbf{I} - \mathbf{P})^{-1}\mathbf{T}$.

Next, let $\mathbf{M}$ be a linear operator on our vector space that moderates the occurrence of events. Then $\mathbf{rM}\boldsymbol{\epsilon}'$ is the instantaneous rate for something to happen. A physical interpretation of what this means is as follows. Suppose that there exists a basis set for Ξ in which $\mathbf{M}$ is diagonal. (It might be quite interesting to explore systems in which this were not possible, although it is not clear what that would mean.) Each basis vector $\mathbf{u}_i$ is referred to as a ***phase*** or ***pure state***, and μ_i, the eigenvalue of $\mathbf{M}$ that goes with $\mathbf{u}_i$, is the formal "probability rate" at which the system leaves state i. The time to leave state i is "exponentially distributed" with exponent μ_i. Note that the $\mu's$ need not be real, so this interpretation may not have physical meaning. As we show presently, this does not lead to any contradictions, as long as physical (i.e., observable) quantities do not depend on the individual components of the vectors in Ξ.

Based on our assumptions about S, only two types of things can happen. We have just seen that either the system changes its internal state according to the linear operator $\mathbf{P}$, or it stops (i.e., the customer leaves), according to the adjoint vector $\mathbf{q}'$. That is, $\mathbf{rMq}'$ is the probability rate that S will have an event that results in a departure. We now examine how the internal status of S evolves in time. Let $\mathbf{r}(t)$ contain that information and have initial value $\mathbf{p} := \mathbf{r}(0)$ such that $\mathbf{p}\boldsymbol{\epsilon}' = 1$. In other words, we assume that whenever S first starts service (at $t = 0$) it will always be represented by the ***initial vector*** or ***entrance vector*** $\mathbf{p}$. Then we have

$$R(t) = \mathbf{r}(t)\boldsymbol{\epsilon}' = \text{probability that } S \text{ is still busy at time } t,$$

and $R(0) = 1$. Now, in some small time interval δ,

$$\mathbf{r}(t)\delta\mathbf{M} + \mathrm{O}(\delta^2) = \text{probability that something will happen.}$$

Then either nothing happens in the interval $[\mathbf{r}(t)(\mathbf{I} - \delta\mathbf{M})]$, or the event results in an internal transition $[\mathbf{r}(t)\delta\mathbf{MP}]$, or there is a departure (no term needed). Thus we have

$$\mathbf{r}(t+\delta) = \mathbf{r}(t)(\mathbf{I} - \delta\mathbf{M}) + \mathbf{r}(t)\delta\mathbf{MP} + \mathbf{O}(\delta^2). \tag{9.2.3a}$$

In the usual way, bring $\mathbf{r}(t)$ to the left-hand side of the equation, divide both sides by δ, and take the limit as δ goes to 0, to get, with the aid of the definition, $\mathbf{B} := \mathbf{M}(\mathbf{I} - \mathbf{P})$,

$$\frac{d\mathbf{r}(t)}{dt} = -\mathbf{r}(t)\mathbf{M}(\mathbf{I} - \mathbf{P}) = -\mathbf{r}(t)\mathbf{B}. \tag{9.2.3b}$$

Even on an abstract vector space, the solution of this differential equation is simple as long as we understand that $\exp(-t\mathbf{B})$ stands for its Maclaurin's series expansion. Given that $\mathbf{p} = \mathbf{r}(0)$, we get

$$\mathbf{r}(t) = \mathbf{p}\exp(-t\mathbf{B}), \tag{9.2.3c}$$

and by postmultiplying with $\boldsymbol{\epsilon}'$, we have

$$R(t) = \mathbf{r}(t)\boldsymbol{\epsilon}' = \Psi\left[\exp(-t\mathbf{B})\right]. \tag{9.2.3d}$$

Given that $b(t) = -R'(t)$, Equation (3.1.7d) directly follows. In fact, all of the equations in Theorem 3.1.1 follow from this if we recognize that $\mathbf{B} = \mathbf{V}^{-1}$, which in turn is true if and only if $\mathbf{T} = \mathbf{M}^{-1}$. Their derivation is almost identical to that which we gave in Chapter 3, except that here we never impose any physical meanings or constraints on the individual components of the matrices.

Equation (9.2.3d) is the primary one that places constraints on $\mathbf{p}$ and $\mathbf{B}$. $R(t)$ is an observable function, therefore it must satisfy the following,

$$t_2 > t_1 \geq 0 \quad \Longrightarrow \quad R(t_1) \geq R(t_2) \geq 0. \tag{9.2.4}$$

If Ξ is finite-dimensional, this constraint is no more or less than requiring that $1 - R(t)$ be a ***matrix exponential*** probability distribution function. In a base-free description, one might ask what the dimensionality of Ξ might be. This has a straightforward answer when one notes that $\boldsymbol{\epsilon}'$ is a unique invariant vector. Therefore, we define the dimension of Ξ' to be the smallest integer for which the family of vectors

$$\boldsymbol{\epsilon}',\ \mathbf{B}\boldsymbol{\epsilon}',\ \mathbf{B}^2\boldsymbol{\epsilon}',\ \mathbf{B}^3\boldsymbol{\epsilon}',\ \ldots,\ \mathbf{B}^n\boldsymbol{\epsilon}',\ \ldots \tag{9.2.5a}$$

is linearly independent. This is a base-free property, even though one usually uses some basis set representation to find that integer. Ξ and Ξ' must have the same dimension (call it m), and because of (9.2.5a), there must exist m linearly independent vectors, $\{\mathbf{r_j}!|1 \leq j \leq m\}$, in Ξ for which

$$\mathbf{r_j}\,\boldsymbol{\epsilon}' = 1, \quad \text{for } j = 1, 2, \ldots, m. \tag{9.2.5b}$$

These (or any independent linear combination of them) can be used as the basis set for Ξ. If we so desired, we could pick an appropriate linear combination that makes $\mathbf{M}$ a diagonal matrix, as discussed in the paragraph following (9.2.2). Note that all bases which satisfy (9.2.5b) must be related to each other by some ***isometric transformation***. Let $\{\mathbf{r_j}\}$ and $\{\tilde{\mathbf{r}}_\mathbf{j}\}$ be two bases for Ξ. Then there exists a matrix (or linear transformation) $\mathbf{S}$ such that

$$\mathbf{r_j}\,\mathbf{S} = \tilde{\mathbf{r}}_\mathbf{j} \quad \text{for } j = 1, 2, \ldots, m, \tag{9.2.5c}$$

and $\mathbf{S}\boldsymbol{\epsilon}' = \boldsymbol{\epsilon}'$.

Having said this, we see that all of the above depend on four independent objects, $\mathbf{p}$, $\mathbf{M}$, $\mathbf{P}$, and $\boldsymbol{\epsilon}'$. There might be a smaller set by combining $\mathbf{M}$ and $\mathbf{P}$ in $\mathbf{B}$. We use $\mathbf{M}$ in describing the interaction of two servers, but even in that more complicated system $\mathbf{M}$ can be absorbed into $\mathbf{B}$, so it remains to be seen if $\mathbf{M}$ is a fundamental object. In any case, we say that S is represented by $\langle\, \mathbf{p}\,,\, \mathbf{B} \,\rangle$ if the pdf for S satisfies Theorem 3.1.1).

9.2.2 Residual Vector and Related Properties

From now on we use the terminology of queueing theory to describe the behavior of servers. Thus S is busy if there is a customer there, and becomes idle when the customer finishes service and leaves. Suppose that instead of leaving forever, the customer immediately returns and starts up again. This parallels what we did in Section 3.5.3. The equation governing this process is directly related to (9.2.3a), except that we must add the term previously ignored, namely that the customer upon leaving $[\mathbf{q}']$ immediately reenters $[\mathbf{p}]$. Thus

$$\mathbf{r}(t+\delta) = \mathbf{r}(t)(\mathbf{I} - \delta\mathbf{M}) + \mathbf{r}(t)\delta\,\mathbf{MP} + \mathbf{r}(t)\delta\,\mathbf{Mq}'\mathbf{p} + \mathrm{O}(\delta^2).$$

Note that $\mathbf{M\,q}'\mathbf{p} = \mathbf{M}(\mathbf{I} - \mathbf{P})\boldsymbol{\epsilon}'\,\mathbf{p} = \mathbf{BQ}$. In the usual way, we get the following differential equation, which is a special case of the Chapman–Kolmogorov equations, (1.3.2b),

$$\frac{d\mathbf{r}(t)}{dt} = -\mathbf{r}(t)[\mathbf{B}(\mathbf{I} - \mathbf{Q})]. \tag{9.2.6}$$

Given that $(\mathbf{I} - \mathbf{Q})\boldsymbol{\epsilon}' = \mathbf{o}'$, we know that a steady-state solution vector $\boldsymbol{\pi}_\mathbf{r} := \lim_{t\to\infty} \mathbf{r}(t)$ exists and satisfies the eigenvector equation:

$$\boldsymbol{\pi}_\mathbf{r}\,\mathbf{B}(\mathbf{I} - \mathbf{Q}) = \mathbf{o}.$$

In Section 3.5 this vector was shown to be [Equation (3.5.10b)],

$$\boldsymbol{\pi}_\mathbf{r} = \frac{\mathbf{pV}}{\mathbf{pV}\,\boldsymbol{\epsilon}'} = \frac{1}{\bar{x}}\mathbf{pV} \tag{9.2.7a}$$

(with $\boldsymbol{\pi}_{\mathbf{r}}\,\boldsymbol{\epsilon}' = 1$). We can say that $\langle \boldsymbol{\pi}_{\mathbf{r}}\,,\, \mathbf{B} \rangle$ generates the residual process, including, for instance, the mean residual time

$$\mathbb{E}(X_r) = \boldsymbol{\pi}_{\mathbf{r}}\,\mathbf{V}\,\boldsymbol{\epsilon}' = \frac{\mathbf{p}\,\mathbf{V}^2\,\boldsymbol{\epsilon}'}{\bar{x}} = \frac{\mathbb{E}(X^2)}{2\bar{x}}. \tag{9.2.7b}$$

X_r is the r.v. denoting the time for service to complete if it is not known when service began.

9.3 Networks of Nonexponential Servers

In Section 8.3.2 we described a token, wandering forever in a closed network of nonexponential servers, emitting packets to the outside world in various prescribed manners. Here we revert to the terminology of Chapter 3 where a customer enters a subsystem and after going from server to server, eventually leaves. As discussed in Definition 8.3.1 we are dealing with three different levels of matrices. The difference is that here the customer eventually leaves. In examining this system, we prove that the mean time spent in the subsystem is independent of the service time distributions of the different servers. We also derive a simple expression for the variance of the time spent in the subsystem. This approach was presented in [KonwarLipSleiman06].

9.3.1 Description of System

Consider a network S with M nonexponential servers as shown in Figure 9.3.1. Recall from Definition 8.3.1 that:

Bold-faced Italic characters such as $\boldsymbol{P}$, $\boldsymbol{p}$, and $\boldsymbol{e}'$ characterize the customer's travel to, and between servers. These operators are M-dimensional,

Bold-faced Roman characters such as $\mathbf{p_i}$, $\mathbf{P_i}$, $\mathbf{B_i}$, $\mathbf{V_i}$, and $\boldsymbol{\epsilon}'_{\mathbf{i}}$ describe the customer's passage into and within server S_i. These operators are m_i-dimensional;

Bold−faced CALIGRAPHIC characters such as $\wp$, $\boldsymbol{\pi}$, $\boldsymbol{\mathcal{B}}$, $\boldsymbol{\mathcal{P}}$, and $\boldsymbol{\mathcal{E}}'$ represent the sum-space composite system. These are M_m-dimensional, where $M_m = \sum_{i=1}^{M} m_i$. We think of $\boldsymbol{\mathcal{W}}$ as an $M \times M$ matrix whose elements are also matrices. Element $(\boldsymbol{\mathcal{W}})_{\mathbf{ij}}$ is an $m_i \times m_j$ matrix.

The ***interserver operators*** are as follows.

$$\boldsymbol{p} = \textit{System entrance vector},$$

whose ith component, $p_i = (\boldsymbol{p})_i$, is the probability that a customer upon entering S goes directly to S_i. Because the customer must go somewhere, $\boldsymbol{p}\boldsymbol{e}' = 1$, where $\boldsymbol{e}'$ is a column M-vector whose components are all equal to 1.

The ***interserver transition matrix*** is $\boldsymbol{P}$, where

$$(\boldsymbol{P})_{ij} = P_{ij}$$

is the probability that the customer, upon leaving S_i goes directly to S_j. Given that the customer must eventually leave S, it must be the case that $(\boldsymbol{I} - \boldsymbol{P})$

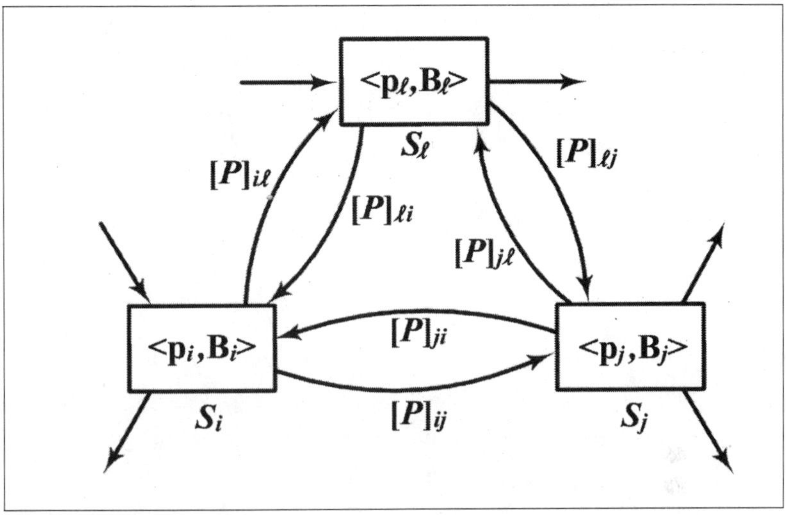

Figure 9.3.1: A network, S, of M nonexponential servers. Each server is represented by the vector-matrix pair $\langle \mathbf{p_j}\,,\ \mathbf{B_j}\rangle$. A customer, upon entering S goes to S_i with probability p_i. $\boldsymbol{P}$ is the transition matrix whose (ij)th component is the probability that the customer, upon leaving S_i, will go to S_j.

has an inverse, and therefore,

$$\boldsymbol{q}' := (\boldsymbol{I} - \boldsymbol{P})^{-1}\boldsymbol{e}'$$

is the ***system exit vector*** whose ith component $q_i = (\boldsymbol{q}')_i$ is the probability that upon leaving S_i the customer leaves S.

The ***intraserver operators*** are as follows. The service time density, $f_i(x)$ for T_i, the time the customer spends in S_i for each visit, is represented by the vector-matrix pair, $\langle \mathbf{p_j}\,,\ \mathbf{B_j}\rangle$. From Chapter 3,

$$f_i(x) = \Psi_i[\exp(-x\mathbf{B_i})\mathbf{B_i}] := \mathbf{p_i}[\exp(-x\mathbf{B_i})\mathbf{B_i}]\boldsymbol{\epsilon}_{\mathbf{i}}', \quad \text{and} \quad \mathbf{V_i} = \mathbf{B_i}^{-1}$$

with $\mathbf{E}[T_i^\ell] = \ell!\,\Psi_i[\mathbf{V_i}^\ell] = \ell!\,\mathbf{p_i}[\mathbf{V_i}^\ell]\boldsymbol{\epsilon}_{\mathbf{i}}'$.

The ***composite-space*** system is constructed exactly as in Section 8.3.2.1. There is a difference in the result. Whereas in Chapter 8 we described a network where a token wandered forever according to $\boldsymbol{\mathcal{Q}}$, here the customer eventually leaves, according to $\boldsymbol{\mathcal{B}}$. That is, here $\boldsymbol{P}$ is substochastic. Many researchers remove the difference between $\boldsymbol{\mathcal{Q}}$ and $\boldsymbol{\mathcal{B}}$ by adding an absorbing state to $\boldsymbol{\mathcal{B}}$, but then one must discard it to find the transient properties of the customer's time spent in the rest of the system. Here, as in the rest of this book, we ignore absorbing states and thereby make a distinction between $\boldsymbol{\mathcal{Q}}$ and $\boldsymbol{\mathcal{B}}$.

First we recall some definitions. Let $\mathbf{W_i}$ be some operator concerning the behavior of the customer while in S_i. Then,

$$\mathcal{W}_\text{o} := \text{Diag}[\mathbf{W_1},\ \mathbf{W_2},\ \cdots,\ \mathbf{W_M}]. \tag{9.3.1}$$

Typical examples we use are: $\boldsymbol{\mathcal{P}}_{\mathrm{o}}$, $\boldsymbol{\mathcal{M}}_{\mathrm{o}}$, $\boldsymbol{\mathcal{B}}_{\mathrm{o}}$, and $\boldsymbol{\mathcal{V}}_{\mathrm{o}}$.

Row (probability) vectors are broken down as follows. Let $\boldsymbol{a} = [a_1, a_2, \ldots, a_M]$ be an M-vector, where a_i can be interpreted as the probability that the customer is at S_i. Further, let $\mathbf{u_i}$ be the conditional probability vector, where $[\mathbf{u_i}]_k$ is the probability that the customer is at phase k of S_i, given that he *is* in S_i. Therefore, $\mathbf{u_i}\,\boldsymbol{\epsilon}'_{\mathbf{i}} = 1$. The sum-space M_m-vector is

$$[a_1\mathbf{u_1},\ a_2\mathbf{u_2},\ \cdots,\ a_M\mathbf{u_M}].$$

If the $\mathbf{u_i}$'s are the entrance vectors ($\mathbf{u_i} = \mathbf{p}_i$) we use the notation from (8.3.4b):

$$\langle \boldsymbol{a} | := [a_1\mathbf{p}_1,\ a_2\mathbf{p}_2,\ \cdots,\ a_M\mathbf{p}_{\mathrm{M}}]. \tag{9.3.2a}$$

Similarly for column vectors: let $\boldsymbol{b}'$ be an M-column vector and $\mathbf{v}'_{\mathbf{i}}$ be an m_i-column vector. Then the composite vector is the transpose of $[b_1\mathbf{v_1},\ b_2\mathbf{v_2},\ \ldots,\ b_M\mathbf{v_M}]$. In particular, if $\mathbf{v}'_{\mathbf{i}} = \boldsymbol{\epsilon}'_{\mathbf{i}}$, we use the notation of (8.3.4c):

$$| \boldsymbol{b}' \rangle := \begin{bmatrix} b_1\boldsymbol{\epsilon}'_{\mathbf{1}} \\ b_2\boldsymbol{\epsilon}'_{\mathbf{2}} \\ \vdots \\ b_M\boldsymbol{\epsilon}'_{\mathbf{M}} \end{bmatrix}. \tag{9.3.2b}$$

It then follows that

$$\langle \boldsymbol{a} |\, | \boldsymbol{b}' \rangle = \boldsymbol{a}\,\boldsymbol{b}' = \sum_{i=1}^{M} a_i\, b_i. \tag{9.3.2c}$$

Two important vectors of this type are

$$\wp = \langle \boldsymbol{p} | \quad \text{and} \quad \boldsymbol{\varepsilon}' = | \boldsymbol{e}' \rangle \tag{9.3.2d}$$

from which it follows that

$$\wp\,\boldsymbol{\varepsilon}' = \langle \boldsymbol{p} |\, | \boldsymbol{e}' \rangle = \boldsymbol{p}\,\boldsymbol{e}' = 1. \tag{9.3.2e}$$

We have shown how M-vectors are embedded into the full space. The extension to $M \times M$ matrices is given by Definition 8.3.2. Thus let $\boldsymbol{W}$ be any $M \times M$ matrix. Then the $M_m \times M_m$ matrix into which it is embedded is

$$\langle \boldsymbol{W} \rangle := \begin{bmatrix} W_{11}\,\boldsymbol{\epsilon}'_{\mathbf{1}}\,\mathbf{p}_1 & W_{12}\,\boldsymbol{\epsilon}'_{\mathbf{1}}\,\mathbf{p}_2 & \cdots & W_{1M}\,\boldsymbol{\epsilon}'_{\mathbf{1}}\,\mathbf{p}_{\mathrm{M}} \\ W_{21}\,\boldsymbol{\epsilon}'_{\mathbf{2}}\,\mathbf{p}_1 & W_{22}\,\boldsymbol{\epsilon}'_{\mathbf{2}}\,\mathbf{p}_2 & \cdots & W_{2M}\,\boldsymbol{\epsilon}'_{\mathbf{2}}\,\mathbf{p}_{\mathrm{M}} \\ \cdots & \cdots & \cdots & \cdots \\ W_{M1}\,\boldsymbol{\epsilon}'_{\mathbf{M}}\,\mathbf{p}_1 & W_{M2}\,\boldsymbol{\epsilon}'_{\mathbf{M}}\,\mathbf{p}_2 & \cdots & W_{MM}\,\boldsymbol{\epsilon}'_{\mathbf{M}}\,\mathbf{p}_{\mathrm{M}} \end{bmatrix}. \tag{9.3.3}$$

These structured matrices have many useful properties to simplify calculations. For instance:

$$\langle \boldsymbol{a} |\, \langle \boldsymbol{W} \rangle = \langle \boldsymbol{a}\boldsymbol{W} | \quad \text{and} \quad \langle \boldsymbol{W} \rangle\, | \boldsymbol{b}' \rangle = | \boldsymbol{W}\boldsymbol{b}' \rangle. \tag{9.3.4a}$$

We just saw how a matrix times a vector reduces to a simpler vector. Here is the obvious reduction to a scalar:

$$\langle \boldsymbol{a} |\, \langle \boldsymbol{W} \rangle\, | \boldsymbol{b}' \rangle = \boldsymbol{a}\,\boldsymbol{W}\,\boldsymbol{b}'. \tag{9.3.4b}$$

The product of two embedded matrices is

$$\langle \boldsymbol{W_1} \rangle \langle \boldsymbol{W_2} \rangle = \langle \boldsymbol{W_1} \boldsymbol{W_2} \rangle, \tag{9.3.4c}$$

and their sum is

$$\langle \boldsymbol{W_1} \rangle + \langle \boldsymbol{W_2} \rangle = \langle \boldsymbol{W_1} + \boldsymbol{W_2} \rangle. \tag{9.3.4d}$$

Furthermore, their commutivity is preserved. That is, each of the following three equations implies the others.

$$\begin{aligned} \langle \boldsymbol{W_1} \rangle \langle \boldsymbol{W_2} \rangle &= \langle \boldsymbol{W_2} \rangle \langle \boldsymbol{W_1} \rangle \\ \langle \boldsymbol{W_1} \boldsymbol{W_2} \rangle &= \langle \boldsymbol{W_2} \boldsymbol{W_1} \rangle \\ \boldsymbol{W_1} \boldsymbol{W_2} &= \boldsymbol{W_2} \boldsymbol{W_1}. \end{aligned} \tag{9.3.4e}$$

Let $\boldsymbol{W_1} = \boldsymbol{W_2} = \boldsymbol{W}$; then it follows that

$$\langle \boldsymbol{W} \rangle^{\ell} = \langle \boldsymbol{W}^{\ell} \rangle. \tag{9.3.4f}$$

The proof for all these relations is by direct computation. We multiply two matrices here. The reader can try out the other equations by working with matrices of dimension $M = 2$. Let us embed two matrices, $\boldsymbol{W_1}$ and $\boldsymbol{W_2}$. Then (we are multiplying by block matrices), noting that $\mathbf{p_k} \boldsymbol{\epsilon}'_{\mathbf{k}} = 1$,

$$\Big[\langle \boldsymbol{W_1} \rangle \langle \boldsymbol{W_2} \rangle\Big]_{\mathbf{ij}} = \sum_{k=1}^{M} \Big[\langle \boldsymbol{W_1} \rangle\Big]_{\mathbf{ik}} \Big[\langle \boldsymbol{W_2} \rangle\Big]_{\mathbf{kj}} = \sum_{k=1}^{M} \boldsymbol{\epsilon}'_{\mathbf{i}} \, [\boldsymbol{W_1}]_{ik} \mathbf{p_k} \, \boldsymbol{\epsilon}'_{\mathbf{k}} \, [\boldsymbol{W_2}]_{kj} \mathbf{p_j}$$

$$= \boldsymbol{\epsilon}'_{\mathbf{i}} \left[\sum_{k=1}^{M} [\boldsymbol{W_1}]_{ik} \, [\boldsymbol{W_2}]_{kj} \right] \mathbf{p_j} = \boldsymbol{\epsilon}'_{\mathbf{i}} [\boldsymbol{W_1} \boldsymbol{W_2}]_{ij} \mathbf{p_j} = \Big[\langle \boldsymbol{W_1} \boldsymbol{W_2} \rangle\Big]_{\mathbf{ij}}.$$

This formulation extends to sum-space matrices that are not the result of embeddings. Let $\boldsymbol{\mathcal{X}}$ be any $M_m \times M_m$ matrix. It can be written in block matrix form:

$$\boldsymbol{\mathcal{X}} = \begin{bmatrix} \mathbf{X_{11}} & \mathbf{X_{12}} & \cdots & \mathbf{X_{1M}} \\ \mathbf{X_{21}} & \mathbf{X_{22}} & \cdots & \mathbf{X_{2M}} \\ \cdots & \cdots & \cdots & \cdots \\ \mathbf{X_{M1}} & \mathbf{X_{M2}} & \cdots & \mathbf{X_{MM}} \end{bmatrix}, \tag{9.3.5a}$$

where $\mathbf{X_{ij}}$ is itself a matrix of dimension $m_i \times m_j$. Next define the matrix $\boldsymbol{X}$ where

$$[\boldsymbol{X}]_{ij} := X_{ij} := \mathbf{p_i} \, \mathbf{X_{ij}} \, \boldsymbol{\epsilon}'_{\mathbf{j}} = \sum_{k=1}^{m_i} \sum_{n=1}^{m_j} [\mathbf{p_i}]_k [\mathbf{X_{ij}}]_{kn}. \tag{9.3.5b}$$

(Note that $\boldsymbol{\mathcal{X}}$, $\mathbf{X_{ij}}$, and $\boldsymbol{X}$ are distinct matrices.) It follows by direct substitution that

$$\langle \boldsymbol{a} \,|\, \boldsymbol{\mathcal{X}} \,|\, \boldsymbol{b}' \rangle = \boldsymbol{a} \, \boldsymbol{X} \, \boldsymbol{b}'. \tag{9.3.5c}$$

Also,

$$\langle \boldsymbol{W_1} \rangle \, \boldsymbol{\mathcal{X}} \, \langle \boldsymbol{W_2} \rangle = \langle \boldsymbol{W_1} \boldsymbol{X} \boldsymbol{W_2} \rangle. \tag{9.3.5d}$$

We have in effect "reduced" $\boldsymbol{\mathcal{X}}$ to the $M \times M$ matrix, $\boldsymbol{X}$. But this reduction and subsequent embedding process is not reversible. That is, in general,

$$\boldsymbol{\mathcal{X}} \neq \langle \boldsymbol{X} \rangle.$$

In any case, we see that the product of three matrices of dimension M_m can be computed by first multiplying three matrices of dimension M, and then embedding.

We now use this notation to find the generator and first two moments of S.

9.3.2 Service Time Distribution

Consider the system in Figure 9.3.1. The (substochastic) transition matrix $\boldsymbol{\mathcal{P}}$ is given by (8.3.3c)

$$\boldsymbol{\mathcal{P}} = \boldsymbol{\mathcal{P}}_o + \begin{bmatrix} \mathbf{q}_1' P_{11} \mathbf{p}_1 & \mathbf{q}_1' P_{12} \mathbf{p}_2 & \cdots & \mathbf{q}_1' P_{1M} \mathbf{p}_M \\ \mathbf{q}_2' P_{21} \mathbf{p}_1 & \mathbf{q}_2' P_{22} \mathbf{p}_2 & \cdots & \mathbf{q}_2' P_{2M} \mathbf{p}_M \\ \cdots & \cdots & \cdots & \cdots \\ \mathbf{q}_M' P_{M1} \mathbf{p}_1 & \mathbf{q}_M' P_{M2} \mathbf{p}_2 & \cdots & \mathbf{q}_M' P_{MM} \mathbf{p}_M \end{bmatrix}. \tag{9.3.6}$$

Then, following (8.3.3d) (where $\boldsymbol{\mathcal{B}}$ replaces $\boldsymbol{\mathcal{Q}}$),

$$\boldsymbol{\mathcal{B}} = \boldsymbol{\mathcal{M}}_o[\boldsymbol{\mathcal{I}} - \boldsymbol{\mathcal{P}}] = \boldsymbol{\mathcal{B}}_o \left[\boldsymbol{\mathcal{I}} - \langle \boldsymbol{P} \rangle\right]. \tag{9.3.7a}$$

For the case where S is made up of a single server ($M = 1$), $\langle \boldsymbol{P} \rangle$ reduces to $\alpha\,\boldsymbol{\epsilon}'\mathbf{p}$ as described in (3.5.9a), and $\boldsymbol{\mathcal{B}} \to \mathbf{B_r}(\alpha)$. If all S_i are exponential servers, then $\boldsymbol{\mathcal{B}}_o \to \mathbf{M}$, $\langle \boldsymbol{P} \rangle \to \mathbf{P}$, and we have a typical ME subsystem.

Let X be the r.v. denoting the time the customer spends in S; then $\langle \wp, \boldsymbol{\mathcal{B}} \rangle$ is the generator of the distribution $F_X(x)$. $\boldsymbol{\mathcal{V}}$ can be found by first getting the inverse of $\left[\boldsymbol{\mathcal{I}} - \langle \boldsymbol{P} \rangle\right]$. This is similar in form to the expression in Lemma 4.2.1 and can be found by expanding it in a power series and using the embedded matrix properties:

$$\begin{aligned} \left[\boldsymbol{\mathcal{I}} - \langle \boldsymbol{P} \rangle\right]^{-1} &= \boldsymbol{\mathcal{I}} + \langle \boldsymbol{P} \rangle + \langle \boldsymbol{P} \rangle^2 + \cdots + \langle \boldsymbol{P} \rangle^\ell + \cdots \\ &= \boldsymbol{\mathcal{I}} + \langle \boldsymbol{P} \rangle + \langle \boldsymbol{P}^2 \rangle + \cdots + \langle \boldsymbol{P}^\ell \rangle + \cdots \\ &= \boldsymbol{\mathcal{I}} + \langle \boldsymbol{P}[\boldsymbol{I} + \boldsymbol{P} + \boldsymbol{P}^2 + \cdots + \boldsymbol{P}^\ell + \cdots] \rangle = \boldsymbol{\mathcal{I}} + \langle \boldsymbol{P}[\boldsymbol{I} - \boldsymbol{P}]^{-1} \rangle. \end{aligned}$$

One needn't accept that the leftmost and rightmost expressions are equal. One need only multiply by $\boldsymbol{\mathcal{I}} - \langle \boldsymbol{P} \rangle$ to verify. The constraint is that $[\boldsymbol{I} - \boldsymbol{P}]^{-1}$ exist, which was assumed in the first place. Therefore,

$$\boldsymbol{\mathcal{V}} = \boldsymbol{\mathcal{B}}^{-1} = \left[\boldsymbol{\mathcal{I}} + \langle \boldsymbol{P}[\boldsymbol{I} - \boldsymbol{P}]^{-1} \rangle\right] \boldsymbol{\mathcal{V}}_o. \tag{9.3.7b}$$

In preparation for finding $\mathbb{E}[X]$, we must look at some properties of $\boldsymbol{\mathcal{V}}_o = \boldsymbol{\mathcal{B}}_o^{-1} = \mathrm{Diag}[\mathbf{V}_1, \mathbf{V}_2, \ldots]$. By direct substitution,

$$\wp \boldsymbol{\mathcal{V}}_o^\ell \boldsymbol{\varepsilon}' = \langle \boldsymbol{p} \,|\, \boldsymbol{\mathcal{V}}_o^\ell \,|\, \boldsymbol{e}' \rangle = \boldsymbol{p} \boldsymbol{T}^{(\ell)} \boldsymbol{e}',$$

where we have defined the diagonal M-matrix

$$[\boldsymbol{T}^{(\ell)}]_{ii} := \mathbf{p_i}\, \mathbf{V_i^\ell}\, \boldsymbol{\epsilon}'_{\mathbf{i}} = \Psi_i[\mathbf{V_i}^\ell] = \frac{1}{\ell\,!}\mathbb{E}[T_i^\ell]. \tag{9.3.8}$$

From this definition, $\boldsymbol{T} = \mathrm{Diag}[\mathbb{E}[T_1],\, \mathbb{E}[T_2],\, \ldots] = \mathrm{Diag}[\bar{t}_1,\, \bar{t}_2,\, \ldots]$. Therefore, $\boldsymbol{T}^\ell = \mathrm{Diag}[\bar{t}_1^\ell,\, \bar{t}_2^\ell,\, \ldots]$. Unfortunately, their definitions imply that $\boldsymbol{T}^{(\ell)} \neq \boldsymbol{T}^\ell$. The equality occurs only when all S_i are exponential, or equivalently, if $m_i = 1$ for all i.

Next look at

$$\wp\mathcal{V} = \langle \boldsymbol{p} \,|\, \mathcal{V} = \langle \boldsymbol{p}[\boldsymbol{I} + \boldsymbol{P}(\boldsymbol{I}-\boldsymbol{P})^{-1}] \,|\, \mathcal{V}_\text{o} = \langle \boldsymbol{p}\,(\boldsymbol{I}-\boldsymbol{P})^{-1} \,|\, \mathcal{V}_\text{o}.$$

Then,

$$\mathbb{E}[X] = \langle \boldsymbol{p} \,|\, \mathcal{V} \,|\, \boldsymbol{e}' \rangle = \langle \boldsymbol{p}(\boldsymbol{I}-\boldsymbol{P})^{-1} \,|\, \mathcal{V}_\text{o} \,|\, \boldsymbol{e}' \rangle = \boldsymbol{p}\left[(\boldsymbol{I}-\boldsymbol{P})^{-1}\right]\boldsymbol{T}\boldsymbol{e}'. \tag{9.3.9a}$$

If all S_i were exponential, this is exactly the expression we would get. Clearly $\mathbb{E}[X]$ does not depend on the details of the servers' distributions. Therefore the mean time spent in S depends only on $\boldsymbol{p}$, $\boldsymbol{P}$, and $(\boldsymbol{T})_{ii} = \bar{t}_i = \mathbf{p_i}\, \mathbf{V_i}\, \boldsymbol{\epsilon}'_{\mathbf{i}}$, where $\bar{t}_i$ is the mean time spent at S_i for each visit. In hopes of making the formulas more transparent, we define

$$\boldsymbol{V_e} := (\boldsymbol{I}-\boldsymbol{P})^{-1}\boldsymbol{T} \tag{9.3.9b}$$

using the subscript $\boldsymbol{e}$ to denote that this is the matrix when all S_i are $\boldsymbol{e}$xponential. Then

$$\mathbb{E}[X] = \boldsymbol{p}\,\boldsymbol{V_e}\,\boldsymbol{e}'. \tag{9.3.9c}$$

This is valid irrespective of the distributions of the S_is.

Before evaluating $\wp\mathcal{V}^2\,\boldsymbol{\varepsilon}'$ we observe that:

$$\mathcal{V}\boldsymbol{\varepsilon}' = \left[\mathcal{I} + \langle\, \boldsymbol{P}[\boldsymbol{I}-\boldsymbol{P}]^{-1} \rangle\right] \mathcal{V}_\text{o} \,|\, \boldsymbol{e}' \rangle$$

$$= \mathcal{V}_\text{o} \,|\, \boldsymbol{e}' \rangle + |\, \boldsymbol{P}(\boldsymbol{I}-\boldsymbol{P})^{-1}\boldsymbol{T}\,\boldsymbol{e}' \rangle = \mathcal{V}_\text{o} \,|\, \boldsymbol{e}' \rangle + |\, \boldsymbol{P}\,\boldsymbol{V_e}\,\boldsymbol{e}' \rangle.$$

Then

$$\wp\mathcal{V}^2\,\boldsymbol{\varepsilon}' = \left[\langle \boldsymbol{p} \,|\, \mathcal{V}\right]\left[\mathcal{V} \,|\, \boldsymbol{e}' \rangle\right] = \left[\langle \boldsymbol{p}\,(\boldsymbol{I}-\boldsymbol{P})^{-1} \,|\, \mathcal{V}_\text{o}\right]\left[\mathcal{V}_\text{o} \,|\, \boldsymbol{e}' \rangle + |\, \boldsymbol{P}\,\boldsymbol{V_e}\,\boldsymbol{e}' \rangle\right]$$

$$= \boldsymbol{p}(\boldsymbol{I}-\boldsymbol{P})^{-1}\boldsymbol{T}^{(\mathbf{2})}\,\boldsymbol{e}' + \boldsymbol{p}\,\boldsymbol{V_e}\,\boldsymbol{P}\,\boldsymbol{V_e}\,\boldsymbol{e}'.$$

It is not hard to show that if all the S_i are exponential, then $\boldsymbol{T}_{\boldsymbol{e}}^{(\mathbf{2})} = T^2$ and $\wp\mathcal{V}^2\,\boldsymbol{\varepsilon}' \to \boldsymbol{p}\,\boldsymbol{V}_{\boldsymbol{e}}^{\mathbf{2}}\,\boldsymbol{e}'$. It is useful to write the expressions relative to what they would be if all servers were exponential. Using $\boldsymbol{T}_{\boldsymbol{e}}^{(\mathbf{2})} = \boldsymbol{T}^2$, the above expression can be written as

$$\wp\mathcal{V}^2\,\boldsymbol{\varepsilon}' = \wp\mathcal{V}_{\mathbf{e}}^2\,\boldsymbol{\varepsilon}' + \boldsymbol{p}(\boldsymbol{I}-\boldsymbol{P})^{-1}[\boldsymbol{T}^{(\mathbf{2})} - \boldsymbol{T}^{\mathbf{2}}]\,\boldsymbol{e}'.$$

We now look at

$$[\boldsymbol{T}^{(\mathbf{2})} - \boldsymbol{T}^2]_{ii} = \Psi_i[\mathbf{V_i}^2] - \bar{t}_i^2.$$

Recall that for any distribution $\sigma^2 = \mathbb{E}[X^2] - \bar{t}^2$, $\mathbb{E}[X^2] = 2\Psi[\mathbf{V}^2]$, and $C^2 = \sigma^2/\bar{t}^2$. These give us

$$[\boldsymbol{T}^{(2)} - \boldsymbol{T}^2]_{ii} = \frac{1}{2}\,\bar{t}_i^2\,[C_i^2 - 1]\,,$$

where C_i^2 is the squared coefficient of variation for S_i. Define the diagonal matrix $\mathbf{\Gamma}$ as

$$[\mathbf{\Gamma}]_{ii} := C_i^2 - 1. \tag{9.3.10}$$

Then

$$[\boldsymbol{T}^{(2)} - \boldsymbol{T}^2] = \frac{1}{2}\boldsymbol{T}^2\,\mathbf{\Gamma}$$

and

$$\wp\,\mathcal{V}^2\,\varepsilon' = \wp\,\mathcal{V}_{\mathrm{e}}^2\,\varepsilon' + \frac{1}{2}\boldsymbol{p}\,\boldsymbol{V_e}\,\boldsymbol{T}\,\mathbf{\Gamma}\,\boldsymbol{e}'.$$

We put all this together and get (finally)

$$\sigma^2 = \sigma_{\mathrm{e}}^2 + \boldsymbol{p}\,\boldsymbol{V_e}\,\boldsymbol{T}\,\mathbf{\Gamma}\,\boldsymbol{e}'. \tag{9.3.11}$$

We summarize some of this in the following theorem.

Theorem 9.3.1: Let S be a system of nonexponential servers where $(\boldsymbol{I} - \boldsymbol{P})$ is invertible. Then the time X spent in S by a single customer has distribution generated by $\langle\,\wp,\,\mathcal{B}\rangle$, where $\mathcal{B}$ is given by (9.3.7a),

$$\mathcal{B} = \mathcal{B}_o\left[\mathcal{I} - \langle\,\boldsymbol{P}\,\rangle\right],$$

with inverse given by (9.3.7b),

$$\mathcal{V} = \mathcal{B}^{-1} = \left[\mathcal{I} + \langle\,\boldsymbol{P}[\boldsymbol{I} - \boldsymbol{P}]^{-1}\,\rangle\right]\mathcal{V}_{\mathrm{o}},$$

and

$$\wp = \langle\,\boldsymbol{p}\,|\,.$$

The mean and variance are given by (9.3.9a) and (9.3.11), respectively:

$$\mathbb{E}[X] = \boldsymbol{p}\left[(\boldsymbol{I} - \boldsymbol{P})^{-1}\right]\boldsymbol{T}\boldsymbol{e}' = \boldsymbol{p}\,\boldsymbol{V_e}\,\boldsymbol{e}',$$

and

$$\sigma^2 = \sigma_{\mathrm{e}}^2 + \boldsymbol{p}\,\boldsymbol{V_e}\,\boldsymbol{T}\,\mathbf{\Gamma}\,\boldsymbol{e}',$$

where $\boldsymbol{V_e} = (\boldsymbol{I} - \boldsymbol{P})^{-1}\boldsymbol{T}$ and $(\mathbf{\Gamma})_{ii} = C_i^2 - 1$. Furthermore, in general, $\mathbb{E}[X^\ell] = \ell!\,\wp\,\mathcal{V}^\ell\,\varepsilon'$, depends only on the first ℓ moments of each of the S_i through $\{\,\boldsymbol{T}^{(k)}\,|\,k \le \ell\,\}$. For instance, after some effort it can be shown that

$$\langle\,\boldsymbol{p}\,|\,\mathcal{V}^3\,|\,\boldsymbol{e}'\,\rangle = \boldsymbol{p}(\boldsymbol{I} - \boldsymbol{P})^{-1}\boldsymbol{T}^{(3)}\,\boldsymbol{e}' + \boldsymbol{p}\,\boldsymbol{V_e}\,\boldsymbol{P}(\boldsymbol{I} - \boldsymbol{P})^{-1}\boldsymbol{T}^{(2)}\,\boldsymbol{e}'$$

$$+\boldsymbol{p}\,(\boldsymbol{I} - \boldsymbol{P})^{-1}\boldsymbol{T}^{(2)}\,\boldsymbol{P}\,\boldsymbol{V_e}\,\boldsymbol{e}'r + \boldsymbol{p}\,\boldsymbol{V_e}\,\boldsymbol{P}\boldsymbol{V_e}\,\boldsymbol{P}\,\boldsymbol{V_e}\,\boldsymbol{e}'.$$

If all servers are exponential, $\boldsymbol{T}_{\boldsymbol{e}}^{(\ell)} \to \boldsymbol{T}^\ell$, and $\langle\,\boldsymbol{p}\,|\,\mathcal{V}^\ell\,|\,\boldsymbol{e}'\,\rangle \to \boldsymbol{p}\,\boldsymbol{V_e}{}^\ell\boldsymbol{e}'$. Could anything be simpler? ■

One might ask if setting up all this mathematical apparatus is worth the effort of this theorem, as well as those in Section 8.3.2. It is hoped that in the future this can be used to explore the behavior of a system where more than one customer can be active at a time. If all the servers have one-dimensional representations, Ξ is one-dimensional and we have a Jackson network, [JACKSON63], [GORDON-NEWELL67], and we have nothing new to contribute. If at least one of the servers needs a higher-dimensional representation, we are into LAQT. If, in particular, exactly one subspace, say S_1, is multidimensional, then the problem may be tractable. But If two or more spaces are multidimensional, one can no longer avoid the problems inherent in product space arithmetic.

9.4 Systems With Two Servers

We have no intention at this time of trying to continue our discussion of many-server systems. Thus let us let $m = 2$ hereafter. Our purpose is to show that many of the known results of queueing theory that have matrix formulations (beyond those we discussed in Section 9.1) are invariant to isometric transformations and can be written in a base-free way. We enumerate some results concerning the G/M/1 and M/G/1 queues and then look momentarily at the G/G/1 queue. Finally, we look at some transient behavior in M/G/1 systems, noting that the procedure is completely generalizable.

In a closed loop, S_1 and S_2 play exactly equivalent roles. But as we have mentioned numerous times before, if the number of customers in the system is so large that one or the other has no likelihood of ever being idle, that subsystem is equivalent to a source of customers to the other. Clearly, for subsystems where only one customer can be served at a time, the one with the smaller maximal throughput will be that subsystem, or server. By convention, we have assumed that S_2 has the longer mean service time for M/G/1 and $G_2/G_1/1$ queues. But for G/M/1 queues S_1 has the longer service time. Let G_i describe the pdf type of server S_i. Then we are looking at $G_2/G_1/1//N$ loops, and their open extensions [i.e., $G_2/G_1/1//(N \to \infty)$ is equivalent to $G_2/G_1/1$].

9.4.1 G/M/1 Queue

We have already shown that the steady-state M/G/1 queue is invariant. The same matrix which governs that system [the matrix $\mathbf{A}$ of (9.1.1)] also has relevance to the open G/M/1 queue, except that now, as in Chapter 5, $\rho = 1/\varrho = \lambda\bar{x} > 1$. For instance, let s and $\hat{\mathbf{u}}$ satisfy the eigenvector equation:

$$\hat{\mathbf{u}}\mathbf{A} = s\hat{\mathbf{u}}, \tag{9.4.1a}$$

where s is the smallest positive eigenvalue of $\mathbf{A}$, and $\hat{\mathbf{u}}\,\boldsymbol{\epsilon}' = 1$. We know that $s < 1$ iff *varrho* < 1 (ϱ is the utilization factor now). In Theorem 5.1.2, we showed the following,

$$r(n) = (1 - s)\varrho s^{n-1}, \qquad n > 0 \tag{9.4.1b}$$

and

$$r(0) = 1 - \varrho. \tag{9.4.1c}$$

Note that the eigenvalues are an invariant property of any matrix. That is, if $\mathbf{X}$ and $\tilde{\mathbf{X}}$ are related by an ***isometric transformation***, they have the same set of eigenvalues. Also, recall from (5.1.6b) that

$$\hat{\mathbf{u}} = \lambda \mathbf{p} \mathbf{V}[\mathbf{I} + \lambda(1-s)\mathbf{V}]^{-1}. \tag{9.4.1d}$$

It follows from Corollary 5.1.2 that $\Psi\left[(\mathbf{I} + \lambda(1-s)\mathbf{V})^{-1}\right] = B^*[\lambda(1-s)] = s$. So we even get the famous relation between the Laplace transform and s without ever knowing what a Riemann–Stieltjes integral is, and from a base-free matrix algebraic formulation.

Next recall two other distributions related to the G/M/1 queue. The first is the interdeparture time distribution we gave in Section 5.2.2, which is generated by $\langle\, \mathbf{p_{2d}}\, ,\, \mathbf{B_{2d}}\,\rangle$ where

$$\mathbf{p_{2d}} := [s\hat{\mathbf{u}},\, 1-s] \quad \text{and} \quad \mathbf{B_{2d}} := \left[\begin{array}{cc} \mathbf{B} & \mathbf{B}\epsilon' \\ \mathbf{o} & \lambda \end{array}\right]\Big\}\,(m+1). \tag{9.4.2}$$

The second distribution describes the arrival time conditioned by departures, which is generated by $\langle\, \hat{\mathbf{u}}\, ,\, \mathbf{B}\,\rangle$. This is rather interesting, for it tells us that the generator of the arrival process is in composite state $\hat{\mathbf{u}}$ at the moment a customer leaves the G/M/1 queue, thus giving us a meaning of the eigenvector of $\mathbf{B}$ belonging to the smallest eigenvalue, s.

System Time for the M/ME/1 Queue

The last process we mention here is the system time for the M/G/1 queue. It is generated by the vector-matrix pair (Section 4.2.3) $\langle\, \mathbf{p_s}\, ,\, \mathbf{B_s}\,\rangle$, where

$$\mathbf{B_s} := \mathbf{B} - \lambda \mathbf{Q} \tag{9.4.3a}$$

and

$$\mathbf{p_s} := (1-\rho)\mathbf{p}(\mathbf{I} - \mathbf{U})^{-1}. \tag{9.4.3b}$$

It is clear that all three distributions

$$\langle\, \hat{\mathbf{u}},\, \mathbf{B}\,\rangle, \quad \langle\, \mathbf{p_d},\, \mathbf{B_d}\,\rangle, \quad \text{and} \quad \langle\, \mathbf{p_s},\, \mathbf{B_s}\,\rangle,$$

are invariant to isometric transformations.

9.4.2 Two Nonexponential Servers

As we have already seen, if the representation of a nonexponential server is m-dimensional, the space required to describe its interaction with exponential servers is also m-dimensional (i.e., there is no increase in dimensionality).[†]

[†]This, by the way, indicates that the concept of an absorbing state interferes with a self-consistent matrix formulation of queueing theory, because then one requires an $(m+1)$–dimensional description.

However, if two servers are nonexponential, one needs a space of $m_1 \cdot m_2$ dimensions. There is no way out of this increase in complexity; it simply reflects the amount of information needed to describe the dynamics of such complex systems. (There is an interesting exception, which we mention in the concluding remarks.)

We first recall the steady-state solution for the closed G/G/1//N loop from Chapter 7. The operators $\mathbf{B_i}$ and $\mathbf{Q_i}$ are defined in the same way for server i as was done in the previous sections. Remember that operators with different subscripts (belonging to different subspaces) automatically commute. When we need a matrix representation of sums of their products, we embed them in the product space, which formally means putting a $\hat{}$ ("hat") on them. Repeating Equations (7.3.5), we have

$$\mathbf{S}^+ := \hat{\mathbf{B}}_\mathbf{1} + \hat{\mathbf{B}}_\mathbf{2} - \hat{\mathbf{B}}_\mathbf{2}\,\hat{\mathbf{Q}}_\mathbf{1}, \tag{9.4.4a}$$

$$\mathbf{S}^- := \hat{\mathbf{B}}_\mathbf{2} + \hat{\mathbf{B}}_\mathbf{1} - \hat{\mathbf{B}}_\mathbf{1}\,\hat{\mathbf{Q}}_\mathbf{2}, \tag{9.4.4b}$$

$$\mathbf{T}^\pm := (\mathbf{S}^\pm)^{-1}, \tag{9.4.4c}$$

and

$$\mathbf{U} := \mathbf{T}^+\mathbf{S}^-. \tag{9.4.4d}$$

It would seem that $\mathbf{S}^+$ and $\mathbf{S}^-$ are the generalizations of $\mathbf{A}$ in (9.1.1) for the M/G/1 queue, but it is not quite that simple. Instead, $\mathbf{U}$ is the direct generalization of the "$\mathbf{U}$" for the M/G/1 queue, with no real analogue for $\mathbf{A}$, for now both servers play symmetric roles in the theory, and $\mathbf{U}^{-1} = \mathbf{T}^-\mathbf{S}^+$. The steady-state solution given by Theorem 7.3.5 is:

$$\mathbf{\Pi}(n,N) = \mathbf{\Pi}(0,N)\,\hat{\mathbf{B}}_\mathbf{2}\,\mathbf{U}^n\,\mathbf{T}^- \quad \text{for } 1 \le n \le N-1, \tag{9.4.5a}$$

$$\mathbf{\Pi}(N,N) = \mathbf{\Pi}(0,N)\hat{\mathbf{B}}_\mathbf{2}\,\mathbf{U}^{N-1}\,\hat{\mathbf{V}}_\mathbf{1}, \tag{9.4.5b}$$

and

$$r(n,N) = \mathbf{\Pi}(n,N)\boldsymbol{\epsilon}'. \tag{9.4.5c}$$

All of these equations are invariant to isometric transformations in the two subspaces, because a transformation in one subspace automatically commutes with matrices in the other space. An interesting research problem would be to study isometric transformations over the product space, an idea that was actually discussed in Chapter 6. There it was shown that if two or more servers are identical and customers are not "marked", then the product space can be reduced to a ***reduced-product space***.

Recall that $\mathbf{Q_i}$ and $\mathbf{B_i}$ do not commute with each other if Ξ_i has dimension greater than 1 (nonexponential). This is what made the M/G/1 queue harder than the M/M/1 queue. But now we have the added problem that $\mathbf{S}^+$ and $\mathbf{S}^-$ do not commute with each other if both Ξ_1 and Ξ_2 are multidimensional, which is what makes the G/G/1 queue harder than the M/G/1 and G/M/1 queues.

9.4.3 Review of Transient Behavior

In the previous chapters, we assumed that there existed a basis set of pure vectors, and that the system could be in one of those pure states initially. By doing so, we appeared to be saying that such states (which we called *phases*) have physical meaning individually. The formulation we are presenting in this chapter treats all vectors on an equal footing. Note that in deriving (9.2.1) and (9.2.2), we talked about operations (linear transformations) on an arbitrary state vector $\mathbf{r}$, and then, given that our intermediate equations were true for all state vectors, we threw $\mathbf{r}$ away. From a rigorous mathematical point of view we said that if an equation of the form $\mathbf{rX} = \mathbf{o}$ is true for m linearly independent vectors, where m is the dimension of the vector space, then it must be true for all $\mathbf{r} \in \Xi$, and furthermore, $\mathbf{X} = \mathbf{O}$. This means that we can pick any m linearly independent vectors from Ξ, and treat them as though they are pure states, even though they may have no independent physical meaning. For instance, we could pick the set discussed in (9.2.5).

The argument goes something like this. Let $\mathbf{r_1}, \mathbf{r_2}, \ldots, \mathbf{r_m}$ be a basis for Ξ. Then any physical vector $\mathbf{r}$ can be written as a linear combination of these basis vectors,

$$\mathbf{r} = \sum_{j=1}^{m} r_j \, \mathbf{r_j}.$$

Every linear operator $\mathbf{X}$ transforms every vector in Ξ to some other vector in Ξ. In particular, $\mathbf{r_j}\,\mathbf{X} \in \Xi$, and thus it can be written as a linear combination of members of the set $\{\mathbf{r_j}\}$. That is,

$$\mathbf{r_j}\,\mathbf{X} = \sum_{k=1}^{m} X_{jk} \, \mathbf{r_k},$$

and thus

$$\mathbf{rX} = \sum_{j=1}^{m} r_j \mathbf{r_j}\,\mathbf{X} = \sum_{j,k=1}^{m} r_j X_{jk} \mathbf{r_k}.$$

In words, if the set of scalars, $\{r_1, r_2, \ldots, r_m\}$, describes $\mathbf{r}$ in terms of the basis set $\{\, \mathbf{r_i} \,\}$, then the set $\{\, \sum r_j\, X_{j1}, \sum r_j X_{j2}, \ldots, \sum r_j X_{jm} \,\}$ describes $\mathbf{rX}$ in the same basis, and X_{jk} is a matrix representation of transformation operator $\mathbf{X}$ in the basis $\mathbf{r_j}$. Note that similarity transformations (which include our isometric transformations) are those that change the basis set.

We can see that dealing with components of vectors and matrices is equivalent to dealing with abstract vectors and transformations. We can do it either way, without implying that the components themselves have any meaning. It is somewhat easier to speak in terms of components. Thus we have been using the notation "$\{i, n\}$" to mean that "S_1 is in state $\mathbf{r_i}$ with queue length n."

In Section 4.5 we considered the process of a queue rising in length. For $n \leq N$, we defined the matrix

$$\mathbf{H_u}(n) := \text{probability matrix of first passage from } n \text{ to } n+1. \qquad (9.4.6a)$$

That is, we said that $[\mathbf{H_u}(n)]_{ij}$ is the probability that S_1 will be in state (phase) j (or $\mathbf{r_j}$) when its queue goes from n to $n+1$ for the first time, given that it started in state i (or $\mathbf{r_i}$) with n customers. Now we would say that if S_1 was initially described by state vector $\mathbf{r}$, with n customers, then when its queue goes from n to $n+1$ for the first time, it will be described by state vector $\mathbf{r}\mathbf{H_u}(n)$. After a while the two viewpoints seem to be synonymous; one no longer notices the difference (are you there yet, dear reader?). By its definition from either viewpoint, the following must be true. After all, the queue must eventually reach every length.

$$\mathbf{H_u}(n)\boldsymbol{\epsilon}' = \boldsymbol{\epsilon}' \quad \text{for } 1 \le n < N. \tag{9.4.6b}$$

$\mathbf{H_u}(n)$ is isometric.

In Section 4.5.1 we derived the recursive equations that $\mathbf{H_u}(n)$ must satisfy; namely

$$\mathbf{H_u}(n) = \lambda[\lambda\mathbf{I} + \mathbf{B} - \mathbf{BQH_u}(n-1)]^{-1}. \tag{9.4.7a}$$

From the definition of $\mathbf{A}$, this can also be written as

$$\mathbf{H_u}(n) = [\mathbf{A} + \mathbf{Q} - \mathbf{AQH_u}(n-1)]^{-1}. \tag{9.4.7b}$$

As with all recursive relations, we must start somewhere, which we did by noting that

$$\mathbf{H_u}(0) = \mathbf{p}, \tag{9.4.8a}$$

and thus

$$\mathbf{H_u}(1) = \lambda[\lambda\mathbf{I} + \mathbf{B} - \mathbf{BQ}]^{-1} = [\mathbf{A} + \mathbf{Q} - \mathbf{AQ}]^{-1}. \tag{9.4.8b}$$

It is easy to show that $\mathbf{H_u}(1)\boldsymbol{\epsilon}' = \boldsymbol{\epsilon}'$, and by induction, using (9.4.7b), prove that (9.4.6b) is true for all n. Note that in general, $\mathbf{H_u}(n)$ changes with n, although the sequence approaches a limit for large n.

From these matrices we found the probability matrices of first passage from n to $n+j$, for any n and j. For instance, the probability matrix (it is actually a vector) of first passage from $0 \to n$ is

$$\mathbf{p_u}(n) := \mathbf{p}\mathbf{H_u}(1)\,\mathbf{H_u}(2) \cdots \mathbf{H_u}(n-1). \tag{9.4.9}$$

These objects may not appear to be very interesting in their own right, but they are needed for calculating first-passage times, as is shown in the next paragraph.

By arguments similar to the preceding, we derived the mean time for the queue to grow from n to $n+1$ for the first time. First we defined the vector $\boldsymbol{\tau}'_{\boldsymbol{u}}(n)$, whose ith component is $[\boldsymbol{\tau}'_{\boldsymbol{u}}(n)]_i :=$ mean first-passage time from n to $n+1$, having started in state $\{i, n\}$. It then followed that

$$\boldsymbol{\tau}'_{\boldsymbol{u}}(n) = \frac{1}{\lambda}\boldsymbol{\epsilon}' + \mathbf{H_u}(n)\,\mathbf{BQ}\,\boldsymbol{\tau}'_{\boldsymbol{u}}(n-1), \quad \text{with } \boldsymbol{\tau}'_{\boldsymbol{u}}(0) := \frac{1}{\lambda}\boldsymbol{\epsilon}'. \tag{9.4.10}$$

The sets of Equations (9.4.7) and (9.4.10) are all that is needed to compute all the vector times. Whether the system is open or closed, irrespective of whether ρ is less than, equal to, or greater than 1, one can then calculate such things as:

1. The mean first-passage time of going from n to $n+1$, given that the customer in service has just begun $[\mathbf{p}\boldsymbol{\tau}'_{\boldsymbol{u}}(n)]$.

2. The mean first-passage time from n to $n+1$, given that the queue was originally empty; see (9.4.9) $[t_u(n) := \mathbf{p_u}(n)\boldsymbol{\tau}'_{\boldsymbol{u}}(n)]$.

3. The mean first-passage time, given that a customer has just arrived and found n customers already there (see Theorem 4.5.2 and its corollaries) $[\boldsymbol{\pi}(n)\boldsymbol{\tau}'_{\boldsymbol{u}}(n)/r(n)]$.

One can even calculate in an efficient way the mean time for a queue to grow to n for the first time given that a customer has just arrived at an empty queue; namely,

$$t(1 \to n) := \sum_{k=1}^{n-1} t_u(k). \tag{9.4.11}$$

Note that this is not the same as the first excursion to n during a busy period (although that too is calculable), because this process allows the queue to empty any number of times before finally reaching its goal.

In like manner one can derive analogous expressions for M/G/C, G/G/1, and even more general systems. The most significant point in this discussion is that all the formulas are expressible in a base-free formulation invariant to isometric transformations. Thus explicit appeal to a "component" interpretation is unnecessary.

9.5 Concluding Remarks

We hope we have shown that an approach which is linear algebraic from beginning to end has great potential for covering material that hitherto has been ignored because of the difficulties involved. The ubiquitousness of such an approach appears to depend on the invariance of formulas to isometric transformations. If this is so, one must be prepared to deal with representations that are distinctly not phase distributions. Only then can one study the purely algebraic properties of various systems using a paradigm that is different from what we have been locked into for 50 years or more. Two such research problems are described below.

1. Consider a G/G/1//N queue. In preparing such a system at say $t = 0$, one must initialize both S_1 and S_2. This would require specifying $m_1 + m_2$ quantities. That is, we have a sum-space description. But as the system evolves in time, the components from each subspace become correlated with those in the other, thus forcing a complete product-space description ($m_1 \cdot m_2$ components). However, as van de Liefvoort has shown [Lief-Lip86], [Liefvoort90], the key matrix for the steady-state solution, $\mathbf{U}$ from (9.4.4d), has $m_1 \cdot m_2 - m_1 - m_2 + 1$ eigenvectors with eigenvalue 1, all of which can be thrown away when calculating the s.s queuelength probabiities $[r(n, N)]$, if one can find an appropriate isometric transformation in the product space (such a transformation exists, finding a general form for it is the problem).

This means that there exists (at least) one sum-space representation of steady-state G/G/1 queues, one that mixes the components of the two subspaces.

2. In describing M/G/C//N-type systems ($N > C$), one must work in spaces that have

$$D := \binom{m + C - 1}{C}$$

components. The steady-state solutions can then be written in terms of matrices that have this dimension. However, when $N \leq C$, the solution is known to be the product-form solution of Jackson networks! What is the relationship between the two? And as in question 1, does there exist a representation of dimension less than D that can be used?

Symbols

□ – End of definition. D1.1.2 [†]
■ – End of Theorem, Lemma, or Corollary. T1.3.2 [¶]
▲ – End of Example. E2.1.1[‖]
$A := B$ – A is defined by B. S1.1.1 [‡]
$\mathbf{A} = \mathbf{I} + \lambda^{-1}\mathbf{B} - \mathbf{Q}$. (4.1.4a)[*]
$\mathbf{a}(n;\, N)$ – S.s. Arrival prob. vector at S_1. D4.1.4
$a(n;\, N) = \mathbf{a}(n;\, N)\boldsymbol{\epsilon}'$ – Scalar prob. associated with $\mathbf{a}(n;\, N)$. D4.1.4
$\mathbf{a_2}(k;\, N)$ – S.s. Arrival prob. vector at S_2. D5.1.3
$a_2(k;\, N) = \mathbf{a_2}(k;\, N)\boldsymbol{\epsilon}'$ – Scalar prob. associated with $\mathbf{a_2}(k;\, N)$. D5.1.3
$a_2(k;\, N \mid C)$ – S.s. Arrival prob. vector at S_2 (ME/M/C//N). D5.4.3
$\mathbf{B} := \mathbf{M}(\mathbf{I} - \mathbf{P})$ – Service rate matrix. (3.1.3)
$\boldsymbol{\mathcal{B}}$ – Generator of interdeparture times for Markov renewal process. S8.2.1
$B(t) = \mathbb{P}\mathbf{r}(T \leq t)$ – Probability Distribution Function (PDF). (1.2.2)
$B^*(s)$ – Laplace transform of $b(t)$. (3.1.10)
$B_d(t;\, N)$ – PDF for inter**d**eparture times (M/ME/1//N). D4.2.3
$B_s(t)$ – PDF for **s**ystem time (M/ME/1). D4.2.1
$b(t) = (d/dt)[B(t)]$ –Probability density function (pdf). (1.2.2)
C – Number of servers at S_1. S5.4, C6[§]
$C_v^2 = \sigma^2/\mathbb{E}[X]^2$ – Squared coefficient of variation. (1.2.4c)
$\mathbf{d}(n;\, N)$ – S.s. Vector as seen by departing cust. in M/G/1//N queue. D4.1.5
$d(n;\, N) = \mathbf{d}(n;\, N)\boldsymbol{\epsilon}'$ – Scalar prob. associated with $\mathbf{d}(n;\, N)$. D4.1.5
$\mathbf{d_2}(k;\, N)$ – S.s. Prob. vector as seen by customer departing S_2. D5.1.2
$d_2(k;\, N) = \mathbf{d_2}(k;\, N)\boldsymbol{\epsilon}'$ – Scalar prob. associated with $\mathbf{d_2}(k;\, N)$. D5.1.2
$\mathbf{d_2}(k;\, N \mid C)$ – S.s. Vector for departure from S_2 (G/M/C//N). D5.4.3
$\mathbb{E}[g(X)] = \int_0^\infty g(x)\, f_X(x)\, dx$ – mean value of $g(x)$. D1.2.3
$\mathbf{H_d}(n;\, N)$ – Prob. mx. of f.p. from n to $n-1$. D4.5.7
$\mathbf{H_{2d}}(k;\, N)$ – Prob. mx. of f.p. at S_2 from k to $k-1$. D5.5.3
$\mathbf{H_{dc}}(n;\, N)$ – Prob. mx. of f.p. from n to $n-1$, where $N \geq n > C$. D6.5.10
$\mathbf{H_{dk}}(N \mid C)$ – Prob. mx. of f.p. from k to $k-1$, where $C \geq x > 0$. D6.5.11
$\mathbf{H_u}(n)$ – Prob. mx. of f.p. from n to $n+1$. D4.5.1
$\mathbf{H_{2u}}(k)$ – Prob. mx. of f.p. at S_2 from k to $k+1$. D5.5.1
$\mathbf{H_u}(n \to n+\ell)$ – Prob. mx. of f.p. from n to $n+\ell$. D4.5.2
$\mathbf{H_{uc}}(n)$ – Prob. mx. of f.p. from n to $n+1$, where $n \geq C$. D6.5.7
$\mathbf{H_{uk}}$ – Related to $\mathbf{X_k}$ by $\mathbf{X_k} = \mathbf{H_{uk}}\,\mathbf{R_{k+1}}$, $k < C$. D6.5.6

[†] Definition number
[¶] Theorem number
[‖] Example number
[‡] Section number
[*] Equation number
[§] Chapter number

$\{j;\ n;\ N\}$ – A state of an M/ME/1//N loop (also ME/M/1//N). D4.1.2
$\mathbf{K}(N) = \mathbf{I} + \mathbf{UK}(N-1)$, where $\mathbf{K}(1) = \mathbf{I} + \lambda\mathbf{V}$. (4.1.6d)
$\mathbf{K} = (\mathbf{I} - \mathbf{U})^{-1}$. (4.2.2)
$\boldsymbol{\mathcal{L}}$ – Instantaneous departure rate matrix for semi-markov processes. D8.2.1
$\mathbf{M}$ – Completion rate matrix. D1.3.6
$\mathbf{M_k}$ – Completion rate matrix for k active servers (M/ME/C). D6.3.2
$N_i(t)$ – Number of departures from S_i in interval, t. D4.4.1
$\mathbf{P}$ – (Substochastic) transition matrix. (3.1.1a)
$\boldsymbol{P}$ – Transition matrix between subsystems ($\boldsymbol{P\epsilon}' = \boldsymbol{\epsilon}'$). D1.3.4, S8.3.2
$\mathbf{P_k}$ – Transition mx. for $k \leq C$ active cust. (M/ME/C). D6.3.6
$P_i(N)$ – S.s. prob. that S_i is busy in a system with N cust. D2.1.2
$\mathbf{p}$ – Entrance vector. S3.1
$\wp = \wp\boldsymbol{\mathcal{Y}}$ – Left eigenvector of $\boldsymbol{\mathcal{Y}}$. (8.2.7)
$\mathbb{P}\mathbf{r}[X]$ – Probability that expression "X" is true. D1.1.2
$\mathbf{p_u}(n)$ – Prob. vector for f.p. from 0 to n (M/ME/1). D4.5.4
$\mathbf{p_{uk}}(n)$ – Prob. vector for f.p. from 0 to n, with k active (M/ME/C). D6.5.8
$\langle\, \mathbf{p}\, ,\ \mathbf{B}\, \rangle$ – Matrix representation of subsystem, S. T3.1.1
$\boldsymbol{Q}$ – Transition rate matrix (Chapter 1 only). (1.3.2c)
$\mathbf{Q} = \boldsymbol{\epsilon}'\mathbf{p}$. L3.5.1‖
$\boldsymbol{\mathcal{Q}} = \boldsymbol{\mathcal{B}} - \boldsymbol{\mathcal{L}}$ – Generator of underlying semi-Markov process (8.2.8a)
$\mathbf{Q_k}$ – Matrix generalization of $\mathbf{q}'$ with k active cust. (M/ME/C). D6.3.5
$\mathbf{q}' = (\mathbf{I} - \mathbf{P})\boldsymbol{\epsilon}'$ – Exit vector. (3.1.1a)
$\bar{q}$ – Mean queue length. (1.1.1c)
$\mathbf{R}(t) = \exp(-t\mathbf{B})$ – Reliability matrix function. D3.1.1
$R(N)$ –Mean response time in a TS system. T6.3.5
$R(t) = \Psi[\mathbf{R}(t)] = 1 - B(t)$ – Reliability function. S1.2.1, (3.1.7d)
$\mathbf{R_k}$ – Matrix generalization of $\mathbf{p}$ for k active cust. (M/ME/C). D6.3.4
$r(n) := \lim_{N\to\infty} r(n;\ N)$ – S.s. prob. for an open M/G/1 system. (4.2.4a)
$r(n,\ N) = \boldsymbol{\pi}(n,\ N)\boldsymbol{\epsilon}'$ – S.s. prob. for n cust. at S_1(M/G/1//N). D4.1.1
$r_k(n,\ N) = \boldsymbol{\pi}_\mathbf{k}(n,\ N)\boldsymbol{\epsilon}'_\mathbf{k}$ – If $n \geq C$, $k{=}C$, else $k{=}n$ (M/G/C//N). D6.3.3
$r_2(k,\ N) = \boldsymbol{\pi}_\mathbf{2}(k,\ N)\boldsymbol{\epsilon}' = r(N-k,\ N)$. D5.1.4
$\mathbf{r}(t) = \mathbf{pR}(t)$ – Reliability vector function. D3.1.2
$\hat{r}(k)$ – Autocorrelation Coefficient, $lag - k$. (8.2.12c)
s – Geom. parameter for G/M/1 queue; smallest eigenvalue of $\mathbf{A}$. T5.1.2
S_i – Subsystem labelled i. S2.1
$t_d(n;\ N)$ – Mean f-p time to drop by 1. D4.5.9
$t_d(k \to 0;\ N)$ – Mean time for k-busy period. D4.5.10
$t_u(n)$ – Mean f-p time for queue to grow from n to $n+1$. D4.5.5
$t_u(0 \to n)$ – Mean f-p time for queue to grow from 0 to n. D4.5.6
$\mathbf{U} = \mathbf{A}^{-1}$. (4.1.4b)
$\hat{\mathbf{u}}$ – Unit eigenvector of $\mathbf{A}$ going with eigenvalue s ($\hat{\mathbf{u}}\boldsymbol{\epsilon}' = 1$). (5.1.4b)
$\mathbf{V} = \mathbf{B}^{-1}$ – Service-time matrix. (3.1.3)
$\boldsymbol{\mathcal{V}} = \boldsymbol{\mathcal{B}}^{-1}$ – Service-time matrix in semi-Markov processes. T8.1.1
$\mathbf{W_d}(n,\ k)$ – Prob. mx. for queue to drop by 1 w.o. exceeding $k \geq n$. D4.5.16
$W_d(n,\ k;\ N)$ – Prob. for queue to drop 1 w.o. exceeding $k{\geq}n$. D2.3.9

‖Lemma number

$\mathbf{W_d}(n \to n-\ell;\ k)$ – Prob. mx. queue will drop by ℓ w.o. exceeding k. D4.5.17
$W_d(k \to 0;\ N)$ – Prob. for queue to drop to 0 w.o. exceeding k. D4.5.17
$W_m(k;\ N)$ – Prob. that queue will reach a max. of k during a b-p. D4.5.17
$\mathbf{W_u}(n) = \mathbf{W_u}(n;\ 0)$ – Prob. mx. for queue to grow by 1 during a b-p. D4.5.14
$\mathbf{W_u}(n;\ k)$ – Prob. mx. for queue to grow by 1 w.o. dropping to k. D4.5.11
$W_u(n;\ k) = \Psi[\mathbf{W_u}(n;\ k)]$. D4.5.12
$\mathbf{W_u}(n \to n+\ell; k)$ – Prob. mx. for growth by ℓ w.o. dropping to k. D4.5.13
$W_u(n)$ – Prob. that queue will grow by 1 during a b-p. D2.3.7
$\mathbf{W_u}(1 \to k)$ – Prob. mx. for queue to grow to k during a b-p. D4.5.13
$W_u(1 \to k) =$ – Prob. that queue will grow to k during a b-p. D2.3.8
$W_u(1 \to k) = \Psi[\mathbf{W_u}(1 \to k)]$. D4.5.13
$\mathbf{w}(n;\ N)$ – S.s. prob. vector between events (M/G/1 queue). D4.1.3
$\mathbf{w_2}(k;\ N)$ – S.s. prob. vector between events, where k is the no. at S_2. D5.4.2
$\mathbf{X_k}$ – Prob. mx. of f.p. from k to $k+1$ active cust., where $k < C$. D6.5.5
$\mathbf{Y_k}$ – Prob. mx. for going from k to $k-1$ active cust., w.o. arrivals. D6.5.2
$\mathbf{Y_k}(\ell)$ – Prob. mx. for going from k to $k-\ell$ active cust., w.o. arrivals. D6.5.3
$\mathcal{Y} = \mathcal{V}\mathcal{L}$ – satisfies $\mathcal{Y}\varepsilon' = \varepsilon'$. (8.2.2)
$\Delta(t)$ – Unit step function. (5.1.12b)
δ_{ij} – Kronecker delta. D1.3.2
$\delta(x)$ – Dirac delta function. (3.2.4), (5.1.12a)
$\kappa = \boldsymbol{\pi}\,\mathcal{L}\varepsilon'$ – Steady-state departure rate in semi-Markov processes. (8.2.8d)
$\Lambda(N)$ – System throughput. D2.1.2
$\mu_\nu(\ell)$ – Load-dependent service rate. D6.3.8
$\mathbf{\Pi}(n;\ N)$ – S.s. vector for n at S_1, and $N-n$ at S_2 (ME/ME/1//N). D7.3.2
$\boldsymbol{\pi}(n;\ N)$ – S.s. prob. vector of finding n cust. at S_1 (M/ME/1//N). D4.1.1
$\boldsymbol{\pi}_\mathbf{2}(k;\ N)$ – S.s. prob. vector of finding k cust. at S_2 (ME/M/1//N). D5.1.4
$\boldsymbol{\pi}_\mathbf{2}(k;\ N \mid C)$ – S.s. prob. vector for a generalized ME/M/C//N queue. D5.4.1
$\boldsymbol{\pi}_\mathbf{2f}(k;\ N)$ – S.s. prob. vector for an ME/M/1/N queue. D5.3.1
$\pi_i(t)$ – Prob. that system will be in state $i \in \Xi$ at time t (Chapter 1). D1.3.2
$\boldsymbol{\pi}_\mathbf{r}(n;\ N)$ – Residual prob. vector (M/ME/1//N). D4.3.1
$\Psi[\mathbf{X}] := \mathbf{p}\,\mathbf{X}\,\boldsymbol{\epsilon}'$ (for any square mx. $\mathbf{X}$). (3.1.5)
ρ – Utilization factor $= \lambda\bar{x}$. (1.1.3), S4.2
ϱ – Utilization factor for G/M/1 queues ($\varrho = \bar{x}_2/\bar{x}_1 = 1\,/\,\rho$) S5.1
$\varrho(X,\ Y)$ – Correlation coefficient. (8.2.11b)
σ^2 – Variance. (1.2.4a)
Ξ – Set of states of system. D1.3.1, D4.1.2, D7.3.1
Ξ_k – Set of states of subsystem, S_k. D6.3.1
$\boldsymbol{\tau}'_\mathbf{d}(n;\ N)$ – Mean f-p time vector for queue to drop by 1. D4.5.8
$\boldsymbol{\tau}'_\mathbf{2d}(k;\ N)$ – Mean f-p time vector for queue at S_2 to drop by 1. D5.5.4
$\tau_d(n;\ N)$ – Mean f-p time for queue to drop by 1 (M/M/1//N). D2.3.4
$\boldsymbol{\tau}'_\mathbf{dk}(n;\ N \mid C)$ – f-p vector for queue to drop by 1 (M/ME/C//N). D6.5.12
$\boldsymbol{\tau}'_\mathbf{u}(n)$ – Mean f-p time vector for queue to grow by 1. D4.5.3
$\tau_u(n)$ – Mean f-p time for queue to grow by 1 (M/M/1). D2.3.2
$\boldsymbol{\tau}'_\mathbf{2u}(k)$ – Mean f-p time vector for queue at S_2 to grow by 1. D5.5.2
$\boldsymbol{\tau}'_\mathbf{uk}(n)$ – Mean f-p vector for queue to increase by 1 (M/ME/C). D6.5.9
$\boldsymbol{\tau}'_\mathbf{k}$ – Departure-time vector with k active cust., w.o. arrivals (ME/C). D6.5.1

Abbreviations

AMAOOMMPP – Alternative Modified Augmented ON-OFF MMPP.
AMMPP – Augmented MMPP
BOP – Buffer Overflow Probability.
b-p – Busy period.
C-K – Chapman-Kolmogorov Equation.
EIEO – Exponential In Exponential Out.
FCFS – First-Come-First-Served.
f.p. – First passage.
LAQT – Linear Algebraic Queueing Theory.
LT – Laplace Transform
MAOOMMPP – Modified, Augmented, ON-OFF MMPP.
MAP – Markov Arrival Process.
MCD – Mean Cell delay.
ME – Matrix Exponential function.
MMPP – Markov Modulated Poisson Process
MPD – Mean Packet delay.
MRDP – Markov Regulated Departure Process.
MRP – Markov Renewal Process.
MTTF – Mean Time To Failure.
mx. – Matrix.
ODE – Ordinary Differential Equation.
OOMMPP – ON-OFF MMPP.
PDF – Probability Distribution Function.
pdf – probability density function.
PH – Phase distribution.
P-K – Pollaczek-Khinchine Formula
PT – Power-Tailed distribution.
QBD – Quasi-Birth-Death Process.
QED – *Quod Erat Demonstrandum*, (which was to be proven)
RLT – Rational Laplace Transform.
RP – Reduced-Product space.
RT – Relaxation Time.
r.v. – random Variable.
SMP – Semi-Markov Process.
s.s. – steady-state.
TPT – Truncated Power-tailed distribution.
TS – Time-Sharing.
w.o. – without.

Bibliography

[ABATECHOUDHURYWHITT96] Abate, J., Choudhury, G.L. and Whitt, W. (1996). On the Laguerre method for numerically inverting Laplace transforms. *INFORMS J. Computing* **8**, 413–427.

[ABRAMOWITZSTEGUN64] Abramowitz, M. and Stegun, I.A. (1964). *Handbook of Mathematical Functions.* U.S. Government Printing Office, Washington D. C.

[ALLEN90] Allen, A.O. (1990). *Probability, Statistics, and Queueing Theory, with Computer Science Applications*, 2nd ed. Academic Press, New York.

[ANTONIOSSCHWEFELLIP07] Antonios, I., Schwefel, H-P, and Lipsky, L. (2007). On the correlation and its relationship to performance for ON/OFF network traffic. Tech. Report, Center for Telecommunications, Aalborg University, Denmark.

[ASMUSSEN03] Asmussen, S. (2003). *Applied Probability and Queues*, 2nd. ed. Springer-Verlag, New York.

[ASMUSSENKLUPPELBERG97] Asmussen, S. and C Kluppelberg (1997). Stationary M/G/1 excursions in the presence of heavy tails, *J. Appl. Prob.* **34**, 208–212.

[BAK96] Bak, Per (1996). *How Nature Works - The Science of Self-Organized Criticality.* Springer-Verlag, New York.

[BASKETETAL75] Baskett, F., Chandy, K.M., Muntz, R.R., and Palacios, F.G. (1975). Open, closed, and mixed networks of queues with different classes of customers. *Journal of the ACM*, **22**, 2, 248–260.

[BEUTLER83] Beutler, F.J. (1983). Mean sojourn times in Markov queueing networks: Little's formula revisited *IEEE Transactions on Information Theory* **29**, 2, March.

[BURKE56] Burke, P.J. (1956). The output of a queueing system. *Operations Research*, **4**, 699–704.

[BUZEN73] Buzen, J.P. (1973). Computational algorithms for closed queueing networks with exponential servers. *Communications of the ACM*, September.

[BUZENDENNING] Buzen, J.P. and Denning, P.J. (1978). The operational analysis of queueing network models. *Computing Surveys*, **10**, 3, 225–261.

[CARROLL79] Carroll, J.L. (1979). *A Study of Closed Queueing Networks with Population Size Constraints.* PhD Dissertation, University of Nebraska, Lincoln.

[CARROLLLIPVDL82] Carroll, J.L., Lipsky, L., and van de Liefvoort, A. (1982). Solutions of M/G/1/N-type loops with extension to M/G/1 and GI/M/1 queues. *Operations Research* **30**, 490–514.

[CHAK-ALFA97] Chakravarthy, S.R. and Alfa, A.S., eds. (1997). *Matrix-Analytic Methods in Stochastic Models* Marcel Dekker, New York.

[COHEN82] Cohen, J.W. (1982). *The Single Server Queue*, 2nd ed. North Holland, New York.

[CONTE-DEBOER80] Conte, S.D. and de Boer, C. (1980). *Elementary Numerical Analysis*, 3rd ed. McGraw-Hill, New York.

[COOPER81] Cooper, R.B. (1981). *Introduction to Queueing Theory.* 2nd ed. Elsevier North Holland, New York.

[COURTOIS77] Courtois, P.J. (1977). *Decomposability; Queueing and Computer System Applications.* Academic Press, New York.

[COX55] Cox, D.R. (1955). Use of complex probabilities in the theory of stochastic processes. *Proceedings of the Cambridge Philosophical Society* **51**, 313–319.

[COX62] Cox, D.R. (1962). *Renewal Theory.* Menthuen, London.

[CROVELLABESTAVROS96] Crovella, M. and Bestavros, A. (1996). Self-similarity in World-Wide-Web traffic: Evidence and possible causes. *Performance Evaluation Review* **24**, *160–169.*

[DENNING78] Denning, P.J., Ed. (1978). Special issue on performance modelling. *Computing Surveys* **10**, 3.

[DING91] Ding, Y. (1991). *On Performance Control of Real-Time Systems.* PhD Dissertation, University of Connecticut, Storrs.

[DISNEYKIESSLER87] Disney, R.L., and Kiessler, P.C. (1987). *Traffic Processes in Queueing Networks: A Markov Renewal Approach.* Johns Hopkins University Press, Batimore.

[DUMOUCHEL71] DuMouchel, W.H. (1971). *Stable Distributions in Statistical Inference.* PhD Thesis. University of Michigan, Ann Arbor.

[EMBR-KLUP-MIK07] Embrechts, P., Klüppelberg, C. and Mikosch, T. (2007–8th printing). *Modelling Extremal Events for Insurance Claims.* Springer, Berlin.

[ERLANG17] Erlang, A.K. (1917). Solution of some problems in the theory of probabilities of significance in automatic telephone exchanges. *The Post Office Electrical Engineer's Journal* **10** 189–197.

[FangLipsky82] Fang, Z. and Lipsky, L. (1982). A note on the persistance of the time-dependent solution of an M/M/1/M queue. Tech. report, Department of Computer Science, University of Nebraska, Lincoln.

[Feller71] Feller, W. (1971). *An Introduction to Probability Theory and Its Applications*, Vol. II., 2nd Ed. John Wiley, New York.

[FioriniLipvdLHsin95] Fiorini, P. M., Lipsky, L., van de Liefvoort, A. and Hsin, W-J (1995). Auto-correlation lag-k for customers departing from semi-Markov processes. Tech. report, Technical University-München, January.

[FioriniLipHatem97] Fiorini, P. M., Lipsky, L. and Hatem, J.E! (1997). Comparison of buffer usage utilizing multiple servers in networks with power-tail distributions. *INFORMS97, Boston, MA*, 30 June-2 July.

[Fiorini98] Fiorini, P.M. (1998). *Modeling Telecommunication Systems with Self-Similar Data Traffic.* PhD thesis, Department of Computer Science, University of Connecticut, May.

[LipGargRobbert92] Lipsky, L., Garg, S and Robbert, M. (1992). The effect of power-tail distributions on response times of time-sharing computer systems. *SIGAPP92 Symposium on Applied Computing* Kansas City, MO, March. Also in *Applied Computing: Technological Challenges of the 1990's*, Vol.II. 719-723. Berghel, H, et al.,Eds., ACM, New York.

[Glynn-Whitt93] Glynn, P.W., and Whitt, W. (1989). Estensions of the queueing relations $L = \lambda W$ and $H = \lambda G$. *Operations Research* **37**, 634–644.

[Gordon-Newell67] Gordon, W.J. and Newell, G.F. (1967). Closed queueing systems with exponential servers. *Operations Research* **15** 254–265.

[Graham81] Graham, A. (1981). *Kronecker Products and Matrix Calculus.* Ellis Horwood, Chichester, England.

[Grein-Job-Lip99] Greiner, M., Jobmann, M. and Lipsky, L. (1999). The importance of power-tail distributions for telecommunication traffic models. *Operations Research* **47**, No.2, 313–326, March.

[Gross-Harris98] Gross, D. and Harris, C.M. (1998). *Fundamentals of Queueing Theory*, 3rd ed. Wiley-Interscience, New York.

[GuptaEtAl07] Gupta, V., Harshol-Balter, M., Sigman, K. and Whitt, W. (2007). Analysis of join-the-shortest-queue routing for web server farms. *Performance Evaluation* **64** 1062-1081.

[Halmos55] Halmos, P.R. (1955). *Finite Dimensional Vector Spaces* Princeton University Press, Princeton, NJ.

[HATEM97] Hatem, J.E! (1997). *Comparison Of Buffer Usage Utilizing Single And Multiple Servers In Network Systems With Power-tail Distributions.* PhD Thesis, Department of Computer Science, University of Connecticut, December.

[HEYMAN-SOBEL82] Heyman, D.P. and Sobel, M.J. (1982). *Stochastic Models in Operations Research*, Vol. 1, McGraw-Hill, New York.

[HORN-JOHNSON85] Horn, R.A. and Johnson, C.R. (1985). *Matrix Analysis.* Cambridge University Press, Cambridge UK.

[JACKSON63] Jackson, J.R. (1963). Jobshop-like queueing systems. *Management Science* **10**, 131–142.

[JENSEN67] Jensen, N.E. (1967). An introduction to Bernoullian utility theory, I: utility functions, *Swedish Journal of Economics* **69**, p.163–83.

[KANT92] Kant, K. (1992). *Introduction to Computer System Performance Evaluation.* McGraw-Hill, New York.

[KEILSON-NUNN79] Keilson, J. and Nunn, W. (1979). Laguerre transformation as a tool for the numerical solution of integral equations of convolution type. *Applied Mathematics and Computation* **5**, 313–359.

[KENDALL52] Kendall, D.G. (1952). Les processus stochastiques de croissance en biologie. *Annales de l'Institut Henri Poincaré*, **13**, 43–108.

[KENDALL53] Kendall, D.G. (1953). Stochastic processes occurring in the theory of queues and their analysis by the method of imbedded Markov chains. *Ann. Math. Statist.* **24**, 338–354.

[KENDALL64] Kendall, D.G. (1964). Some recent work and further problems in the theory of queues. *Theory of Probability and Its Applications* **9**, 1–15.

[KHINCHINE32] Khinchine, A.Y. (1932). Mathematical theory of stationary queues. *Mat. Sbornik* **39**, 73–84.

[KHINCHINE60] Khinchine, A.Y. (1960). *Mathematical Methods in the Theory of Queueing* Griffin, London.

[KINGMAN72] Kingman, J. F.C. (1972). *Regenerative Phenomena.* John Wiley, New York.

[KLEINROCK75] Kleinrock, L. (1975). *Queueing Systems, Volume I: Theory.* John Wiley, New York.

[KLINGER97] Klinger, W. (1997). *On the Convergence of Sums of Power-Tail Samples to their α-Stable Distributions.* MS Thesis, Department of Computer Science, University of Connecticut, August.

[KLINGERETAL97] Klinger, W., Greiner, M., Crovella, M., Lipsky, L., Jobmann, M., Fiorini, P. and Schwefel, H-P. (1997). How to model telecommunications (and other) systems where power-Tail behavior is observed: (Background Review and Research Proposal). Technical Report, CSE/BRC, University of Connecticut, May, 1997.

[KONWARLIPSLEIMAN06] Konwar, K. M., Lipsky, L. and Sleiman, M. (2006). Moments of memory access time for systems with hierarchical memories. *21st International Conference on Computers and their Applications* (CATA-2006), Seattle WA, March.

[LATOUCHETAYLOR00] Latouche, G. and Taylor, P., eds. (2000). *Advances in Algorithmic Methods for Stochastic Models.* Notable Publications, New Jersey, 2000.

[LATOUCHE-RAM99] Latouche, G. and Ramaswami, V. (1999). *Introduction to Matrix Analytic Methods in Stochastic Modeling.* SIAM/ASA, Philadelphia Pa.

[LAZOWSKAETAL84] Lazowska, E.D., Zahorjan, J., Graham, G.S., and Sevcik, K.C. (1984). *Quantitative System Performance - Computer System Analysis Using Queueing Network Models.* Prentice Hall, Englewood Cliffs, NJ.

[LEE-LIEF-WALLACE00] Lee, Y. D., van de Liefvoort, A. and Wallace, V.L. (2000). Modelling correlated traffic with a generalized ipp *Performance Evaluation* **40**, 99–114.

[LELAND-OTT86] Leland, W. E. and T. Ott (1986). UNIX processor behavior and load balancing among loosely coupled computers. In *Teletraffic Analysis and Computer Performance Evaluation*, O.J. Boxma, J.W. Cohen, and H.C. Tijms, Eds, 191–208, Elsevier, NY.

[LELANDETAL94] Leland, W.E., Taqqu, M., Willinger, W., and Wilson, D.V. (1994). On the self-similar nature of ethernet traffic (extended version). *Proc. of IEEE/ACM Trans. on Networking*, **2**, 1–15, February.

[LIEFVOORT82] van de Liefvoort, A. (1982). *An Algebraic Approach to the Steady-state Solution of G/G/1//N-Type Loops*, PhD Thesis, University of Nebraska, Lincoln.

[LIEF-LIP86] van de Liefvoort, A., and Lipsky, L. (1986). A matrix-algebraic solution to two K_m servers in a loop, *Journal of the ACM* **33**, 1, 207–223.

[LIEFVOORT87] van de Liefvoort, A. (1987). A sum-space characterization of G/G/1/N-type queues. Technical Report TR-87-5, Computer Science Department, University of Kansas, Lawrence.

[LIEFVOORT90] van de Liefvoort, A. (1990). The waiting-time distribution and its moments of the Ph/Ph/1 queue. *Operations Research Letters*, **9**, 261–269.

[LIPSKY-CHURCH77] Lipsky, L. and Church, J.D. (1977). Applications of a queueing network model for a computer system. *Computing Surveys*, **9**, 205–221, September.

[LIPSKY80] Lipsky, L. (1980). A study of time-sharing systems considered as queueing networks of exponential servers. *Computer Journal* **23**, 290–297.

[LIPTEHRVDLLIEU82] Lipsky, L., Tehranipour, A., van de Liefvoort, A. and Lieu, H. (1982). On the asymptotic behavior of time-sharing systems. *Communications of the ACM* **25**, 707–714, October.

[LIPSKY-RAM85] Lipsky, L. and Ramaswami, V. (1985). A unique minimal representation of Coxian service centers. Technical report, Department of Computer Science, University of Nebraska, Lincoln.

[LIPSKY86] Lipsky, L. (1986). A heuristic fit of an unusual set of data BELCOR Research Report, January.

[LIPSKY-FANG86] Lipsky, L. and Fang, Z. (1986). Classification of functions with rational Laplace transforms *Summer Simulation Conference*, Las Vegas, NV, July.

[LITTLE61] Little, J.D.C. (1961). A proof of the queueing formula $L = \lambda W$. *Operations Research* **9**, 383–387.

[LOWRIE-LIP93] Lowry, W. and Lipsky, L. (1993). A model for the probability distribution of medical expenses *Conference of Actuaries in Public Practice.*

[MARKOV07] Markov, A.A. (1907). Extension of the limit theorems of probabiltiy theory to a sum of variables connected in a chain. *The Notes of the Imperial Academy of Science of St. Petersburg* **XXII**, 9, Physio-Mathematical College.

[MEIER-FISCHER92] Meier-Hellstern, K. and Fischer, W. (1992). MMPP cookbook. *Performance Evaluation* **18**, 149–171.

[MELAMEDWHITT90] Melamed, B. and Whitt, W. (1990). On arrivals that see time averages. *Operations Research*, **38**, 156–172.

[MOHAMED04] Mohamed, A.M.A-R. (2004). *Performance Based Cluster Architecture: Analytic Modelling and Analysis.* PhD Thesis, Department of Computer Science, University of Connecticut.

[MOLLOY89] Molloy, M.K. (1989). *Fundamentals of Performance Modeling.* Macmillan, New York.

[MORSE58] Morse, P.M. (1958). *Queues, Inventories and Maintenance.* John Wiley, New York.

[NEUTS75] Neuts, M.F. (1975). Probability distributions of phase type. *Liber Amicorum Prof. Emeritus H. Florin*, Department of Mathematics, University of Louvain, Belgium, 173–206.

[NEUTS77] Neuts, M.F. (1977). The mythology of the steady state. In *Joint National ORSA-TIMS Meeting*, Atlanta.

[NEUTS81] Neuts, M.F. (1981). *Matrix-Geometric Solutions in Stochastic Models - An Algorithmic Approach.* Johns Hopkins University Press, Baltimore.

[NEUTS82] Neuts, M.F. (1982). Explicit steady-state solutions to some elementary queueing models. *Operations Research* **30** 480–489.

[NEUTS89] Neuts, M.F. (1989). *Structured Stochastic Matrices of M/G/1 Type and Their Applications.* Marcel Dekker, New York.

[O'CINNEIDE91] O'Cinneide, C.A. (1991). Personal communication. See also Asmussen, S. and O'Cinneide, C.A. (1999). Matrix exponential distributions, *Encyclopedia of Statistical Sciences, Update Volume*, **3**, 435–440, Wiley.

[PALM43] Palm, C. (1943). Intensitätsschwankungen im fernsprechverkehr. *Ericsson Technics* **44**(3), 189.

[PARK-WILL00] Park, K. and Willinger, W., Eds. (2000). *Self-Similar Network Traffic and Performance Evaluation.* Wiley-Interscience, New York.

[PERROS94] Perros, H. (1994). *Queueing Networks with Blocking: Exact and Approximate Solutions.* Oxford University Press.

[PHILLIPS02] Phillips, K. (2002). *Wealth and Democracy.* Broadway Books, New York.

[POLLACZEK30] Pollaczek, F. (1930). Über eine Aufgabe der Wahrscheinlichkeitstheorie, I und II. *Mathematische Zeitschrift* **32**, 64–100, 729–750.

[RAMASWAMI80] Ramaswami, V. (1980). The N/G/1 queue and its detailed analysis. *Adv. in Appl. Prob.*, **12**, 222–261.

[ROSS92] Ross, S. M. (1992). *Applied Probabiity Models with Optimization Applications.* Dover, New York.

[ROSS96] Ross, S. M. (1996). *Stochastic Processes*, 2nd Ed. Wiley, New York.

[SAITO90] Saito, Hiroshi (1990). The departure process of an N/G/1 queue. *Performance Evaluation* **11**, 241–251.

[SAM-TAQQU94] Samorodnitsky, G. and Taqqu, M.S. (1994). *Stable Non-Gaussian Random Processes.* Chapman and Hall, New York.

[SCHWEFEL00] Schwefel, H-P. (2000). *Performance Analysis of Intermediate Systems Serving Aggregated ON/OFF Traffic with Long-Range Dependent Properties.* PhD Thesis, School of Informatics, Technical University, Munich, Germany, September.

[SCHWEFEL-LIP01] Schwefel, H-P, and Lipsky, L. (2001). Impact of aggregated, self-similar ON/OFF traffic on delay in stationary queueing models (extended version). *Performance Evaluaton* **43**, 203–221.

[STEWART95] Stewart, W. J., Ed. (1995). *Computations with Markov Chains.* Klewer Academic Publishers, Boston.

[STIDHAM74] Stidham, S.,Jr. (1974). A last word on $L = \lambda W$. *Operations Research* **22**, 417–421.

[TAKACS62] Takacs, L. (1962). *Introduction to the Theory of Queues.* Oxford University Press, New York.

[TEHRANIPOUR83] Tehranipour, A. (1983). *Explicit Solutions of Generalized M/G/C//N Systems Including an Analysis of Their Transient Behavior.* Ph.D. Thesis, University of Nebraska, Lincoln, December.

[TEHRANIPOURVDLLIP89] Tehranipour, A., van de Liefvoort, A., and Lipsky, L. (1989). Residual lifetimes as a function of queue length for M/G/1//N loops. *Joint ACM-IEEE Workshop on Applied Computing '89*, Stillwater, OK.

[TRIVEDI82] Trivedi, K.S. (1982). *Probability and Statistics with Reliability, Queueing, and Computer Science Applications.* Prentice Hall, Englewood Cliffs, New Jersey.

[TRIVEDI02] Trivedi, K.S. (2002). *Probability and Statistics with Reliability, Queueing, and Computer Science Applications*, 2nd Ed. Wiley-Interscience, New York.

[WALLACE69] Wallace, V.L. (1969). *The Solution of Quasi-Birth and Death Processes Arising from Multiple Access Computer Systems.* PhD Dissertation, University of Michigan, Ann Arbor.

[WALLACE72] Wallace, V.L. (1972). Toward an algebraic theory of Markovian networks. *Proceedings of the Symposium on Computer Communications Networks and Teletraffic*, 397–408.

[SHERMANMORRISON50] Sherman, J., and Morrison, W.J. (1950) Adjustment of an inverse marix corresponding to a change in one element of a given matrix. *Annals of Mathematical Statistics*, **21**, 1, 124–127.

[WOLFF82] Wolff, R.W. (1982). Poisson arrivals see time averages. *Operations Research*, **30**, 223–231.

[ZHANG07] Zhang, F. (2007). *Modelling Restricted Processor Sharing in a Computer System with Non-Exponential Service Times.* PhD Thesis, Department of Computer Science, University of Connecticut, December.

[ZOLOTAREV86] Zolotarev, V.M. (1986). *One-Dimensional Stable Distributions*, V. 65. Translations of Mathematical Monographs, AMS.

Index

Q

R

S

T

U

V

W

Z